Using Total Worker Health® to Advance Worker Health and Safety

Using Total Worker Health® to Advance Worker Health and Safety

Special Issue Editors

Diane S. Rohlman
Kevin M. Kelly

MDPI • Basel • Beijing • Wuhan • Barcelona • Belgrade

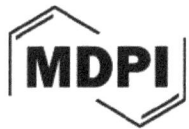

Special Issue Editors
Diane S. Rohlman
Healthier Workforce Center of the Midwest
University of Iowa
USA

Kevin M. Kelly
Healthier Workforce Center of the Midwest
University of Iowa
USA

Editorial Office
MDPI
St. Alban-Anlage 66
4052 Basel, Switzerland

This is a reprint of articles from the Special Issue published online in the open access journal *International Journal of Environmental Research and Public Health* (ISSN 1660-4601) from 2018 to 2019 (available at: https://www.mdpi.com/journal/ijerph/special_issues/advance_worker).

For citation purposes, cite each article independently as indicated on the article page online and as indicated below:

LastName, A.A.; LastName, B.B.; LastName, C.C. Article Title. *Journal Name* **Year**, *Article Number*, Page Range.

ISBN 978-3-03921-992-6 (Hbk)
ISBN 978-3-03921-993-3 (PDF)

Cover image courtesy of Roman Slabach and Michael Guhin.

© 2020 by the authors. Articles in this book are Open Access and distributed under the Creative Commons Attribution (CC BY) license, which allows users to download, copy and build upon published articles, as long as the author and publisher are properly credited, which ensures maximum dissemination and a wider impact of our publications.
The book as a whole is distributed by MDPI under the terms and conditions of the Creative Commons license CC BY-NC-ND.

Contents

About the Special Issue Editors ix

Preface to "Using Total Worker Health® to Advance Worker Health and Safety" xi

Sara L. Tamers, L. Casey Chosewood, Adele Childress, Heidi Hudson, Jeannie Nigam and Chia-Chia Chang
Total Worker Health® 2014–2018: The Novel Approach to Worker Safety, Health, and Well-Being Evolves
Reprinted from: *IJERPH* **2019**, *16*, 321, doi:10.3390/ijerph16030321 1

Tessa Bonney, Christina Welter, Elizabeth Jarpe-Ratner and Lorraine M. Conroy
Understanding the Role of Academic Partners as Technical Assistance Providers: Results from an Exploratory Study to Address Precarious Work
Reprinted from: *IJERPH* **2019**, *16*, 3903, doi:10.3390/ijerph16203903 20

Aileen Hoge, Anna T. Ehmann, Monika A. Rieger and Achim Siegel
Caring for Workers' Health: Do German Employers Follow a Comprehensive Approach Similar to the Total Worker Health Concept? Results of a Survey in an Economically Powerful Region in Germany
Reprinted from: *IJERPH* **2019**, *16*, 726, doi:0.3390/ijerph16050726 38

Janalee Thompson, Natalie V. Schwatka, Liliana Tenney and Lee S. Newman
Total Worker Health: A Small Business Leader Perspective
Reprinted from: *IJERPH* **2018**, *15*, 2416, doi:10.3390/ijerph15112416 53

Ami Sedani, Derry Stover, Brian Coyle and Rajvi J. Wani
Assessing Workplace Health and Safety Strategies, Trends, and Barriers through a Statewide Worksite Survey
Reprinted from: *IJERPH* **2019**, *16*, 2475, doi:10.3390/ijerph16142475 68

José Joaquín Del Pozo-Antúnez, Antonio Ariza-Montes, Francisco Fernández-Navarro and Horacio Molina-Sánchez
Effect of a Job Demand-Control-Social Support Model on Accounting Professionals' Health Perception
Reprinted from: *IJERPH* **2018**, *15*, 2437, doi:10.3390/ijerph15112437 82

Sophie-Charlotte Meyer and Lena Hünefeld
Challenging Cognitive Demands at Work, Related Working Conditions, and Employee Well-Being
Reprinted from: *IJERPH* **2018**, *15*, 2911, doi:10.3390/ijerph15122911 98

Aviroop Biswas, Colette N. Severin, Peter M. Smith, Ivan A. Steenstra, Lynda S. Robson and Benjamin C. Amick III
Larger Workplaces, People-Oriented Culture, and Specific Industry Sectors Are Associated with Co-Occurring Health Protection and Wellness Activities
Reprinted from: *IJERPH* **2018**, *15*, 2739, doi:/10.3390/ijerph15122739 112

María del Carmen Pérez-Fuentes, María del Mar Molero Jurado, África Martos Martínez and José Jesús Gázquez Linares
New Burnout Evaluation Model Based on the Brief Burnout Questionnaire: Psychometric Properties for Nursing
Reprinted from: *IJERPH* **2018**, *15*, 2718, doi:10.3390/ijerph15122718 125

Tamara D. Street, Sarah J. Lacey and Klaire Somoray
Employee Stress, Reduced Productivity, and Interest in a Workplace Health Program: A Case Study from the Australian Mining Industry
Reprinted from: *IJERPH* **2019**, *16*, 94, doi:10.3390/ijerph16010094 137

Nathan C. Huizinga, Jonathan A. Davis, Fred Gerr and Nathan B. Fethke
Association between Occupational Injury and Subsequent Employment Termination among Newly Hired Manufacturing Workers
Reprinted from: *IJERPH* **2019**, *16*, 433, doi:10.3390/ijerph16030433 150

Gyesook Yoo and Soomi Lee
It Doesn't End There: Workplace Bullying, Work-to-Family Conflict, and Employee Well-Being in Korea
Reprinted from: *IJERPH* **2018**, *15*, 1548, doi:10.3390/ijerph15071548 162

Eric A. Lauer, Karla Armenti, Margaret Henning and Lissa Sirois
Identifying Barriers and Supports to Breastfeeding in the Workplace Experienced by Mothers in the New Hampshire Special Supplemental Nutrition Program for Women, Infants, and Children Utilizing the Total Worker Health Framework
Reprinted from: *IJERPH* **2019**, *16*, 529, doi:10.3390/ijerph16040529 175

Susan E. Peters, Michael P. Grant, Justin Rodgers, Justin Manjourides, Cassandra A. Okechukwu and Jack T. Dennerlein
A Cluster Randomized Controlled Trial of a Total Worker Health® Intervention on Commercial Construction Sites
Reprinted from: *IJERPH* **2018**, *15*, 2354, doi:10.3390/ijerph15112354 192

Ryan Olson, Jennifer A. Hess, Kelsey N. Parker, Sharon V. Thompson, Anjali Rameshbabu, Kristy Luther Rhoten and Miguel Marino
From Research-to-Practice: An Adaptation and Dissemination of the COMPASS Program for Home Care Workers
Reprinted from: *IJERPH* **2018**, *15*, 2777, doi:10.3390/ijerph15122777 212

Jaime R. Strickland, Anna M. Kinghorn, Bradley A. Evanoff and Ann Marie Dale
Implementation of the Healthy Workplace Participatory Program in a Retail Setting: A Feasibility Study and Framework for Evaluation
Reprinted from: *IJERPH* **2019**, *16*, 590, doi:10.3390/ijerph16040590 231

Rajashree Kotejoshyer, Yuan Zhang, Marian Flum, Jane Fleishman and Laura Punnett
Prospective Evaluation of Fidelity, Impact and Sustainability of Participatory Workplace Health Teams in Skilled Nursing Facilities
Reprinted from: *IJERPH* **2019**, *16*, 1494, doi:10.3390/ijerph16091494 248

Ashamsa Aryal, Megan Parish and Diane Rohlman
Generalizability of Total Worker Health® Online Training for Young Workers
Reprinted from: *IJERPH* **2019**, *16*, 577, doi:10.3390/ijerph16040577 265

Onno Bouwmeester and Tessa Elisabeth Kok
Moral or Dirty Leadership: A Qualitative Study on How Juniors Are Managed in Dutch Consultancies
Reprinted from: *IJERPH* **2018**, *15*, 2506, doi:10.3390/ijerph15112506 275

Tariku Ayana Abdi, José M. Peiró, Yarid Ayala and Salvatore Zappalà
Four Wellbeing Patterns and their Antecedents in Millennials at Work
Reprinted from: *IJERPH* **2019**, *16*, 25, doi:10.3390/ijerph16010025 297

Eva M. Shipp, Sharon P. Cooper, Luohua Jiang, Amber B. Trueblood and Jennifer Ross
Influence of Work on Elevated Blood Pressure in Hispanic Adolescents in South Texas
Reprinted from: *IJERPH* **2019**, *16*, 1096, doi:10.3390/ijerph16071096 . . . . **314**

José M. Peiró, Malgorzata W. Kozusznik, Isabel Rodríguez-Molina and Núria Tordera
The Happy-Productive Worker Model and Beyond: Patterns of Wellbeing and Performance at Work
Reprinted from: *IJERPH* **2019**, *16*, 479, doi:10.3390/ijerph16030479 . . . . **326**

Toni Alterman, Rebecca Tsai, Jun Ju and Kevin M. Kelly
Trust in the Work Environment and Cardiovascular Disease Risk: Findings from the Gallup-Sharecare Well-Being Index
Reprinted from: *IJERPH* **2019**, *16*, 230, doi:10.3390/ijerph16020230 . . . . **346**

About the Special Issue Editors

Diane Rohlman (Professor): Diane Rohlman is Center Director of the Healthier Workforce Center of the Midwest, and Professor in the Department of Occupational and Environmental Health at the University of Iowa, Iowa City, Iowa, as well as Director of the Agricultural Safety and Health Training Program in the University of Iowa's Heartland Center for Occupational Health and Safety. She received her Master's degree and PhD in Experimental Psychology from Bowling Green State University in Ohio. Her research focuses on both basic and applied research designed to identify, characterize, and prevent occupational and environmental illness and injury in high-risk populations.

Kevin Kelly (Associate Research Scientist/Adjunct Associate Professor): Kevin Kelly is the Deputy Director, and Director of Evaluation, at the Healthier Workforce Center of the Midwest, and Adjunct Associate Professor in the Department of Anthropology at the University of Iowa, Iowa City, Iowa. He received his Master's degree and PhD in Anthropology from the University of Illinois at Urbana-Champaign. His research interests are in the biological and cultural aspects of human health and variations. He has conducted research in diverse settings, and has applied a broad set of quantitative, qualitative and mixed methods to that research.

Preface to "Using Total Worker Health® to Advance Worker Health and Safety"

It is now recognized that workplace aspects (scheduling, shift work, physically demanding work, chemical exposure) not only increase the risk of injury and illness, but also impact health behaviors (smoking, physical activity) and health outcomes (sleep disorders and fatigue, obesity, musculoskeletal disorders). In turn, ill health and chronic conditions can affect performance at work, increasing risk for injury, absenteeism, and reduced productivity. In the past few decades, programs that expand the traditional focus of occupational safety and health to consider nontraditional work-related sources of health and well-being have been shown to be more effective than programs that separately address these issues. This Total Worker Health® approach has been recognized by the National Institute for Occupational Safety and Health (NIOSH) as a method for protecting the safety and health of workers, while also advancing the overall well-being of these workers by addressing work conditions.

This Special Issue is devoted to "Advancing Worker Health and Safety". It includes basic and applied research relevant to programs, policies, and practices that promote holistic approaches to worker well-being. The volume begins with an overview of the NIOSH Total Worker Health program, describing the history of the program and identifying new challenges with the rapidly changing nature of work. The international importance of this topic is demonstrated by research addressing working populations in the United States, Australia, Korea, Canada, and countries in the European Union who are employed in worksites as varied as manufacturing, retail, healthcare, accounting, construction, and mining.

Several articles address new workers to the workplace. These focus on providing training and encouraging young workers to communicate about health and safety, the importance of preventing injuries to reduce retention, and how supervisor support and clear work organization and policies can help reduce stress among junior employees. Other articles describe the evaluation of interventions among construction workers, young workers, and homecare workers. Required components for the successful development, implementation, and adoption of interventions promoting worker safety and well-being are identified (e.g., the elimination of hazards, leadership support, participatory approaches in the design and delivery of programs, and evaluation metrics). Not surprisingly, implementation differs across industries and by organization size.

This compendium presents work from an international collection of scholars exploring the relationship between workplace factors and worker safety, health, and well-being. It provides guidance for improving the organization and design of work environments, innovative strategies for promoting worker well-being, and novel methods for exposing underlying occupational causes of chronic disease.

We would like to thank all of the authors that took the time to contribute to this Special Issue, and the editors and reviewers for their assistance.

Diane S. Rohlman, Kevin M. Kelly
Special Issue Editors

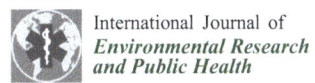

Review

Total Worker Health® 2014–2018: The Novel Approach to Worker Safety, Health, and Well-Being Evolves

Sara L. Tamers [1,*], L. Casey Chosewood [2], Adele Childress [1], Heidi Hudson [3], Jeannie Nigam [3] and Chia-Chia Chang [1]

1. Centers for Disease Control and Prevention, National Institute for Occupational Safety and Health, 395 E St. SW, Washington, DC 20201, USA; ahc0@cdc.gov (A.C.); cuc8@cdc.gov (C.-C.C.)
2. Centers for Disease Control and Prevention, National Institute for Occupational Safety and Health, 1600 Clifton Rd., Atlanta, GA 30329, USA; ahx6@cdc.gov
3. Centers for Disease Control and Prevention, National Institute for Occupational Safety and Health, 1150 Tusculum Ave, Cincinnati, OH 45226, USA; cvv2@cdc.gov (H.H.); zgy1@cdc.gov (J.N.)
* Correspondence: stamers@cdc.gov

Received: 11 December 2018; Accepted: 22 January 2019; Published: 24 January 2019

Abstract: *Background*: The objective of this article is to provide an overview of and update on the Office for *Total Worker Health*® (TWH) program of the Centers for Disease Control and Prevention's National Institute for Occupational Safety and Health (CDC/NIOSH). *Methods*: This article describes the evolution of the TWH program from 2014 to 2018 and future steps and directions. *Results*: The TWH framework is defined as policies, programs, and practices that integrate protection from work-related safety and health hazards with promotion of injury and illness prevention efforts to advance worker well-being. *Conclusions*: The CDC/NIOSH TWH program continues to evolve in order to respond to demands for research, practice, policy, and capacity building information and solutions to the safety, health, and well-being challenges that workers and their employers face.

Keywords: *Total Worker Health*®; occupational safety and health; worker well-being

1. Introduction

The mission of the United States (U.S.) Centers for Disease Control and Prevention's National Institute for Occupational Safety and Health (CDC/NIOSH) is rooted in its dedication to preserving and enhancing the total health of workers. This mission—to generate knowledge in the field of occupational safety and health and to transfer that knowledge into practice for the betterment of workers—generated the *Total Worker Health*® (TWH) program. As of 2015, the TWH framework is defined as policies, programs, and practices that integrate protection from work-related safety and health hazards with promotion of injury and illness prevention efforts to advance worker well-being [1]. TWH efforts protect the safety and health of workers and advance their well-being by fostering safer and healthier workplaces and by addressing work organization, employment and supervisory practices, and workplace culture. Integration can ensue through collaboration and coordinated programming around organizational leadership and commitment; supportive organizational policies and practices; management and employee engagement strategies; supportive benefits and incentives; accountability and training; and integrated real-time evaluation and surveillance that bring about corrective action where required [2]. Frameworks and models have been published to help describe what integration is like in practice [3–5].

The original emergence of the TWH approach at NIOSH began years prior with the Steps to a Healthier U.S. Workforce Initiative in 2003, which explored the benefits of integrating worker safety and health protection efforts with health promoting ones [6]. As research developed and implementation increased, the focus on the integration of health protection and health promotion expanded to a framework with a greater appreciation of (and demand for) a growing set of worker well-being determinants that impact safety and health. In 2014, as initiatives evolved and more research and information became available, NIOSH launched the Office for TWH Coordination and Research Support (Office for TWH) to coordinate and advance research, programs, policy, and training in collaboration with intramural and extramural partners [7]. A comprehensive history on the evolution of the TWH program prior to 2014 is available elsewhere [6,8].

Some traditional occupational safety and health (OSH) and worksite wellness programs (that is, non-integrated, stand-alone, siloed approaches) have had a favorable impact. However, scientific evidence has increasingly found that for tackling the wide-ranging, complex concerns of workers, integrating OSH protection activities with health-enhancing ones may be more efficacious than concentrating on either of these activities alone [2,8–10]. More specifically, studies have shown that emphasizing a TWH or integrated approach to jointly and comprehensively address work-related hazards and other exposures addresses the synergistic risks that exist, engendering more promising efforts and results [8].

There has been much headway in the field of TWH over the past several years, and the TWH program has continued to develop. Integration efforts have expanded to consider the synergistic opportunities between and among the health of workers at and away from work and a broader look at the interplay of work and non-work factors and influences on the well-being of workers. This article provides an update on the TWH program since the 2013 publication by Schill and Chosewood [6] and describes its evolution from 2014 to 2018—including major program accomplishments and stakeholder and partnership activities—as well as highlights of future directions.

2. Discussion

2.1. The 1st International Symposium to Advance Total Worker Health®

A vital and key event in the maturation of the TWH field was the convening of a TWH scientific conference. Building on prior initiatives and symposia, the Office for TWH held the 1st International Symposium to Advance *Total Worker Health*® in 2014, at the U.S. National Institutes of Health (NIH) [11]. Given that this was the very first symposium of its kind, the theme was "Total Worker Health," and these were its goals:

- Showcase current research that advances the concept of TWH;
- Connect stakeholders who share an interest in TWH;
- Provide resources and strategies for practitioners working to improve the health, safety and well-being of workers; and
- Inform a future research agenda to expand the evidence-base for TWH.

The symposium brought together over 17 partner organizations and more than 350 national and international scientists and practitioners. These participants represented academia, labor, industry, and government, including workplace health, human resources, employee benefits, employee assistance, health promotion, organized labor, workers' compensation, disability management, emergency response, public health, health policy, health economics, organizational and occupational health psychology, industrial hygiene, and related disciplines.

Over the course of two days, attendees explored topics and issues relevant to a TWH perspective, such as TWH frameworks, research methods, integrated approaches, implementation, evaluation, and practical toolkits. Sessions highlighted high-risk industries such as construction, transportation, and health care, particularly in the areas of work stress and psychosocial factors, obesity, and musculoskeletal conditions. They also emphasized examples of integrated interventions for a changing workforce, new employment patterns, physical/built environment, community/workplace supports, advances in return-to-work policies, and disability and rehabilitation management.

2.2. The National Total Worker Health® Agenda

A prime feature of the 1st International Symposium to Advance *Total Worker Health®* was the launch of the National *Total Worker Health®* Agenda draft, another important and major step forward in the growth of the TWH approach [12].

Over 20 years ago, NIOSH partnered with wide-ranging stakeholders to pinpoint and establish national priorities for the most significant issues affecting workers across varied occupations and industries, by means of an OSH research framework known as the National Occupational Research Agenda (NORA), now in its third decade. The goal of the first NORA in TWH (National *Total Worker Health®* Agenda) was to encourage and motivate diverse stakeholders dedicated to concurrently protecting workers from hazards in the workplace and advancing their well-being. These stakeholders include OSH practitioners, labor organizations, health promotion and wellness professionals, researchers, workers, employers, educators, policymakers, health care providers, and many others. In line with NORA tradition, NIOSH sought extensive stakeholder input during the development of the National *Total Worker Health®* Agenda. This ensured that it emphasized stakeholder priority areas not only explicitly in TWH research but also in practice, policy, and capacity building.

To that end, in 2014, NIOSH announced in the Federal Register that a draft version of the TWH NORA, entitled "Proposed National *Total Worker Health®* Agenda," was available for stakeholder review. The Office for TWH subsequently reviewed, synthesized, and responded to all comments and critiques received [13]. On the basis of those comments, the Office for TWH added and further developed goals, and it refocused the TWH definition and approach. Refining the description ensured a better understanding of the program priorities and further differentiated the approach from traditional worksite health promotion programming that does not integrate worker safety and protection elements. Prioritizing a foundation of safety first, and then integrating workplace policies, programs, and practices that grow health, creates greater worker well-being and is the cornerstone of the TWH framework.

The National *Total Worker Health®* Agenda goals reflect not only stakeholder comments but also sources in the peer-reviewed literature [6,8,14–16] and two workshops. The latter were *Total Worker Health*™: Promising and Best Practices in the Integration of Occupational Safety and Health Protection with Health Promotion in the Workplace—A Workshop [17] and the Pathways to Prevention Workshop, *Total Worker Health®*: What's Work Got to Do With It? [18].

Four strategic goals, each supported by several intermediate and activity/output goals, comprise the following domains: research, practice, policy, and capacity building.

1. Research: Advance and conduct etiologic, surveillance, and intervention research that builds the evidence base for effectively integrating protection from work-related safety and health hazards with promotion of injury and illness prevention efforts to advance worker well-being.
2. Practice: Increase the implementation of evidence-based programs and practices that integrate protection from work-related safety and health hazards with promotion of injury and illness prevention efforts to advance worker well-being.
3. Policy: Increase adoption of policies that integrate protection from work-related safety and health hazards with promotion of injury and illness prevention efforts to advance worker well-being.
4. Capacity Building: Build capacity to strengthen the TWH workforce and TWH field to support the development, growth, and maintenance of policies, programs, and practices that integrate protection from work-related safety and health hazards with promotion of injury and illness prevention efforts to advance worker well-being.

The continued fulfillment of these goals by stakeholders over the next years (2016–2026) will better safeguard the safety, health, and well-being of workers, support overall workforce vitality, and foster economic prosperity.

2.3. Advances in TWH Research

The research goals in the National *Total Worker Health®* Agenda focus on advancing and conducting etiologic, surveillance, and intervention research activities that build the evidence base [12].

Though the research base has grown, the field will benefit from further exploration of current and new research areas to solidify the evidence base and advance the field [19]. This led the Office for TWH to develop the intramural research program and coordinate research-related activities, both intramurally and extramurally, targeting priority topics and working populations [6]. At NIOSH, researchers are engaged in varied TWH activities such as conducting research, participating on the TWH steering committee, providing support activities, presenting at seminars and in webinars, publishing peer-reviewed papers, and engaging in collaborative stakeholder and partnership research efforts.

2.3.1. Issues Relevant to Advancing Worker Well-Being through *Total Worker Health*®

NIOSH has accomplished its goal of developing and publishing the research-centric National *Total Worker Health*® Agenda [12]. Another objective of the Office for TWH was to update a summarized list of seminal and current issues relevant to TWH and to the future of the workforce, to advance the scientific research focus and direction. Aside from the more customary workplace hazards that organizations have long faced, such as chemical exposures, traumatic injury, and shift work, workers and employers are also now navigating changing workforce demographics, growing work/life balance challenges, a multi-generational and aging workforce, and rising levels of work-related stress [20]. What is more, new work arrangements such as precarious or contingent work are often entrenched with increased exposure to hazardous work, little or no job security, minimal advancement and training, and a higher proportion of health insurance costs shouldered by the worker [20,21]. Therefore, in 2015, to highlight critical concerns to worker health and well-being, the Office for TWH published a list of these key issues that are relevant to advancing worker well-being through TWH (Figure 1) [20].

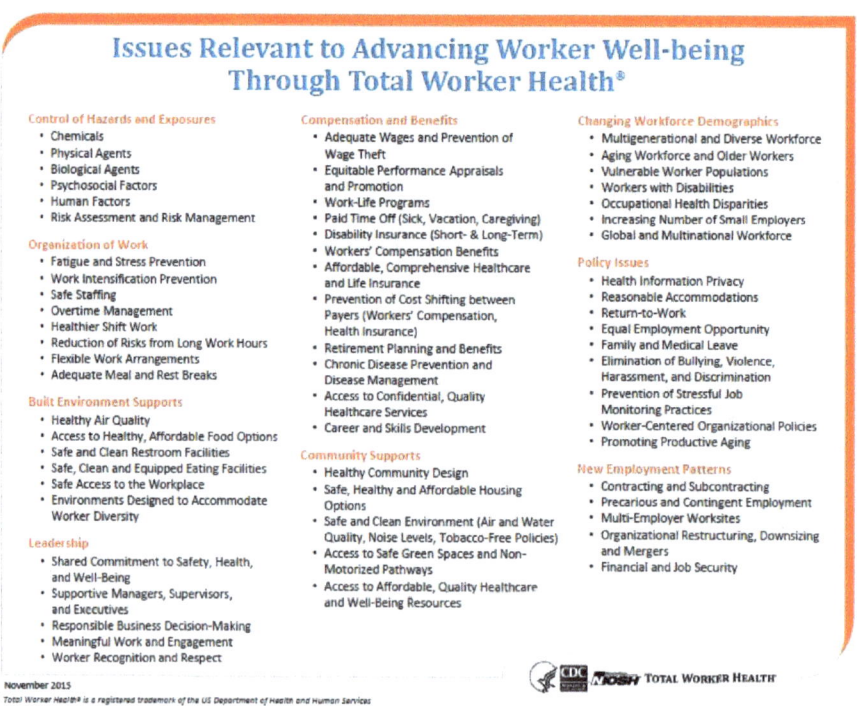

Figure 1. Issues relevant to advancing worker well-being through *Total Worker Health*®.

2.3.2. NIOSH Centers of Excellence for TWH

In addition to NIOSH TWH research activity, the bulk of TWH research is conducted by NIOSH-funded extramural Centers of Excellence for TWH (Figure 2), located in the U.S.; each of their websites provides a wealth of information, tools, resources, and peer-reviewed papers on the effectiveness of TWH [22]. These centers are uniquely qualified to be among the leaders in the field of TWH and are crucial to gaining knowledge that can help workers, employers, and communities.

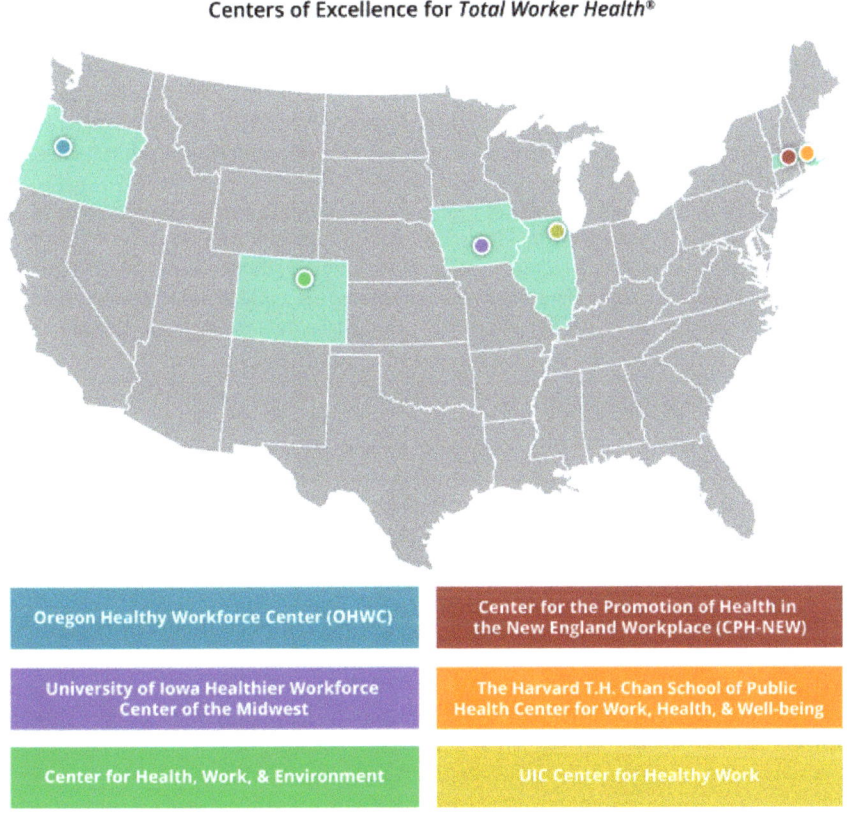

Figure 2. NIOSH Centers of Excellence for *Total Worker Health*®.

In 2006 and 2007, NIOSH funded three centers: the Healthier Workforce Center of the Midwest (University of Iowa), the Center for the Promotion of Health in the New England Workplace (University of Massachusetts—Lowell and University of Connecticut), and the Harvard T.H. Chan School of Public Health's Center for Work, Health, and Well-Being (Harvard University). In 2011, NIOSH funded a fourth center: the Oregon Healthy Workforce Center (Oregon Health and Science University). In 2016, NIOSH funded two more centers: the Center for Health, Work & Environment (University of Colorado); and the Center for Healthy Work (University of Illinois–Chicago). Ongoing coordination with the Centers of Excellence for TWH in the areas of mutual interest continues to be a critical partnership to complement intramural efforts.

2.3.3. Total Worker Health® Research Methodology Workshop

One such recent and vital effort that NIOSH, the NIOSH-funded Centers of Excellence for TWH, and several other external partners undertook was to assess methodological and measurement issues for TWH intervention research and establish concrete examples of how challenges can be overcome to drive research practices in the field of TWH. There were multiple goals for the workshop. The first was to respond to two of the eight recommendations put forth by the Independent Panel of the Pathways to Prevention 2015 Meeting, co-sponsored by NIH and NIOSH: *Total Worker Health®: What's Work Got to Do With It?* [18]: (1) expand research and evaluation design options to include a range of rigorous methodologies; and (2) develop a core set of measures and outcomes that are incorporated into all integrated intervention studies. The second was to respond to the intermediate and activity/output goals (Sections 1.3; 1.3.2–1.3.6) to apply and develop rigorous, standardized methods for TWH interventions, as outlined in the National *Total Worker Health®* Agenda [12]. More detail on the impetuses and need for such a workshop have been previously published in publicly available papers [12,19,23].

Accordingly, in 2017, the University of Iowa's College of Public Health and Healthier Workforce Center of the Midwest hosted the *Total Worker Health®* Research Methodology Workshop. An open-access peer-reviewed article summarizing this workshop, by Tamers et al. (2018), highlights the TWH research methodological and measurement approaches currently in use and suggests others that the workshop experts believe have the potential to advance the field through rigorous and repeatable TWH intervention research [24].

2.3.4. Worker Well-Being Framework

Another key TWH accomplishment in recent years is NIOSH's partnership with the Research ANd Development (RAND) Corporation to develop a framework for worker well-being and its subsequent still-in-development survey instrument. The framework was published in 2018 [25] and will serve as a conceptual model for future research on worker well-being. The continued work of NIOSH and RAND to develop the survey will be useful in advancing the understanding of issues related to worker well-being.

2.4. Advances in TWH Practice

The practice goals in the National *Total Worker Health®* Agenda center on the need to increase the implementation of evidence-based programs and practices [12]. Although the scientific evidence base is relatively new, the uptake of the integrated concept of TWH has gained substantial traction among leaders and practitioners in safety and health [26]. A testament that advancements in worker safety, health, and well-being are not entirely an academic enterprise is also demonstrated by industry and other private sector interest in TWH strategies [27,28].

2.4.1. Tools and Resources

A number of tool-kits, actionable guidance, web-based training, continuing education courses, and other practice-based resources that have been developed in recent years are available on the NIOSH TWH website and on the Centers of Excellence for TWH websites [22]. An increasing community of stakeholders receive information about these tools and resources regularly through a multitude of dissemination channels (i.e., social media, e-newsletters, and other media outlets) and through other outreach efforts and engagement programs. One of the most widely consumed outputs of NIOSH's communication efforts has been an electronic newsletter, *TWH in Action!* [29]. Published quarterly since 2012, this e-newsletter now has more than 80,000 subscribers. Another highly popular resource is the NIOSH *Total Worker Health®* Webinar series [30]. This free, online training platform features the latest research and practice in the field of TWH and has provided continuing education credits to more than 1000 physicians, nurses, health educators, and others.

2.4.2. Hierarchy of Controls Applied to NIOSH *Total Worker Health*®

In 2015, the Office for TWH published the *Hierarchy of Controls Applied to NIOSH Total Worker Health*® (Figure 3)—adapted from the Hierarchy of Controls framework used in OSH—to strengthen the link between traditional OSH approaches and TWH and to further illustrate the value of this kind of approach to practitioners who are quite familiar with this means toward risk mitigation [31]. As in the traditional hierarchy, the controls and strategies are in descending order of likely effectiveness and protectiveness. The emphasis on addressing system-level or environmental determinants of health before individual-level approaches is a key tenet of the TWH approach.

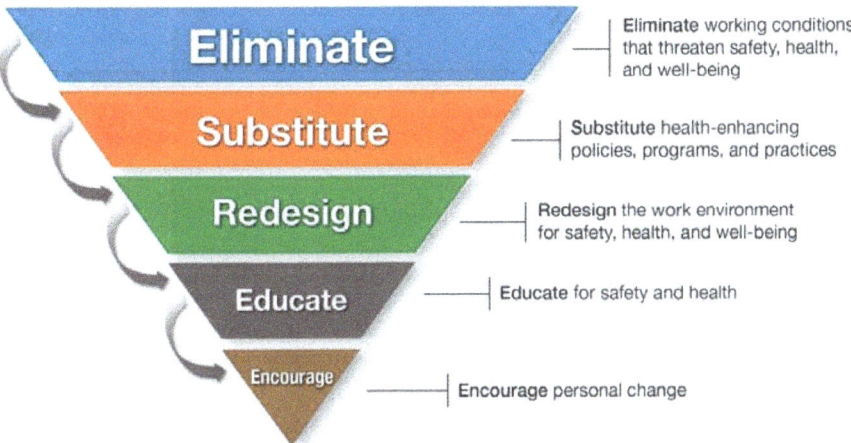

Figure 3. Hierarchy of Controls Applied to NIOSH *Total Worker Health*®.

2.4.3. Fundamentals of *Total Worker Health*® Approaches

A central practice-based tool developed by the Office for TWH and published in 2016 is the Fundamentals of *Total Worker Health*® Approaches: Essential Elements for Advancing Worker Safety, Health, and Well-Being [32]. To help organizations launch and sustain their own programs, the Office for TWH developed this workbook centered on five fundamental steps essential to the TWH approach. These five defining elements of TWH are guiding principles that provide practical direction for organizations seeking to develop workplace policies, programs, and practices that contribute to worker safety, health, and well-being:

1. Demonstrate leadership commitment;
2. Eliminate hazards and promote well-being;
3. Engage workers in program design and delivery;
4. Ensure confidentiality and privacy; and
5. Integrate systems effectively.

2.4.4. Edited Volume on TWH

Forthcoming is an edited volume on TWH [33]. This book will bring together state-of-the-art research and practice in comprehensive, integrated prevention strategies from the most accomplished scholars and practitioners in the field. The book will serve as premier guidance for interested professionals on the foundations of TWH, to further prevent adverse worker safety and health outcomes from contemporary work and work environments.

2.5. Advances in TWH Policy

The policy goals in the National *Total Worker Health*® Agenda aim to increase the adoption of TWH and related policies, mostly by external entities [12]. There has been growing interest in organizational policies that integrate OSH with business strategy and practices. In particular, topics covered by guidance include responsible organizational and worker sustainability; small- and medium-sized businesses; and risk management and workers' compensation.

2.5.1. Partner and Stakeholder Efforts

Over the past few years, several initiatives have contributed to the National *Total Worker Health*® Agenda's intermediate goal of "implementing policy guidance developed from evidence-based research and consensus statements to promote worker safety, health, and well-being" and activity/output goals focused on promoting responsible organizational policies and sustainability of workers. These have been led by a number of stakeholders and partners, some with direct and some with indirect or no firm affiliation to the Office for TWH.

For instance, the theme of the 11th International Conference on Occupational Stress and Health in 2015, which NIOSH co-hosted along with the American Psychological Association and the Society for Occupational Health Psychology, was Sustainable Work, Sustainable Health, Sustainable Organizations [34]. During the conference, researchers and practitioners discussed how sustainable work and worker well-being can affect economic growth and organizational health. The relevance of OSH to sustainability was recognized by the U.S. Occupational Safety and Health Administration (OSHA) in its report based on interviews with stakeholders, *Sustainability in the Workplace: A New Approach for Advancing Worker Safety and Health* [35]. To facilitate implementation of policy guidance, OSHA identified opportunities in shareholder engagement, recognition of OSH as a business innovation, rankings of businesses, and materiality of factors that affect business performance.

Similarly, the Center for Safety and Health Sustainability (CSHS), which represents more than 70,000 OSH professionals in over 70 countries, has developed guidance supporting worker sustainability [36]. CSHS recommended integrated reporting of both financial and non-financial information, such as environmental, social, and governance (ESG) issues, including human, intellectual, social, and relationship capital. To facilitate sustainability policies that take into consideration worker well-being, CSHS highlighted the need to understand how organizations create value for their stakeholders through various types of capital. In 2016, CSHS outlined guidance for OSH in sustainability reports and key performance metrics to provide information on corporate performance. The Vitality Institute created a different approach, which recognized employee health as a crucial input to organizational success and proposed a comprehensive scorecard for sustainability reporting, to use for making decisions and tracking progress. By reporting on job satisfaction and turnover, health status, assessment of health risk, physical environment, corporate capacity, strategic communications, health policies/programs/practices, population health, corporate climate, leadership, and community relations, organizations can ensure that policies are supportive of worker well-being [37].

2.5.2. Small- and Medium-Sized Businesses

A further area of progress in policy implementation is the targeting of small- and medium-sized companies and incorporation of TWH approaches within workers' compensation systems, which are additional activity/output goals in the National *Total Worker Health*® Agenda. To gather evidence to guide organizational policies, NIOSH and the U.S. National Academy of Medicine convened a public workshop noted earlier (*Total Worker Health*™: Promising and Best Practices in the Integration of Occupational Safety and Health Protection with Health Promotion in the Workplace) to identify prevalent and best practices in small, medium, and large workplaces. The summary report from this workshop, which included recommendations from experts on the workshop's concluding reactors panel, was published in 2014 [17]. Common elements identified include the importance of leader recognition and prioritization of TWH in a business culture, a "comprehensive perspective" on safety, and attention to activities that can help workers be healthier and more satisfied, which in turn can positively impact businesses. Later in 2017, NIOSH and the Colorado School of Public Health's Center for Health, Work & Environment sponsored the International Understanding Small Enterprises conference [38]. The conference enabled small business owners, researchers specializing in small businesses, representatives from chambers of commerce, workers, and other stakeholders to share policy strategies for engaging workers and increasing happiness and productivity by creating safer and healthier workplaces.

A newly developed key small-business resource is a series of videos created by the Healthier Workforce Center of the Midwest. This center interviewed small businesses to identify gaps where it would be useful to provide guidance, and the resulting videos have shed light on useful policies for small businesses that seek to implement TWH approaches. Additionally, implementation of TWH approaches in workers' compensation programs has occurred by way of two NIOSH TWH Affiliates: the Ohio Bureau of Workers' Compensation (OBWC) and the State Accident Insurance Fund (SAIF), a workers' compensation company in Oregon. The OBWC created a program to support the health and well-being of workers for their client policyholders. SAIF shares the TWH approach with its policyholders and offers free consulting services to facilitate adoption of TWH policies. Furthermore, SAIF partnered with the Oregon OSHA and the Oregon Healthy Workforce Center to create a statewide alliance to encourage the updating of TWH policies in workplaces.

2.5.3. Voluntary Standards

For general policies, voluntary standards are useful for widespread adoption of a TWH approach. In 2018, the International Organization for Standardization (ISO) finalized the voluntary standard *ISO 45001—Occupational Health and Safety*. Although the guidance does not specify requirements for responsible business practices, it enables integration of OSH management systems with other systems, including those related to worker well-being [39]. Another related policy effort well-aligned with the TWH approach is the National Standard of Canada for Psychological Health and Safety in the Workplace; this could serve as a useful template for other nations seeking to improve working conditions. Adoption of the Canadian voluntary standard, developed in 2013, has increased and the standard has served as useful guidance internationally [40].

2.6. Advances in TWH Capacity Building

The capacity building goals in the National *Total Worker Health*® Agenda emphasize the need to build and strengthen the TWH workforce and field [12]. Multidisciplinary and comprehensively trained OSH professionals are essential to apply a TWH approach that addresses complex current and future workplace challenges, such as existing and emerging hazards and exposures, a multigenerational workforce, and rapid changes in technology. An important focus since the establishment of the Office for TWH has been to develop and equip OSH professionals as well as allied workplace professionals with the knowledge, skills, and training to prevent worker injury and illness and to advance health and well-being.

2.6.1. NIOSH Workforce Development Framework Guidance

The NIOSH Workforce Development Framework Guidance, which is an unpublished NIOSH-led document, explores approaches to build capacity and identifies competencies and training professionals need to apply an integrated approach that addresses the diverse needs of the U.S. workforce. In 2014, the Office for TWH shared this guidance with stakeholders and partners. This was an opportunity to identify current training needs and approaches, foster partnerships with research and training centers, and identify additional organizations and collaborators (Schools of Business,

Engineering, Nursing, Occupational Medicine Residency Programs, Public Health, and others). The guidance includes five broad foci necessary for professionals to apply a more comprehensive TWH approach, as well as recommendations for accomplishing this goal:

1. Identify training and professional development needs;
2. Develop a list of current TWH training programs;
3. Establish a TWH workforce development committee of interested stakeholders to discuss and provide guidance on building capacity for a TWH workforce;
4. Develop a list of TWH competencies; and
5. Identify effective methods of training and standardize a TWH curriculum.

Key internal/external stakeholders and partners who are in a position to lead this charge include professionals from academia, labor, OSH and health promotion, the private sector, human resources, and international partners and governments. Work in this area by the Office for TWH and myriad partners, some of which is highlighted in this article, is ongoing.

2.6.2. TWH Training and Certificate Programs

During the 1st International Symposium to Advance *Total Worker Health*® [11], a plenary session consisting of research and training experts from the NIOSH-funded Centers of Excellence for TWH, NIOSH-funded Education Research Centers (ERCs), and NIOSH TWH Affiliates covered current training initiatives, plans to formally solicit external input and engage key stakeholders, curricular reform, and integration of TWH into NIOSH-funded ERCs. During this session, speakers and participants confirmed a growing need to increase the knowledge and skills of researchers and practitioners to implement an integrated TWH approach through interdisciplinary education of the existing and future workforce. Currently, a number of differing types of continuing education and certificate programs are available or in development; such programs could include TWH approaches in already existent OSH or health promotion programs, or create new ones altogether. These include the University of Colorado [41]; the University of North Carolina—Chapel Hill; Oregon and Portland State Universities in collaboration with SAIF; Northern Kentucky University; and Western Kentucky University.

2.6.3. TWH Workforce Development Roundtable

Another key accomplishment in 2017 was the Office for TWH's collaboration with the University of North Carolina–Chapel Hill and Harvard University to convene a roundtable discussion with partners from the NIOSH-funded Centers of Excellence for TWH, ERCs, organized labor, NIOSH-funded OSH training institutions, state health departments, professional societies, workplace-wellness training vendors, and other experts in the field. The roundtable discussion explored training that could be incorporated into existing core OSH degree programs such as occupational health nursing, occupational medicine, and industrial hygiene. The focus of the roundtable was to identify the highest priority audiences; perform needs assessments; identify competencies for TWH; and suggest effective training approaches and programs (certificate, continuing education, and others). Key findings and recommendations from a 2017 report by the University of Colorado (Uncovering Training Needs for *Total Worker Health*® Professionals: Results of a National Continuing Education Survey [unpublished data]) were also reviewed at the meeting and influenced future directions. Of individuals working within the OSH and peripheral fields (human resources, benefits, wellness), survey results found that 2.8% indicated TWH as their primary profession, 14% indicated TWH as a secondary work task, and 75% identified a need for basic and advanced TWH training ($n = 1501$).

2.7. The 2nd International Symposium to Advance Total Worker Health®

The 2nd International Symposium to Advance *Total Worker Health®* was held four years after the first, in 2018, at NIH [11]. The theme of the symposium was "Work & Well-Being: How Safer, Healthier Work Can Enhance Well-Being," and these were its goals:

- Reaffirm TWH dedication and commitment to the safety and health of workers by prioritizing safety in all jobs;
- Redesign the organization of work to promote a workplace environment that optimizes healthy opportunities through leadership, management, and supervision;
- Reveal new strategies to redesign work to improve worker well-being through new links and solutions for work and chronic disease risks; and
- Introduce novel research methods and interventions for advancing TWH.

More than 100 partners and affiliate organizations and nearly 400 participants from 37 states and 15 countries attended the symposium, highlighting both a national and international demand for critical TWH research, training, and implementation in the workplace.

Presenters from nonprofit, government, private, and academic institutions shared their perspectives and research findings on TWH, as well as demonstrations of successful practical applications. Sessions included themes and topics on integrated TWH methods, approaches, interventions, evaluations, results, and recommendations from the NIOSH-funded Centers of Excellence for TWH, NIOSH researchers, and other experts in the field. High-risk industries and occupations, such as transportation, agriculture, firefighting and first response, manufacturing, health care, and law enforcement and corrections were the focus of many presentations. Speakers highlighted risks, exposures, and health conditions facing many workers in these fields, such as acute and chronic diseases, stress and mental health, fatigue, and violence.

Additional topics focused on the needs of small businesses, special populations, and government workers; strategies for optimizing community collaborations, integration, organizational policies and practices, supervision, and employee relations practices; and ways to enhance the work-life continuum and work design. Featured speakers covered worker health and well-being through the lens of new technologies, the current opioid crisis, globalization, and the rapidly evolving domestic and international economy. Finally, an important highlight was the launch of the Vision Zero Campaign for North America, organized by the International Social Security Association, to engage partners, institutions, and organizations worldwide in reducing occupational accidents and diseases by focusing on responsible leadership and investing in healthy workplaces and a motivated workforce [42].

2.8. TWH Partnership and Stakeholder Involvement

As discussed throughout this article, partnership and stakeholder involvement across multiple factions and disciplines has been and continues to be critical in advancing TWH research, practice, policy, and capacity building. To move the field of TWH forward, all stakeholders must work together, take ownership, and contribute.

Fundamental but sometimes challenging is demonstrating the value that a TWH approach brings to long-term sustainability of employers, industry, and society. Perhaps one of the most critical developments is inspiring the gatekeepers of worker health—professionals in labor, healthcare, and public health—to engage in new ways that bring greater visibility to the value of an integrated approach to worker safety and health [26,43,44]. Scholars believe this high-level engagement could stimulate more alignment of the field with long-standing and current social movements (such as labor rights, worker advocacy, sustainability-related responsible business practices, and paid family leave) and encourage broader collaboration among and within labor, academia, government, and industry [45]. For example, novel solutions to access worker populations could develop with new or better engagement with economic development [46], community-based, and labor organizations. The relationship between health and economic prosperity and national security is a priority of the U.S. Surgeon General [47].

In addition, new models of interventions at the workplace, community, industry, and society levels could establish the results sought for simultaneously addressing work- and non-work-related risks. Many of these actions involve expanding the role of professionals who protect worker safety, health, and well-being. Examples of NIOSH successes in increasing recognition of the relationship between work and health, as well as the role of community partnerships, include TWH participation in the U.S. National Academies Action Collaborative on Business Engagement in Building Healthy Communities and the U.S. National Academies of Medicine Action Collaborative on Clinician Well-Being and Resilience [48,49].

Finally, a significant accomplishment in the development of new partners in recent years was the Office for TWH's co-sponsorship with the NIH Office of Disease Prevention and the National Heart, Lung, and Blood Institute (NHLBI) to convene the 2015 NIH Pathways to Prevention Workshop *Total Worker Health*®: What's Work Got to Do With It? [18]. Approval for the conference's TWH theme required buy-in from several other NIH offices/institutes and U.S. federal agencies, making this a noteworthy TWH partnership achievement in raising awareness of the importance of TWH issues across U.S. federal agencies. The workshop had over 700 registered attendees, making it the largest TWH event to date. Outcomes include a review of the literature on research gaps and an independent panel report on future research priorities [23,50] as well as a new partnership with the American Heart Association and NHLBI to plan a meeting on workplace health.

NIOSH TWH Affiliates

In addition to work done within NIOSH, the NIOSH-funded Centers of Excellence for TWH, and the NIOSH-funded ERCs, TWH activities are shaped by the NIOSH TWH Affiliate program. The Office for TWH established this partnership program in 2014 to recognize not-for-profit, labor, academic, and government organizations that are advancing the TWH approach [28].

The program presently includes 45 NIOSH TWH Affiliates (Figure 4). Though the NIOSH TWH Affiliates do not receive funding from NIOSH, they are critical to all of the activities discussed in this article, each in their own way. The academic NIOSH TWH Affiliates conduct valuable research on systems approaches to worker well-being, organization of work, and workplace exposures and are leaders in the concept of an integrated framework for worker safety and health [28]. Some NIOSH TWH Affiliates provide training to professionals and students in TWH and have been instrumental in research and intervention evaluations in work settings. Several also collaborate with businesses to assess the effectiveness of workplace policies and practices. Labor union NIOSH TWH Affiliates are vital to ensure that worker involvement and outreach are embedded in TWH translation, education, and communication activities. Not-for-profit NIOSH TWH Affiliates are key in sharing TWH messages with local employer organizations and in facilitating regional outreach. The professional association/society NIOSH TWH Affiliates help translate research findings into training materials, share the latest promising practices, and provide continuing education to practitioners. Finally, employer-organization NIOSH TWH Affiliates help implement the TWH approach and, in doing so, provide successful TWH case studies from which other interested employers have learned. Relaying of ongoing NIOSH TWH Affiliate activities and development of collaborative efforts with NIOSH have also taken place during NIOSH TWH Affiliate-specific and other expert colloquia hosted annually by the Office for TWH since 2014.

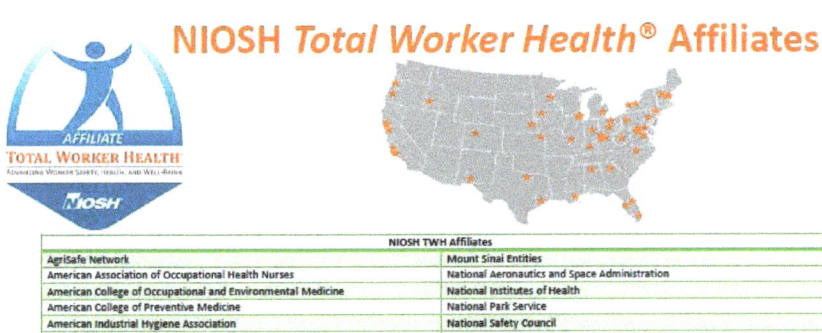

Figure 4. NIOSH *Total Worker Health*® Affiliates.

2.9. The Future of TWH

2.9.1. Research, Practice, Policy, and Capacity Building

Notwithstanding key efforts accomplished between 2014 and 2018 by the Office for TWH, along with its internal and external partners and stakeholders, as outlined in this article, continued developments are necessary for the TWH field to evolve even further.

More research is vital, not only in the intervention space but particularly also in the area of basic, etiologic, and surveillance research. Investment in a more developed understanding of the overall implementation of TWH research into practice and policy is additionally imperative. Much can be drawn from the emerging field of implementation science for insight regarding factors that influence adoption of evidence into practice and how research can be applied to drive policy change [51]. This is relevant for the increasing prevalence of workers in nonstandard work arrangements, a population segment typically more difficult to reach. There is similarly a distinct need to translate research on known work-related risks (such as work-family conflict) and to bring awareness of those risks to other related disciplines (such as human resources). Subsequently, gained knowledge should be used to inform practice-based research. For best practices to develop in this area, an agenda for dissemination and implementation research is essential [52,53]. These developments could help accelerate the adoption of evidence-based programs and move industries and communities along a continuum of integrated practices and policies, with implications for future research and comprehensive training of tomorrow's TWH workforce.

Finally, increased attention on evaluating the TWH approach is imperative. Anger et al. (2015) published an evaluation of the effectiveness of TWH interventions and found that TWH interventions covering both injuries and chronic diseases can improve worker safety and health; however, the authors found only 17 interventions that met their criteria for review [19]. Feltner et al. (2016) concluded that TWH interventions may improve health behaviors, although the authors were unable to draw conclusions about the interventions' impact on injuries and overall quality of life because of differences in measures used [23]. Similarly, Loeppke et al. (2015) assessed seven national and international guidelines aimed at worker safety, health, and well-being and concluded that there was promise but considerable variation in the guidelines on strategies, evidence, and strategic elements [26].

2.9.2. Healthy Work Design and Well-Being

In addition to forthcoming critical work by external TWH stakeholders and partners, NIOSH continues to make considerable headway. The TWH program has had a widespread impact on other NIOSH programs through the recognition of well-being as an imperative component of the NIOSH intramural research program structure. Indeed, the Office for TWH influenced the overall research trajectory of NIOSH, bringing to life the construct of worker well-being [25] into the decades-old NORA portfolio. This included enhancing future collaborations and deepening connections in the area of improved work design and well-being across NIOSH.

The programmatic synthesis of elements of three separate and independent programs: TWH, economics, and work organization and stress-related disorders is evident in a newly developed program entitled, Healthy Work Design and Well-Being (HWD). HWD is one of only seven NORA cross-sector programs in the third decade of NORA. The HWD program seeks to improve the design of work, work environments, and management practices in order to advance worker safety, health, and well-being. This program works with partners in labor, industry, trade associations, professional organizations, and academia to accomplish its goals.

Work design has implications for the safety, health, well-being, and functioning of individuals, families, groups, organizations, and communities. Like the TWH approach, the HWD program views workplaces as settings not only to impact work-related risks, such as unsafe working conditions, high job demands, and low control, but also to promote workplace programs and conditions that provide support for workers' health and well-being, such as smoking cessation or promotion of healthy physical activity [54]. The close alignment and potential for synergy with TWH efforts is apparent, rich, and compelling.

Healthy work design efforts include primary-level interventions that change the design of both the physical workspace and work processes to reduce sedentary behavior and increase physical activity during the work day. Furthermore, these efforts collectively serve another critical function, which is to support the overall well-being of workers. Worker well-being characterizes quality of life with respect to an individual's health and work-related environmental, organizational, and psychosocial factors [25]. Organizational practices that focus on prevention of safety and health hazards and promotion of well-being typically involve multi-level approaches that include commitment and involvement from management as well as worker input on identification of effective strategies.

Going forward, the HWD program, along with TWH professionals and other partners, will further our understanding of healthy work design and advance worker well-being through researching, implementing interventions, and translating findings into practice.

2.9.3. New Workforce Challenges

As time goes on, the Office for TWH will strive to bring credible solutions to not only on-going but also new challenges facing workers and employers. One such pressing example the CDC is prioritizing—as is the Office for TWH—is the need for comprehensive remedies to the U.S. opioid epidemic, from which the workplace and workers are not immune.

The U.S. Bureau of Labor Statistics reported that overdose deaths at work from non-medical use of drugs or alcohol increased by at least 38% annually between 2013 and 2016. The 217 workplace overdose deaths reported in 2016 accounted for 4.2% of occupational injury deaths that year, compared with 1.8% in 2013 [55]. Opioids are often initially prescribed to manage pain arising from a work injury though workers can develop a subsequent non-work injury related dependence, making this a critical issue for all those involved in worker safety, health, and well-being. Though opioid use/misuse rates are higher in certain occupations/industries, there are some commonplace factors associated with use/misuse; these include heavy workloads; hazards causing slips, trips, and falls; job insecurity;

job loss; and high-demand/low-control jobs [56]. Further, rates are higher in occupations with lower availability of paid sick leave, suggesting that the need to return to work soon after an injury may contribute to high rates of opioid-related overdose deaths [57,58].

Whether they involve examining antecedents of drug use or developing strategies for those returning to the workplace while recovering from addiction, TWH strategies can offer guidance for employers to follow. Briefly, using NIOSH- and the Office for TWH-developed resources [31,32,59], early efforts would focus on eliminating or minimizing working conditions that may predispose to worker injury or illness or that lead to increased levels of worker stress or excessive work demands. Next, educating occupational health providers, onsite and community-wide, of the organization's policies related to return-to-work after an injury and after the prescribing of opioids would be imperative. Additional steps would be taken to educate and train leaders, managers, and supervisors about likely red flags to observe, and how to effectively, efficiently, and compassionately address these. Careful examination of the impacts, risks, and considerations of safety-sensitive jobs and particular worker duties would occur, as well as of pre-employment/ongoing requirements. Finally, workers and their families would be provided with the necessary education on the proper and safe use of opioids, both at work and away from work. The Office for TWH and others across NIOSH are diligently working on actionable guidance and recommendations, materials, and resources to help address the opioid crisis affecting workers and employers [60].

No matter the complex, multi-faceted, or new challenge facing the future workforce, the Office for TWH will continue to work with its partners and stakeholders to effectively tackle issues amenable to integrated and comprehensive solutions that account for work and non-work factors.

3. Conclusions

The TWH framework, while rooted in the bedrock of worker health protection and prevention, must be a living, breathing entity, responding to the changing needs of workers, organizations, and the U.S. economy. Perennial challenges of the work environment, such as safety hazards, work stress, mental health, substance misuse, and chronic disease, are prime targets for integrated, holistic approaches rather than the more limited, siloed ones of the past. Where worker health issues cross the boundaries of work and home, affecting the lives of workers in and out of the workplace, there will be a place for TWH strategies that bridge this distance.

Author Contributions: Conceptualization, S.L.T., L.C.C., A.C., H.H., J.N. and C.-C.C.; Supervision, S.L.T.; Writing—original draft, S.L.T., L.C.C., A.C., H.H., J.N. and C.-C.C.; Writing—review & editing, S.L.T., L.C.C., A.C., H.H., J.N. and C.-C.C. All authors read and approved the final manuscript.

Funding: This research received no external funding.

Acknowledgments: The authors express their thanks to Harpriya Kaur, Sara Luckhaupt, Anita Schill, Reid Richards, and Seleen Collins for reviewing and editing the manuscript. The findings and conclusions in this paper are those of the authors and do not necessarily represent the official position of the National Institute for Occupational Safety and Health, Centers for Disease Control and Prevention.

Conflicts of Interest: The authors declare no conflict of interest.

References

1. National Institute for Occupational Safety and Health. What Is Total Worker Health? Available online: https://www.cdc.gov/niosh/twh/totalhealth.html (accessed on 8 March 2018).
2. Sorensen, G.; McLellan, D.; Dennerlein, J.T.; Pronk, N.P.; Allen, J.D.; Boden, L.I.; Okechukwu, C.A.; Hashimoto, D.; Stoddard, A.; Wagner, G.R. Integration of health protection and health promotion: Rationale, indicators, and metrics. *J. Occup. Environ. Med.* **2013**, *55* (Suppl. 12), S12–S18. [CrossRef] [PubMed]
3. Institute of Medicine. Integrating Employee Health: A Model Program for NASA. 2005. Available online: https://www.nap.edu/catalog/11290/integrating-employee-health-a-model-program-for-nasa (accessed on 22 September 2018).

4. Pronk, N. Integrated worker health protection and promotion programs: Overview and perspectives on health and economic outcomes. *J. Occup. Environ. Med.* **2013**, *55* (Suppl. 12), S30–S37. [CrossRef] [PubMed]
5. Punnett, L.; Cherniack, M.; Henning, R.; Morse, T.; Faghri, P.; Team, C.-N.R. A conceptual framework for integrating workplace health promotion and occupational ergonomics programs. *Public Health Rep.* **2009**, *124* (Suppl. 1), 16–25. [CrossRef] [PubMed]
6. Schill, A.L.; Chosewood, L.C. The NIOSH Total Worker Health program: An overview. *J. Occup. Environ. Med.* **2013**, *55* (Suppl. 12), S8–S11. [CrossRef] [PubMed]
7. National Institute for Occupational Safety and Health. Total Worker Health. Available online: https://www.cdc.gov/niosh/twh/ (accessed on 3 August 2018).
8. National Institute for Occupational Safety and Health. *Research Compendium; The NIOSH Total Worker Health™ Program: Seminal Research Papers 2012*; DHHS (NIOSH) Publication No. 2012-146; U.S. Department of Health and Human Services, Centers for Disease Control and Prevention, National Institute for Occupational Safety and Health: Cincinnati, OH, USA, 2012.
9. DeJoy, D.; Southern, D. An integrative perspective on work-site health promotion. *J. Occup. Med.* **1993**, *35*, 1221–1230. [PubMed]
10. Sauter, S.L. Integrative approaches to safeguarding the health and safety of workers. *Ind. Health* **2013**, *51*, 559–561. [CrossRef] [PubMed]
11. National Institute for Occupational Safety and Health. 1st and 2nd International Symposia to Advance Total Worker Health®. Available online: https://www.cdc.gov/niosh/TWH/symposium.html (accessed on 30 October 2018).
12. National Institute for Occupational Safety and Health. *National Occupational Research Agenda (NORA)/National Total Worker Health® Agenda (2016–2026): A National Agenda to Advance Total Worker Health® Research, Practice, Policy, and Capacity*; DHHS (NIOSH) Publication 2016-114; U.S. Department of Health and Human Services, Centers for Disease Control and Prevention, National Institute for Occupational Safety and Health: Cincinnati, OH, USA, 2016.
13. National Institute for Occupational Safety and Health. NIOSH Response to Summarized Stakeholders' Comments. Available online: https://www.cdc.gov/niosh/twh/pdfs/NIOSH-Response-to-Summarized-Stakeholders-Comments_4_12_16.pdf (accessed on 27 December 2018).
14. Cherniack, M.; Henning, R.; Merchant, J.; Punnett, L.; Sorensen, G.; Wagner, G. Statement on National WorkLife Priorities. *Am. J. Ind. Med.* **2010**, *54*, 10–20. [CrossRef]
15. Hymel, P.A.; Loeppke, R.R.; Baase, C.M.; Burton, W.N.; Hartenbaum, N.P.; Hudson, T.W.; McLellan, R.K.; Mueller, K.L.; Roberts, M.A.; Yarborough, C.M.; et al. Workplace health protection and promotion: A new pathway for a healthier—And safer—Workforce. *J. Occup. Environ. Med.* **2011**, *53*, 695–702. [CrossRef]
16. Sorensen, G.; Landsbergis, P.; Hammer, L.; Amick, B.C., 3rd; Linnan, L.; Yancey, A.; Welch, L.S.; Goetzel, R.Z.; Flannery, K.M.; Pratt, C.; et al. Preventing chronic disease in the workplace: A workshop report and recommendations. *Am. J. Public Health* **2011**, *101* (Suppl. 1), S196–S207. [CrossRef]
17. Institute of Medicine. *Promising and Best Practices in Total Worker Health: Workshop Summary*; The National Academies Press: Washington, DC, USA, 2014; Available online: http://www.iom.edu/Activities/Environment/TotalWorkerHealth/2014-MAY-22.aspx (accessed on 22 September 2018).
18. National Institutes of Health and National Institute for Occupational Safety and Health Pathways to Prevention Workshop. Total Worker Health: What's Work Got to Do with It? Available online: https://prevention.nih.gov/programs-events/pathways-to-prevention/workshops/total-worker-health (accessed on 22 February 2018).
19. Anger, W.K.; Elliot, D.L.; Bodner, T.; Olson, R.; Rohlman, D.S.; Truxillo, D.M.; Kuehl, K.S.; Hammer, L.B.; Montgomery, D. Effectiveness of total worker health interventions. *J. Occup. Health Psychol.* **2015**, *20*, 226–247. [CrossRef]
20. National Institute for Occupational Safety and Health. Issues Relevant to Advancing Worker Well-Being through Total Worker Health. Available online: https://www.cdc.gov/niosh/twh/pdfs/TWH-Issues-4x3_10282015_final.pdf (accessed on 27 January 2018).
21. McLellan, R.K. Work, Health, And Worker Well-Being: Roles and Opportunities For Employers. *Health Aff. (Millwood)* **2017**, *36*, 206–213. [CrossRef] [PubMed]
22. National Institute for Occupational Safety and Health. Centers of Excellence. Available online: https://www.cdc.gov/niosh/twh/centers.html (accessed on 11 October 2018).

23. Feltner, C.; Peterson, K.; Palmieri Weber, R.; Cluff, L.; Coker-Schwimmer, E.; Viswanathan, M.; Lohr, K.N. The Effectiveness of Total Worker Health Interventions: A Systematic Review for a National Institutes of Health Pathways to Prevention Workshop. *Ann. Intern. Med.* **2016**, *165*, 262–269. [CrossRef] [PubMed]
24. Tamers, S.L.; Goetzel, R.; Kelly, K.M.; Luckhaupt, S.; Nigam, J.; Pronk, N.P.; Rohlman, D.S.; Baron, S.; Brosseau, L.M.; Bushnell, T.; et al. Research Methodologies for Total Worker Health®: Proceedings from a Workshop. *J. Occup. Environ. Med.* **2018**, *60*, 968–978. [CrossRef] [PubMed]
25. Chari, R.; Chang, C.C.; Sauter, S.L.; Sayers, E.L.P.; Cerully, J.L.; Schulte, P.; Schill, A.L.; Uscher-Pines, L. Expanding the Paradigm of Occupational Safety and Health: A New Framework for Worker Well-Being. *J. Occup. Environ. Med.* **2018**, *60*, 589–593. [CrossRef] [PubMed]
26. Loeppke, R.R.; Hohn, T.; Baase, C.; Bunn, W.B.; Burton, W.N.; Eisenberg, B.S.; Ennis, T.; Fabius, R.; Hawkins, R.J.; Hudson, T.W.; et al. Integrating health and safety in the workplace: How closely aligning health and safety strategies can yield measurable benefits. *J. Occup. Environ. Med.* **2015**, *57*, 585–597. [CrossRef] [PubMed]
27. National Institute for Occupational Safety and Health. Promising Practices for Total Worker Health. Available online: https://www.cdc.gov/niosh/twh/practices.html (accessed on 12 September 2018).
28. National Institute for Occupational Safety and Health. Total Worker Health Affiliates. Available online: https://www.cdc.gov/niosh/twh/affiliate.html (accessed on 2 September 2018).
29. National Institute for Occupational Safety and Health. TWH in Action! eNewsletter. Available online: https://www.cdc.gov/niosh/twh/newsletter/default.html (accessed on 6 December 2018).
30. National Institute for Occupational Safety and Health. Total Worker Health Webinar Series. Available online: https://www.cdc.gov/niosh/twh/webinar.html (accessed on 6 December 2018).
31. National Institute for Occupational Safety and Health. The Hierarchy of Controls Applied to Total Worker Health. Available online: https://www.cdc.gov/niosh/twh/letsgetstarted.html (accessed on 22 September 2017).
32. Lee, M.P.; Hudson, H.; Richards, R.; Chang, C.C.; Chosewood, L.C.; Schill, A.L. *Fundamentals of Total Worker Health Approaches: Essential Elements for Advancing Worker Safety, Health, and Well-Being*; DHHS (NIOSH) Publication No. 2017-112; U.S. Department of Health and Human Services, Centers for Disease Control and Prevention, National Institute for Occupational Safety and Health: Cincinnati, OH, USA, 2016.
33. Hudson, H.L.; Nigam, J.S.; Sauter, S.L.; Chosewood, L.C.; Schill, A.S.; Howard, J. *Total Worker Health: Integrative Approaches to Safety, Health, and Well-Being*; American Psychological Association: Washington, DC, USA, 2018; in press.
34. American Psychological Association Work, Stress and Health. 2015: Sustainable Work, Sustainable Health, Sustainable Organizations. Available online: https://www.apa.org/wsh/past/2015/index.aspx (accessed on 2 October 2018).
35. Occupational Safety & Health Administration. Sustainability in the Workplace: A New Approach for Advancing Worker Safety and Health. Available online: www.osha.gov/sustainability (accessed on 2 October 2018).
36. Center for Safety and Health Sustainability. Center for Safety and Health Sustainability. Available online: http://www.centershs.org/aboutus.php (accessed on 20 September 2018).
37. Vitality Institute. Reporting on Health: A Roadmap for Investors, Companies, and Reporting Platforms. Available online: www.thevitalityinstitute.org/healthreporting (accessed on 3 September 2018).
38. National Institute for Occupational Safety and Health. *Understanding small enterprises: proceedings from the 2017 conferenc*; Cunningham, T., Schulte, P., Jacklitsch, B., Burnett, G., Newman, L., Brown, C., Haan, M., Eds.; DHHS (NIOSH) Publication No. 2019-108; U.S. Department of Health and Human Services, Centers for Disease Control and Prevention, National Institute for Occupational Safety and Health: Cincinnati, OH, USA, 2018.
39. International Organization for Standardization. Occupational Health and Safety Management Systems—Requirements with Guidance for Use. Available online: https://www.iso.org/obp/ui/#iso:std:iso:45001:ed-1:v1:en (accessed on 11 October 2018).
40. Mental Health Commission of Canada National Standard of Canada for Psychological Health and Safety in the Workplace. Available online: https://www.mentalhealthcommission.ca/English/what-we-do/workplace/national-standard (accessed on 4 September 2018).

41. University of Colorado. Certificate in Total Worker Health. Available online: http://www.ucdenver.edu/academics/colleges/PublicHealth/Academics/degreesandprograms/certificate/Pages/TotalWorkerHealth.aspx (accessed on 2 October 2018).
42. International Society Security Association. Vision Zero. Available online: http://visionzero.global/ (accessed on 2 October 2018).
43. Black, C. Working for a Healthier Tomorrow. 2008. Available online: https://www.rnib.org.uk/sites/default/files/Working_for_a_healthier_tomorrow.pdf (accessed on 10 October 2018).
44. Sepulveda, M.J. From worker health to citizen health: Moving upstream. *J. Occup. Environ. Med.* **2013**, *55* (Suppl. 12), S52–S57. [CrossRef] [PubMed]
45. Peckham, T.K.; Baker, M.G.; Camp, J.E.; Kaufman, J.D.; Seixas, N.S. Creating a future for occupational health. *Ann. Work Expo. Health* **2017**, *61*, 3–15.
46. Adams, J.M. The Value of Wellness. *Public Health Rep.* **2018**, *133*, 127–129.
47. U.S. Department of Health and Human Services. The Surgeon General's Priorities. Available online: https://www.surgeongeneral.gov/priorities/index.html#econ (accessed on 6 December 2018).
48. National Academies of Sciences, Engineering and Medicine, Action Collaborative on Business Engagement Building Healthy Communities. Available online: http://www.nationalacademies.org/hmd/Activities/PublicHealth/~{}/link.aspx?_id=3DEB3B97AEDA43FCBDBF4AB2091E1A87&_z=z (accessed on 6 December 2018).
49. National Academy of Medicine. Action Collaborative on Clinician Well-Being and Resilience. Available online: https://nam.edu/initiatives/clinician-resilience-and-well-being/ (accessed on 6 December 2018).
50. Curry, S.; Bradley, C.; Grossman, D.; Hubbard, R.; Ortega, A. NIH Pathways to Prevention Workshop Total Worker Health®: What's Work Got to Do with It? 2015. Available online: https://prevention.nih.gov/sites/default/files/documents/twh/twh-final-report-2016.pdf (accessed on 7 October 2018).
51. Bradley, C.J.; Grossman, D.C.; Hubbard, R.A.; Ortega, A.N.; Curry, S.J. Integrated Interventions for Improving Total Worker Health: A Panel Report From the National Institutes of Health Pathways to Prevention Workshop: Total Worker Health-What's Work Got to Do With It? *Ann. Intern. Med.* **2016**, *165*, 279–283. [CrossRef]
52. Dugan, A.G.; Farr, D.A.; Namazi, S.; Henning, R.A.; Wallace, K.N.; El Ghaziri, M.; Punnett, L.; Dussetschleger, J.L.; Cherniack, M.G. Process evaluation of two participatory approaches: Implementing total worker health(R) interventions in a correctional workforce. *Am. J. Ind. Med.* **2016**, *59*, 897–918. [CrossRef]
53. Schulte, P.A.; Cunningham, T.R.; Nickels, L.; Felknor, S.; Guerin, R.; Blosser, F.; Chang, C.C.; Check, P.; Eggerth, D.; Flynn, M.; et al. Translation research in occupational safety and health: A proposed framework. *Am. J. Ind. Med.* **2017**, *60*, 1011–1022. [CrossRef] [PubMed]
54. Sorensen, G.; Stoddard, A.; Quintiliani, L.; Ebbeling, C.; Nagler, E.; Yang, M.; Pereira, L.; Wallace, L. Tobacco use cessation and weight management among motor freight workers: Results of the gear up for health study. *Cancer Causes Control* **2010**, *21*, 2113–2122. [CrossRef] [PubMed]
55. Bureau of Labor Statistics. *Economic News Release: Census of Fatal Occupational Injuries Summary, 2017*; Bureau of Labor Statistics: Washington, DC, USA, 2017. Available online: https://www.bls.gov/news.release/cfoi.nr0.htm (accessed on 12 September 2018).
56. Kowalski-McGraw, M.; Green-McKenzie, J.; Pandalai, S.P.; Schulte, P.A. Characterizing the Interrelationships of Prescription Opioid and Benzodiazepine Drugs with Worker Health and Workplace Hazards. *J. Occup. Environ. Med.* **2017**, *59*, 1114–1126. [CrossRef] [PubMed]
57. Massachusetts Department of Public Health. *Opioid-Related Overdose Deaths in Massachusetts by Industry and Occupation, 2011–2015*; MDPH Occupational Health Surveillance Program: Boston, MA, USA, 2018. Available online: https://www.mass.gov/files/documents/2018/08/15/opioid-industry-occupation.pdf (accessed on 1 November 2018).
58. Centers for Disease Control and Prevention. *Occupational Patterns in Unintentional and Undetermined Drug-Involved and Opioid-Involved Overdose Deaths—United States, 2007–2012*; U.S. Department of Health and Human Services, Centers for Disease Control and Prevention: Atlanta, GA, USA, 2018. Available online: https://www.cdc.gov/mmwr/volumes/67/wr/mm6733a3.htm?s_cid=mm6733a3_e (accessed on 1 November 2018).

59. National Institute for Occupational Safety and Health. Total Worker Health Tools: Let's Get Started. Available online: https://www.cdc.gov/niosh/twh/letsgetstarted.html (accessed on 22 September 2017).
60. National Institute for Occupational Safety and Health. Opioids. Available online: https://www.cdc.gov/niosh/topics/opioids/default.html (accessed on 3 January 2019).

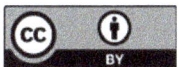

© 2019 by the authors. Licensee MDPI, Basel, Switzerland. This article is an open access article distributed under the terms and conditions of the Creative Commons Attribution (CC BY) license (http://creativecommons.org/licenses/by/4.0/).

International Journal of
Environmental Research and Public Health

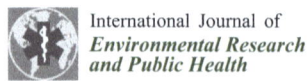

Article

Understanding the Role of Academic Partners as Technical Assistance Providers: Results from an Exploratory Study to Address Precarious Work

Tessa Bonney *, Christina Welter, Elizabeth Jarpe-Ratner[ID] and Lorraine M. Conroy

Environmental and Occupational Health Sciences, School of Public Health, University of Illinois at Chicago, Chicago, IL 60607, USA
* Correspondence: tbonne5@uic.edu

Received: 23 September 2019; Accepted: 12 October 2019; Published: 15 October 2019

Abstract: Universities may be well poised to support knowledge, skill, and capacity-building efforts to foster the development of multi-level interventions to address complex problems. Researchers at the University of Illinois at Chicago (UIC) engaged organizations interested in developing policy- and systems-level initiatives to address the drivers of precarious work in a six-meeting Action Learning (AL) process, in which the researchers served as technical assistance (TA) providers focused on facilitating learning and promoting critical thinking among participants. This exploratory qualitative study examined the role, facilitators, challenges, and impacts of university facilitation in this context. A total of 22 individuals participated in this study, including UIC TA providers, content expert TA providers from labor-focused organizations, and TA recipients from health-focused organizations. Results from interviews and a focus group highlight the utility of a university connecting organizations from different disciplines that do not traditionally work together, and suggest that the TA provided by UIC helped participants think concretely about precarious work and ways in which their organizations might work collaboratively to bring about sustainable change. Findings from this study suggest that university facilitation using an AL approach may be effective in increasing knowledge to action.

Keywords: precarious work; action learning; technical assistance; community-university partnership; policy, systems, and environmental (PSE) change

---

1. Introduction

In recent years, the National Institute for Occupational Safety and Health (NIOSH) has funded several *Total Worker Health*® Centers for Excellence at universities across the United States with the goal of building scientific evidence around innovative approaches to address complex problems faced by workers in the United States [1]. Occupational safety and health researchers and practitioners are increasingly called to navigate the complexities of a changing work landscape, in which work arrangements have increasingly shifted away from standard, full-time employment with benefits toward non-standard, "atypical", and precarious work arrangements such as employment in temporary or contract jobs [2]. The University of Illinois at Chicago (UIC) Center for Healthy Work, one of the NIOSH Total Worker Health (TWH) Centers for Excellence, has focused its efforts on understanding the barriers faced by workers in these precarious jobs in Illinois, and building evidence around the development of interventions to remove those barriers [3].

Over the past several years, a subset of researchers at the UIC Center for Healthy Work have engaged with individuals and organizations in Chicago and across the state of Illinois to better understand the causes and consequences of precarious work and initiatives that are already underway to address them. One of the Center for Healthy Work's aims is to work with a variety of organizational partners, across sectors and levels, to build organizations' capacities to develop and implement interventions to address the barriers to healthy work. While some studies have examined the value and impacts of community–university engagement in research and practice partnerships [4–6], existing studies have not focused on universities as a convener for processes focused heavily on planning and preparing for action, and focused less on traditional research methodology. The UIC Center for Healthy Work is examining the role that a university can play in supporting knowledge, skills, and overall capacity-building efforts to foster the development of multi-level initiatives to address precarious work.

1.1. Precarious Work and the Healthy Work Collaborative Initiative

The term "precarious work" has been used to describe work that is "uncertain, unpredictable, and risky from the point of view of the worker" [7]. The rise in precarious work in the US can be linked to macroeconomic changes that resulted in increased global competition, which led to outsourcing of labor, weakened labor unions, and deregulation of the labor market [7]. Employers have sought to minimize costs by shifting jobs away from standard, full-time work arrangements toward a more flexible labor market. These more flexible, precarious work arrangements are characterized by low wages, a lack of protection from termination, variable work schedules, disproportionate exposure to health and safety hazards in the workplace, and working conditions that cause high psychosocial stress [2,8–10]. Without intervention, a growing share of workers in the US will experience precarious employment conditions, regardless of occupation [11].

Although studies increasingly show that these highly precarious work arrangements adversely affect the health of workers [12–15], interventions that improve the health of workers in these jobs are difficult to design and implement, given the nature of their work arrangements [16]. There is a substantial body of literature that posits that public health interventions that create the social and environmental conditions to promote and facilitate health are likely to be most effective and impactful on a population level [17–19]. Since many of the features of precarious work are not unique to a single occupation or to a single workplace, interventions aimed at addressing the causes of precarious work must be implemented at these broadly impactful social ecological levels. These types of interventions, typically in the form of policy, systems, and environmental (PSE) changes, are most effective when a diverse group of stakeholders are involved in intervention development and implementation, and when these stakeholders understand the problem and relevant power dynamics [17,20,21].

While there are several examples of successful, cross-sectoral PSE interventions to address public health issues, including tobacco control and measures to reduce automotive crashes [19], there is little evidence in the literature of similar strategies to address precarious work. Given the absence of existing best practices or evidence-based initiatives in this area, researchers at the UIC Center for Healthy Work engaged a group of multi-disciplinary stakeholders in a process designed to understand and begin to develop upstream action to address drivers of precarious work. This process, known as the Healthy Work Collaborative Initiative, involved a six-session series of instructional and planning-based activities for organizations that were interested in addressing precarious work.

The six session Healthy Work Collaborative (HWC) was part of a larger project in the UIC Center for Healthy Work. The overarching aim of this larger project was to use an action research framework to understand and address precarious work through cycles of inquiry and action planning [22]. The HWC was a component of this larger project, which was designed with an intent to increase stakeholders' individual and organizational capacities to apply PSE strategies to address drivers of precarious work. The primary goal of the HWC was to bring together health and labor organizations to explore initiatives that may address health in the context of precarious employment. The goal of this manuscript is to report on a study that examined the role of university-based facilitation in this HWC process, conceptualized as technical assistance (TA) provided by UIC researchers. The HWC and TA in the HWC are further described below.

UIC researchers recruited Chicago- and Illinois-based public health and healthcare organizations and their partners to participate in the six in-person HWC sessions; many participants were recruited through existing relationships between the School of Public Health researchers and representatives of these organizations. The researchers also recruited representatives of labor organizations, including Chicago-based worker centers and labor advocacy groups, to share content expertise with participants during the HWC sessions. All labor organizations represented in the HWC also had longstanding relationships with researchers in the UIC School of Public Health. All six in-person HWC sessions took place within a 10-week period in the spring and summer of 2018.

Collaborations between university groups and outside partner organizations have been described in various contexts in the literature. Much of the existing literature on community–university partnerships focuses on opportunities for knowledge translation, or the application of research findings in the community, and service-learning and community-based research [4,6]. While the HWC model shares some of the features of community–university partnerships highlighted in the literature, such as an opportunity to co-create knowledge and develop shared research and action agendas [4], the purpose of the HWC was primarily to drive action rather than to generate knowledge.

The researchers designed the HWC using an Action Learning (AL) approach, which is an approach to problem solving that emphasizes learning through action and reflection on the results of that action [23]. AL was originally conceptualized by Reg Revans in the early 1980s, but has been adapted by others to better suit emerging learning and action needs in different contexts. One of these adaptations is that of Marquardt et al., in which AL is used with the intent to build and sustain systems-level change [24]. Similar to Revan's original AL approach, that described by Marquardt et al. uses an iterative, participatory process, which combines scientific knowledge with evidence derived from learners' experiences to solve complex problems [24,25]. However, unlike Revan's approach, Marquardt et al.'s AL approach relies on AL "coaches", or facilitators who promote critical thinking through the probing and prompting of learners throughout a process. In the HWC, UIC researchers served in this facilitator role, which is further described below.

Activities within each HWC session were designed to build upon one another so that participants would leave with foundational knowledge and skills to begin to plan for and take action to address the drivers of precarious work. The HWC sessions were grouped into three phases (Table 1), all of which incorporated AL tools: (1) Understanding; (2) System, strategies, and approaches; and (3) Planning for action. A fourth phase, the Action phase, was not included in the HWC sessions. Each phase included two sessions. Table 1 details the purpose of each phase and the activities that were included in that phase's sessions.

Small stipends were provided to HWC participants to compensate for their time spent preparing for and participating in the sessions. This aligns with the community–university partnership literature that suggests that funding community engagement in university-sponsored activities both supports community involvement and demonstrates the value that the university places on community engagement [6]. Funding was also provided to representatives from local worker centers and other labor advocacy and educational organizations who served as TA providers in the HWC sessions. The various participant roles in the HWC are further described below.

Table 1. Healthy Work Collaborative (HWC) Initiative.

Phase	Purpose of Cycle in the HWC	Aligning HWC Activities
Understanding	Gather information and begin to develop a shared understanding of precarious work.	Presentations and Q&A with panel of experts * Root cause analysis and creation of a rich picture diagram (systems map).
System, strategies, and approaches	Analyze and interpret data from the "Understanding" phase and further develop a shared understanding of precarious work and approaches to address it.	Framing and stakeholder exercises. Power analysis and mapping exercise.
Planning for action	Begin to develop a plan for action to address drivers of precarious work based on the shared understanding of precarious work from the previous cycles.	Past, current, and future state exercise. Development of a Theory of Change.
Action	Implement the plan for action developed during the previous phase. The "Action" phase was not part of the HWC sessions.	The "Action" phase was not part of the HWC sessions, but data collection for this study occurred during this phase.

* Experts included representatives from local worker centers and other labor advocacy organizations, as well as labor-focused academic partners from outside of the University of Illinois at Chicago (UIC) Center for Healthy Work. These experts are further described under "Technical Assistance (TA) in the Healthy Work Collaborative (HWC)".

1.2. Participant Roles in the Healthy Work Collaborative (HWC)

Participants in the HWC sessions fell into three categories: (1) the UIC researchers who organized and facilitated the overall HWC process and served as AL facilitators; (2) representatives from labor organizing, labor advocacy organizations, and labor-focused academic organizations who attended select HWC sessions and led HWC activities during those sessions; and (3) representatives from primarily public health and healthcare organizations who attended and participated in all six HWC sessions.

The first two groups, the UIC researchers and the representatives from labor organizations, were termed "technical assistance (TA) providers" for the HWC. Together, these TA providers engaged the largely non-labor and non-academic health-focused participants in the various HWC activities. The TA providers also engaged with individuals or small groups in other capacities within and outside of the in-person sessions as they grappled with the issue of precarious work and plans for action in their own organizational or partnership-based contexts. The role of labor expert TA is examined elsewhere (manuscript in preparation).

While there is no empirical research pointing to an ideal structure for a TA process for moving recipients toward action, some studies point to features of TA–recipient models that make them more effective than others. Effective TA models integrate several theoretical principles, including theories of change, adult learning, consultation, and facilitation [26–28]. Using these principles, researchers and practitioners in several fields have conceptualized TA as a multi-tiered approach to build the capacity of individuals or organizations to achieve substantial change [29,30].

TA has also been classified along a continuum from less intensive, content-driven TA, to more intensive, relationship-based TA [26,29]. The intensity of TA provided to a recipient typically depends on the recipient's needs and their desired project outcomes. Less intensive TA typically involves sharing of content or skill knowledge with the TA recipient, which is most useful when the recipient already has structures and policies in place to support PSE change [31]. This type of TA often involves fewer, less intensive TA–recipient encounters in which TA providers present information to the recipients, but do not engage in longer-term collaborative work. More intensive TA, on the other hand, requires a more sophisticated relationship between the TA provider and the recipient. In this instance, the TA provider engages in sustained, in-depth work in partnership with the TA recipient, and takes on more responsibility for the outcomes of the program that they are supporting [29].

In the HWC, TA provided by UIC researchers was conceptualized as more intensive, relationship-based TA, focused on facilitating behavior and systems change, while TA provided by labor experts was conceptualized as more content-driven, focused on the transfer of knowledge to participants. For the duration of the HWC, UIC TA providers divided themselves up between TA recipient groups, helping to guide TA recipients through each of the HWC activities and exercises. UIC TA providers also followed up with their TA recipient groups between HWC sessions, pointing them in the direction of resources, clarifying content from the sessions, and pushing them toward actionable next steps. This type of higher intensity TA, focused on the facilitation of learning and action planning, aligned with the role of an AL "coach" described in the AL literature [32,33]. There is some evidence that higher intensity TA, facilitation, or coaching, involving frequent check-ins and tailored supports and feedback, increases the sustained engagement of learners, or TA recipients, in later implementation or action phases [26,34]. With the HWC, UIC researchers positioned themselves in a way to both connect practitioners in different disciplines who do not already work together, and support engagement between those practitioners as they move to bring about sustainable change. Little is known about universities operating in this role, and this study aims to contribute knowledge to this gap.

This study explores the role of TA provided by UIC researchers in the HWC process. Specifically, this study seeks to understand UIC TA providers' perceptions of their own roles in the HWC process, facilitators, and challenges associated with these roles, and any outcomes of the HWC process that they attribute to these roles. This study also seeks to understand the perceptions of other HWC participants, including labor expert TA providers and health-focused TA recipients, regarding these same concepts. Given that TA and university–community partnerships have been identified as important mechanisms to close the "knowledge to action" gap, this study seeks to explore the importance of these factors in facilitating the learning and development of PSE change interventions in the context of the HWC.

2. Materials and Methods

UIC researchers used a mixed-methods approach to evaluate the overall HWC process. For this study, researchers used an exploratory qualitative study design with focus group and interview methodology to examine HWC participants' perceptions of the role of TA provided by UIC in the HWC, including during the period leading up to the six sessions, the periods between sessions, and the period after the sessions. The UIC Institutional Review Board approved this study in 2018.

All 31 individuals who participated in the HWC in some capacity were invited to participate in this study. Information about the HWC participants is included in Table 2. Seven UIC TA providers participated in the HWC sessions, including two UIC faculty members, three staff members, and two student research assistants. Seven labor expert TA providers participated in at least one HWC session, and five participated in two or more sessions. Four of these labor expert TA providers represented Chicago-area worker centers, two represented national labor advocacy organizations, and one represented a labor-focused academic research center at UIC that is not part of the UIC Center for Healthy Work. A total of 17 representatives of other organizations participated in the HWC sessions as TA recipients, including representatives from local health departments (LHDs), public health and other health advocacy organizations, a hospital system, an academic institution other than UIC, a local board of health, two worker centers, and a labor union.

Of these TA recipients, 14 came to the HWC with other partners (see the TA Recipient Groups in Table 2). These TA recipient groups focused on action planning with their partners. The remaining three TA recipients attended the HWC sessions as individual representatives of their organization, and focused their efforts on action planning within their own organization's purview. Each TA recipient group or individual organization joined the HWC with a pre-determined focus for action planning. These foci are briefly described in Table 2.

Several instruments were developed to obtain information about UIC TA providers' roles in the HWC from the various HWC participants. A semi-structured focus group guide was developed to collect perspectives from the UIC facilitators immediately following the conclusion of the HWC. One semi-structured interview guide was designed to collect perspectives from the labor experts, who served as TA providers in the HWC sessions, immediately following their involvement in the HWC, and another semi-structured interview guide was designed to collect perspectives from non-labor, primarily health-focused TA recipients three months after the conclusion of the HWC sessions. Notably, both of the interview guides included questions aimed at understanding other features of the HWC and impacts of participating in the sessions. The results reported in this study focus on the aforementioned concepts around TA provided by UIC. Table 3 compares the content relevant to this study included in the interview guides and the focus group guide, all of which are further described below.

UIC TA providers were invited to participate in an in-person focus group in the days immediately following the final HWC session. The focus group guide was designed to capture UIC TA provider's perceptions of what TA recipients gained from the HWC process, perceptions of UIC TA providers' own roles inside and outside of the HWC sessions, and perceptions of impacts that the HWC process had on UIC TA providers' own thinking. Labor expert TA providers were invited to participate in a follow-up phone interview in this same time frame. All TA recipients were invited to participate in a phone interview approximately three months after the final HWC session, as were TA providers who had continued to engage with TA recipients beyond the formal HWC six-meeting period. The immediate post-HWC guide and the three-month post-HWC interview guide were designed to capture labor experts' and TA recipients' perceptions of the same concepts as the UIC TA provider focus group guide, as well as their impressions of the HWC process more generally. TA recipients were interviewed at the three-month time point instead of immediately post-HWC to better capture ways in which the TA recipients had applied what they had learned from the HWC since the conclusion of the sessions, and any implementation of activities planned during the HWC sessions.

Analysis

A preliminary codebook for this study was developed prior to data collection with template codes based on the study's research questions and relevant technical assistance literature similar to the code manual development described by Fereday and Muir Cochrane [35]. Four broad code categories were included in this a priori codebook: perception of TA role, intensity of TA, impact of TA, and importance of TA. These broad categories and sub-codes within each category were included in the a priori codebook with a definition and description of each code. Emergent codes were added during the preliminary analysis steps, and are described below. The codebook used for this study was separate to that used for the overall evaluation of the HWC process.

The in-person focus group with UIC TA providers and all phone interviews with labor expert TA providers and TA recipients were audio recorded and professionally transcribed. The transcripts were analyzed using a hybrid approach that involved both inductive and deductive coding and theme development, similar to the approach described by Fereday and Muir-Cochrane [35]. Dedoose software (Dedoose Version 7.0.23, web application for managing, analyzing, and presenting qualitative and mixed method research data, SocioCultural Research Consultants LLC, Los Angeles, CA, USA) was used for all qualitative analyses in this study.

Table 2. HWC Participants. TA: technical assistance, UIC: University of Illinois at Chicago.

TA Provider	Individuals/Organizations Represented (N Individual Representatives)	Focus of TA Provision
UIC TA Providers	Faculty (2) Staff (3) Students (2)	Process TA; organized HWC process and engaged TA recipients directly in in-depth discussions and action-planning activities using an AL approach. Clarified content and pushed TA recipients to move toward action.
Labor Expert TA Providers	Worker Centers (4) * Advocacy Orgs (2) Academic Orgs (1)	Content-focused TA; focused on the transfer of knowledge to TA recipients. Engaged TA recipients in presentations and discussions about precarious work and skills and strategies to address it.
TA Recipient Groups	Individuals/Organizations Represented (N individual representatives)	Focus for Action Planning
Rural	Local Health Department (LHD) (2), workforce development org (1), government representative (1)	Develop interventions to support health and well-being of precarious workers in rural county.
Hospital–Legal–Labor	Hospital system (1), legal organization (1), worker center (1) *	Identify precarious workers who enter hospital system and connect with appropriate legal and other support services.
Public Health Advocacy–Academic	Public health advocacy organization (1), academic institution (1)	Improve community health worker employment structures across the state of Illinois.
LHD-Labor 1	LHD (1), worker center (1)	Develop strategies to enforce minimum wage and sick-leave ordinances at county level.
LHD-Labor 2	LHD (1), worker center (1) *	Develop strategies for LHD's enforcement of labor standards during routine restaurant inspections.
TA Recipient Individuals	Individuals/Organizations Represented (N individual representatives)	Focus for Action Planning
Health Advocacy 1	Health advocacy organization (1)	Develop paid internship model focused on equity and inclusion.
Health Advocacy 2	Health advocacy organization (1)	Explore strategies to include precarious workers in workplace wellness programs.
Labor Union	Labor union (1)	Develop strategies to organize low-wage healthcare workers.

* Note: Two of the worker center representatives served in both labor expert presenter roles and participant team roles in the HWC initiative.

Table 3. Data Collection Instruments.

Instrument	Intended Audience	Key Constructs for this Study
Immediate Post-HWC Focus Group Guide	UIC TA providers (process facilitators).	Observed impacts of UIC TA provider engagement with other participants. Perceptions of value of UIC TA provider role. Challenges and facilitators to HWC TA providers–recipient model. Opportunities for engagement beyond HWC.
Immediate Post-HWC Interview Guide	Labor expert TA providers (content experts).	Experiences with UIC TA providers; observed and experienced impacts of all participants' engagement with UIC TA providers. Perceptions of value of UIC TA provider role. Challenges and facilitators to HWC TA providers–recipient model. Opportunities for engagement beyond HWC.
Three-Month Post-HWC Interview Guide	All non-TA provider participants (TA recipients). Labor expert TA providers involved with TA recipients beyond HWC sessions.	Experiences with UIC TA providers; impacts of engagement with UIC TA providers. Perceptions of value of UIC TA provider role. Challenges and facilitators to HWC TA providers–recipient model. Opportunities for engagement beyond HWC.

Immediate post-HWC interviews with labor expert TA providers and the focus group with UIC TA providers were coded by a single coder. For each transcribed interview, the following analysis protocol was used:

(1) Each full interview and the focus group transcript was read and key points were summarized in a memo. At this point, additional codes were added to the codebook based on new categories that emerged from the textual data.

(2) Then, a priori codes and emergent codes were applied to the interview text where text segments were considered representative of and matched the definition of an individual code.

(3) As segments of text were coded, each new excerpt was compared with segments that had previously been assigned the same code. In the event that a code did not seem to fit for both segments, a new code was added to the codebook, and relevant sections of the transcribed interview were recoded.

(4) After all interviews were coded and additions to and refinements of the codebook were complete, a new cycle of coding began. Each interview was re-coded using the updated codebook.

(5) After the second coding cycle, final coded segments were read and subjected to a process of clustering around similar patterns. Themes were identified when all data supporting a given pattern were clustered and saturation was reached. At this stage, differences in themes across interviewees were examined.

Three-month follow-up interviews were coded by two separate coders, and a slightly different analysis protocol was used. Steps 1 and 2 from the baseline and immediate post-HWC interview protocol were followed, as described above, with both coders reading and summarizing transcribed interviews and collaboratively making additions to the codebook. Then, the following steps were completed by the two coders in lieu of steps 3–5 from the baseline and immediate post-HWC analysis protocol: After each transcribed interview was coded by both coders, coded segments were compared for agreement. In the event that the two coders did not agree on coding for a particular segment, they discussed the segment and attempted to come to agreement as to which code(s) should be applied. In the event that the two coders could not come to agreement, a third coder was asked to code the interview and discuss applied codes with the original two coders. Additionally, in the event that no codes seemed to fit a given segment, a new code was added to the codebook, and relevant sections of the transcribed interview were recoded. Both coders reviewed already coded interviews for a comparison of applied codes and recoded those interviews as needed to reflect codebook updates. Final coded segments were read and a process of clustering around similar patterns and themes began. At this stage, differences in themes across participant type were examined.

3. Results

A total of 22 HWC participants (71%) participated in either the in-person focus group or at least one follow-up phone interview after the conclusion of the HWC. The immediate post-HWC focus group lasted approximately 90 minutes and was conducted in person, while the immediate post-HWC and three-month post-HWC follow-up interviews lasted approximately 60 min and were conducted by phone.

Seven UIC TA providers participated in the immediate post-HWC focus group, representing all but one of the UIC representatives who helped to facilitate the HWC process. One UIC representative (the first author on this paper) facilitated but did not participate in the focus group. Five labor expert TA providers participated in interviews immediately post-HWC, and two of these TA providers also participated in three-month post-HWC follow-up interviews. The two TA providers who participated in three-month follow-up interviews had substantial, continued involvement with at least one other non-TA HWC participant beyond the six HWC sessions, either in the form of more tailored and intensive TA provision or in the form a formalized partnership. Ten non-labor, primarily health-focused TA recipients also participated in three-month post-HWC follow-up interviews.

UIC TA providers, labor expert TA providers, and TA recipients shared a variety of perceptions of UIC TA in the HWC. Findings from the focus group and interviews are organized under the following broad categories: UIC's role in the HWC, facilitators and challenges associated with UIC's role, impacts of UIC's provision of TA, and future roles for UIC beyond the HWC.

3.1. Role of UIC TA in the HWC

All participants, including UIC TA providers, labor expert TA providers, and TA recipients reflected on the utility of UIC researchers as TA providers in the HWC. Three main themes emerged from the focus group and interview data: (1) the value of UIC's role as a convener of the HWC; (2) UIC TA providers' ability to facilitate learning by guiding TA recipients through the HWC activities and holding them accountable to the next steps; and (3) UIC researchers' ability to both fill a gap in the literature and aid in the development of actions to address a complex issue. Each of these themes is further described below.

3.1.1. UIC's Role in Convening the HWC

In individual interviews, TA recipients and labor expert TA providers shared their perspectives of UIC's role as a convener of the HWC. Generally, interviewees noted that UIC was an appropriate connector and host for such a process, given the value that UIC as an institution places on community engagement. Interviewees described their own experiences interacting with faculty and staff at the university, and several highlighted explicit value statements put forth by university groups that reinforce UIC's commitment to community-engaged activities. One TA recipient mentioned the UIC School of Public Health, which houses the Center for Healthy Work, as being particularly committed to community engagement:

> *"So I think that one of the public health school's missions, or part of the mission, is to be engaged with the community. And I think that this is one very strong way of doing it."—TA recipient.*

Interviewees also highlighted the rigor that a university can bring to an initiative such as the HWC. Several interviewees noted the reputation of the UIC School of Public Health and its recognition as a leading research institution in Chicago. At least one interviewee described the value of having a public health perspective when planning for action around upstream issues such as work:

> *"I think there is certain rigor to having it, in a public health perspective, that maybe in a limited way could have come from some of the other participants in the collaborative ... [UIC TA providers] brought that."—TA recipient.*

3.1.2. UIC's Role in Facilitating Learning

An important observation of UIC TA providers' own role in the HWC was that of facilitating a shared language and fostering opportunities for open dialogue about the issues related to precarious work for all participants. UIC TA providers generally agreed that establishing a definition of precarious work early on in the HWC sessions helped to facilitate engagement in subsequent HWC activities and deeper dialogue between the various participants. One UIC TA provider described both UIC and labor expert TA providers' role in establishing this shared language:

"So I think it was a skill that people were able to find a shared language, and I think we helped facilitate that along with the TA providers, to be able to talk to one another."—UIC TA provider.

UIC TA providers further described their role as "pushing" or "coaching" TA recipients toward action as they progressed through the HWC sessions. Several UIC TA providers shared examples of ways in which they had helped TA recipients develop action steps based on what they had learned or created in HWC session activities; for example, one UIC TA provider had helped their group build a small action plan based on the Theory of Change that the group had developed during one of the HWC sessions. Several UIC TA providers noted that TA recipients were seemingly appreciative of this type of TA-led facilitation and encouragement, as summarized by one UIC TA provider below:

"I did hear quite a bit that having somebody to push them to help them focus, give them that extra support ... They wouldn't be doing it, without that push. They need the push. They need the ... And, I don't mean pushing them out the door. But, th ... to help encourage, to build their self-advocacy/capacity."—UIC TA provider.

In interviews, many TA recipients shared similar reflections of the utility of UIC TA providers' facilitation or "pushing" of TA recipients throughout the HWC process. Several TA recipients described specific interactions with UIC TA providers during or between HWC sessions in which the TA provider had helped them to further refine or develop tools or plans to move the recipients toward action. One TA recipient described their experience as follows:

"I liked the idea that you had a staff person that was sort of assigned to each group, because it really kept us together, and then you organized us. You made sure we had meetings, and we decided to have a little pre-meeting before the actual training sessions, and you really facilitated sort of all of the logistics, as well as providing leadership in the groups. And I think we loved working with the folks that we were working with."—TA recipient.

TA recipients also recognized UIC TA providers' roles in guiding them toward a more profound understanding of precarious work and TA recipients' own roles in addressing its drivers. Several TA recipients noted the ways in which UIC TA providers helped TA recipients to think about the issues without being overly prescriptive or forceful in what their takeaways should be. One TA recipient described their experiences with UIC TA providers as follows:

"One of the things I liked is that with [the] UIC facilitator and UIC facilitator and everybody, you all guided. You don't imprint on it ... And it's a great way to learn. And you helped guide people to where, I think where we should have gotten to without saying, you know, you let us have a learning experience, that's what I guess I'm trying to say, without handing us a syllabus and saying, 'You're going to be at this point, this point,' you know what I'm saying? And so I really liked that approach. And it's really very beneficial."—TA recipient.

3.1.3. UIC's Role in Contributing Evidence and Facilitating Action

In the focus group, UIC TA providers reflected on the factors that made their role in organizing and coordinating the HWC feasible and appropriate. Several UIC TA providers described the gap in the literature around PSE strategies to address the drivers of precarious work, and how this gap presented an opportunity for the researchers in the UIC Center for Healthy Work to gather contributing evidence in this arena via the HWC. One UIC TA provider summarized these sentiments below:

> "... it's about building the evidence that doesn't exist, there is not good evidence around how to do PSE change around in particular precarious work for sustainable change, and that's what we've been trying to do and we are documenting it, we're building evidence, we're adapting theory based on feedback for practice and integrating it to do something we hope is impactful."—UIC TA provider.

UIC TA providers also engaged in a discussion around academic expectations and needs for evidence building that allow for the dedicated time and funding to support an initiative such as the HWC. At least one UIC TA provider mentioned the need to respond to the expectations of the funding agency for the Center for Healthy Work by collecting data and producing products for dissemination, which is made possible through the engagement of other stakeholders in the HWC.

> "... we have to keep the funders in mind and research and building evidence in mind ... So having a product, something that can be disseminated widely or policy change, environmental change, having something happen that can be counted, that's [the funder's] perspective."—UIC TA provider.

3.2. Facilitators and Challenges Associated with UIC TA Role

Several themes emerged from the data regarding facilitators and challenges associated with the TA role that UIC researchers played in the HWC. Existing relationships between UIC researchers and representatives from the organization that participated in the HWC, and UIC's knowledge of the participants' needs and related opportunities emerged as facilitators associated with the UIC researchers' role; in contrast, constraints related to time, content, planning, and limitations to TA control emerged as challenges associated with this role. These facilitators and challenges are described below.

3.2.1. Existing Relationships

Labor expert TA providers and TA recipients described their existing relationships with UIC researchers as a catalyst to their involvement in the HWC. All labor expert TA providers described longstanding relationships with UIC faculty and staff in the Environmental and Occupational Health Division of the School of Public Health, while most of the non-labor TA recipients described existing relationships with faculty and staff at the MidAmerica Center for Public Health Practice, also in the School of Public Health, which provided training to public health professionals. Representatives from both School of Public Health groups were involved in the planning and coordinating of the HWC. One TA recipient described their relationship with UIC and their decision to participate in the HWC:

> "We're fortunate enough to have a long-standing working relationship with UIC ... So I heard about the collaborative from [UIC facilitators], and we talked about some of the work that was going to be done and what the overall, I guess what the health outcomes might be. There was [sic] some issues that I've kind of wanted to work on, and so I just said, yeah, I kind of was interested in pursuing this."—TA recipient.

Several interviewees indicated that they felt UIC researchers had their organization's best interests and needs in mind when soliciting their involvement in something such as the HWC. A labor expert TA provider summarized this sentiment:

> "... we have relationships with individuals and the departments that span all my time here ... we already have an idea of what kind of things that it would involve, or yeah, there's less uncertainty about, "Well, would this be a good use of my time?" That sort of thing 'cause we already have the relationship and are accustomed to working together. I think part of it is just experience is a factor in our decision making here to engage, being that we already have experience together."—Labor expert TA provider.

3.2.2. UIC's Capacity to Recognize Needs and Opportunities

Additionally, several interviewees described the university's unique capacity to recognize the need for and engage a diverse group of stakeholders to collaboratively learn about and plan for upstream action to address drivers of precarious work. Several interviewees described the unique features of the university as a convener, including its commitment to community engagement and its existing relationships with community organizations (further described below) that made the HWC especially impactful in a way that it would not have been without UIC's involvement. One interviewee summarized these sentiments below:

"I doubt we would have had the same kind of people, diversity of entities in the room and in conversation. Without you all ... I doubt the conversation would have happened without the (HWC), the grant funding which all happened behind it."—TA recipient.

At least one TA recipient also noted that the representatives in the HWC would not have had the opportunity to connect if it were not for the convening of the HWC.

"It is really helpful to bring groups together who haven't worked together before and who we may not always think of—and see how it ties back to our work—unless we get connected and seek it out on our own, which we don't really have time for, we don't have access to these new relationships."—Labor expert TA provider.

3.2.3. Time and Content Balance

Despite the many touted benefits of UIC's TA provision in the HWC, participants described some of the limitations, challenges, and opportunities for change given their experience in this HWC process. Many of the TA recipients, in particular, described the challenges of digesting so much new content in such a short period of time. Some TA recipients also felt that there was not enough time built in to reflect upon and apply what they had learned in the HWC sessions. One TA recipient summarized these sentiments below:

"It was super structured and a lot of stuff over a short timeline. There was a balance that it needed to be structured so it didn't lose the thread ... But it still was quite a bit."—TA recipient.

Several UIC TA providers also attributed challenges in timing with what TA recipients were able to accomplish through the HWC process. UIC TA providers felt that the readiness of TA recipients to both engage with a complex new issue such as precarious work and actively plan implementable interventions outside of the HWC sessions varied between groups and individual TA recipients. One UIC TA provider noted that the timing of the HWC was based solely on UIC researchers' own needs and not on the needs of participants, including both the readiness piece and the amount of time participants, including TA recipients and labor expert TA providers, needed in between sessions to digest information and prepare for subsequent sessions. One UIC TA provider summarized these observations below:

"I think the timing issue was really a very important factor in influencing what went on and what went well for some and what didn't go well for others."—UIC TA provider.

3.2.4. Time and Planning Constraints

UIC TA providers noted some of the challenges related to the tight HWC timeline, both in terms of what content could be covered in the sessions and in terms of limitations in time to plan the sessions. Several UIC TA providers shared the challenges that stemmed from working within a time-bound grant structure, in which funds allocated to activities such as the HWC needed to be spent down within a short time frame. This presented problems with HWC planning, limiting UIC TA providers' abilities to engage labor expert TA providers in much of the planning in advance of the meetings themselves:

" ... ultimately we only had so much time to devote to developing this curriculum and structuring these meetings that there are certain things with the curriculum that I think we may have done differently that would facilitate learning in a different way. I wonder if we had brought in all of the ... if they had the capacity to do this, if we had brought in all of the TA providers from the get go to develop a curriculum in a more collaborative way."—UIC TA provider.

3.2.5. Limitations of UIC TA Role

Beyond the challenges related to content load and timing, UIC TA providers shared several limitations of what they as TA providers were able to bring about through the HWC process. Although they were able to provide tools to TA recipients, follow up with them between sessions, and push them to focus on particularly relevant content or action steps, UIC TA providers could not force TA recipients to actually move toward action. Many UIC TA providers described an obvious shift in TA recipients' thinking over the course of the HWC sessions, but in many cases felt that it was not apparent how those TA recipients will actually move toward action post-process. One UIC TA provider described this challenge below:

"The "doing" part in their case, I struggled with ... so I don't know what else I could have done or you could have done. We literally handed them a lot of stuff and I couldn't get them to really put a plan together ultimately, in terms of what was next."—UIC TA provider.

Another limitation encountered by UIC TA providers was their ability to promote diverse partnerships between TA recipients in the HWC. While some TA recipients entered the HWC with pre-determined partners (e.g., representatives of other organizations interested in developing interventions to address issues of shared interest), others began and ended the HWC process as individual representatives of their own organizations. One UIC TA provider, who worked primarily with one such individual, described this as an observed limitation during the HWC process:

"I think [what] the other groups show was that coming in with a team with a diversity of voices really does make a difference, that that can foster learning ... I think he had some shift in his ideas but I don't it was as much as with the groups where people came in as a diverse team."—UIC TA provider.

3.3. Impacts of UIC TA Provision

Despite some limitations to UIC TA providers' roles in the HWC process, UIC TA providers, labor expert TA providers, and TA recipients were able to articulate a number of impacts attributed to TA provision by UIC researchers in the HWC. Two themes that emerged from the data included pushing TA recipients toward a more concrete understanding of precarious work and holding TA recipients accountable to next steps throughout the HWC process. Both themes are described below.

3.3.1. Shifts from Abstract to Concrete Understanding of Precarious Work

In the focus group, UIC TA providers described the various ways in which they helped guide TA recipients toward a deeper understanding of the drivers and manifestations of precarious work, both within the HWC sessions and in follow-up calls with TA recipients between sessions. One UIC TA provider observed the most significant changes in TA recipients' understanding of the issues when debriefing the previous week's session by phone:

"I think for some of the groups that I was working with, it was a big transition between abstraction and like recognizing, "Yeah, this is an issue," and then putting pen to paper and actually devising a plan and having concrete ways to talk about it and to address it. I think that those changes have been the most in our individual phone calls with them."—UIC TA provider.

3.3.2. Accountability and Resultant Shifts toward Action

In addition to encouraging or "pushing" TA recipients toward actionable next steps, UIC TA providers and TA recipients agreed that UIC TA also helped hold individuals and groups accountable to those next steps. Several UIC TA providers described the utility in scheduling follow-up conversations, typically by phone, in between HWC sessions as means to check in with TA recipients about agreed upon next steps. One UIC TA provider highlighted this accountability role as particularly impactful for a TA recipient they were working with:

"I think having someone to hold him accountable and I feel like the same as the case with the other team too, being held accountable for something made a big difference."—UIC TA provider.

3.4. Role of UIC beyond HWC

Focus group and interview data revealed a range of anticipated needs for UIC TA provision post-HWC. In the focus group, which took place several days after the conclusion of the HWC, several UIC TA providers speculated that going forward, many of the TA recipients would need additional supports as they continued to both digest information from the HWC and move forward in their plans for action. At least one UIC TA provider expressed a feeling that TA recipients would require little content-related TA beyond the HWC sessions, but would instead require substantial guidance and continued structure and encouragement from UIC TA providers:

"I think going forward, it seems to me as though there may have to be less of a desire for the other TA providers and more of a desire for things that we can do. Which is sort of helping them navigate things and connect them to other resources that may not be one of our TA providers . . . "—UIC TA provider.

TA recipients echoed these sentiments in their interviews, indicating that they would value and benefit from additional facilitation and related supports from UIC TA providers moving forward. Some TA recipients went so far as to describe a specific role for UIC in the implementation of their planned actions, with some describing UIC TA providers serving in coordination and evaluative capacity. One TA recipient commented on the utility of having UIC TA support beyond the HWC:

"I think just having [UIC] as technical assistance providers as we move our project forward . . . it would be really helpful if our team doesn't have to develop the next phases on our own or come up with the ideas . . . I think our group is open enough to your feedback on the direction to take the project."—TA recipient.

4. Discussion

This study examined the perceptions of HWC participants, including UIC TA providers, labor expert TA providers, and TA recipients of UIC researchers' TA role throughout the HWC process. The findings centered on HWC participants' perceptions of the appropriateness and utility of UIC's role as TA in the HWC, challenges encountered in this TA provider–recipient model, and potential next steps for UIC's involvement with TA recipients beyond the HWC sessions. The findings provide insight into the role of a university, such as UIC, in convening a learning and action planning initiative such as the HWC, and highlight the impacts of UIC TA providers' engagement with other participants throughout the HWC process. UIC's experience in convening and facilitating the HWC sheds light on factors that contributed to participants' perceptions of the success of the university-facilitated TA provider–recipient model for learning and action development, which may be useful to other universities or similarly positioned organizations interested in engaging diverse stakeholders with the aim of facilitating PSE change. Data from this study suggest that this unique model helped to prepare representatives of various organizations to develop PSE change initiatives to address the complexities of precarious work.

This study provides important insight into how universities, such as UIC, can position themselves to support non-academic organizations across sectors and levels to facilitate evidence-informed development and the implementation of actions to address complex problems such as precarious work. The data from this study highlight the utility of having a community-engaged university bring together organizations that have existing relationships with the university, but do not necessarily have existing relationships with one another. The data also highlight the benefits and challenges of having university researchers play a TA role in a process such as the HWC, and suggest ways in which university researchers might be involved beyond initial capacity building activities to support the implementation of PSE change.

Findings that highlight the value that HWC participants placed on UIC's role as a research-focused and community-engaged institution offer support to UIC's decision to organize the HWC and convene its various participants in six in-person sessions. These findings align with much of the community–university partnership literature, which details community engagement with university researchers as a means for knowledge translation and the development of shared action agendas [4]. This supports UIC's role in putting together an initiative that has the potential to help close a knowledge-to-action gap, although this initiative differs from many of the examples in the literature. Unlike other community–university partnerships, the HWC relied on the expertise of outside TA providers, in this case labor experts, to share knowledge with the groups who are well positioned to implement interventions to address a complex problem, in this case the multi-faceted drivers of precarious work. UIC researchers' roles as facilitators differs from the more traditional knowledge-sharing role described in much of this literature.

Due to longstanding relationships with individuals involved in occupational health research and public health practice groups at UIC, labor expert TA providers and TA recipients described a level of trust and reciprocity that were vital to their decisions to participate in the HWC. These findings indicate that UIC was uniquely positioned to convene and facilitate the HWC, suggesting that the HWC participants may not have otherwise willingly participated in such an initiative. It is unlikely that without the HWC, participants would have interacted with one another at all, further highlighting the importance of UIC's role in supporting important steps toward PSE change. Without strong, pre-existing relationships between UIC researchers and members of the various organizations that were represented in the HWC, these representatives may not have decided to commit the time and resources to participate the inaugural HWC initiative. The time and effort that UIC researchers put into developing and maintaining their relationships with the labor- and health-focused organizations that ultimately agreed to participate in the HWC, either as TA providers or TA recipients, cannot be overlooked as an important step in facilitating diverse engagement and commitment to participate in a pilot initiative such as the HWC.

In addition to UIC's role as a convener of the HWC, data from the focus group and interviews reveal several perceptions of the function of UIC TA in the HWC sessions. These functions, from providing guidance, facilitation, encouragement, and accountability to TA recipients, display the range of intensity of TA provided by UIC researchers in the HWC model. This intensity differed from that described in the TA literature, with UIC TA providers serving in a capacity that might be likened to that of a coach or accountability manager instead of a role in which the TA provider takes on responsibility for some of the work. The HWC model seemed nevertheless effective for TA recipients, many of whom attributed their progress in digesting HWC content and planning for next steps of the involvement of UIC TA providers. This suggests that TA as it is described in the literature does not fit the HWC's model, and perhaps an expanded definition of TA is needed. Further, this suggests that university facilitation using AL, in a model such as the HWC, may be effective in increasing knowledge to action. This aligns with calls for capacity-building initiatives to foster more effective public health practice to address complex issues such as precarious work [36].

These findings did highlight some of the limitations of this UIC TA model. Many of the limitations described by participants revolved around the the timing and tight timeline of the HWC, both of which resulted from constraints of operating within a time-bound grant period. UIC TA providers described the challenges of planning and developing the HWC curriculum in such a short time period, which limited opportunities for cooperative planning between UIC and labor expert TA providers. Likewise, labor expert TA providers noted the challenges of not being involved in the planning of each session. This particular issue highlights the limitations of having a university group, which relies on grant funding, designing, and hosting such an initiative, given many of the factors, such as timing and funding, are determined by the funder and are out of their immediate control.

Finally, findings from the focus group and interviews suggested that TA recipients would value and benefit from UIC TA beyond the HWC sessions. This finding highlights some of the ways in which TA recipient organizations were underprepared for action following the HWC, likely requiring additional guidance and supports to move their plans forward. This finding also highlights the importance of sustained engagement between university groups, such as the UIC TA providers in the HWC, and community groups, which is mirrored in the community–university partnership literature [4].

While this manuscript describes the role of university-provided TA in developing strategies for addressing precarious work, evaluation of the HWC in promoting sustainable relationships and partnerships is ongoing. The impact of the HWC on organizational priorities and on process and systems change to better address precarious employment is also an area of ongoing and future research.

Limitations

There are a number of limitations in this study, including low participation in study components and the involvement of the author in the HWC process. Since the HWC process was a pilot, there was only a small number of representatives in both TA provider and TA recipient roles who participated in this study, and approximately 30% did not participate in interviews. Since the TA provider sample was especially small (seven UIC TA providers and seven labor expert TA providers), attempts were made to accommodate varying schedules and allow for participation in interviews or the focus group at times that best suited the TA providers. For TA recipients, similar efforts were made to ensure that at least one representative from each team (see Table 1) was interviewed to capture the team's experiences. An additional limitation was there were no opportunities to compare findings from this study to another similar collaborative process with multiple TA providers and TA recipients, as similar examples of TA provider–recipient models were not found in the literature.

Another potential limitation of this study is the author's involvement in the HWC as one of the UIC TA providers who helped with the design and facilitation of the HWC process. This presents a potential bias, both due to the author's own involvement and perceptions of the HWC and the potential bias in interviewees' responses to interview questions, given their knowledge of my role in the HWC process. To partially address this limitation, assurances were made to participants that their data would be both de-identified and reported in the aggregate, and would not be shared outside of the UIC research team. Further, another UIC TA provider conducted interviews with the TA recipients who the author interacted with most directly in the HWC sessions. Although the author did facilitate the focus group with other UIC TA providers, she did not participate in the focus group herself (i.e., she did not share her own perceptions of the HWC process and the role of TA). The author worked with an external colleague to code and debrief transcribed data to both reflect upon and document potential biases and subjectivities.

5. Conclusions

The complex problems that workers face, especially those in precarious work arrangements, demand innovative and comprehensive solutions. The *Total Worker Health*® model recognizes the need for research and practice to improve the health of workers, and TWH Centers for Excellence, such as the Center for Healthy Work at UIC, are tasked with understanding the conditions that workers face and developing strategies to improve those conditions through multi-disciplinary projects. The findings from this study, which focuses on an initiative at the UIC Center for Healthy Work, highlight the utility of university facilitation in engaging diverse stakeholders in learning and action planning, in the context of a process rooted in Action Learning, to promote action to address drivers of precarious work.

Author Contributions: Conceptualization: T.B., C.W., and E.J.-R.; methodology, T.B., C.W., and E.J.-R.; formal analysis, T.B.; investigation: T.B. and E.J.-R.; writing—original draft preparation, T.B.; writing—review and editing, C.W., E.J.-R., and L.M.C.; supervision, C.W. and L.M.C.; funding acquisition, C.W. and L.M.C.

Funding: The UIC Center for Healthy Work is supported by grant number U190H011232 from the National Institute for Occupational Safety and Health (CDC). The views expressed in written materials or do not necessarily reflect the official policies of the Department of Health and Human Services, nor does the mention of trade names, commercial practices, or organizations imply endorsement by the U.S. Government. Total Worker Health® is a registered trademark of the U.S. Department of Health and Human Services (HHS). Participation by the UIC Center for Healthy Work does not imply endorsement by HHS, the Centers for Disease Control and Prevention, or the National Institute for Occupational Safety and Health. Tessa Bonney was also supported by the Illinois Education and Research Center, grant number T42/OH008672 from the National Institute for Occupational Safety and Health (CDC). The work is solely the responsibility of the authors and does not necessarily represent the official views of the National Institute for Occupational Safety and Health.

Acknowledgments: Nandini Deb, research assistant; Elizabeth Fisher, Devangna Kapadia, Marsha Love, Eve Pinsker, Anna Yankelev, and Joseph Zanoni from the UIC Center for Healthy Work; and all Healthy Work Collaborative participants.

Conflicts of Interest: The authors declare no conflict of interest. The funders had no role in the design of the study; in the collection, analyses, or interpretation of data; in the writing of the manuscript, or in the decision to publish the results.

References

1. National Institute for Occupational Safety and Health (NIOSH). Total Worker Health. Available online: https://www.cdc.gov/niosh/twh/totalhealth.html (accessed on 20 July 2019).
2. Benach, J.; Muntaner, C. Precarious employment and health: Developing a research agenda. *J. Epidemiol. Community Health* **2007**, *61*, 276–277. [CrossRef] [PubMed]
3. University of Illinois at Chicago School of Public Health. Center for Healthy Work. Available online: http://publichealth.uic.edu/healthywork (accessed on 20 July 2019).
4. Shannon, J.; Wang, T. A Model for University-Community Engagement: Continuing Education's Role as Convener. *J. Contin. High. Educ.* **2010**, *58*, 108–112. [CrossRef]
5. Drabble, L.; Lemon, K.; D'Andrade, A.; Donoviel, B.; Le, J. Child welfare partnership for research and training: A Title IV-E university/community collaborative research model. *J. Public Child Welf.* **2013**, *7*, 411–429. [CrossRef]
6. Leisey, M.; Holton, V.; Davey, T.L. Community engagement grants: Assessing the impact of university funding and engagements. *J. Community Engagem.* **2012**, *5*, 6.
7. Kalleberg, A. Precarious Work, Insecure Workers: Employment Relations in Transition. *Am. Sociol. Rev.* **2009**, *74*, 1–22. [CrossRef]
8. National Employment Law Project (NELP). Unregulated Work: Research and Public Policy for an Emerging Trend in the U.S. Labor Market. 2009. Available online: http://nelp.org/content/uploads/2015/03/UnregulatedWorkResearchPublicPolicy509.pdf (accessed on 20 July 2019).
9. Hadden, W.; Muntaner, C.; Benach, J.; Gimeno, D.; Benavides, F. A glossary for the social epidemiology of work organisation: Part 3, Terms from the sociology of labour markets. *J. Epidemiol. Community Health* **2007**, *61*, 6–8. [CrossRef]
10. Weil, D. Rethinking the regulation of vulnerable work in the USA: A sector-based approach. *J. Ind. Relat.* **2009**, *51*, 411–430. [CrossRef]
11. Weil, D. *The Fissured Workplace*; Harvard University Press: Cambridge, MA, USA, 2014.
12. Benach, J.; Muntaner, C.; Santana, V. Employment Conditions and Health Inequalities Final Report to the WHO Commission on Social Determinants of Health (CSDH) Employment Conditions Knowledge Network (EMCONET). 2007. Available online: http://www.who.int/social_determinants/resources/articles/emconet_who_report.pdf?ua=1 (accessed on 20 July 2019).
13. Azaroff, L.; Levenstein, C.; Wegman, D. Occupational injury and illness surveillance: Conceptual filters explain underreporting. *Am. J. Public Health* **2002**, *92*, 1421–1429. [CrossRef]

14. Park, Y.; Butler, R. The safety costs of contingent work: Evidence from Minnesota. *J. Labor Res.* **2001**, *22*, 831–849. [CrossRef]
15. Benavides, F.; Delclos, G. Flexible employment and health inequalities. *J. Epidemiol. Community Health* **2005**. [CrossRef]
16. Baron, S.; Beard, S.; Davis, L.; Delp, L.; Forst, L.; Kidd-Taylor, A.; Liebman, A.K.; Linnan, L.; Punnett, L.; Welch, L.S. Promoting integrated approaches to reducing health inequities among low-income workers: Applying a social ecological framework. *Am. J. Ind. Med.* **2014**, *57*, 539–556. [CrossRef] [PubMed]
17. Golden, S.; McLeroy, K.; Green, L.; Earp, J.; Lieberman, L. Upending the Social Ecological Model to Guide Health Promotion Efforts Toward Policy and Environmental Change. *Health Educ. Behav.* **2015**, *42*, 8S–14S. [CrossRef] [PubMed]
18. Phelan, J.C.; Link, B.G.; Tehranifar, P. Social conditions as fundamental causes of health inequalities: Theory, evidence, and policy implications. *J. Health Soc. Behav.* **2010**, *51*, S28–S40. [CrossRef] [PubMed]
19. Allegrante, J. Policy and Environmental Approaches in Health Promotion. *Health Educ. Behav.* **2015**, *42*, 5S–7S. [CrossRef]
20. Freudenberg, N.; Franzosa, E.; Chisholm, J.; Libman, K. New Approaches for Moving Upstream. *Health Educ. Behav.* **2015**, *42*, 46S–56S. [CrossRef]
21. Freudenberg, N.; Silver, M.; Hirsch, L.; Cohen, N. The Good Food Jobs Nexus: A Strategy for Promoting Health, Employment, and Economic Development. *J. Agric. Food Syst. Community Dev.* **2016**, *6*, 1–19. [CrossRef]
22. Stringer, E. *Action Research*; Sage Publications: Thousand Oaks, CA, USA, 2013.
23. Revans, R. Action Learning: Its origins and nature. *High. Educ. Rev.* **1982**, *15*, 20–29.
24. Marquardt, M.; Leonard, H.; Freedman, A.; Hill, C. *Action Learning for Developing Leaders and Organizations: Principles, Strategies, and Cases*; American Psychological Association: Washington, DC, USA, 2009.
25. Hawe, P.; Noort, M.; King, L.; Jordens, C. Multiplying health gains: The critical role of capacity-building within health promotion programs. *Health Policy* **1997**, *39*, 29–42. [CrossRef]
26. Le, L.; Anthony, B.; Bronheim, S.; Holland, C.; Perry, D. A Technical Assistance Model for Guiding Service and Systems Change. *J. Behav. Health Serv. Res.* **2016**, *43*, 380–395. [CrossRef]
27. De Silva, M.; Breuer, E.; Lee, L.; Asher, L.; Chowdhary, N.; Lund, C.; Patel, V. Theory of Change: A theory-driven approach to enhance the Medical Research Council's framework for complex interventions. *Trials* **2014**, *15*, 267. [CrossRef]
28. Trohanis TA Project. Guiding Principles for Effective Technical Assistance. 2014. Available online: http://ectacenter.org/~{}pdfs/trohanis/trohanis_guiding_principles.pdf (accessed on 20 July 2019).
29. Fixsen, D.; Blasé, K.; Horner, R.; Sugai, G. Intensive Technical Assistance. Scaling-Up Brief. Number 2. *FPG Child Dev. Inst. ERIC* **2009**, *2*, 1–4.
30. Chilenski, S.; Welsh, J.; Olson, J.; Hoffman, L.; Perkins, D.; Feinberg, M. Examining the Highs and Lows of the Collaborative Relationship between Technical Assistance Providers and Prevention Implementers. *Prev. Sci.* **2018**, *19*, 250–259. [CrossRef] [PubMed]
31. Rushovich, B.; Bartley, L.; Steward, R.; Bright, C. Technical Assistance: A Comparison between Providers and Recipients. *Hum. Serv. Organ. Manag. Leadersh. Gov.* **2015**, *39*, 362–379. [CrossRef]
32. Marquardt, M. Action learning and leadership. *Learn. Organ.* **2000**, *7*, 233–241. [CrossRef]
33. Marsick, V.; O'Neil, J. The many faces of action learning. *Manag. Learn.* **1999**, *30*, 159–176. [CrossRef]
34. Noell, G.; Witt, J.; Slider, N.; Connell, J.; Gatti, S.; Williams, K.; Koenig, J.L.; Resetar, J.L.; Duhon, G.J. Treatment implementation following behavioral consultation in schools: A comparison of three follow-up strategies. *School Psychol. Rev.* **2005**, *34*, 87–106.
35. Fereday, J.; Muir-Cochrane, E. Demonstrating rigor using thematic analysis: A hybrid approach of inductive and deductive coding and theme development. *Int. J. Qual. Methods* **2006**, *5*, 80–92. [CrossRef]
36. Brownson, R.; Fielding, J.; Green, L. Building capacity for evidence-based public health: Reconciling the pulls of practice and the push of research. *Annu. Rev. Public Health Annu. Rev.* **2018**, *39*, 27–53. [CrossRef]

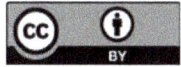

© 2019 by the authors. Licensee MDPI, Basel, Switzerland. This article is an open access article distributed under the terms and conditions of the Creative Commons Attribution (CC BY) license (http://creativecommons.org/licenses/by/4.0/).

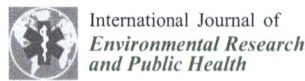

Article

Caring for Workers' Health: Do German Employers Follow a Comprehensive Approach Similar to the Total Worker Health Concept? Results of a Survey in an Economically Powerful Region in Germany

Aileen Hoge [†], Anna T. Ehmann [†], Monika A. Rieger [‡] and Achim Siegel [*,‡]

Institute of Occupational Medicine, Social Medicine and Health Services Research, University Hospital Tübingen, Wilhelmstraße 27, 72074 Tübingen, Germany; Aileen.Hoge@student.uni-tuebingen.de (A.H.); Anna.Ehmann@med.uni-tuebingen.de (A.T.E.); Monika.Rieger@med.uni-tuebingen.de (M.A.R.)

* Correspondence: Achim.Siegel@med.uni-tuebingen.de; Tel.: +49-7071-29-86812
† Equal contribution (shared first).
‡ Equal contribution (shared last).

Received: 30 January 2019; Accepted: 26 February 2019; Published: 28 February 2019

Abstract: Similar to 'Total Worker Health' in the United States (USA), 'Workplace Health Management' in Germany is a holistic strategy to protect, promote, and manage employees' health at the workplace. It consists of four subcategories. While the subcategories 'occupational health and safety' and 'reintegration management' contain measures prescribed by law, 'workplace health promotion' and 'personnel development' can be designed more individually by the companies. The present study focused on the current implementation of voluntary and legally required measures of the four subcategories, as well as companies' satisfaction with the implementation. A total of N = 222/906 companies (small, medium, and big enterprises of one German county) answered a standardized questionnaire addressing the implementation of health-related measures, satisfaction with the implementation, and several company characteristics. In the subcategory 'occupational health and safety', 23.9% of the companies fulfilled all of the legally required measures, whereas in the category 'reintegration management', that rate amounted to 50.9%. There was a positive correlation between company size and the implementation grade, and as well between company size and the fulfilling of measures required by law. Companies tended to be more satisfied with higher implementation grades. Nevertheless, a surprisingly high proportion of the companies with poor implementation indicated satisfaction with the measures' implementation.

Keywords: workplace health management; total worker health; workplace health promotion; occupational health and safety; company reintegration management; return to work; cross-sectional survey; Germany

1. Introduction

Similar to many other high-income countries, Germany currently faces two trends that have a serious impact on its economy and workforce. First of all, the composition of the working population is shifting toward older age groups, which is a process that will probably be accompanied by an increase in the burden of non-communicable diseases among the workforce [1,2]. Secondly, many branches of the German economy are confronted with an acute shortage of skilled workers and qualified staff, which is a situation that has persisted for years, and recently deteriorated [3,4]. Against this background, stakeholders are increasingly recognizing activities that strengthen the workability and employability of the workforce and promote the good health of workers [2,5]. Thus, it comes as no surprise that during the last few decades, a strategy called 'workplace health management' (in German

'Betriebliches Gesundheitsmanagement') has gained popularity in Germany [6–8]. 'Workplace health management' is very similar to the 'Total Worker Health' approach in the USA [9–19]. The National Institute for Occupational Safety and Health (NIOSH) defined 'total worker health' as activities integrating protection from work-related safety and health hazards with the promotion of injury and illness prevention efforts in order to advance worker well-being [12,13]. The German 'workplace health management' approach pursues a similarly holistic strategy. It is commonly defined as the integration and management of all operational processes (in an enterprise) so as to create healthy working conditions and promote the health of its employees [5,20]. Workplace health management can be differentiated into four components or subcategories: (1) occupational health and safety measures, (2) management of the return to work process of employees who have been on long-term sickness absence (in short: 'reintegration management'), (3) workplace health promotion, and (4) a corresponding personnel development. In Germany, these components differ as to their legal status: whereas many occupational health and safety measures as well as some reintegration management activities are required by law, measures in the areas of workplace health promotion and personnel development are voluntary (cf., in greater detail below).

While the importance of comprehensive workplace health management in Germany seems to be commonly recognized in public discourse, a quite different question is whether and to what extent enterprises actually follow the concept in practice. From several surveys we know that in small and medium enterprises (with up to 250 employees, or—according to another common categorization—with up to 500 employees), workplace health management is often neglected. The ability or willingness to implement workplace health management measures seems to depend linearly on company size. The smaller the company, the less likely it is that a comprehensive workplace health management will be implemented [21–24]. Small enterprises with up to 50 employees seem to have implementation deficits even with regard to occupational health and safety measures that are required by law [25]. Thus, as to small and medium enterprises (SMEs), the situation in Germany seems to be comparable to the United States (USA) and other European countries [26,27].

In light of these former surveys we wanted to find out the current situation in a German region in which the social and economic environment for health-related measures is comparably good, i.e., clearly above average. If the results of such a survey show that the implementation of workplace health management measures is still as poor as previous surveys suggest, we may conclude and confirm that serious implementation problems persist also within an above-average social and economic environment. Thus, we designed a short survey of health-related measures in small, medium, and big enterprises in the county of Reutlingen (Landkreis Reutlingen). As far as socio-economic strength and population health is concerned, the County of Reutlingen is well above the German average. In 2015, e.g., the unemployment rate in the county was 3.7% (Germany: 6.4%), the average monthly household income per inhabitant amounted to 1946 €, i.e., about 2208 USD (Germany: 1787 €, i.e., about 2028 USD), and the gross domestic product per inhabitant was 38,400 €, i.e., about 43,574 USD (Germany: 36,900 €, i.e., about 41,872 USD) [28]. At the same time, the average life expectancy in the county was 82.69 years (Germany: 80.89 years). At the end of 2015, the county had 282,000 inhabitants. Furthermore, five out of 26 municipalities in the county have been certificated as 'healthy communities' because of their commitment to promote physical activity and population health.

In our survey, we addressed only companies that had a minimum size of 10 employees in craft enterprises or 20 employees respectively in non-craft enterprises (cf., further details in the next section). Craft enterprises are enterprises that do not produce industrial mass goods, but generally work to order or provide services on demand (such as carpenters, painters, etc.). As we know from previous studies that the implementation of health-related measures in micro enterprises is very poor or virtually non-existent [21–24], we concentrated—for economic reasons—on enterprises that had a certain minimum size. Thus, our focus on small, medium, and big enterprises (leaving aside micro, i.e., very small enterprises) and on the county of Reutlingen sets the framework for the following argument. If the degree of implementation of workplace health management measures in the companies we surveyed is good or acceptable, we should not conclude that this is the same (or similar) on average in Germany. On the other hand, if the degree of implementation is poor even in the companies we surveyed, we can conclude that this probably also applies to the German average.

In this context, we will answer the following research questions (RQs):

RQ 1: *What is the current state as to the implementation of various workplace health management measures in the companies we addressed in our survey?*

RQ 2: *Do enterprises generally comply with legal requirements in the areas of occupational health and safety and reintegration management?*

RQ 3: *What influence does the size of the company have on implementation status?*

RQ 4: *How satisfied are company representatives with the implementation status as to the above-mentioned four components of workplace health management? How aware are the company representatives of inadequate implementation?*

2. Materials and Methods

2.1. Data Collection

In July 2017, $N = 906$ enterprises in the county of Reutlingen in southwestern Germany were determined as potential respondents of the survey. This number contained all of the enterprises in the county, except for the very small ones: we excluded craft businesses with less than 10 employees and non-craft enterprises with less than 20 employees.

At the end of July and the beginning of August 2017, we sent a standardized questionnaire to these 906 enterprises. Craft businesses received our letter via the local chamber of crafts, which supported the survey; non-craft enterprises received the questionnaire directly from our institute, as we were able to use the complete address data record of the county's enterprises that was available from a marketing agency (Creditreform [29]). An enclosed leaflet included the request to hand out the questionnaire either to the managing director or to a member of the personnel department. Fourteen days after the first invitation to participate in the survey, a reminder was sent to all of the potential participants, regardless of whether some of them had already returned the questionnaire.

A formal ethical approval from the ethical committee at the University Hospital Tübingen was not required. Study participants were informed that the study was voluntary, and that all of the data were analyzed anonymously.

2.2. Questionnaire

The questionnaire was based on previous studies and current literature [24,30–33]. It was developed, discussed, and formulated in a multidisciplinary team consisting of a specialist in occupational medicine (MAR), a sociologist and public health researcher (AS), and a medical student (AH). After a pretest with $N = 24$ participants (senior employees of the personnel departments of different enterprises of the metal and electrical industry in southwestern Germany), the questionnaire was partially modified and supplemented to ensure good comprehensibility.

Based on a self-developed questionnaire for a similar survey of companies in Constance County that was conducted in 2015 [34], questions covered the implementation status of four categories of health-related measures within the enterprise, referring to the above-mentioned four components of workplace health management. Each category was assessed by several items depicting typical measures (cf., Table 1). Answers regarding the implementation of individual measures in the company within the last two years could be given on a three-point Likert scale (zero = 'no', one = 'no, but in concrete planning', two = 'yes'). Hereby, the order of the four categories was as following: workplace health promotion (six items and one possibility for free-text indication), occupational health and safety (seven items and one free-text indication), personnel development (five items and one free-text indication), and reintegration management for employees on long-term sickness absence (eight items and one free-text indication) (cf., Table 1 for all items).

Table 1. Surveyed measures (items) regarding workplace health promotion, occupational health and safety, personnel development, and reintegration management.

Categories and Items	Median	Mean	Standard Deviation	Min–Max
Workplace Health Promotion				
Measures to promote and maintain work-related health (e.g., stress management, back health, courses or advice on general workplace health issues)	1	0.96	0.94	0–2
Measures to promote and maintain health that go beyond workplace-related health (e.g., addiction prevention, sports and exercise, healthy nutrition)	0	0.76	0.91	0–2
Employee counseling for psychological complaints	0	0.57	0.87	0–2
Introduction of preventive measures of the German pension insurance (e.g., programs such as Betsi, Balance plus)	0	0.20	0.55	0–2
Info material/brochures on work-related health	2	1.08	0.96	0–2
Info material/brochures on health without a particular reference to work	0	0.82	0.97	0–2
Occupational Health and Safety				
Occupational medical check-ups for early detection and prevention of work-related disorders	2	1.34	0.92	0–2
Implementation of occupational health and safety rules (e.g., risk assessment of activities or workplaces, regular instruction of employees according to the Occupational Health and Safety Act)	2	1.89	0.40	0–2
Health-friendly design of working conditions (e.g., adaptation of the working environment, ergonomic improvement of workplaces, improvement of work processes, organization of working time, adherence of working hours)	2	1.85	0.47	0–2
Causal analysis of accidents at work and on the way to and from work	2	1.06	0.98	0–2
Derivation of protective measures on the basis of analyzed accidents at work	1	1.05	0.96	0–2
Analysis of the causes of work-related complaints by employees	2	1.13	0.95	0–2
Derivation of measures on the basis of work-related complaints by employees	2	1.18	0.93	0–2
Personnel Development				
Management training/supervision/coaching/consulting (e.g., with regard to mobbing, communication, conflict management)	2	1.28	0.89	0–2
Systematic further training of employees	2	1.64	0.71	0–2
Regular staff appraisals (e.g., for personnel development)	2	1.77	0.54	0–2
Support in reconciling private and professional life (e.g., home office, company kindergarten)	2	1.19	0.96	0–2
Use of demographic counseling (e.g., survey on the age structure of employees, planning strategies to keep older employees healthy, etc.)	0	0.28	0.63	0–2
Reintegration Management				
Observe the duration of sick leave to notice prolonged and repeated incapacity to work	2	1.58	0.79	0–2
Procedure for addressing employees with long or repeated incapacities to work	2	1.22	0.90	0–2
Procedure for the inclusion of the health insurance fund in the event of long or repeated incapacity to work	0	0.71	0.90	0–2
Structured approach to the planning of occupational reintegration in the event of long or repeated incapacity for work	2	1.21	0.93	0–2
Appointment of a representative for reintegration management in the company	0	0.58	0.84	0–2
Cooperation with the German pension insurance for benefits for participation in working life	0	0.42	0.79	0–2
Cooperation with the Federal Employment Agency for benefits for participation in working life	0	0.58	0.88	0–2
Contact the joint rehabilitation service center	0	0.24	0.59	0–2

Explications regarding Table 1: Fields in italics: in general legally required according to German laws. The question in the questionnaire had read: 'Which of the listed measures have taken place in your company in the last two years? (Please also take into account offers that took place outside the company but were (co)financed by the company.)'. Answers were given on a 3-point Likert scale: 0 = 'no', 1 = 'no, but in concrete planning', 2 = 'yes'.

Next, the participants were asked about their satisfaction with the current implementation of the four categories of measures. Here, a four-point Likert scale was used (zero = 'very dissatisfied', one = 'rather dissatisfied', two = 'rather satisfied', and three = 'very satisfied').

At the end of the questionnaire, sociodemographic data of the respondents and company characteristics were gathered (branch, number of employees, availability of occupational health and safety experts, and number of employees addressed in reintegration management during the last two years).

2.3. Statistical Analysis

For each category of measures a score, ranging from 'zero' to '10', was calculated to represent a standardized implementation grade. This score was only calculated if at most one entry per category was missing. A score of 'zero' points corresponded to no offered measures and no measures in concrete planning, while a score of '10' stood for the complete implementation of all the listed measures in a given category. The legal requirements in a given category were considered 'fulfilled' if all of the legally required measures of that category had been implemented. All seven measures listed in the category 'occupational safety and health' were legally required due to regulations in the "Arbeitsschutzgesetz" ([Act on the Implementation of Measures of Occupational Safety and Health to Encourage Improvements in the Safety and Health Protection of Workers at Work]—ArbSchG (1996) [35]), in the "Verordnung über die arbeitsmedizinische Vorsorge" ([Ordinance on Occupational Health Care]—ArbMedVV (2008) [36]), in the "Arbeitssicherheitsgesetz" ([Act on Occupational Physicians, Safety Engineers, and Other Occupational Safety Specialists]—ASiG (1973) [37]), in the "DGUV Vorschrift 1" ([DGUV Regulation 1 "Principles of prevention"] (2013) [38]) and the "DGUV Vorschrift 2" ([DGUV Regulation 2 "Occupational physicians and OSH professionals"] (2011) [39]), and the first two measures listed in the category 'reintegration management' were legally required due to the respective regulations in "Book Nine of the Social Code" (Sozialgesetzbuch) (§ 167 SGB "Prevention" [40]) (cf., Table 1).

Rank correlation (Spearman's r) coefficients were calculated to analyze relationships between ordinal variables (such as, e.g., satisfaction with a given implementation status) and metrically scaled variables or when metrical variables were not normally distributed. Thus, e.g., Spearman's r was calculated to compare companies of different sizes, which were measured by their number of employees, in terms of adherence of legal requirements (categorized as either 'yes'/'fulfilled' or 'no'/'not fulfilled'). To analyze relationships between metrically scaled and normally distributed variables, we calculated Pearson's correlation coefficients. Coefficients up to 0.3 were classified as low, those between 0.3–0.5 were classified as moderate, and those from 0.5 on were classified as high [41]. The level of significance was set to $p < 0.05$.

As part of a non-responder analysis, responding and non-responding companies were compared concerning their company size. For this purpose, we used an ordinal five-point scale of company size that had been delivered by the Reutlingen Chamber of Crafts for craft enterprises, and thus was available for both responders and non-responders. We proceeded similarly with regard to the non-craft enterprises.

All of the analyses were performed with SPSS, version 24 (IBM Analytics, IBM Corporation, Armonk, NY, USA).

3. Results

3.1. Participants

The response rate to the questionnaire was all in all 24.5% ($N = 222/906$). On average, there were less than 5% missing values in each category of the questionnaire. The response was above average in medium-sized companies (cf., Table 2) with 101 to 500 employees (31.5% and 32.3%), whereas it was clearly below average in small enterprises with up to 50 employees (22.1%) and in big companies with more than 500 employees (23.1%). Then, the correlation between response and company size seems to be of the inverted u-shaped type. About half of the companies (48.2%) indicated the availability of an occupational health physician, with a range from 29.4% (small companies with up to 50 employees) to 85.0% (companies with 201 to 500 employees). The presence of an occupational safety engineer was reported by 76.8% of all the participating companies (cf., in greater detail in Table 2).

Table 2. Company characteristics of participating companies according to company size.

Company Size	10–50 Employees	51–100 Employees	101–200 Employees	201–500 Employees	>500 Employees
Number of companies addressed	N = 570	N = 159	N = 89	N = 62	N = 26
Response (%/n)	22.3% n = 127	25.8% n = 41	31.5% n = 28	32.3% n = 20	23.1% n = 6
Occupational health physician available (%/n)*	29.1% n = 37	63.4% n = 26	78.6% n = 22	85.0% n = 17	83.3% n = 5
Occupational safety engineer available (%/n)‡	63.0% n = 80	85.4% n = 35	100.0% n = 28	100.0% n = 20	100.0% n = 6

* Occupational medical check-ups according to the relevant legal regulation (ArbMedVV [36]) (e.g., screen work, handling of hazardous substances, or noisy work places) have to be available to all employees in Germany. According to another regulation [39], an occupational health physician has to be available in all enterprises with more than 50 employees (in some branches, this limit is lower), and in the smaller enterprises in case the employer feels the need for occupational health counseling (so-called "alternative, demand-based supervision"). ‡ An occupational safety engineer has to be available in all enterprises with more than 50 employees (in some branches, this limit is lower), and in the smaller enterprises in case the employer feels the need for occupational health counseling (so-called "alternative, demand-based supervision"). In small enterprises (max. 50 employees), the employer can receive special training with regard to occupational health and safety by the statutory accident insurance in order to reduce the need for support by occupational safety engineers [39].

In enterprises with up to 50 employees (the maximum number differs between individual branches due to the respective accident prevention regulation of the respective statutory accident insurance), the employer can participate in a specific occupational health and safety training that entitles him to utilize the service of an occupational safety engineer only when necessary (so-called "Unternehmermodell"). This was indicated by 32/127 enterprises (missing n = 5) with up to 50 employees.

As to the sectoral affiliation of the participating companies, almost one third (30.2%; n = 67) of the participating companies belonged to the manufacturing industry, and 16.7% (n = 37) belonged to the construction industry. Another 15.3% (n =3 4) and 14.0% (n = 31) can be attributed to services and trade, respectively. The remaining 24% of participating companies were distributed among the following sectors: hospitality industry, agriculture and forestry, maintenance and repair, banking and insurance, transport/storage/communication, public administration, mining and quarrying, education, and energy and water supply.

The sociodemographic characteristics of the responding persons in the companies are shown in Table 3. As to the position of the respondents, 52.7% of these were managing directors, 34.7% were from the personnel department, and 11.7% were other employees (cf., Table 3).

Table 3. Sociodemographic characteristics of respondents.

Characteristic		% (n)
Position of respondent	Managing director	52.7% (n = 117)
	Member of personnel department	34.7% (n = 77)
	Other	11.7% (n = 26)
	Missing	0.9% (n = 2)
Gender of respondent	Male	54.1% (n = 120)
	Female	45.0% (n = 100)
	Missing	0.9% (n = 2)

Table 3. Cont.

Characteristic		% (n)
Age of respondent (in years)	Mean	50.3
	Median	52.0
	Standard deviation	10.6
	Min–Max	25-82

3.2. Current State of Implementation of Health-Related Measures in the Companies

In this subsection, we consecutively present the results of the first three research questions (RQ 1, RQ 2, and RQ 3, as explicated in the Introduction).

RQ 1: The average implementation grade of health-related measures in companies as assessed by scores was highest in the category 'occupational health and safety' (6.75 points on a scale between zeo and a maximum of 10 points), followed by 'personnel development' (6.11 points), 'reintegration management' (4.06 points), and finally 'workplace health promotion' (3.63 points) (cf., in detail Table 4).

Table 4. Average standardized implementation grade (implementation scale mean) in four categories of health-related measures (total sample, N = 222).

Category	Workplace Health Promotion (n = 217)	Occupational Health and Safety (n = 215)	Personnel Development (n = 217)	Reintegration Management (n = 213)
Mean	3.63	6.75	6.11	4.06
Standard Deviation	2.87	2.81	2.40	2.75

Explications regarding Table 4: Theoretical range of the standardized implementation grade in all four categories: zero to 10. The 'n' of the individual columns represents the valid number in each case.

RQ 2: All health-related measures that are required by law were fulfilled by 23.9% (n = 53) of the companies in the category 'occupational health and safety' and by 50.9% (n = 113) in the category 'reintegration management'.

RQ 3: There is a positive correlation between company size and implementation grade in the four categories of health-related measures. This means for all four categories of health-related measures, the bigger the company, the more measures have been implemented. In the category 'reintegration management', the correlation is the most pronounced (Pearson's r = 0.35, $p < 0.001$), followed by 'workplace health promotion' (Pearson's r = 0.26, $p < 0.001$), 'occupational health and safety' (Pearson's r = 0.23, $p < 0.001$), and 'personnel development' (Pearson's r = 0.21, $p = 0.002$).

There is also a positive correlation between company size and the fulfilling of measures required by law (occupational health and safety: Spearman's r = 0.35, $p < 0.001$; reintegration management: Spearman's r = 0.38, $p < 0.001$).

In the next subsection, we present the results of the fourth research question (RQ 4, as explicated in the Introduction).

3.3. Satisfaction with Implementation Status

In case important—or even legally required—health-related measures are lacking, it is important to know whether and to what extent these companies are aware of this deficiency before planning any interventions.

In the present survey, company representatives generally tended to be more satisfied with the implementation of a given category of health-related measures the higher the implementation score of their company was in that category. Thus, correlation analyses showed that satisfaction—as measured by the four-point Likert scale—was positively associated with the implementation score value in the categories 'workplace health promotion' (Spearman's r = 0.34, $p < 0.001$), 'occupational health and safety' (Spearman's r = 0.16, p = 0.022), 'personnel development' (Spearman's r = 0.21, p = 0.002), and 'reintegration management' (Spearman's r = 0.25, p < 0.001).

To get further hints on the above-mentioned awareness of company representatives, we furthermore checked how satisfied those company representatives were whose enterprises had a comparably low implementation score in a given category. We defined having a 'low implementation score' as belonging to the lowest quartile of the respective scores. In the category 'workplace health promotion', n = 81 companies (37.3%) belonged to the lowest implementation quartile, and in the category 'occupational health and safety', n = 62 (28.8%) companies belonged to the lowest implementation. In the category 'personnel development', n = 58 (26.7%) enterprises belonged to the lowest implementation quartile, while in 'reintegration management' this was true for n = 57 (26.8%) companies. Within each of these groups of enterprises with a comparably poor implementation of corresponding measures, a substantial proportion of company representatives were nevertheless satisfied (either 'rather satisfied' or 'very satisfied') with the implementation status (cf., in detail Table 5). With regard to the current situation in the domain 'workplace health promotion', n = 33 (40.7% of those companies that belonged to the lowest implementation score quartile) company representatives were satisfied. As to the domain 'occupational health and safety', n = 55 (88.7%) company representatives were satisfied in spite of their comparably poor implementation grade. As to 'personnel development', n = 39 (67.2%) company representatives were satisfied, despite the relatively poor implementation status of their companies, and regarding the category 'reintegration management', n = 25 (43.9%) of company representatives were satisfied, although they had a poor implementation record in this category. Thus, a substantial proportion—if not the majority—of 'under-performing' enterprises (those belonging to the lowest score quartile) seemed to be satisfied despite a comparably poor implementation.

Table 5. Satisfaction with implementation status in all enterprises vs. enterprises with poor implementation status (enterprises in the lowest implementation score quartile).

Degree of Satisfaction	Workplace Health Promotion (N = 217)	Occupational Health and Safety (N = 215)	Personnel Development (N = 217)	Reintegration Management (N = 213)
	Enterprises in the lowest implementation score quartile			
	n = 81	n = 62	n = 58	n = 57
Dissatisfied: n (%)	38 (46.9)	6 (9.7)	18 (31.0)	20 (35.1)
Satisfied: n (%)	33 (40.7)	55 (88.7)	39 (67.2)	25 (43.9)
Missing: n (%)	10 (12.3)	1 (2.8)	1 (1.7)	12 (21.1)
	Enterprises in the upper three implementation score quartiles			
	n = 136	n = 153	n = 159	n = 156
Dissatisfied: n (%)	25 (18.4)	7 (4.6)	24 (15.1)	30 (19.2)
Satisfied: n (%)	110 (80.9)	145 (94.8)	134 (84.3)	119 (76.3)
Missing: n (%)	1 (0.7)	1 (0.7)	1 (0.6)	7 (4.5)

Explication of Table 5: For the sake of clarity, the response categories 'very dissatisfied' and 'rather dissatisfied' were combined to form the 'dissatisfied' category, while the response categories 'very satisfied' and 'rather satisfied' were combined to form the 'satisfied' category.

Turning to the association between satisfaction and the fulfillment of legally required measures in a given domain, the results were as follows (cf., Table 6). Among those companies that did not comply with all of the legal occupational health and safety requirements as assessed in this study (n = 155), 92.3% (n = 143) were satisfied with the current status of their company's occupational health and safety implementation. This proportion was nearly as high as within the group of company representatives whose companies fulfilled the listed legal requirements (96.2%). Correspondingly, there was no significant correlation between satisfaction (dichotomously grouped into 'satisfied' versus 'dissatisfied') and the fulfillment of legally required measures in that domain (Chi^2 test p = 0.383; Fisher's exact test p = 0.522). As to the category of 'reintegration management' (cf., Table 6), among those companies that did not comply with all of the listed legal requirements (n = 101), 53.5% (n = 54) were satisfied with the current situation of their company's reintegration management implementation. As to this domain, there was a significant but low correlation between satisfaction (grouped into 'satisfied' versus 'dissatisfied') and the fulfillment of the legally prescribed measures (Spearman's r = 0.22; p = 0.002). Nevertheless, in both domains, a majority of respondents representing companies that did not fully comply with legal requirements were satisfied (either 'very' or 'rather satisfied'); as to the occupational health and safety domain, this majority seemed to be overwhelming (92.3%).

Table 6. Satisfaction with implementation status in the domains 'occupational health and safety' and 'reintegration management' according to compliance with legal requirements in a given domain.

Degree of Satisfaction	Occupational Health and Safety (N = 208)	Reintegration Management (N = 214)
	Enterprises that do not fully comply with legal requirements	
	n = 155	n = 101
Dissatisfied: n (%)	11 (7.1)	32 (31.7)
Satisfied: n (%)	143 (92.3)	54 (53.5)
Missing: n (%)	1 (0.6)	15 (14.9)
	Enterprises that fully comply with legal requirements	
	n = 53	n = 113
Dissatisfied: n (%)	2 (3.8)	19 (16.8)
Satisfied: n (%)	51 (96.2)	90 (79.6)
Missing: n (%)	-	4 (3.5)

Explication of Table 6: For the sake of clarity, the response categories 'very dissatisfied' and 'rather dissatisfied' were combined to form the 'dissatisfied' category, while the response categories 'very satisfied' and 'rather satisfied' were combined to form the 'satisfied' category.

4. Discussion

The aim of the study was to provide an assessment of the implementation (RQ 1 and RQ 2) and satisfaction with workplace health management activities (RQ 4) in enterprises in the economically very strong county of Reutlingen. In addition, relationships between company size and implementation (RQ 3) as well as between implementation and satisfaction were to be analyzed and discussed.

4.1. Study Design, Questionnaire, Response Rate, and Data Quality

We performed an almost complete cross-sectional survey where only enterprises with less than 10 (craft enterprises) or 20 employees (non-craft enterprises) were not included. Yet, due to the cross-sectional design, no causal relationships can be described.

The questionnaire items were developed to retrieve as many typical health-related measures as possible because of the wide range of measures in workplace health management. The respondents' low utilization of an offered blank text field for further possible "other measures" that had not been presented as listed items suggests that the lists were practically complete.

The response rate of the survey was 24.5%. The response rate is within the range of the common rates for studies of this type [42–44]. The non-responder analysis showed that the response rate was the highest in medium-sized companies, whereas it was lower in both small enterprises (with up to 100 employees) and big companies (with more than 500 employees). An average of less than 5% missing answers indicates a high data quality.

The study results show a large deficit regarding the compliance with legal requirements according to the participants' indications. Less than 25% of the responding enterprises indicated that their company fulfilled all of the listed legally required measures in the category 'occupational health and safety'; in the category 'reintegration management', about half of the surveyed companies (50.9%) indicated the implementation of all the legally required measures. These comparably low compliance rates might be due to several shortcomings. First of all, companies might be not sufficiently informed about their obligations as employers with regard to all aspects of occupational health and safety (legally required since 1973 [37] and 1996 [35], but with major modifications concerning the defined need for occupational health physicians and occupational safety engineers in 2008 and 2011 [36]) and the implementation of reintegration management (legally required since 2001 [40]). Second, the people who indicated the status of the respective measures in the questionnaire might not have been aware of all the activities implemented in the enterprise. One reason for this could be that some of the activities that were surveyed might be implemented more or less in an implicit manner, but not be spoken of explicitly, especially if the occasion (i.e., an accident or work-related health complaint of an employee) is rather rare. Another reason could be that occupational health physicians, occupational safety engineers, and other experts are available and take care of the implementation without the management noticing much of it. Thus, the respective measures might well be implemented, but not known. Fourth, enterprises are not encouraged strongly enough to follow the legal requirements, as there is not enough compliance monitoring by the respective institutions in Germany (government and statutory accident insurances).

Particularly in the category 'reintegration management', small enterprises might not see the need for the implementation of methods of reintegration management, because they may not have needed it yet. Possibly in some small enterprises, individual occupational health and safety measures might be taken now and then according to need, but not on a regular basis [45], which would in part explain the low proportion of companies fulfilling all of the listed occupational health and safety measures. Yet, there is no satisfying explanation for only 29.1% to 85.0% of the study participants indicating the availability of an occupational health physician (cf., Table 2), other than the current shortage of occupational health physicians in Germany [46]. The availability of occupational safety engineers in only 63.0% of the small enterprises (10–50 employees) can well be explained by the regulation that the employer himself can participate in an occupational health and safety training offered by the statutory accident insurance with the consequence that usually no occupational safety engineer is necessary (so-called "Unternehmermodell"). The proportion of only 85.4% of enterprises indicating the availability of an occupational safety engineer in companies with 51–100 employees may either be related to the current lack of occupational safety engineers and other occupational health and safety experts in Germany [47] or due to underreporting, which may also explain the figures reported with regard to occupational health physicians.

Taking these aspects together, the lack of implementation, especially in the area of occupational health and safety, may be somewhat overestimated in this survey. However, the findings do point to the need for supportive measures for a better implementation of legally required measures in German enterprises. The same is true for some measures of workplace health promotion in the majority of enterprises, especially with regard to general, rather than work-related, health (median = 0, cf., Table 1).

Due to the positive correlation between company size and the implementation of the components of workplace health management, we may suppose that the real implementation in all of the companies in the county of Reutlingen is even lower than implied in our study, because very small enterprises—where implementation is generally poor [21–24]—did not participate in this survey. This assumption applies both to legally required measures and voluntary measures. Furthermore, it should be kept in mind that the county of Reutlingen is a German district with an above-average social and economic environment, as has been shown in the Introduction. Then, we have to assume that in other districts with less favorable economic conditions the situation is probably not better or even worse.

Although there is a positive correlation between satisfaction and implementation grade in the four categories, there is still a surprisingly high satisfaction in enterprises with poor implementation (cf., Tables 5 and 6). This might indicate that many measures, including those required by law, are not considered necessary (or are not perceived as being required by law). This result, as surprising as it is, needs to be taken into account before planning any interventions to improve the implementation of workplace health management measures.

The results of our study seem to show—once again—that the effectiveness of a top–down approach to the implementation of comprehensive health-related measures in enterprises is rather limited, at least in the context of Western, liberal–capitalist social systems. Even (or just?) in Germany, where there is a long tradition of occupational health and safety legislation, this seems evident. Perhaps a different, less top–down approach is more promising in contemporary Western social systems. The demonstration and publication of success stories of companies that have benefited economically from the implementation of comprehensive health management approaches and the dissemination of corresponding best practice models could possibly stimulate more willingness and motivation on the part of companies to adopt such approaches in the mid and long term.

4.2. The Significance of the Study in Comparison with Previous Implementation Research in Germany

Compared with previous studies, this study has several special features. Most previous surveys, particularly those in Germany, were focused on workplace health promotion, while this study differentiates between four categories of workplace health management in order to gain detailed data on each category. The correlation between implementation grade and company size is already well evidenced by literature on Germany as well as other high-income countries [21,22,24–27,48–50]. In addition, our study enables the analysis of new relationships such as the correlation between implementation status and satisfaction of company representatives with their implementation status [30].

To get a holistic overview of the current situation of workplace health management, one must move on from the scope of our survey. It is not only important what companies do, but also how they do it and, first of all, to what extent health-related measures actually reach the employees. Subjective perceptions of working conditions and appreciation of employees by managers play an important role in employee health and well-being in companies, as has been shown for the prevention of psychological and psychosomatic disorders in employees in our recent research [44]. Therefore, further research should also integrate this dimension.

5. Conclusions

The implementation of health-related measures among companies of one county in southwestern Germany is heterogeneous. There are major shortcomings regarding compliance with legal requirements, as well as specifically in the domain of occupational health and safety measures. Although there is a positive correlation between implementation and satisfaction, surprisingly many companies are satisfied despite a comparably poor implementation of single measures of workplace health management. These conditions—even in a country where occupational health and safety as well as reintegration management for employees are legally required—must be taken into account before planning interventions to improve workers' health through a comprehensive approach.

Author Contributions: A.H., A.E., M.A.R., and A.S. drafted the manuscript. A.H., A.S., and M.A.R. developed the study design; A.H., A.S., and M.A.R. developed the questionnaire; and A.S. performed the pre-test. A.H., A.S., and M.A.R. planned the data collection, wrote the study protocol, and performed the survey. A.H. and A.E. performed the statistical analysis and received valuable advice from A.S. and M.A.R. All of the authors read and approved the final manuscript.

Funding: The survey was financed by the institute's own resources. The work of the Institute of Occupational and Social Medicine and Health Services Research Tübingen is supported by an unrestricted grant of the Employers' Association of the Metal and Electric Industry Baden-Württemberg (Südwestmetall). We acknowledge additional financial support by the German Research Foundation and the Open Access Publishing Fund of the University of Tübingen. This study is also part of the lead author's (A.H.) work toward a doctoral degree.

Acknowledgments: The authors thank all the participating enterprises and the local chamber of crafts for support of the survey. Parts of the questionnaire were based on a survey among enterprises in the Constance County in 2015 [30] that was funded by the Sozialministerium (Ministry of Social Affairs) Baden-Württemberg (lead author: Martina Michaelis (Institute of Occupational and Social Medicine and Health Services Research Tübingen and Research Centre for Occupational and Social Medicine (FFAS), Freiburg).

Conflicts of Interest: The authors declare no conflict of interest.

References

1. World Economic Forum. *The Global Risks Report 2016*, 11th ed.; World Economic Forum: Cologny/Geneva, Switzerland, 2016.
2. Bundesministerium für Arbeit und Soziales. [Preservation of Employability. Occupational Health Recommendation] Erhalt der Beschäftigungsfähigkeit, Arbeitsmedizinische Empfehlung. 2018. Available online: http://www.bmas.de/SharedDocs/Downloads/DE/PDF-Publikationen-DinA4/a452-erhalt-beschaeftigungsfaehigkeit.pdf?__blob=publicationFile (accessed on 20 December 2018).
3. Deutscher Industrie- und Handelskammertag. [Key Findings of the DIHK Business Survey at the Beginning of 2018.] Die wesentlichen Ergebnisse der DIHK-Konjunkturumfrage Jahresbeginn 2018. Available online: https://www.dihk.de/themenfelder/wirtschaftspolitik/konjunktur-und-wachstum/umfragen-und-prognosen/konjunkturumfrage-jahresbeginn-2018/ergebnisse-02-18 (accessed on 20 December 2018).
4. Bundesministerium für Wirtschaft und Energie. [Skilled Personnel for Germany] Fachkräfte für Deutschland. 2018. Available online: https://www.bmwi.de/Redaktion/DE/Dossier/fachkraeftesicherung.html (accessed on 20 December 2018).
5. Südwestmetall. [Guidelines for Workplace Health Management] Leitfaden Betriebliches Gesundheitsmanagement. 2014. Available online: https://www.suedwestmetall.de/SWM/medien.nsf/gfx/55FF5BE6D485B790C1257D5B00342E95/$file/BGM%20Leitfaden.pdf (accessed on 20 December 2018).
6. Badura, B.; Ducki, A.; Schröder, H.; Klose, J.; Meyer, M. [*Absenteeism Report 2018. Experience Sense—Work and Health*] *Fehlzeiten-Report 2018: Sinn erleben—Arbeit und Gesundheit*; Springer: Berlin/Heidelberg, Germany, 2018.
7. Badura, B. [*Work and Health in the 21st Century. Employee Retention through Cultural Development*] *Arbeit und Gesundheit im 21. Jahrhundert: Mitarbeiterbindung durch Kulturentwicklung*; Springer: Berlin/Heidelberg, Germany, 2017.
8. Badura, B.; Ducki, A.; Schröder, H.; Klose, J.; Meyer, M. [*Absenteeism Report 2016. Corporate Culture and Health—Challenges and Opportunities*] *Fehlzeiten-Report 2016: Unternehmenskultur und Gesundheit—Herausforderungen und Chancen*; Springer: Berlin/Heidelberg, Germany, 2016.
9. Anger, W.K.; Elliot, D.L.; Bodner, T.; Olson, R.; Rohlman, D.S.; Truxillo, D.M.; Kuehl, K.S.; Hammer, L.B.; Montgomery, D. Effectiveness of total worker health interventions. *J. Occup. Health Psychol.* **2015**, *20*, 226–247. [CrossRef] [PubMed]
10. Bradley, C.J.; Grossman, D.C.; Hubbard, R.A.; Ortega, A.N.; Curry, S.J. Integrated Interventions for Improving Total Worker Health: A Panel Report from the National Institutes of Health Pathways to Prevention Workshop: Total Worker Health-What's Work Got to Do with It? *Ann. Intern. Med.* **2016**, *165*, 279–283. [CrossRef] [PubMed]
11. Feltner, C.; Peterson, K.; Palmieri Weber, R.; Cluff, L.; Coker-Schwimmer, E.; Viswanathan, M.; Lohr, K.N. *Total Worker Health®175: Comparative Effectiveness Review Number*; Agency for Healthcare Research and Quality: Rockville, MD, USA, 2016.
12. Feltner, C.; Peterson, K.; Palmieri Weber, R.; Cluff, L.; Coker-Schwimmer, E.; Viswanathan, M.; Lohr, K.N. The Effectiveness of Total Worker Health Interventions: A Systematic Review for a National Institutes of Health Pathways to Prevention Workshop. *Ann. Intern. Med.* **2016**, *165*, 262–269. [CrossRef] [PubMed]
13. Faghri, P.D.; Punnett, L. Inclusion of 'Total Worker Health®' a program by NIOSH. *Health Promot. Int.* **2018**. [CrossRef] [PubMed]
14. Rohlman, D.S.; Campo, S.; Hall, J.; Robinson, E.L.; Kelly, K.M. What Could Total Worker Health® Look Like in Small Enterprises? *Ann. Work Expo. Health* **2018**, *62*, 34–41. [CrossRef] [PubMed]
15. Thompson, J.; Schwatka, N.V.; Tenney, L.; Newman, L.S. Total Worker Health: A Small Business Leader Perspective. *Int. J. Environ. Res. Public Health* **2018**, *15*, 2416. [CrossRef] [PubMed]
16. Tamers, S.L.; Goetzel, R.; Kelly, K.M.; Luckhaupt, S.; Nigam, J.; Pronk, N.P.; Rohlman, D.S.; Baron, S.; Brosseau, L.M.; Bushnell, T.; et al. Research Methodologies for Total Worker Health®: Proceedings from a Workshop. *J. Occup. Environ. Med.* **2018**, *60*, 968–978. [CrossRef] [PubMed]
17. Schill, A.L.; Chosewood, L.C. The NIOSH Total Worker Health™ program: An overview. *J. Occup. Environ. Med.* **2013**, *55*, 8–11. [CrossRef] [PubMed]
18. Schill, A.L.; Chosewood, L.C. Total Worker Health®: More Implications for the Occupational Health Nurse. *Workplace Health Saf.* **2016**, *64*, 4–5. [CrossRef] [PubMed]

19. Schill, A.L. Advancing Well-Being Through Total Worker Health®. *Workplace Health Saf.* **2017**, *65*, 158–163. [CrossRef] [PubMed]
20. Drexler, H.; Letzel, S.; Nesseler, T. [Occupational medicine 4.0: Theses of Occupational Medicine on the Status and Development Needs of Occupational Prevention and Health Promotion in Germany.] Arbeitsmedizin 4.0, Thesen der Arbeitsmedizin zum Stand und zum Entwicklungsbedarf der betrieblichen Prävention und Gesundheitsförderung in Deutschland; Stellungnahme der Deutschen Gesellschaft für Arbeitsmedizin und Umweltmedizin, DGAUM. Available online: https://www.arbeitenviernull.de/fileadmin/user_upload/Arbeitsmedizin_4.0_Broschuere_final.pdf (accessed on 27 February 2019).
21. European Agency for Safety and Health at Work. Motivation for Employers to Carry out Workplace Health Promotion, Literature Review. Available online: https://osha.europa.eu/en/tools-and-publications/publications/literature_reviews/motivation-for-employers-to-carry-out-workplace-health-promotion (accessed on 20 December 2018).
22. Ahlers, E. [Demand and Reality of Workplace Health Managment in a Changing Working Environment.] Anspruch und Wirklichkeit des Betrieblichen Gesundheitsmanagements in Einer sich Verändernden Arbeitswelt. In *Absenteeism Report 2015*; Badura, B., Ducki, A., Schröder , H., Klose, J., Meyer, M., Eds.; Springer: Berlin/Heidelberg, Germany, 2015; pp. 39–47.
23. Kiesche, E. *[Workplace Health Management.] Betriebliches Gesundheitsmanagement*; Bund-Verlag: Frankfurt am Main, Germany, 2013.
24. Bechmann, S.; Jäckle, R.; Lück, P.; Herdegen, R. [Motives and Barriers for Worksite Health Management. Survey and Recommendation.] Motive und Hemmnisse für Betriebliches Gesundheitsmanagement (BGM), Umfrage und Empfehlungen. 2011. Available online: https://www.iga-info.de/fileadmin/redakteur/Veroeffentlichungen/iga_Reporte/Dokumente/iga-Report_20_Umfrage_BGM_KMU_final_2011.pdf (accessed on 27 February 2019).
25. Beck, D. *[Modern Health Policy in Micro and Small Enterprises. Inhibiting and Promoting Conditions] Zeitgemäße Gesundheitspolitik in Kleinst- und Kleinbetrieben: Hemmende und fördernde Bedingungen*, 1st ed.; Sigma: Berlin, Germany, 2011.
26. Linnan, L.; Bowling, M.; Childress, J.; Lindsay, G.; Blakey, C.; Pronk, S.; Wieker, S.; Royall, P. Results of the 2004 National Worksite Health Promotion Survey. *Am. J. Public Health* **2008**, *98*, 1503–1509. [CrossRef] [PubMed]
27. Tremblay, P.A.; Nobrega, S.; Davis, L.; Erck, E.; Punnett, L. Healthy workplaces? A survey of Massachusetts employers. *Am. J. Health Promot.* **2013**, *27*, 390–400. [CrossRef] [PubMed]
28. Bundesinstitut für Bau-, Stadt- und Raumforschung. [Indicators and Maps for Territorial and Urban Development] Indikatoren und Karten zur Raum- und Stadtentwicklung. 2018. Available online: https://www.inkar.de (accessed on 20 August 2018).
29. Federation of Creditreform Associations. Services, Marketing Data from the Information Expert. 2019. Available online: https://www.creditreform.com/en/services/marketing-data.html (accessed on 29 January 2019).
30. Michaelis, M.; Rieger, M.A. [Scientific Support and Conducting of the Survey to Determine the Needs with Regard to "Workplace Health Management (BGM) in the Lake of Konstanz county"] Wissenschaftliche Begleitung und Durchführung der Befragung zur Bedarfsermittlung "Betriebliches Gesundheitsmanagement (BGM) im Landkreis Konstanz". In *[Unpublished final report on the research project "Scientific Monitoring of the Model Phase I Dialogue on Work and Health" for submission to the "Work and Health" department, Ministry of Economics, Labour and Housing Baden-Württemberg] Unveröffentlichter Abschlussbericht zum Forschungsvorhaben "Wissenschaftliche Begleitung der Modellphase I Dialog Arbeit und Gesundheit" zur Vorlage beim Referat "Arbeit und Gesundheit", Ministerium für Wirtschaft, Arbeit und Wohnungsbau Baden-Württemberg*; Rieger, M.A., Ed.; Tübingen, Germany, 2017; pp. 11–29.
31. Rieger, M.A.; Hildenbrand, S.; Nesseler, T.; Letzel, S.; Nowak, D. *[Prevention and Health Promotion at the Interface between Curative Medicine and Occupational Medicine: A Compendium for Occupational Health Management.] Prävention und Gesundheitsförderung an der Schnittstelle zwischen kurativer Medizin und Arbeitsmedizin: Ein Kompendium für das Betriebliche Gesundheitsmanagement*; Ecomed Medizin: Landsberg am Lech, Germany, 2016.

32. Bräunig, D.; Haupt, J.; Kohstall, T.; Kramer, I.; Pieper, C.; Schröer, S. [Effectiveness and Benefits of Occupational Prevention.] Wirksamkeit und Nutzen betrieblicher Prävention, iga-Report.28. Available online: https://www.iga-info.de/fileadmin/redakteur/Veroeffentlichungen/iga_Reporte/Dokumente/iga-Report_28_Wirksamkeit_Nutzen_betrieblicher_Praevention.pdf (accessed on 27 February 2019).
33. Knoche, K.; Sochert, R. [Company Reintegration Management.] Betriebliches Eingliederungsmanagement, Iga.Report 24. 2013. Available online: https://www.iga-info.de/fileadmin/redakteur/Veroeffentlichungen/iga_Reporte/Dokumente/iga-Report_24_Betriebliches_Eingliederungsmanagement.pdf (accessed on 27 February 2019).
34. Rieger, M.A. [Scientific support and implementation of the survey to determine the needs of 'Workplace Health Management in the Constance County'.] Wissenschaftliche Begleitung und Durchführung der Befragung zur Bedarfsermittlung 'Betriebliches Gesundheitsmanagement (BGM) im Landkreis Konstanz'. In *[Unpublished final report on the research project "Scientific Monitoring of the Model Phase I Dialogue on Work and Health" for submission to the "Work and Health" department, Ministry of Economics, Labour and Housing Baden-Württemberg] Unveröffentlichter Abschlussbericht zum Forschungsvorhaben "Wissenschaftliche Begleitung der Modellphase I Dialog Arbeit und Gesundheit" zur Vorlage beim Referat "Arbeit und Gesundheit", Ministerium für Wirtschaft, Arbeit und Wohnungsbau Baden-Württemberg*; Rieger, M.A., Ed.; Tübingen, Germany, 2017; pp. 4–6.
35. Arbeitsschutzgesetz [Act on the Implementation of Measures of Occupational Safety and Health to Encourage Improvements in the Safety and Health Protection of Workers at Work]: *ArbSchG*. 1996. Available online: http://www.gesetze-im-internet.de/englisch_arbschg/ (accessed on 28 February 2019).
36. Verordnung über die arbeitsmedizinische Vorsorge [Ordinance on Occupational Health Care]: *ArbMedVV*. 2008. Available online: https://www.gesetze-im-internet.de/englisch_arbmedvv/englisch_arbmedvv.html (accessed on 28 February 2019).
37. Arbeitssicherheitsgesetz [Act on Occupational Physicians, Safety Engineers and Other Occupational Safety Specialists]: *ASiG*. 1973. Available online: https://www.gesetze-im-internet.de/englisch_asig/englisch_asig.html (accessed on 28 February 2019).
38. Deutsche Gesetzliche Unfallversicherung. DGUV Regulation 1, Accident Prevention Regulation. Principles of Prevention. 2013. Available online: https://www.dguv.de/medien/inhalt/praevention/vorschriften_regeln/vorschrift_1_en.pdf (accessed on 28 January 2019).
39. Deutsche Gesetzliche Unfallversicherung. DGUV Regulation 2, Accident Prevention Regulation. Occupational Physicians and OSH Professionals. Available online: https://www.dguv.de/medien/inhalt/praevention/vorschriften_regeln/regulation_2_en.pdf (accessed on 28 January 2019).
40. Sozialgesetzbuch (SGB IX) Neuntes Buch Rehabilitation und Teilhabe von Menschen mit Behinderungen [Book Nine of the Social Code (§ 167 SGB "Prevention")]: *§ 167 SGB IX "Prevention"*. 2018. Available online: https://www.gesetze-im-internet.de/sgb_9_2018/__167.html (accessed on 28 February 2019).
41. Cohen, J. *Statistical Power Analysis for the Behavioral Sciences*, 2nd ed.; Erlbaum: Hillsdale, MI, USA, 1988.
42. Völter-Mahlknecht, S.; Michaelis, M.; Preiser, C.; Blomberg, N.; Rieger, M.A. Research Report 448. Utilization of Medical Check-ups in the Field of Occupational Medicine. Available online: http://www.bmas.de/SharedDocs/Downloads/DE/PDF-Publikationen/forschungsbericht-f448.pdf;jsessionid=DA7F8539671B556D67B3FC0A659C634D?__blob=publicationFile (accessed on 28 January 2019).
43. Michaelis, M.; Lange, R.; Junne, F.; Rothermund, E.; Zipfel, S.; Gündel, H.; Rieger, M.A. Prevention of common mental disorders in employees—Conception, study design and sample characteristics of a multi-target survey. *Ment. Health Prev.* **2016**, *4*, 88–95. [CrossRef]
44. Junne, F.; Michaelis, M.; Rothermund, E.; Stuber, F.; Gündel, H.; Zipfel, S.; Rieger, M.A. The Role of Work-Related Factors in the Development of Psychological Distress and Associated Mental Disorders: Differential Views of Human Resource Managers, Occupational Physicians, Primary Care Physicians and Psychotherapists in Germany. *Int. J. Environ. Res. Public Health* **2018**, *15*, 559. [CrossRef] [PubMed]
45. Schuller, K. ["Good we talked about this . . . ?!"—Methodological challenges for the risk assessment of psychological stress in SMEs] "Gut, dass wir mal darüber geredet haben . . . ?!"—Methodische Herausforderungen für die Gefährdungsbeurteilung psychischer Belastung in KMU. *Arbeitsmedizin Sozialmedizin Umweltmedizin* **2018**, *53*, 790–797.
46. Barth, C.; Hamacher, W.; Blanco-Trillo, S. [Occupational health care needs in Germany] Arbeitsmedizinischer Betreuungsbedarf in Deutschland. 2014. Available online: https://www.baua.de/DE/Angebote/Publikationen/Berichte/F2326.pdf?__blob=publicationFile&v=5 (accessed on 29 January 2019).

47. Barth, C.; Eickholt, C.; Hamacher, W.; Schmauder, M. [Need for occupational safety specialists in Germany] Bedarf an Fachkräften für Arbeitssicherheit in Deutschland. Available online: https://www.baua.de/DE/Angebote/Publikationen/Berichte/F2388.pdf?__blob=publicationFile&v=4 (accessed on 29 January 2019).
48. Harris, J.R.; Hannon, P.A.; Beresford, S.A.A.; Linnan, L.A.; McLellan, D.L. Health promotion in smaller workplaces in the United States. *Annu. Rev. Public Health* **2014**, *35*, 327–342. [CrossRef] [PubMed]
49. Beck, D.; Lenhardt, U. [Workplace Health Promotion in Germany: Prevalence and Utilisation. Analyses on Labour Force Surveys of the Federal Institute for Occupational Safety and Health in 2006 and 2012.] Betriebliche Gesundheitsförderung in Deutschland: Verbreitung und Inanspruchnahme. Ergebnisse der BIBB/BAuA-Erwerbstätigenbefragungen 2006 und 2012. *Gesundheitswesen* **2016**, *78*, 56–62. [PubMed]
50. Faller, G. [Implementation of Workplace Health Promotion/Workplace Health Management in Germany: State-of-the Art and Need for Further Research.] Umsetzung Betrieblicher Gesundheitsförderung/Betrieblichen Gesundheitsmanagements in Deutschland: Stand und Entwicklungsbedarfe der einschlägigen Forschung. *Gesundheitswesen* **2018**, *80*, 278–285. [PubMed]

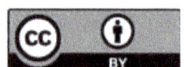

© 2019 by the authors. Licensee MDPI, Basel, Switzerland. This article is an open access article distributed under the terms and conditions of the Creative Commons Attribution (CC BY) license (http://creativecommons.org/licenses/by/4.0/).

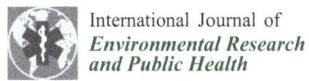

Article

Total Worker Health: A Small Business Leader Perspective

Janalee Thompson [1], Natalie V. Schwatka [1,2,*], Liliana Tenney [1,2] and Lee S. Newman [1,2,3,4]

1. Center for Health, Work & Environment, Colorado School of Public Health, University of Colorado, Anschutz Medical Campus, 13001 E. 17th Pl., 3rd Floor, Mail Stop B119 HSC, Aurora, CO 80045, USA; janaleethompson7@gmail.com (J.T.); liliana.tenney@ucdenver.edu (L.T.); lee.newman@ucdenver.edu (L.S.N.)
2. Department of Environmental and Occupational Health, Colorado School of Public Health, University of Colorado, Anschutz Medical Campus, 13001 E. 17th Pl., 3rd Floor, Mail Stop B119 HSC, Aurora, CO 80045, USA
3. Department of Epidemiology, Colorado School of Public Health, University of Colorado, Anschutz Medical Campus, 13001 E. 17th Pl., 3rd Floor, Mail Stop B119 HSC, Aurora, CO 80045, USA
4. Division of Pulmonary Science and Critical Care Medicine, Department of Medicine, School of Medicine, University of Colorado, Anschutz Medical Campus, 13001 E 17th Pl., Aurora, CO 80045, USA
* Correspondence: Natalie.Schwatka@ucdenver.edu; Tel.: +1-303-724-4607

Received: 28 September 2018; Accepted: 28 October 2018; Published: 31 October 2018

Abstract: Total Worker Health® (TWH) frameworks call for attention to organizational leadership in the implementation and effectiveness of TWH approaches. It is especially important to study this within in the small business environment where employees face significant health, safety, and well-being concerns and employers face barriers to addressing these concerns. The purpose of this study was to gain a better understanding of how small business leaders perceive employee health, safety, and well-being in the context of their own actions. We conducted semi-structured interviews with 18 small business senior leaders and used a qualitative coding approach to analyze the transcripts to determine the frequency with which leaders discussed each code. When we asked leaders about their leadership practices for health, safety, and well-being, leaders reflected upon their business (65%), themselves (28%), and their employees (7%). Leaders rarely discussed the ways in which they integrate health, safety, and well-being. The interviews demonstrate that small business leaders care about the health of their employees, but because of the perceived value to their business, not to employees or themselves. Thus, they may lack the knowledge and skills to be successful TWH leaders. The present study supports a need for continued small business TWH leadership research.

Keywords: workplace safety; safety leadership; health promoting leadership; safety programs; health promotion; health protection; leadership; qualitative study

1. Introduction

Total Worker Health® (TWH) is defined as policies, programs, and practice that integrate protection from work-related safety and health hazards with promotion of injury and illness prevention efforts to advance worker well-being [1]. As the field of TWH gains research and practice support, it is important to study the role of organizational leadership. Several TWH frameworks call for attention to organizational leadership in the implementation and effectiveness of TWH approaches [2–4]. However, to date, leadership research has rarely integrated both health promoting leadership and safety leadership. Doing so can improve our understanding of how to assess and improve TWH-specific leadership practices to ensure TWH system effectiveness [5]. This is especially important in the small business environment where employees face significant health, safety, and well-being concerns [6,7] and employers face barriers to addressing these concerns (e.g., resources) [6,8]. Therefore, as a first step, the purpose of this study was to improve our understanding of how small business leaders perceive employee health, safety, and well-being in the context of their own actions.

The field of leadership research has grown substantially over the past few decades. Dinh et al. [9] found 66 leadership theory domains in their review of the leadership literature. While the evidence base for each of these theories varies, it is generally agreed that leadership is a significant contributor to organizational culture and ultimately, organizational success [10]. Successful organizations primarily have leaders who adopt several leadership characteristics to best meet organizational needs [11]. A healthy business culture is derived from integrating leadership theories that align employee and organizational goals [12], though some leaders who use some styles of leadership have been more effective in promoting health than others.

Building positive relationships, empowerment and the ability to view the organization from an employee viewpoint are characteristics of successful leaders. Servant leaders are known for their supportive nature and how they achieve organizational goals by prioritizing needs of employees first [13]. Similarly, leaders who employ high quality relationships (leader-member exchange (LMX)) leverage employee relationships to meet organizational ambitions [14]. Successful leaders also place value in employee perceptions of meaningful work and contribution to the larger picture. Sirota's Three Factor Theory argues for building and maintaining employee enthusiasm through equal treatment, employee belief that work is meaningful, and camaraderie. Sirota's theory describes that when leaders champion these factors, workers will be enthusiastic and motivated to produce more, while enjoying what they do [15].

Leadership has an impact on employee physical and psychological health. Transformational leadership, specifically, has been positively associated with psychological well-being [16], stress [17], depression [18], and sleep quality [19]. In terms of safety-specific outcomes, several meta-analyses demonstrate that leadership (generally defined) and transformational leadership are related to better safety climate, better safety practices, and fewer occupational injuries [20–22]. However, employee health can also be compromised as a result of poor leadership. Researchers have found associations between poor management support and ischemic heart disease [23], elevated blood pressure [24], problem drinking [25], smoking [26], as well as mental health issues related to affective well-being [27] and job well-being [16,28,29]. For example, Skakon et al. found that when leaders have high stress and poor affective well-being, their subordinates also have high stress levels and poor well-being [27].

Recently, researchers have begun to investigate health promoting leadership. Health promoting leadership theory involves leadership characteristics that encourage wellness at work [30]. Research has shown that leaders who promote workplace health are hands-on, supportive [31], demonstrate health awareness, and value community and fairness [32,33]. It has also been suggested that work-related stress may be reduced when specific, health promoting transformational leadership skills are demonstrated at work [34]. Though research may be limited, all health promoting leadership studies suggest that health promoting leadership characteristics are likely to produce positive health outcomes. However, in the context of TWH, health promoting leadership fails to consider the role of safety leadership.

In contrast, the theory and evidence base for safety leadership gained traction over fifteen years ago [35]. The majority of the safety-specific literature focuses on Bass's multifactor leadership theory [36]. Some researchers developed safety-specific assessments of transformational and passive leadership and found them to be more associated with safety outcomes than general forms of leadership [37]. Studies have shown that the passive form of transactional safety leadership negatively impacts safety outcomes (e.g., injury rates) whereas transformational safety leadership positively impacts safety outcomes [38]. However, other more active forms of transactional leadership, contingent reward and active management-by-exception, have been linked to positive safety outcomes [39]. Safety leadership intervention studies have suggested that training leaders on transformational safety leadership skills can lead to positive safety outcomes [40,41]. Other researchers applied the LMX theory [42] and empowering leadership theory [43] to workplace safety and found both to be related to positive safety outcomes. Although, similar to the singular focus of HP leadership, safety leadership research has focused solely on safety and has rarely included research on other outcomes.

The literature illustrates the segmented nature of leadership research in the employee health promotion and safety contexts. Health promoting and safety leadership are both "best practices" to support worker health and safety but we are unaware of a concerted effort to evaluate their use in synchrony. Furthermore, we are aware of only one study that assessed health promotion and safety leadership support amongst small businesses. They found that small business leaders who advocate for TWH have higher integration scores than leaders who do not [44]. However, this study did not define TWH leadership support or describe the ways in which TWH leaders advocate. Thus, while there is some indication that TWH leadership is important amongst small businesses, it is unclear how small businesses leaders can demonstrate support for TWH. For this reason, as a first step in understanding TWH leadership development needs, we sought to interview small business leaders to understand how they discuss their use of practices that demonstrate a commitment to health, safety, and well-being.

2. Materials and Methods

We conducted a qualitative study with small business leaders to understand their current approach to leadership for employee health, safety, and well-being (Appendix A). We recruited small business leaders (<500 employees) in Colorado and Wyoming from a variety of industries by phone and email from May 2017 to August 2017. Businesses were identified through existing networks including a workers' compensation insurer, chambers of commerce, and a community-based program, Health Links™. Leaders were eligible to participate if they had significant decision-making power in the organization (e.g., owner, senior executive, or CEO).

The first author conducted 30-min, semi-structured interviews in-person or by phone asking each leader how they perceive health, safety, and well-being in their organization and their role in shaping it. The authors generated eleven interview questions based on the following themes related to key theories used in previous health promotion or safety leadership research: organizational mission, organizational culture, leading by example as well as employee advancement, feedback, and recognition [11,15,37,45–47]. We chose these theories because they reflect important leader characteristics and actions for employee health, safety, and well-being. Beyond the transformational style commonly studied in safety leadership [11,37], other styles layer in important leadership aspects, including openness, ethics [45], equity [15], focus on follower needs [47], and relationships [46]. In keeping with the TWH framework, all questions inquired about leader actions associated with health, safety and well-being together. In keeping with leadership frameworks, all questions asked them about their own practices, not their general business practices. If the interview lasted less than 30 min, the first author asked additional follow-up questions. Follow-up questions were developed a priori, however they were chosen by the interviewer based on participant answers to main survey items. The interview questions can be read in the supplementary material. All interviews were recorded. We obtained verbal permission from all participants prior to recording. The first author transcribed the interview by hand in Microsoft Word and then imported it into Dedoose, qualitative data analysis software [48]. Our protocol and all study procedures were approved by the Colorado Multiple Institutional Review Board.

Analysis

The first and second authors analyzed the interview data using a qualitative coding approach described by Saldana [49]. We used descriptive codes to summarize content line by line into concise themes. The authors initially coded two transcripts individually with codes that best represented the interview content, allowing the codes to emerge from the content. The authors then met to compare codes and determine which codes best represented the content. Manuscripts were coded two at a time until all coding was complete. During this initial coding phase, three overarching themes became apparent. Thus, the authors decided to categorize all codes into one of three overarching themes. First, a *business* overarching theme included transactional policies, programs, and practices. To be coded within this overarching theme, the leader must have spoken about how their business operates in general and not specific to either what they do or say or what their employees do or say in a health and safety context. Second, an *employee* overarching theme represented a discussion of health, safety, and well-being from their employee's perspective. Finally, a *self* overarching theme represented a discussion of what they personally do for health, safety, and well-being.

The pair met after initial coding to compare and discuss their respective coding scheme. Codes were structured as: parent code (three overarching themes), child code (sub-code), grandchild code (sub-sub-code). It was agreed upon a priori that lines of code could be simultaneously coded as more than one code, if deemed necessary. When codes differed between investigators, a discussion took place and the most agreeable code was assigned. After each combined coding session, we transferred the finalized codes into Dedoose [48]. This process was followed until all transcripts were coded. Once the coding phase was completed, we extracted the coded data from Dedoose to Microsoft Excel. Finally, we conducted a descriptive, quantitative analysis of the overall frequency of codes.

3. Results

In total, we interviewed 18 small business leaders from diverse industries based on the 10 Occupational Safety and Health Administration (OSHA) industry divisions. Industries were represented as follows: (A). Agriculture, Forestry, Fishing, 4; (B). Mining, 1; (C). Construction, 2; (D). Manufacturing, 1; (E). Transportation, Communications, Electric, Gas, Sanitary Services, 2; (G). Retail trade, 1; (H). Finance, Insurance, Real Estate, 1; and (I). Services, 6. About half of the leaders were female (n = 8.44%). Overall, the most common overarching theme discussed was their business, which represented 66% of total codes. Leaders discussed themselves and their employees much less frequently (see Figure 1). In the following sections, we describe each of these three overarching themes by highlighting the top five child codes within each theme. There were no qualitative differences in responses by the gender of the leader.

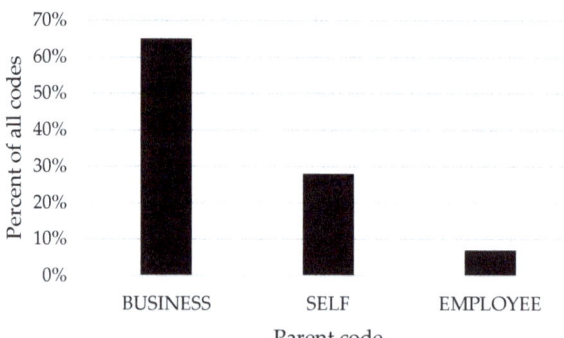

Figure 1. Percent of total codes mentioned by parent code.

3.1. Business

Small business leaders primarily talked about health, safety and well-being in the context of the business they owned or worked for. The most frequent child codes in a business context, in order from most to least frequently mentioned, included health and safety programs, organizational barriers to doing TWH, gathering employee feedback on health and safety, communicating the importance of health, and program evaluation (see Table 1).

Table 1. Percent of child codes mentioned in leader interviews by parent code.

Parent Code	Child Code	Description	Percent of Total Parent Code
Business	Health and safety programs	Program in general or specific program components, such as incentives, biometrics or training	38%
	Organizational barriers	Business barriers that hinder success of health and safety program, such as multi-site work environments	10%
	Employee feedback	Systematic efforts to collect employee feedback on the health and safety program, such as during an annual review	9%
	Health communication	Communicating the importance of health in general and the health and safety program specifically via different channels, such as email	9%
	Program evaluation	Efforts to evaluate their health and safety program and adjust as needed, such as tracking flu shot uptake during a campaign to get employees to take their flu shot	7%
Self	Lead by example	Talking and acting in ways that are consistent with their health and safety program, such as modeling good work/life balance	25%
	Individual consideration	Efforts to personally attend to individual employee's needs, such as regular one-on-one check-ins	20%
	Helpful strategies	Mention of a specific thing they say or do that they have found to be particularly helpful	12%
	Outcome	Perceived outcome of personally being involved in the health and safety programs, such as a better relationship with their employees	8%
	Health value	Personal value for health, safety, and well-being	6%
Employee	Employee barrier	Employee-specific barriers that hinder success of health and safety program, such as employees already having too much to do	26%
	Family	Recognition that employees have a family outside of work, family participation in health and safety program, or employees taking health and safety program home to their family	20%
	Employee leadership	Ways in which employees demonstrate leadership in the health and safety program, such as employees identifying hazards and working to control them	17%
	Program participation	Mention of a percent engagement in the health and safety program or ways in which employees participate	15%
	Personal accountability	Employees needing to take care of themselves and leaving health decisions ultimately up to the employee	6%

Within this overarching theme, health and safety programs were overwhelmingly referenced the most with leaders mentioning a variety of program elements. The most common element was employee incentives. Most small business leaders either discussed the current use of incentives, or desire to implement incentives to increase employee participation in health and wellness activities.

"We tied it to an incentive program. So we pay out incentives three times a year … we are one of the few remaining family-owned businesses that still pay full benefits for our 30 management team members and their entire family … if someone can't participate in one of the platforms that we choose and they can't take and invest that time for themselves and go get a health assessment and be active, that maybe they don't get an incentive".

"For participating in a lot of these activities, just by signing up to do yoga or signing up to give blood, we do random drawings for gift cards ... After the event, we publicize how many people participated and who got the gift card".

Other common, but less frequently mentioned, grand-child codes under health and safety programs included safety and wellness meetings and/or committees as well as health insurance offerings, such as benefits and biometric screenings. Compared to larger businesses, it is not as common for small businesses to offer health insurance benefits to employees, however, a few of the leaders in our study did mention offering these benefits to their white-collar workforce (see quote above under incentives).

"We also conduct monthly safety meetings in the field and all of the employees in the field attend. We do keep attendance at it and we've begun to integrate a variety of things. [There is an] enhanced level awareness and knowledge base at those meetings".

"Through our benefits program ... once a year or twice a year we have the third party come in and do the health assessments where they do the blood pressure, cholesterol levels and readings and it's interesting because you can see the history through the years ... it's just interesting just to see how that changes throughout a period of time".

"We started to, about a year and a half ago, provide some of our more management level positions and some of our full-time employees with health insurance".

It is worth noting that leaders rarely discussed health, safety, and well-being practices from an integrated perspective. Leaders mentioned a variety of program elements from paid time off to job hazard analyses processes, but only one leader mentioned that they took steps to integrate these efforts. Another leader recognized the need for their business to integrate their efforts to protect and promote employee health. However, it was somewhat common for leaders to compare their safety and health promotion programs. About one-third of the leaders mentioned that one program was in better shape than the other.

"We definitely separate health and safety. When we think about safety, we think about workplace accidents only. We don't connect the two, so I think one of the future things I would like to do is find an overlap of them".

Within this overarching theme, leaders also discussed organizational barriers associated with doing TWH. Leaders mentioned barriers such as an offsite workforce (e.g., easier to give office employees resources than field workers), difficulty obtaining employee engagement (e.g., challenge of designing programs that reach employees), and generational differences (e.g., millennials being perceived as unreliable and not working as hard as older generations). However, if they are able to successfully implement programs, some leaders (7% of all business child codes) mentioned some perceived beneficial business outcomes of adopting TWH, including better employee health and improved employee engagement.

Leaders also discussed the ways in which their business communicates health information to their employees and gathers employee feedback on health and safety programs. When discussing health communication, leaders frequently mentioned different modes of communication such as email, newsletters, and postings on wall boards. When discussing the ways in which their business goes about gathering feedback, leaders mentioned surveys, annual performance reviews, direct communication between the safety/wellness committee and employees, near miss injury reporting programs, etc. Some leaders also discussed efforts to evaluate their programs and take action to improve their programs, for example, not only asking for employee feedback, but also taking steps to act upon that feedback.

"Then we have a newsletter that goes out to all of our employees and again, there is something in there about safety, something in there about your health and other things".

"Information that we get through the near-miss program can also show us what employees are looking for and what they're needing and just kind of assessing that and prioritizing that and seeing if there's something that we can do about it".

3.2. Self

About one-third of the time, leaders spoke about workplace health, safety, and well-being from their own perspective. In order from most to least frequently mentioned, included leading by example, demonstrating individual consideration, helpful strategies for engaging employees, outcomes they perceive by personally engaging in TWH-focused leadership practices, and value for health. Leading by example was most commonly expressed as the leader participating in health and wellness initiatives or activities. Notably, "participate" was a grandchild code of "lead by example" and represented 15% of the "lead by example" codes. Individual consideration was denoted when a leader gave an example of how they paid special attention to individual employee to check-in or to help them. Some leaders specifically mentioned having an open-door policy to provide a safe place for employees to talk about both work and non-related work issues. Others also stressed the importance of connecting with employees on an individual level.

"You can't expect people to pull away from their desks and come participate in something if it's not important enough for you to do it yourself".

"I hope that my actions positively affect the behaviors of my employees . . . if I come into the office in a bad mood, others are also in a bad mood. If I come into the office psyched and engaged, others are psyched and engaged. As a leader, I get that people mirror and model my behavior".

"One thing that I tried to do over the years able to listen to my coworkers and just, you know be willing to hear them and how they're doing and be able to help in any way that I can".

" . . . we have an open-door policy . . . if you're struggling whether or not it's work-related or outside of work . . . you know we are here for you. We get life . . . we [upper management] tried to take our own personal experiences and reach out with regards to how we can involve our employees".

"But there are tremendous opportunities when you do connect with someone . . . they know you understand what they're doing and that you have their best interest in mind. You can make a really meaningful change by simply helping someone do something the right way so they don't get hurt, or helping them achieve a professional development goal that they've always wanted to do, whether it's a training, or a certification . . . "

Of the few times leaders mentioned their health values, they spoke from a couple of perspectives. For example, some mentioned it terms of a personal value while others mentioned it in relation to their work team.

"And another thing I'd add is that I truly care about the well-being of the people that I work with and that are my co-workers. From a human perspective, it just matters to me that they feel as good as they can".

"I think it's important from a personal perspective not only for ourselves, but also for our employees and that they conduct themselves in a safe manner so that they return to their families safely and be healthy and be able to provide for their families".

On several occasions, leaders mentioned strategies they found to be helpful as they personally worked to promote employee health, safety, and well-being.

"First and foremost, it's building a trust level".

"We have an advantage because we are small, and I think it's critical in a small business environment that you need to develop a structure that tunes it for each individual employee".

When leaders spoke about perceived outcomes of their personal efforts to engage in TWH, they most commonly referred to better employee/leader relationship and employee engagement.

"I think that I have so many people that want to work with us and with me, and with my partners just because they see us doing what we're doing".

3.3. Employee

In order from most to least frequently mentioned, leaders mentioned employees as a barrier to program effectiveness, employees who are treated like family, employees demonstrating leadership in the program, employees participating in workplace health and safety programs, and individual accountability. Leaders mentioned difficulty in getting employees engaged in the programs for several reasons, such as adding more work to their busy schedules and cultural differences.

"The reality is that everyone is juggling things like having a family, getting their work done ... having a hard time finding time to fit it exercise or gardening or all of the great stuff that we'd do if we only worked 30-h weeks".

"It matters from an employee perspective obviously because we have got a small workforce ... We wear a lot of different hats".

"Our employee base is mostly Latino based and in most cases there is a difference of cultures between their originating country and here in the United States".

Business leaders also expressed an understanding that employees have other non-work responsibilities, like family. Some even promoted family inclusion to increase participation in health and wellness initiatives.

" ... people can bring their families and their pets".

Some leaders mentioned that their employees demonstrate leadership. For example, leaders mentioned instances in which employees identify hazards and help to control them, help build safety and/or wellness programs, and senior employees who voluntarily coach newer employees until they become familiar with safe work processes.

"I think it's important to involve employees in that decision-making process and development of programs".

"So we take somebody who is extremely knowledgeable and skilled and they have to oversee someone actually executing on a procedure before they sign off that they are competent to do that".

Finally, as it pertains to health in general, some leaders mentioned that ultimately employees have to make the decision to be healthy.

"We just try to leave it up to the individual to make their own decisions about what they are comfortable with".

4. Discussion

We sought to understand TWH from the small business leader perspective. When we asked leaders about their leadership practices for health, safety, and well-being, leaders reflected upon their business 65% of the time, on themselves 28% of the time, and their employees 7% of the time. These findings demonstrate that small business leaders primarily communicate about TWH through the lens of their business policies and programs. Within each of these three overarching themes, leaders most commonly discussed elements of their TWH programs followed by the ways in which they lead by example within these programs and the employee barriers to TWH program effectiveness. Leaders rarely discussed the ways in which they integrate health, safety, and well-being.

Historically, leadership research focused on individual leader qualities and practices. The leaders in our study mentioned several times that they lead by example and considered the individual needs of their workforce, both of which were previously linked to health and safety outcomes [39]. However, other positive leadership characteristics such as empowering employees, coaching and teaching, motivating and inspiring, being authentic and ethical, and sharing or distributing leadership were rarely mentioned in the interviews [36,45,47,50,51]. Leaders mentioned business practices to encourage employee growth (i.e., training), solicit employee feedback, and communicate health messages. However, they did not specifically mention the ways in which they personally engaged in these practices.

Present day leadership research expands the concept of leadership from the individual leader to followers, the work environment, culture, etc. [52]. Our finding that small business leaders overwhelmingly discuss health, safety and well-being in the context of their business when asked about TWH leadership practices highlights the importance of considering leadership in a more comprehensive context. Similar to other qualitative studies on management perceptions of safety or health promotion programs [53,54], leaders mentioned a variety of policies and programs they have for their employees, as well as barriers to program effectiveness and outcomes of the program if successful. This perspective focuses on what Burke et al. [55] would call a transactional rather than transformational perspective. A transactional perspective focuses on management issues (e.g., TWH structures and systems), whereas a transformational perspective focuses on leadership, culture, and overall organizational mission and vision. Both are important aspects of a business's TWH strategy [7]. Our findings point to an opportunity to study leadership practices in the context of existing TWH systems, especially as it pertains to integration. It also demonstrates a need to help small business leaders connect their own practices to their business's TWH structures and systems in practice [52].

In our study, leaders rarely talked about their employees' perspective of health, safety, and well-being. When leaders did, they talked about employees in the context of barriers to program effectiveness. Small businesses leaders who wish to increase employee engagement must be able to understand and describe their employee's perceptions of the TWH program. Safety climate research demonstrates the importance of employee perception, showing that employees often report worse perceptions of organizational or management commitment to safety than managers [56,57]. Huang et al. [56] argues that this difference can result in management failing to act to improve safety conditions, and as a result that more weight should be placed on the employee than management perspective when making program decisions. Furthermore, TWH researchers argue for a participatory approach to program development and management [58]. Thus, if small business leaders are primarily focused on TWH in a business context, as found in the present study, there are likely substantial gaps between TWH programs and employee needs and interests.

In practice, these finding suggests that small business leaders may be more receptive to TWH leadership practices if it is communicated through the lens of their business. To obtain leadership support for TWH, academics and practitioners should build an argument for why and how consideration of their employees perspective as well as their own perspective on TWH contributes to business operations and overall business success.

It is worth noting that there may be some alternative explanations for the code frequencies we observed. As mentioned above, leaders rarely talked about specific leadership practices. However, this does not mean they do not display them in their daily work activities. It may mean that they do not naturally discuss them. We may have observed different results had we structured our questions differently. For example, we did not preface the interview with an explanation of what leadership is nor did we explain what TWH is. The latter may have helped leaders better understand of the aim of the interview and resulted in more description of their leadership practices. The former may have contributed to our finding that small business leaders primarily discussed health, safety, and well-being separately. Leaders may have interpreted the questions as asking for non-integrative responses.

4.1. Future Research

The present study adds to the literature on leadership support for TWH business practices [59] by being the first to begin to understand what leadership support means from small business leaders' own words. This follows previous calls by leadership researchers for more mixed methods leadership research to better understand leadership in context [52]. Building upon the present study, future qualitative research should consider focusing interview questions on TWH as an integrative concept to better understand the ways leadership practices are used to simultaneously influence health, safety, and well-being. Additionally, concrete questions should be used to hone in on specific leadership practices such as coaching or ethics. An important next step in this research will also be to study small business TWH leadership from the employee perspective to learn whether they observe their leaders engaging in leadership practices. As described above, employee and management perceptions often differ.

Next, a quantitative needs assessment that employs a larger sample of small business leaders is needed to quantify opportunities for TWH leadership development. This should investigate which leadership styles, or combination of styles, elicit the best health, safety, and well-being outcomes including organizational-level indicators of TWH [60] as well as employee-level health, safety, and well-being outcomes. It will be important to assess TWH leadership from multiple perspectives, such as management, health and safety manager, human resources manager, and employee. Finally, future research on this topic should consider how contextual factors including business size, industry, business structure, geographic location, ownership, and other factors are associated with leadership. Other factors, including leaders' age, gender, race, ethnicity, and identifying workforce information (e.g., diversity, industry sector, part-time, full-time) should be considered as well.

Another next step is to investigate TWH leadership development strategies. Leadership development research for health promotion and safety has historically been siloed. Thus, an important next step will be to investigate the ways in which leadership development can be a means of improving TWH. We are currently investigating a TWH leadership development program described in Schwatka et al. [7] by structuring the learning content based on the three themes learned in this qualitative study: their business's TWH policies and practices, their employee's perspective of these policies and practices, and their own perspective via key leadership practices curated from multiple leadership theories. Our aim is to help small business leaders place their business practices in the context of their employees TWH needs as well as their own leadership practices.

4.2. Limitations

The present study had a few limitations. First, small business leaders who agreed to be interviewed may represent leaders who are more interested in TWH than all small business leaders. Results of the present study also reflect the small business leader perspectives of only 18 leaders from two states. Leaders from other states may approach health, safety and well-being differently. However, our sample was diverse in terms of industry and gender, which may strengthen the generalizability of our findings. The study findings would be strengthened if we had also interviewed small business employees. Finally, due to the way the questions were worded, we cannot say for sure whether leaders' responses reflect the TWH integrated framework or whether they were reflecting upon what they do for health, safety, and well-being separately.

5. Conclusions

Leadership is a critical to TWH system effectiveness in small business. In this qualitative study we aimed to integrate both health promoting leadership and safety leadership to begin to understand small business leadership practices that protect and promote employee health. The interviews demonstrate that small business leaders care about the health of their employees, but because of the perceived value to their business, not to employees or themselves. Thus, they may lack the knowledge and skills to be successful TWH leaders. The present study supports a need for continued TWH leadership research in a small business context, including mixed methods research to understand and quantify TWH leadership practices from the small business leader and employee perspectives, as well as the development and evaluation of TWH leadership development strategies.

Author Contributions: Each author contributed to this paper. Conceptualization: J.T., N.V.S., L.T., and L.S.N.; Methodology: J.T. and N.V.S.; Software: J.T. and N.V.S.; Validation: J.T. and N.V.S.; Formal analysis: J.T. and N.V.S.; Investigation: J.T., N.V.S., L.T., and L.S.N.; Resources: N.V.S., L.T., and L.S.N.; data Curation: J.T.; Writing—original draft preparation: J.T. and N.V.S.; Writing—review and editing: J.T., N.V.S., L.T., L.S.N.; Visualization: J.T. and N.V.S.; Supervision: N.V.S.; Project administration: J.T.; Funding acquisition: L.S.N., L.T., and N.V.S.

Funding: This study was funded by a Total Worker Health Center of Excellence Cooperative Agreement 1 U19 OH 011227-01, funded by the Centers for Disease Control and Prevention and the National Institute for Occupational Safety and Health. Its contents are solely the responsibility of the authors and do not necessarily represent the official views of the National Institute for Occupational Safety and Health, Centers for Disease Control and Prevention, or the Department of Health and Human Services.

Conflicts of Interest: The authors declare no conflict of interest.

Appendix A. Small Business Leader Interview Questions

Appendix A.1. Organizational Mission and Vision

1. Why does health, safety, and well-being matter to you? For both your own health, safety, and well-being but also for your employees. How did you come to this understanding?
2. What does employee health, safety, and well-being look like today in your organization?
3. Now that we've talked about what employee health, safety, and well-being looks like today, how do you determine what the future of employee health, safety, and well-being looks like in your organization?

Follow-up Questions

How do you communicate your vision for employee health, safety, and well-being?
Do you spend time talking to your employees about health and safety in your organization?—Can you give me an example of when you did this?

Appendix A.2. Organizational Culture

4. Every organization has its own unique culture of health and safety that develops over time based on what's said and what's done. What does your organization do to set the culture for healthy work? How do you involve employees?
5. Do you find it challenging, or difficult to engage your employees around health, safety, and wellness?—How do you approach this?

Follow-up Question

How do you encourage your employees to provide feedback for health and wellness in your organization?

When one of your employees provides feedback on health and wellness policies or programs, how do you react?

Have you ever incorporated employee suggestions into policies or standards? How did you do this?

Can you give me an example of how you have inspired your employees or how your employees have inspired each other to be healthier and safer in the workplace?

Appendix A.3. Lead Yourself

6. How do you lead by example in your organization when it comes to health, safety, and well-being?
7. How do you think your actions affect the behaviors of employees? Can you provide an example?

Follow-up Question

Do you ask for feedback on how you're leading by example from your employees? If so, how do you do it?

Employee Advancement

8. How do you go about identifying opportunities for supporting the values and goals of your employees?
9. Can you describe the opportunities and challenges you have experienced when initiating changes to improve employee health, safety and well-being?

Appendix A.4. Feedback and Recognition

10. What methods do you use to hold yourself and your employees accountable for sustaining good health, safety and wellness practices?
11. What are some ways that you recognize your employees for prioritizing health, safety, and wellness? For example, do you use rewards, praise, celebrate?

Follow-up Questions

How do you provide feedback, whether it's good or needs improvement, to your employees when it comes to health, safety, and wellness in your organization?

How do you solicit and receive feedback from other leaders and employees about prioritizing health, safety, and well-being in your organization?

Have you ever encountered opposition to change around employee health, safety, and well-being? How did you deal with it?

References

1. NIOSH. What Is Total Worker Health? 2018. Available online: https://www.cdc.gov/niosh/twh/default.html (accessed on 15 October 2018).
2. McLellan, D.; Moore, W.; Nagler, E.; Sorensen, G. *Implementing an Integrated Approach: Weaving Employee Health, Safety, and Well-Being into the Fabric of Your Organization*; Harvard, T.H., Ed.; Chan School of Public Health Center for Work, Health, and Well-Being: Boston, MA, USA, 2017.
3. Sorensen, G.; McLellan, D.; Dennerlein, J.T.; Pronk, N.P.; Allen, J.D.; Boden, L.I.; Okechukwu, C.A.; Hashimoto, D.; Stoddard, A.; Wagner, G.R. Integration of health protection and health promotion rationale, indicators, and metrics. *J. Occup. Environ. Med.* **2013**, *55*, S12–S18. [CrossRef] [PubMed]
4. Sorensen, G.; McLellan, D.; Sabbath, E.; Dennerlein, J.; Nagler, E.; Hurtado, D.; Pronk, N.; Wagner, G. Integrating worksite health protection and health promotion: A conceptual model for intervention and research. *Prev. Med.* **2016**, *91*, 188–196. [CrossRef] [PubMed]
5. Kelloway, E.K.; Barling, J. Leadership development as an intervention in occupational health psychology. *Work Stress* **2010**, *24*, 260–279. [CrossRef]

6. McCoy, K.; Stinson, K.; Scott, K.; Tenney, L.; Newman, L.S. Health promotion in small business: A systematic review of factors influencing adoption and effectiveness of worksite wellness programs. *J. Occup. Environ. Med.* **2014**, *56*, 579–587. [CrossRef] [PubMed]
7. Schwatka, N.; Tenney, L.; Dally, M.; Scott, J.; Brown, C.; Weitzenkamp, D.; Shore, E.; Newman, L. Small business total worker health: A conceptual and methodological approach to facilitating organizational change. *Occup. Health Sci.* **2018**, *2*, 25–41. [CrossRef]
8. Cunningham, T.R.; Sinclair, R.; Schulte, P. Better understanding the small business construct to advance research on delivering workplace health and safety. *Small Enterp. Res.* **2014**, *21*, 148–160. [CrossRef]
9. Dinh, J.E.; Lord, R.G.; Gardner, W.L.; Meuser, J.D.; Liden, R.C.; Hu, J. Leadership theory and research in the new millennium: Current theoretical trends and changing perspectives. *Leadersh. Q.* **2014**, *25*, 36–62. [CrossRef]
10. Alvesson, M. The culture perspective on organizations: Instrumental values and basic features of culture. *Scand. J. Manag.* **1989**, *5*, 123–136. [CrossRef]
11. Kouzes, J.M.; Posner, B.Z. *The Leadership Challenge: How to MAke Extraordinary Things Happen in Organizations*, 5th ed.; Wiley: San Francisco, CA, USA, 2012.
12. Hogan, R.; Kaiser, R.B. What we know about leadership. *Rev. Gen. Psychol.* **2005**, *9*, 169–180. [CrossRef]
13. Allen, G.P.; Moore, W.M.; Moser, L.R.; Neill, K.K.; Sambamoorthi, U.; Bell, H.S. The role of servant leadership and transformational leadership in academic pharmacy. *Am. J. Pharm. Educ.* **2016**, *80*, 113. [PubMed]
14. Graen, G.B.; Uhl-Bien, M. Relationship-based approach to leadership: Development of leader-member exchange (lmx) theory of leadership over 25 years: Applying a multi-level multi-domain perspective. *Leadersh. Q.* **1995**, *6*, 219–247. [CrossRef]
15. Sirota, D.; Mischkind, L.; Meltzer, M. *The Enthusiastic Employee: How Companies Profit by Giving Workers What They Want*; Wharton School Publishing: Upper Saddle River, NJ, USA, 2005.
16. Arnold, K.A.; Turner, N.; Barling, J.; Kelloway, E.K.; McKee, M.C. Transformational leadership and psychological well-being: The mediating role of meaningful work. *J. Occup. Health Psychol.* **2007**, *12*, 193–203. [CrossRef] [PubMed]
17. Sosik, J.; Godshalk, V. Leadership styles, mentoring functions received, and job-related stress: A conceptual model and preliminary study. *J. Organ. Behav.* **2000**, *21*, 365–390. [CrossRef]
18. Munir, F.; Nielsen, K.; Carneiro, I.G. Transformational leadership and depressive symptoms: A prospective study. *J. Affect. Disord.* **2010**, *120*, 235–239. [CrossRef] [PubMed]
19. Munir, F.; Nielsen, K. Does self-efficacy mediate the relationship between transformational leadership behaviours and healthcare workers' sleep quality? A longitudinal study. *J. Adv. Nurs.* **2009**, *65*, 1833–1843. [CrossRef] [PubMed]
20. Clarke, S. Safety leadership: A meta-analytic review of transformational and transactional leadership styles as antecedents of safety behaviours. *J. Occup. Organ. Psychol.* **2013**, *86*, 22–49. [CrossRef]
21. Nahrgang, J.D.; Morgeson, F.P.; Hofmann, D.A. Safety at work: A meta-analytic investigation of the link between job demands, job resources, burnout, engagement, and safety outcomes. *J. Appl. Psychol.* **2011**, *96*, 71–94. [CrossRef] [PubMed]
22. Christian, M.S.; Bradley, J.C.; Wallace, J.C.; Burke, M.J. Workplace safety: A meta-analysis of the roles of person and situation factors. *J. Appl. Psychol.* **2009**, *94*, 1103–1127. [CrossRef] [PubMed]
23. Nyberg, A.; Alfredsson, L.; Theorell, T.; Westerlund, H.; Vahtera, J.; Kivimaki, M. Managerial leadership and ischaemic heart disease among employees: The swedish wolf study. *Occup. Environ. Med.* **2009**, *66*, 51–55. [CrossRef] [PubMed]
24. Karlin, W.; Brondolo, E.; Schwartz, J. Workplace social support and ambulatory cardiovascular activity in new york city traffic agents. *Psychosom. Med.* **2003**, *65*, 67–176. [CrossRef]
25. Bamberger, P.A.; Bacharach, S.B. Abusive supervision and subordinate problem drinking: Taking resistance, stress, and subordinate personality into account. *Hum. Relat.* **2006**, *59*, 723–752. [CrossRef]
26. Erikson, W. Work factors as predictors of smoking relapse in nurses' aides. *Int. Arch. Occup. Environ. Health* **2005**, *79*, 244–250. [CrossRef] [PubMed]
27. Skakon, J.; Nielsen, K.; Borg, V.; Guzman, J. Are leaders' well-being, behaviours and style associated with the affective well-being of their employees? A systematic review of three decades of research. *Work Stress* **2010**, *24*, 107–139. [CrossRef]

28. Colquitt, J.A.; Conlon, D.E.; Wesson, M.J.; Porter, C.O.L.H.; Ng, K.Y. Justice at the milleninium: A meta-analytic review of 25 years of organizational justice research. *J. Appl. Psychol.* **2001**, *86*, 425–445. [CrossRef] [PubMed]
29. Nielsen, K.; Randall, R.; Yarker, J.; Brenner, S.-O. The effects of transformational leadership on followers' perceived work characteristics and psychological well-being: A longitudinal study. *Work Stress* **2008**, *22*, 16–32. [CrossRef]
30. Eriksson, A.; Axelsson, R.; Bihari Axelsson, S. Health promoting leadership—Different views of the concept. *Work J. Prev. Assess. Rehabil.* **2011**, *40*, 75–86.
31. Skarholt, K.; Bli, E.; Sandsund, M.; Andersen, T. Health promoting leadership practices in four norweigan industries. *Health Promot. Int.* **2016**, *31*, 936–945. [PubMed]
32. Jiménez, P.; Winkler, B.; Dunkl, A. Creating a healthy working environment with leadership: The concept of health-promoting leadership. *Int. J. Hum. Resour. Manag.* **2016**, *28*, 2430–2448. [CrossRef]
33. Winkler, E.; Busch, C.; Clasen, J.; Vowinkel, J. Leaderhsip behavior as a health-promoting resoruces for workers in low-skillsed jobs and the moderating role of power distance orientation. *Ger. J. Hum. Resour. Manag.* **2014**, *28*, 96–116. [CrossRef]
34. Dunkl, A.; Jimenez, P.; Sarotar Zizek, S.; Milfeiner, B.; Kallus, W.K. Similarities and differences of health-promoting leadership and transformational leadership. *Our Econ.* **2015**, *61*, 3–13. [CrossRef]
35. Hofmann, D.A.; Morgeson, F.P. *The Role of Leadership in Safety*; Barling, J., Frone, M., Eds.; American Psychological Association: Washington, DC, USA, 2004; pp. 159–180.
36. Bass, B. *Leadership and Performance Beyond Expectations*; Free Press: New York, NY, USA, 1985.
37. Barling, J.; Loughlin, C.; Kelloway, E.K. Development and test of a model linking safety-specific transformational leadership and occupational safety. *J. Appl. Psychol.* **2002**, *87*, 488–496. [CrossRef] [PubMed]
38. Kelloway, E.; Mullen, J.; Francis, L. Divergent effects of transformational and passive leadership on employee safety. *J. Occup. Health Psychol.* **2006**, *11*, 76–86. [CrossRef] [PubMed]
39. Hoffmeister, K.; Gibbons, A.M.; Johnson, S.K.; Cigularov, K.P.; Chen, P.Y.; Rosecrance, J.C. The differential effects of transformational leadership facets on employee safety. *Saf. Sci.* **2014**, *62*, 68–78. [CrossRef]
40. Mullen, J.; Kelloway, E. Safety leadership: A longitudinal study of the effects of transformational leadership on safety outcomes. *J. Occup. Organ. Psychol.* **2009**, *82*, 253–272. [CrossRef]
41. von Thiele Schwarz, U.; Augustsson, H.; Hasson, H.; Stenfors-Hayes, T. Promoting employee health by integrating health protection, health promotion, and continuous improvement. *J. Occup. Environ. Med.* **2015**, *57*, 217–225. [CrossRef] [PubMed]
42. Hofmann, D.; Morgeson, F.; Gerras, S. Climate as a moderator of the relationship between leader-member exchange and content specific citizenship: Safety climate as an exemplar. *J. Appl. Psychol.* **2003**, *88*, 170–178. [CrossRef] [PubMed]
43. Martínez-Córcoles, M.; Schöbel, M.; Gracia, F.J.; Tomás, I.; Peiró, J.M. Linking empowering leadership to safety participation in nuclear power plants: A structural equation model. *J. Saf. Res.* **2012**, *43*, 215–221. [CrossRef] [PubMed]
44. McLellan, D.L.; Williams, J.A.; Katz, J.N.; Pronk, N.P.; Wagner, G.R.; Caban-Martinez, A.J.; Nelson, C.C.; Sorensen, G. Key organizational characteristics for integrated approaches to protect and promote worker health in smaller enterprises. *J. Occup. Environ. Med* **2017**, *59*, 289–294. [CrossRef] [PubMed]
45. Avolio, B.J.; Gardner, W.L. Authentic leadership development: Getting to the root of positive forms of leadership. *Leadersh. Q.* **2005**, *16*, 315–338. [CrossRef]
46. Uhl-Bien, M. Relational leadership theory: Exploring the social processes of leadership and organizing. *Leadersh. Q.* **2006**, *17*, 654–676. [CrossRef]
47. van Dierendonck, D. Servant leadership: A review and synthesis. *J. Manag.* **2011**, *37*, 1228–1261. [CrossRef]
48. *Dedoose*; Version 7.0.23; Web Application for Managing, Analyzing, and Presenting Qualitative and Mixed Method Research Data; SocioCultural Research Consultants, LLC: Los Angeles, CA, USA, 2016.
49. Saldana, J. *The coding Manual for Qualitative Researchers*, 2nd ed.; Sage Publications Ltd.: Thousand Oaks, CA, USA, 2012.
50. Bolden, R. Distributed leadership in organizations: A review of theory and research. *Int. J. Manag. Rev.* **2011**, *13*, 251–269. [CrossRef]
51. Brown, M.E.; Treviño, L.K. Ethical leadership: A review and future directions. *Leadersh. Q.* **2006**, *17*, 595–616. [CrossRef]

52. Avolio, B.J.; Walumbwa, F.O.; Weber, T.J. Leadership: Current theories, research, and future directions. *Annu. Rev. Psychol.* **2009**, *60*, 421–449. [CrossRef] [PubMed]
53. Huang, Y.H.; Leamon, T.B.; Courtney, T.K.; Chen, P.Y.; DeArmond, S. Corporate financial decision-makers: Perceptions of workplace safety. *Accid. Anal. Prev.* **2007**, *39*, 767–775. [CrossRef] [PubMed]
54. Pescud, M.; Teal, R.; Shilton, T.; Slevin, T.; Ledger, M.; Waterworth, P.; Rosenberg, M. Employers' views on the promotion of workplace health and wellbeing: A qualitative study. *BMC Public Health* **2015**, *15*, 642. [CrossRef] [PubMed]
55. Burke, W.; Litwin, G. A causal model of organizational performance. *J. Manag.* **1992**, *18*, 532–545.
56. Huang, Y.-H.; Robertson, M.M.; Lee, J.; Rineer, J.; Murphy, L.A.; Garabet, A.; Dainoff, M.J. Supervisory interpretation of safety climate versus employee safety climate perception: Association with safety behavior and outcomes for lone workers. *Transp. Res. Part F Traffic Psychol. Behav.* **2014**, *26*, 348–360. [CrossRef]
57. Gittleman, J.L.; Gardner, P.C.; Haile, E.; Sampson, J.M.; Cigularov, K.P.; Ermann, E.D.; Stafford, P.; Chen, P.Y. Citycenter and cosmopolitan construction projects, las vegas, nevada: Lessons learned from the use of multiple sources and mixed methods in a safety needs assessment. *J. Saf. Res.* **2010**, *41*, 263–281. [CrossRef] [PubMed]
58. Punnett, L.; Warren, N.; Henning, R.; Nobrega, S.; Cherniack, M.; CPH-NEW Research Team. Participatory ergonomics as a model for integrated programs to prevent chronic disease. *J. Occup. Environ. Med.* **2013**, *55*, S19–S24. [CrossRef] [PubMed]
59. McLellan, D.L.; Caban-Martinez, A.J.; Nelson, C.C.; Pronk, N.P.; Katz, J.N.; Allen, J.D.; Davis, K.L.; Wagner, G.R.; Sorensen, G. Organizational characteristics influence implementation of worksite health protection and promotion programs. *J. Occup. Environ. Med.* **2015**, *57*, 1009–1016. [CrossRef] [PubMed]
60. Williams, J.A.R.; Nelson, C.C.; Caban-Martinez, A.J.; Katz, J.N.; Wagner, G.R.; Pronk, N.P.; Sorensen, G.; McLellan, D.L. Validation of a new metric for assessing the integration of health protection and health promotion in a sample of small- and medium-sized employer groups. *J. Occup. Environ. Med.* **2015**, *57*, 1017–1021. [CrossRef] [PubMed]

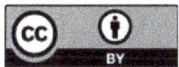

© 2018 by the authors. Licensee MDPI, Basel, Switzerland. This article is an open access article distributed under the terms and conditions of the Creative Commons Attribution (CC BY) license (http://creativecommons.org/licenses/by/4.0/).

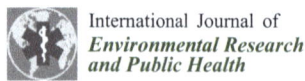

Article

Assessing Workplace Health and Safety Strategies, Trends, and Barriers through a Statewide Worksite Survey

Ami Sedani [1], Derry Stover [2,*], Brian Coyle [2] and Rajvi J. Wani [2]

[1] Department of Biostatistics and Epidemiology, Hudson College of Public Health, University of Oklahoma Health Sciences Center, Oklahoma City, OK 73104, USA
[2] Division of Public Health, Nebraska Department of Health and Human Services, Lincoln, NE 68509, USA
* Correspondence: derry.stover@nebraska.gov

Received: 8 April 2019; Accepted: 9 July 2019; Published: 11 July 2019

Abstract: Chronic diseases have added to the economic burden of the U.S. healthcare system. Most Americans spend most of their waking time at work, thereby, presenting employers with an opportunity to protect and promote health. The purpose of this study was to assess the implementation of workplace health governance and safety strategies among worksites in the State of Nebraska, over time and by industry sector using a randomized survey. Weighted percentages were compared by year, industry sector, and worksite size. Over the three study periods, 4784 responses were collected from worksite representatives. Adoption of workplace health governance and planning strategies increased over time and significantly varied across industry sector groups. Organizational safety policies varied by industry sector and were more commonly reported than workplace health governance and planning strategies. Time constraints were the most common barrier among worksites of all sizes, and stress was reported as the leading employee health issue that negatively impacts business. Results suggest that opportunities exist to integrate workplace health and safety initiatives, especially in blue-collar industry sectors and small businesses.

Keywords: workplace health; wellness; governance; planning; barriers; survey; industry; ACA

1. Introduction

Chronic diseases remain the leading cause of death and disability in the United States, as well as the leading contributor to the nation's healthcare cost [1–3]. More than 150 million Americans are workers with most spending more than half of their waking time at work [4]. Maintaining a healthier workforce can lower direct costs to the business (e.g., insurance premiums and workers' compensation claims) as well as indirect costs (e.g., absenteeism, return on investment, and worker productivity) [5–9]. With changes in the workforce population, chronic health conditions have become a growing concern for employees and businesses [10]. Worksite health and wellness programs offer an important population health strategy to address the increase in chronic diseases [11–13].

While adoption of workplace health programs have increased in the U.S. in recent years, there is still variation in uptake by business size and industries [14–16]. Many workplaces also lack a comprehensive, integrated approach that addresses multiple risk factors and health conditions. Successful worksite health programs are tailored to their employee population, thus making it difficult to evaluate initiatives across multiple businesses. However, all successful programs should be built on a solid foundation. According to the Centers for Disease Control and Prevention (CDC) Workplace Health Model, this foundation requires a basic organizational governance infrastructure to administer and manage health promotion activities [17].

Organizational factors are important for other aspects of worker health, including worker safety and occupational injury and illness prevention [18]. Employers have many opportunities for promoting safety and occupational injury and illness prevention at the organizational level [19]. One example is the Total Worker Health® (TWH) framework, which involves organizational-level strategies aimed at integration of worksite injury prevention and health promotion activities [20]. TWH is defined as policies, programs, and practice that integrate protection from work-related safety and health hazards with promotion of injury and illness prevention efforts to advance worker well-being [21].

While many organizational approaches exist to improve worker health and safety through workplace initiatives, there is a need to better understand the adoption of these initiatives among employers. Findings have the potential to yield useful information when developing public health policies and prevention activities for improving worker health, safety, and well-being. The primary aim of this study is to assess the implementation of workplace health governance and safety strategies among worksites in the largely rural State of Nebraska, over time and by industry sector. Secondary aims include describing employer perception of barriers related to implementing workplace health strategies and employee health issues that negatively impact business. Responses on the Nebraska Worksite Wellness Surveys from 2010, 2013, and 2016 were utilized for the study.

2. Materials and Methods

Three point-in-time surveys were conducted among worksites in Nebraska to test our central hypothesis that the prevalence of reported health promotion and safety strategies did not vary across years or industry sectors. The sample frames for all survey years (2010, 2013, and 2016) were generated from an employer database of establishments provided by the Nebraska Department of Labor. The sample frame data included worksite name, number of employees per worksite, worksite address, and industry code. Establishments were coded and grouped using the 2-digit industry sector according to the North American Industry Classification System (NAICS) ((Health Care and Social Assistance (62); Wholesale and Retail Trade (42, 44–45); Information, Finance, and Management services (51–55); Other Services (56, 71, 72, 81); Education Services (61); Construction (23); Manufacturing (31–33); Public Administration (92); Transportation and Warehousing (48–49); All Other Sectors (11, 21, 22)).

Worksites in the sample frame were defined as establishments with a Nebraska worksite address and 10 or more employees. In order to ensure worksites of all sizes were represented in the survey data, each sample was stratified by business size: Small (10 to 49 employees), medium (50 to 199 employees), and large (200 or more employees). Disproportionate stratification was used to allow for oversampling. All large businesses in the State were included in samples ($N = 503$ in 2010; $N = 523$ in 2013; and $N = 525$ in 2016). For small and medium-sized businesses, random samples were included ($N = 1500$ in 2010 and 2013, and $N = 2010$ in 2016 for both sizes). In 2016, two priority industry sectors with low responses in the 2013 survey, 'Construction' and 'Transportation and Warehousing', were oversampled. The sampling design allowed some businesses being surveyed across all three study periods, but none of the businesses were repeated within the same time period.

The survey questions were developed by the Division of Public Health, Nebraska Department of Health and Human Services (NDHHS) in consultation with the Bureau of Sociological Research (BOSR), University of Nebraska—Lincoln. Questions were adapted from a variety of sources, and a small pilot of the survey instrument was conducted with businesses randomly selected from the sample. Because these were point-in-time surveys, worksites were asked to report current workplace practices (i.e., if they have a specific health promotion policy or program in place) and perceived barriers in each survey year. The majority of questions remained unchanged across survey years to ensure comparability over time. Survey questions pertaining to this study are in Supplementary Materials (Table S1).

The 2010, 2013, and 2016 surveys were mailed to worksites, which included a cover letter, the survey, and a postage-paid envelope. The small and medium size surveys were addressed to the business owner or manager, while the surveys for large businesses were addressed to the human resource representative. For the 2016 survey, we provided an option in 2016 for businesses to visit a website and complete the survey via a web-based questionnaire.

Results were weighted to adjust for the business size differences found between the overall sample frame and the final compilation of businesses who are represented in the completed survey data. A weighting variable was calculated by applying the appropriate sampling weights and then also adjusting for nonresponse by strata [22].

A bivariable analysis was conducted to examine the prevalence of workplace governance and safety strategies among worksites over time, by industry sector and by worksite size. Weighted percentages and confidence limits were calculated. The Rao–Scott χ^2 statistic was used to assess differences according to year and industry sector. Effect modification was assessed by refitting the model multiple times, once for each of the main effects which was generated from the stepwise selection process. Point estimates and 95% confidence limits were calculated for multivariable analysis. The Wald χ^2 statistic was used to compare multivariable models fit to sectors with and without a workplace governance and safety strategies. Significance levels were set at $\alpha < 0.05$. All data analyses were conducted using PROC SURVEYFREQ and PROC LOGISTIC commands in SAS version 9.4 (SAS Institute Inc., Cary, NC, USA).

3. Results

3.1. Survey Responses

A total of 4784 responses were collected in 2010 ($n = 1512$; response rate: 47.4%), 2013 ($n = 1352$; response rate: 42.1%), and 2016 ($n = 1920$; response rate: 38.6%). A total of 4784 responses were collected in 2010 ($n = 1512$; response rate: 47.4%), 2013 ($n = 1352$; response rate: 42.1%), and 2016 ($n = 1920$; response rate: 38.6%). Overall, small and medium worksites were less likely to respond to the survey (response rate 39.2% and 36.3%, respectively) than large worksites (response rate: 47.3%). Over the three study periods, response rates were consistent among medium size worksites but increased among large and small worksites ($p < 0.0001$). The response rate decreased among large worksites from 54.5% in 2010 to 38.1% in 2016. Among small worksites, the response rate decreased from 43.4% in 2010 to 31.0% in 2016 (Table S2).

Table 1 presents the characteristics of participating worksites by size and industry sector grouping over the three study periods (2010, 2013, and 2016). Small (10–49 employees) and medium (50–199 employees) worksites comprised more than three-quarters of the respondents across the years. Specifically, in 2010, the majority (46%) of respondents were medium size worksites, whereas as in 2013 and 2016, the majority of respondents were small worksites (43.1% and 45.9%, respectively). Worksites in the 'Health Care and Social Assistance' industry sector were the most represented sector in all survey years (17–20%), followed by 'Wholesale and Retail Trade' (14–16%) and 'Information, Finance, and Management Services' (13–14%).

3.2. Workplace Health Governance and Planning Strategies

Increases in the weighted percentage of worksites responding "yes" to implementing workplace health governance and planning strategies were observed (Table 2). There were statistically significant differences across years in responses among questions pertaining to having an assigned coordinator for employee health promotion or wellness ($p = 0.04$), having a staff responsible for employee health promotion or wellness ($p = 0.02$), and including funding for health promotion or wellness in the worksite's budget (in the past month) ($p = 0.04$). Among all worksites, all of the six strategies assessed were reported in less than twenty percent of worksites. All of the reported governance and planning strategies assessed significantly varied across industry sectors ($p < 0.001$). The 'Construction' sector reported the lowest adoption of five of the six governance and planning strategies, including having a health promotion or wellness committee (4.4%) and having a coordinator responsible for employee health promotion or wellness (6.2%). Other sectors that reported lower uptake of strategies include

'Other Services', 'Transportation and Warehousing', 'Wholesale and Retail Trade', and 'Health Care and Social Assistance'. Conversely, the 'Educational Services' sector had the highest adoption of strategies, followed by 'Public Administration' and 'Information, Finance, and Management Services'.

Table 1. Participating worksites by size and industry sector by year (2010, 2013, and 2016).

	2010 (n = 1512)		2013 (n = 1352)		2016 (n = 1920)	
	n	(%)	n	(%)	n	(%)
Worksite Size *						
Small (10 to 49 employees)	574	(38.0)	582	(43.1)	881	(45.9)
Medium (50 to 199 employees)	695	(46.0)	510	(37.7)	839	(43.7)
Large (more than 200 employees)	243	(16.1)	260	(19.2)	200	(10.4)
Industry Sector *						
Health Care and Social Assistance	262	(17.3)	260	(19.6)	342	(17.8)
Wholesale and Retail Trade	237	(15.7)	197	(14.8)	269	(14.0)
Information, Finance, and Management Services	189	(12.5)	188	(14.2)	236	(12.3)
Other Services	225	(14.9)	185	(13.9)	219	(11.4)
Educational Services	148	(9.8)	149	(11.2)	183	(9.5)
Construction	92	(6.1)	58	(4.4)	180	(9.4)
Manufacturing	169	(11.2)	141	(10.6)	171	(8.9)
Public Administration	113	(7.5)	80	(6.0)	130	(6.8)
Transportation and Warehousing	42	(2.8)	37	(2.8)	143	(7.5)
All Other Sectors	35	(2.3)	34	(2.6)	47	(2.5)

Note: Unweighted sample. Industry classified and grouped by NAICS 2-digit sector codes: Health Care and Social Assistance (62); Wholesale and Retail Trade (42, 44–45); Information, Finance, and Management Services (51–55); Other Services (56, 71, 72, 81); Education Services (61); Construction (23); Manufacturing (31–33); Public Administration (92); Transportation and Warehousing (48–49); All Other Sectors (11, 21, 22); * statistically significant using chi-square test, $p < 0.0001$.

Table 2. Weighted percentage of worksite responses to implementing workplace health strategies by industry sectors, survey years and worksite sizes.

	Health Promotion Committee *,†	Coordinator Responsible for Employee Health Promotion *,†,‡	Staff Responsible for Employee Health Promotion *,†,‡	Funding for Health Promotion in Budget *,†	Written Objectives for Employee Health *,‡	Stated Mission or Goal Regarding Employee Health *,‡
	% (CI)	% (CI)	% (CI)	% (CI)	% (CI)	% (CI)
Industry Sector						
Wholesale and Retail Trade	12.6 (9.8–15.4)	15.2 (12.1–18.3)	10.9 (8.3–13.5)	10.5 (7.9–13.1)	10.6 (7.9–13.2)	10.3 (7.7–12.9)
All Other Sectors	29.9 (19.8–39.9)	27.4 (17.8–37.1)	22.6 (13.6–31.7)	27.4 (17.8–37.0)	15.1 (8.2–21.9)	11.0 (5.1–16.9)
Construction	6.2 (3.3–9.0)	4.4 (2.3–6.6)	2.6 (1.0–4.2)	5.2 (2.4–8.1)	5.0 (2.3–7.7)	2.9 (0.6–5.1)
Educational Services	64.3 (58.1–70.4)	57.8 (51.5–64.0)	47.5 (41.3–53.8)	19.6 (14.7–24.5)	22.8 (17.8–27.9)	24.0 (18.7–29.3)
Health Care and Social Assistance	16.9 (13.9–20.0)	16.8 (13.7–19.9)	16.3 (13.2–19.3)	12.9 (10.2–15.6)	11.1 (8.6–13.7)	11.2 (8.7–13.8)
Information, Finance, and Management Services	24 (20.0–28.0)	25.2 (21.1–29.3)	18.5 (15.0–22.1)	21.6 (17.8–25.4)	13.4 (10.4–16.4)	13.1 (10.2–16.0)
Manufacturing	21.6 (17.1–26.2)	23.8 (19.1–28.6)	20.7 (16.1–25.4)	19.8 (15.5–24.0)	15 (11.1–19.0)	12.3 (8.8–15.7)
Other Services	7.7 (5.4–10.1)	7.9 (5.5–10.2)	7.4 (5.0–9.7)	5.2 (3.3–7.2)	4.8 (3.0–6.6)	5.4 (3.4–7.4)
Public Administration	26.0 (19.8–32.3)	21.1 (15.4–26.9)	19.5 (13.9–25.2)	21.1 (15.2–27.0)	17.1 (11.6–22.7)	16.4 (11.0–21.9)
Transportation and Warehousing	12.7 (7.7–17.6)	14.9 (9.7–20.1)	11.1 (6.3–15.8)	8.2 (4.4–12.1)	9.5 (5.5–13.5)	8.5 (4.6–12.4)
Year						
2010	16.2 (14.0–18.3)	15.7 (13.6–17.8)	12.6 (10.7–14.5)	11.1 (9.3–12.9)	10.1 (8.3–11.8)	9.2 (7.5–10.9)
2013	20.0 (17.0–22.6)	19.7 (17.2–22.2)	15.7 (13.4–18.0)	13.3 (11.2–15.4)	11.9 (9.9–13.9)	11.3 (9.4–13.2)
2016	21.2 (18.9–23.5)	21.4 (19.2–23.7)	18.5 (16.4–20.7)	15.6 (13.6–17.7)	12.2 (10.5–14.0)	12.1 (10.3–13.9)
Worksite Size						
Small	13.8 (12.2–15.4)	14.3 (12.7–15.9)	11.5 (10.0–13.0)	9.8 (8.4–11.2)	8.2 (6.9–9.5)	7.9 (6.6–9.1)
Medium	33.1 (30.6–35.5)	30.8 (28.4–33.2)	25.9 (23.7–28.2)	21.2 (19.2–23.2)	18.1 (16.2–19.9)	17.3 (15.4–19.2)
Large	65.1 (60.3–69.8)	64.0 (59.0–69.0)	57.2 (52.3–62.0)	53.5 (48.7–58.3)	45.8 (41.1–50.4)	43.5 (38.9–48.1)
Total	19.4 (18.1–20.7)	19.3 (17.9–20.6)	15.9 (14.7–17.1)	13.6 (12.4–14.7)	11.4 (10.4–12.5)	11.0 (10.4–12.5)

Note: Weighted percentage (95% confidence limits); * Significant Differences for Sector, † Significant Differences for Year, ‡ Significant Differences for Size.

3.3. Workplace Health Governance and Planning Strategies: Multivariable Analysis

The adjusted model further illustrated the significant differences in implementation of workplace health strategies between sectors. In 2016, 'Educational Services' were estimated to have the greatest odds of having a coordinator responsible for employee health promotion/wellness (OR = 17.44, 95% CL: 8.85–30.56), health promotion/wellness committee (OR = 23.41, 95% CL: 13.09–41.87), staff responsible for employee health promotion/wellness (OR = 14.01, 95% CL: 8.25–23.81), funding for health promotion/wellness in budget (OR = 3.36, 95% CL: 1.97–5.71), written objectives for employee wellness/health (OR = 3.33, 95% CL: 1.95–5.69), and stated mission or goal regarding improvement or employee health status (OR = 3.32, 95% CL: 1.95–5.68), compared to 'Wholesale and Retail Trade' (Table 3).

Table 3. Multivariable adjusted odds of implementing workplace health strategies stratified by year and industry sector.

Workplace Health Strategy	Industry Sector	2010 Estimate (95% CL)	2013 Estimate (95% CL)	2016 Estimate (95% CL)
Coordinator responsible for employee health promotion/wellness	Wholesale and Retail Trade (Ref)	1.00	1.00	1.00
	All Other Sectors	3.01 (1.29–7.03)	3.33 (1.38–8.07)	1.70 (0.92–3.14)
	Construction	0.09 (0.02–0.38)	0.60 (0.23–1.56)	0.27 (0.12–0.61)
	Educational Services	2.87 (1.69–4.88)	11.16 (6.48–19.25)	17.44 (9.95–30.56)
	Health Care and Social Assistance	1.07 (0.65–1.76)	1.08 (0.62–1.88)	1.12 (0.75–1.66)
	Information, Finance, and Management Services	1.73 (1.08–2.79)	2.07 (1.23–3.51)	1.68 (1.14–2.47)
	Manufacturing	1.40 (0.81–2.44)	2.02 (1.07–3.81)	1.80 (1.10–2.95)
	Other Services	0.22 (0.11–0.45)	0.95 (0.54–1.68)	0.50 (0.30–0.82)
	Public Administration	1.44 (0.80–2.59)	2.23 (1.10–4.52)	1.26 (0.73–2.18)
	Transportation and Warehousing	0.22 (0.04–1.28)	1.31 (0.50–3.44)	1.43 (0.73–2.82)
Health promotion/wellness committee	Wholesale and Retail Trade (Ref)	1.00	1.00	1.00
	All Other Sectors	3.72 (1.58–8.77)	5.38 (2.27–12.76)	2.30 (1.25–4.26)
	Construction	0.36 (0.14–0.92)	0.723 (0.29–1.82)	0.42 (0.20–0.87)
	Educational Services	8.00 (4.65–13.75)	13.68 (7.78–24.03)	23.41 (13.09–41.87)
	Health Care and Social Assistance	1.51 (0.89–2.58)	1.21 (0.68–2.14)	1.40 (0.93–2.10)
	Information, Finance, and Management Services	2.00 (1.19–3.38)	2.17 (1.26–3.73)	2.17 (1.46–3.25)
	Manufacturing	1.55 (0.84–2.85)	2.16 (1.13–4.15)	2.02 (1.21–3.37)
	Other Services	0.37 (0.19–0.75)	0.94 (0.52–1.71)	0.60 (0.36–1.00)
	Public Administration	2.57 (1.43–4.61)	3.77 (1.92–7.38)	1.89 (1.10–3.25)
	Transportation and Warehousing	0.44 (0.10–2.01)	1.48 (0.56–3.92)	1.16 (0.54–2.48)
Staff responsible for employee health promotion/wellness	Wholesale and Retail Trade (Ref)	1.00	1.00	1.00
	All Other Sectors	4.14 (1.73–9.87)	2.82 (1.04–7.65)	1.93 (0.991–3.757)
	Construction	0.08 (0.01–0.55)	0.42 (0.12–1.50)	0.24 (0.09–0.632)
	Educational Services	3.52 (1.96–6.33)	9.04 (5.06–16.16)	14.01 (8.25–23.81)
	Health Care and Social Assistance	1.78 (1.03–3.06)	1.50 (0.82–2.73)	1.44 (0.94–2.20)
	Information, Finance, and Management Services	1.87 (1.07–3.25)	1.52 (0.82–2.83)	1.86 (1.22–2.85)
	Manufacturing	1.62 (0.86–3.04)	2.88 (1.47–5.64)	2.09 (1.23–3.54)
	Other Services	0.22 (0.09–0.54)	1.13 (0.60–2.13)	0.78 (0.48–1.30)
	Public Administration	2.16 (1.14–4.09)	2.79 (1.32–5.89)	1.61 (0.90–2.87)
	Transportation and Warehousing	0.15 (0.01–2.07)	1.70 (0.62–4.71)	1.25 (0.57–2.73)
Funding for health promotion/wellness in budget	Wholesale and Retail Trade (Ref)	1.00	1.00	1.00
	All Other Sectors	6.03 (2.51–14.52)	6.56 (2.66–16.16)	2.18 (1.12–4.25)
	Construction	0.36 (0.13–1.02)	1.20 (0.51–2.86)	0.26 (0.10–0.67)
	Educational Services	0.94 (0.41–2.12)	2.36 (1.24–4.49)	3.36 (1.97–5.71)
	Health Care and Social Assistance	1.56 (0.87–2.79)	0.91 (0.48–1.73)	1.19 (0.76–1.85)
	Information, Finance, and Management Services	2.76 (1.59–4.80)	1.92 (1.07–3.47)	2.31 (1.51–3.54)
	Manufacturing	1.86 (0.98–3.53)	3.13 (1.63–6.02)	1.55 (0.88–2.74)
	Other Services	0.27 (0.12–0.64)	0.69 (0.35–1.37)	0.50 (0.28–0.88)
	Public Administration	1.93 (0.98–3.80)	3.29 (1.60–6.77)	2.30 (1.32–4.02)
	Transportation and Warehousing	0.05 (<0.001–5.29)	0.94 (0.29–3.12)	1.05 (0.46–2.41)
Written objectives for employee wellness/health	Wholesale and Retail Trade (Ref)	1.00	1.00	1.00
	All Other Sectors	3.21 (1.28–8.04)	5.32 (2.11–13.43)	0.39 (0.12–1.25)
	Construction	0.19 (0.05–0.72)	1.43 (0.62–3.34)	0.28 (0.11–0.70)
	Educational Services	1.83 (0.93–3.61)	3.06 (1.64–5.73)	3.33 (1.95–5.69)
	Health Care and Social Assistance	1.31 (0.73–2.37)	0.73 (0.36–1.46)	1.05 (0.67–1.65)
	Information, Finance, and Management Services	1.47 (0.82–2.63)	1.27 (0.67–2.42)	1.17 (0.73–1.86)
	Manufacturing	1.23 (0.62–2.433)	1.94 (0.94–3.99)	1.36 (0.76–2.44)
	Other Services	0.24 (0.10–0.58)	0.93 (0.482–1.80)	0.34 (0.18–0.65)
	Public Administration	2.17 (1.12–4.19)	2.13 (0.97–4.69)	1.52 (0.83–2.77)
	Transportation and Warehousing	0.59 (0.14–2.53)	0.94 (0.27–3.23)	1.07 (0.47–2.45)
Stated mission or goal regarding improvement or employee health status	Wholesale and Retail Trade (Ref)	1.00	1.00	1.00
	All Other Sectors	1.56 (0.50–4.84)	3.52 (1.33–9.35)	0.47 (0.16–1.38)
	Construction	0.17 (0.04–0.70)	0.97 (0.37–2.50)	0.08 (0.01–0.40)
	Educational Services	2.35 (1.23–4.46)	2.95 (1.58–5.51)	3.32 (1.95–5.68)
	Health Care and Social Assistance	1.37 (0.76–2.48)	0.96 (0.50–1.83)	0.98 (0.61–1.56)
	Information, Finance, and Management Services	1.19 (0.64–2.20)	1.24 (0.65–2.37)	1.34 (0.84–2.13)
	Manufacturing	0.93 (0.44–1.95)	1.54 (0.72–3.30)	1.21 (0.66–2.23)
	Other Services	0.25 (0.10–0.59)	0.77 (0.39–1.53)	0.59 (0.34–1.03)
	Public Administration	1.73 (0.87–3.43)	2.41 (1.12–5.19)	1.47 (0.80–2.71)
	Transportation and Warehousing	0.32 (0.05–2.15)	0.88 (0.25–3.08)	1.13 (0.49–2.61)

3.4. Workplace Safety Policies

Table 4 represents the weighted proportion of worksites by industry sector that reported implementing workplace safety policies for survey years 2013 and 2016 (questions not asked in 2010). Among all industries, the most commonly reported safety policies were having a worksite safety committee (62.5%), requiring seatbelts while driving (61.5%), and having a return to work program (55.5%). Significant variation in reported safety policies across industry sectors was found among all policies assessed ($p < 0.001$). Both 'Construction' and 'Transportation and Warehousing' sectors reported the highest adoption of policies related to seatbelt use and restrictions on cell phone use and texting. Sectors reporting the highest adoption of a worksite safety committee were 'Manufacturing', 'Construction', and 'Educational Services'. Generally, lower adoption of safety policies were reported among the sectors 'Information, Finance, and Management Services', 'Health Care and Social Assistance', 'Wholesale and Retail Trade', and those classified as 'Other Services'.

Table 4. Weighted percentage of worksites that responded "Yes" to implementing workplace safety policies, by industry sectors, survey years, and worksite sizes.

	Require Seatbelts While Driving *,‡	Require Refrain from Talking on Cell Phone While Driving *,†,‡	Require Refrain from Texting While Driving *,‡	Promotes Off-The-Job Safety for Employee and Family *,‡	Return to Work Program *,‡	Worksite Safety Committee *,‡
	% (CI)	% (CI)	% (CI)	% (CI)	% (CI)	% (CI)
Industry Sector						
Wholesale and Retail Trade	67.7 (62.4–73.0)	54.5 (48.9–60.1)	60.5 (55.0–66.0)	28.8 (23.8–33.9)	59.2 (53.6–64.8)	62.7 (57.2–68.2)
All Other Sectors	76.0 (64.0–87.9)	65.1 (51.9–78.4)	66.7 (79.8–79.8)	36.5 (23.8–49.2)	68.1 (55.2–81.0)	75.5 (63.7–87.3)
Construction	91.6 (88.0–95.2)	69.9 (63.4–76.4)	82.2 (77.0–87.3)	45.3 (38.2–52.3)	73.1 (66.7–79.5)	84.6 (79.4–89.8)
Educational Services	71.8 (64.5–79.0)	63.2 (55.8–70.6)	66.7 (59.5–73.9)	42.8 (35.2–50.4)	46.6 (39.0–54.3)	83.1 (77.2–89.0)
Health Care and Social Assistance	51.6 (46.2–57.1)	46.2 (40.8–51.6)	47.6 (42.2–52.9)	33.2 (28.2–38.2)	53.6 (48.2–59.1)	60.6 (55.2–66.1)
Information, Finance, and Management Services	45.1 (39.0–51.1)	36.6 (30.8–42.4)	41.1 (35.1–47.0)	19.0 (14.5–23.4)	42.1 (36.1–48.1)	48.2 (42.1–54.3)
Manufacturing	74.0 (66.5–81.5)	61.6 (53.5–69.6)	64.1 (56.2–72.1)	41.4 (33.6–49.2)	72.6 (64.7–80.6)	90.4 (84.9–95.9)
Other Services	45.2 (39.3–51.1)	37.5 (31.8–43.2)	39.6 (33.9–45.3)	25.8 (20.7–30.9)	48.3 (42.4–54.1)	40.7 (35.0–46.4)
Public Administration	73.8 (65.2–82.3)	48.4 (39.0–57.8)	50.2 (40.7–59.6)	33.4 (24.6–42.1)	55.8 (46.4–65.3)	74.3 (65.5–83.1)
Transportation and Warehousing	91.5 (86.8–96.3)	88.0 (82.8–93.3)	89.4 (84.4–94.4)	49.8 (40.6–59.0)	77.8 (70.8–84.7)	66.7 (57.8–75.6)
By Year						
2010	56.9 (53.7–60.2)	41.7 (38.5–44.9)	-	-	-	-
2013	61.3 (58.0–64.7)	50.3 (46.9–53.7)	54.4 (51.0–57.9)	30.7 (27.6–33.8)	55.7 (52.3–59.2)	63.0 (59.7–66.4)
2016	61.9 (58.9–64.9)	51.2 (48.3–54.2)	54.7 (51.7–57.7)	32.5 (29.8–35.2)	55.2 (52.2–58.2)	62.1 (59.1–65.1)
Worksite Size						
Small	56.9 (54.6–59.2)	45.0 (42.7–47.2)	51.8 (49.1–54.5)	28.5 (26.1–30.9)	51.1 (48.4–53.9)	57.2 (54.5–59.9)
Medium	69.8 (67.2–72.4)	57.1 (54.4–59.9)	66.2 (63.7–68.8)	42.5 (39.8–45.3)	72.7 (70.2–75.1)	84.6 (82.6–86.5)
Large	78.0 (74.6–81.4)	62.4 (57.9–66.9)	68.3 (63.9–72.8)	61.2 (56.5–65.9)	80.4 (76.6–84.3)	89.5 (86.5–92.5)
Total	61.5 (59.3–63.8)	50.8 (48.6–53.1)	54.6 (52.4–56.9)	31.8 (29.7–33.8)	55.5 (53.2–57.8)	62.5 (60.2–64.7)

Note: Weighted percentage (95% Confidence limits); * Significant Differences for Sector, † Significant Differences for Year, ‡ Significant Differences for Size.

3.5. Workplace Safety Policies: Multivariable Analysis

The adjusted model showed that sites in the 'Information, Finance, and Management' sector were significantly least likely to have policies that require seatbelts while driving, promote off the job safety for employee and family, and have a return to work program for both years that these questions were asked (2013, 2016). Sites in 'Construction' were most likely to require seatbelts while driving in 2013 and 2016, and in 2013 they were most likely to require refraining from texting while driving. In 2013, sites in 'Manufacturing' were 7.88 times more likely to have a worksite safety committee than sites in 'Wholesale and Retail Trade' (95% CL: 2.94–21.11). In 2016, worksites in 'Manufacturing' were only 3.93 times more likely to have a worksite safety committee than sites in 'Wholesale and Retail Trade' (95% CL: 1.93–8.00) (Table 5).

Table 5. Multivariable regression model of implementing workplace safety policies by sector, stratified by year and industry sector.

Workplace Safety Policy	Industry Sector	2013 Estimate (95% CL)	2016 Estimate (95% CL)
Require seatbelts while driving	Wholesale and Retail Trade (Ref)	1.00	1.00
	All Other Sectors	1.58 (0.51–4.96)	1.84 (0.781–4.34)
	Construction	29.49 (2.18–398.55)	3.07 (1.50–6.24)
	Educational Services	1.08 (0.59–1.98)	0.88 (0.50–1.56)
	Health Care and Social Assistance	0.36 (0.23–0.58)	0.42 (0.29–0.61)
	Information, Finance, and Management Services	0.33 (0.20–0.53)	0.23 (0.16–0.34)
	Manufacturing	1.26 (0.62–2.55)	1.518 (0.8–2.88)
	Other Services	0.35 (0.22–0.56)	0.47 (0.31–0.70)
	Public Administration	0.84 (0.41–1.73)	1.23 (0.67–2.24)
	Transportation and Warehousing	4.98 (1.11–22.43)	2.71 (1.04–7.03)
Require refrain from talking on cell phone while driving	Wholesale and Retail Trade (Ref)	1.00	1.00
	All Other Sectors	2.20 (0.83–5.79)	1.632 (0.842–3.162)
	Construction	2.26 (1.14–4.48)	1.395 (0.888–2.191)
	Educational Services	1.67 (0.97–2.89)	1.502 (0.892–2.529)
	Health Care and Social Assistance	0.63 (0.41–0.97)	0.745 (0.531–1.046)
	Information, Finance, and Management Services	0.54 (0.35–0.84)	0.328 (0.23–0.469)
	Manufacturing	1.12 (0.64–1.97)	1.36 (0.83–2.23)
	Other Services	0.54 (0.35–0.84)	0.62 (0.43–0.88)
	Public Administration	0.65 (0.35–1.20)	0.70 (0.44–1.13)
	Transportation and Warehousing	8.34 (2.22–31.32)	4.69 (1.95–11.26)
Require refrain from texting while driving	Wholesale and Retail Trade (Ref)	1.00	1.00
	All Other Sectors	2.29 (0.74–7.10)	1.26 (0.65–2.45)
	Construction	8.07 (2.37–27.46)	1.91 (1.15–3.18)
	Educational Services	1.11 (0.64–1.94)	1.46 (0.85–2.52)
	Health Care and Social Assistance	0.39 (0.25–0.60)	0.65 (0.46–0.92)
	Information, Finance, and Management Services	0.44 (0.28–0.69)	0.31 (0.22–0.44)
	Manufacturing	0.67 (0.38–1.19)	1.40 (0.83–2.35)
	Other Services	0.40 (0.25–0.62)	0.55 (0.38–0.79)
	Public Administration	0.38 (0.20–0.70)	0.65 (0.40–1.06)
	Transportation and Warehousing	5.76 (1.46–22.70)	4.58 (1.78–11.77)
Promotes off-the-job safety for employee and family	Wholesale and Retail Trade (Ref)	1.00	1.00
	All Other Sectors	1.89 (0.85–4.24)	1.39 (0.77–2.53)
	Construction	2.20 (1.22–3.96)	1.96 (1.28–3.00)
	Educational Services	1.58 (0.97–2.56)	2.14 (1.34–3.42)
	Health Care and Social Assistance	1.08 (0.712–1.63)	1.06 (0.76–1.48)
	Information, Finance, and Management Services	0.44 (0.27–0.73)	0.54 (0.37–0.79)
	Manufacturing	1.72 (1.01–2.92)	1.62 (1.02–2.55)
	Other Services	0.83 (0.53–1.28)	1.03 (0.72–1.49)
	Public Administration	0.93 (0.50–1.74)	1.37 (0.85–2.21)
	Transportation and Warehousing	2.87 (1.39–5.92)	2.15 (1.20–3.86)
Return to work program	Wholesale and Retail Trade (Ref)	1.00	1.00
	All Other Sectors	2.58 (0.88–7.60)	4.09 (1.50–11.16)
	Construction	3.24 (1.55–6.78)	1.23 (0.77–1.98)
	Educational Services	0.65 (0.40–1.06)	0.61 (0.37–1.01)
	Health Care and Social Assistance	1.07 (0.70–1.61)	0.53 (0.37–0.74)
	Information, Finance, and Management Services	0.56 (0.37–0.85)	0.43 (0.30–0.63)
	Manufacturing	3.27 (1.67–6.41)	1.29 (0.76–2.19)
	Other Services	0.95 (0.63–1.43)	0.56 (0.39–0.81)
	Public Administration	1.24 (0.66–2.32)	0.64 (0.39–1.04)
	Transportation and Warehousing	4.46 (1.62–12.30)	1.68 (0.82–3.46)
Worksite safety committee	Wholesale and Retail Trade (Ref)	1.00	1.00
	All Other Sectors	1.31 (0.54–3.19)	2.23 (1.04–4.72)
	Construction	2.54 (1.22–5.30)	2.61 (1.48–4.59)
	Educational Services	3.21 (1.71–6.04)	2.39 (1.28–4.50)
	Health Care and Social Assistance	0.68 (0.45–1.03)	0.73 (0.52–1.03)
	Information, Finance, and Management Services	0.60 (0.39–0.92)	0.38 (0.27–0.55)
	Manufacturing	7.88 (2.9–21.11)	3.93 (1.93–8.00)
	Other Services	0.36 (0.24–0.53)	0.36 (0.25–0.51)
	Public Administration	1.86 (0.91–3.78)	1.29 (0.76–2.18)
	Transportation and Warehousing	1.10 (0.50–2.41)	1.17 (0.61–2.26)

3.6. Negative Impacts of Employee Health Issues

Figure 1 represents the weighted percentage of worksites that indicated specific employee health issues having a negative impact on business in 2016. Among health issues which employers noted as "very severely", "severely", or "moderately" having a negative impact on the worksite, stress (53%) was listed as the top issue. Obesity (34%) and lack of physical activity/exercise/fitness (33%) were the second and third most frequently cited health issues that negatively impacted business. When results were restricted to health issues that "very severely" impacted the worksite, injuries at the worksite (5%) was the most frequent health issue reported, followed by stress (4%) and alcohol/other drug habits (4%).

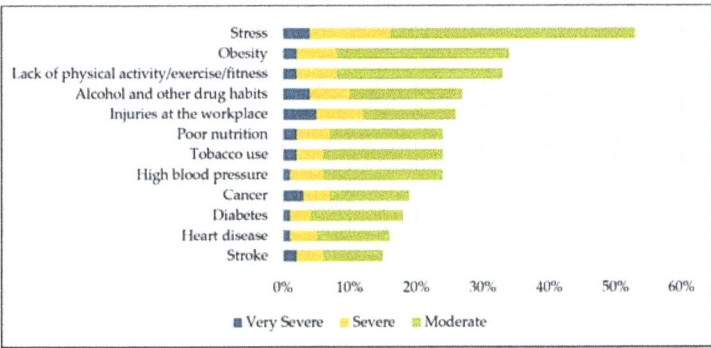

Figure 1. Percentage of Nebraska worksites that reported selected employee health issues negatively impacted business, 2016.

3.7. Barriers in Implementing Workplace Health and Wellness Strategies

Worksites indicated perceived barriers to implementing workplace health and wellness programs and policies (Figure 2). Differences in barriers were examined based on worksite size. Time constraints were the most reported barrier, regardless of worksite size. In 2016, more than half of all worksites reported time constraints as a barrier, which was lowest in small worksites (49%). Large worksites were least likely to identify staff to organize worksite health and wellness as a barrier (4%), while small worksites were least likely to identify lack of management support as a barrier (18%). More than half of large worksites reported lack of participation by high-risk employees as a barrier (56%), which was comparably lower than for small businesses (30%).

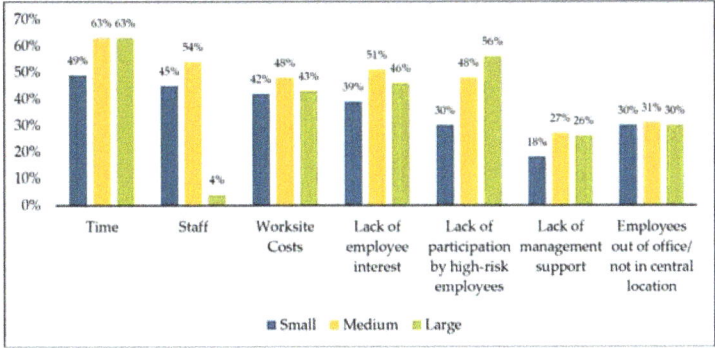

Figure 2. Weighted percentage of Nebraska worksites that indicated the following as barriers to implementing worksite health and wellness programs by worksite size, 2016.

4. Discussion

Due to the growing burden of chronic diseases on employee health and well-being, coupled with the cost of health care coverage, businesses are adopting a wide variety of workplace health promotion initiatives. A comprehensive workplace health program consists of essential components such as: Health education, supportive physical and social environments, integration of the worksite program into the organization's structure, linkage to related programs, and worksite screening programs [17,23]. At the same time, occupational health regulatory requirements compel employers to adopt employee safety policies aimed at injury and illness prevention. Studies highlight the important role of organizational capacity and workplace policies in the prevention of injury, illness, and chronic disease [18,24–26]. This study sought to learn more about the implementation of workplace health governance and planning strategies and organizational safety policies among employers in a largely rural state through a worksite survey.

When compared across survey years, we found an increase in the implementation of all the six workplace health planning and governance strategies measured. The comprehensive U.S. health care reform law was enacted in March 2010, which happened to be during the first year of our study. The Prevention and Public Health Fund (PPHF), under the ACA, includes a provision for creating employer-based wellness programs [11,27]. Peer-reviewed research on the effectiveness of the ACA's employer-based wellness programs is limited [28]. While we did not directly assess impact of the ACA's wellness incentives, the results of our study suggest an increase over time in the implementation of workplace health governance and planning strategies.

When results were combined over multiple study periods, we found adoption of workplace health governance and planning strategies among all worksites was relatively low (less than 20%) and varied widely across industry sectors. Higher adoption found in the 'Educational Services' sector was consistent with Hannon et al. who assessed workplace health capacity among mid-sized employers [29]. Comparably low implementation of governance and planning strategies was found among 'Other Services', 'Construction', and 'Transportation and Warehousing' industries. Studies have shown participation and availability of workplace health initiatives are generally lower among workers in blue-collar and low-wage industries [18,30,31].

Overall, the presence of selected organizational safety policies was higher than governance and planning strategies, a result consistent with similar studies [18,32]. The observed higher adoption of policies related to seatbelt use and cell phone/texting while driving in the 'Construction' and 'Transportation and Warehousing' sectors was expected considering these workers are more likely to engage in work-related travel. Among all worksites, 62.5% reported having a worksite safety committee, a similar result found in a survey among small businesses by McLellan et al. [18]. The presence of a safety committee and a return to work program was lower than expected in some sectors. For example, less than two-thirds of worksites in the 'Health Care and Social Assistance' sector reported having safety committees and return to work programs, despite the fact that these workers experience significant risk for occupational injuries [33].

The discordance between the adoption of governance, planning, and safety strategies and policies highlights the opportunity for integrating prevention programs at the organizational level and within specific sectors. Workers, especially in labor-intensive and blue-collar industries, face unique behavioral and occupational hazards and outcomes as evidenced by data from health behavior surveys and occupational injury surveillance [34–39]. For example, truck driving workers face environmental factors that both influence unhealthy eating patterns and excess weight gain and result in higher risks of occupational injuries and illnesses [40–42]. The combined health hazards and risks make workers in blue-collar worksites prime candidates for comprehensive programs which integrate injury prevention, employee safety, and worker well-being initiatives.

One approach for integrating health protection with health promotion is the TWH framework. Research supports the potential of integrated workplace approaches to improve worker health, safety, and well-being by addressing overlapping risk factors [43–45]. While evaluating the impacts of TWH framework is an emerging field, several studies have shown that TWH interventions can effectively address injuries and chronic diseases in specific worker populations [46–50]. While the current study did not evaluate specific integrated TWH interventions or programs, in our 2016 survey we found that only 15.6% of worksites reported a coordinated program for occupational health and safety with health promotion (data not shown).

Our findings on the impact of employer's perceived health issues demonstrate a business case for TWH approaches. We found stress, obesity, physical activity, alcohol/drug use, and workplace injuries were the top five employee health issues reported by worksites which negatively affect business. These results highlight the complex and interconnected worker health dynamic which could be addressed with an integrated approach. Worksite stress, for example, is associated with negative health outcomes such as increased risk of cardiovascular disease and metabolic syndrome [51,52]. Evidence also supports the relationship between workplace injuries and chronic disease [36,53–55].

Our results regarding barriers suggest challenges in implementing workplace health initiatives can be attributed to both the employers and the employees, similar to other studies [14,25]. More than half of businesses stated that time constraints were a barrier to successful workplace health and wellness at their worksite. For these worksites, having a coordinator who is responsible for employee health promotion or a health promotion/wellness committee could help to provide a platform for employee engagement and collaboration to drive effective worksite health planning and implementation efforts.

Generally, small worksites were less likely to report barriers; no barrier was reported higher than 50% among small worksites. Worksite costs and time barriers were less likely to be reported among small worksites, which was a similar result in a survey among Australian workplaces [56]. There are many opportunities for workplace health and wellness programs in small businesses to be successful and well-accepted among employees. For example, the process of implementing new initiatives is comparatively less bureaucratic and easier to implement, a greater proportion of employees' preferences may be incorporated, and employees may have greater personal accountability [14].

There were several limitations to this study. Given the self-report nature of the worksite survey, this study was susceptible to selection bias. Large worksites were more likely to complete the survey compared to small and medium sized worksites, and these large worksites may be more likely to have certain workplace health or safety initiatives. Furthermore, nonresponse rates increased over time among large and small businesses which was unexplained. This nonresponse increase could account for the significant increase in trends observed in Table 2. To mitigate selection bias, reminders were sent to potential respondents during all three years of survey collection. Weighting was also performed to adjust for the effect of nonresponses across worksite size (Table S3).

The relationship between worksite size and industry sector should be considered when interpreting the results. Generally, certain industries like 'Construction' tend to be smaller establishments while industries such as 'Manufacturing' tend to be larger. This association held true between worksite size and industry sector in our sample ($p < 0.0001$) (Table S4). Additionally, surveys were addressed to either the business owner, manager, or human resource representative, but the worksite information collected may result in misclassification if the representative was not the most appropriate respondent. Lastly, the data represents the views of a single worksite, thus caution is warranted when interpreting our results since evidence suggests that employees' perceptions may vary from employers' [57].

Despite these limitations, the findings can be used to guide recommendations for future workplace health and safety promotion research and practice. To our knowledge, this is the first study to describe the adoption and trends of specific workplace health governance and planning strategies using multiple point-in-time surveys. The data also fill a critical gap which no recent, publicly available, and existing data on workplace health governance and planning strategies and organizational safety policies by detailed industry sector. Lastly, our study had a relatively large sample size, especially for just one state.

The scope of this study did not allow for assessing the employee utilization of workplace health programs, thus observational studies are needed to verify the validity of these survey results. Furthermore, employee outcome data as well as employees' perspectives need to be taken into consideration. While disparities in uptake of workplace health initiatives have been observed in this study as well as others, further research is needed to examine how to better engage high risk and underserved worker populations [14,30]. The majority of small businesses in Nebraska are in rural settings; therefore, a follow-up study on the urban and rural differences in the adoption of workplace health and safety strategies is warranted.

5. Conclusions

Results of this multi-year worksite survey show progress in workplace health initiatives among businesses in Nebraska. Our findings support the need for targeted approaches to building organizational capacity for comprehensive, integrated workplace health and safety programs in industries most impacted by chronic diseases and workplace injuries. The opportunity to advance worker health, safety, and well-being using TWH strategies is greater in blue-collar industries where adoption of governance and planning strategies were low. Public health practitioners should focus on how businesses can address the most common barriers to implementation relative to business size. Targeting promotion of workplace health programs in small business may be fruitful as they may face fewer obstacles.

Supplementary Materials: The following are available online at http://www.mdpi.com/1660-4601/16/14/2475/s1, Table S1: Survey questions on workplace health governance, planning, and safety policies., Table S2. Worksite sizes related to response rates., Table S3. Testing responses of worksites associated over time with nonresponse., Table S4. Industry sector by worksite size among respondents.

Author Contributions: Conceptualization, A.S., D.S. and R.W.; Methodology, R.W, A.S and D.S.; Software, D.S. and A.S.; Validation, D.S. and B.C.; Formal Analysis, D.S. and A.S.; Investigation, B.C.; Resources, B.C.; Data Curation, A.S, D.S. and B.C.; Writing—Original Draft Preparation, D.S., A.S. and R.W.; Writing—Review & Editing, D.S., A.S. and R.W.; Supervision, R.W.; Project Administration, D.S.; Funding Acquisition, D.S., A.S. and B.C.

Funding: This project was supported by Cooperative Agreement Numbers 2B01OT00936, NU58DP004819, and 5U60OH010897, funded by the Centers for Disease Control and Prevention, as well as by the Nebraska Department of Health and Human Services, Tobacco Free Nebraska Program as a result of the Tobacco Master Settlement Agreement. Its contents are solely the responsibility of the authors and do not necessarily represent the official views of the Centers for Disease Control and Prevention, the Department of Health and Human Services, or the Nebraska Department of Health and Human Services.

Acknowledgments: We would like to thank the Nebraska Department Labor for their assistance in identifying sample frame information. We also thank the Bureau of Sociological Research (BOSR), University of Nebraska—Lincoln for their contributions to survey design, collection, weighting, and data management.

Conflicts of Interest: The authors declare no conflict of interest.

References

1. Kochanek, K.D.; Murphy, S.L.; Xu, J. Deaths: Final data for 2011. *Natl. Vital Stat. Rep.* **2015**, *63*, 1–120. [PubMed]
2. Gerteis, J.; Izrael, D.; LeRoy, L.; Deitz, D.; Ricciardi, R.; Miller, T.; Basu, J. *Multiple Chronic Conditions Chartbook*; Agency for Healthcare Research and Quality: Rockville, MD, USA, 2014.
3. National Center for Chronic Disease Prevention and Health Promotion. The Power of Prevention: Chronic Disease ... the Public Health Challenge of the 21st Century 2009. Available online: https://www.cdc.gov/chronicdisease/pdf/2009-Power-of-Prevention.pdf (accessed on 19 January 2019).
4. U.S. Bureau of Labor Statistics. Current Population Survey: Labor Force Statistics. Available online: https://data.bls.gov/timeseries/LNS12000000 (accessed on 4 April 2019).
5. Aldana, S.G. Financial impact of health promotion programs: A comprehensive review of the literature. *Am. J. Health Promot. AJHP* **2001**, *15*, 296–320. [CrossRef] [PubMed]
6. Soler, R.E.; Leeks, K.D.; Razi, S.; Hopkins, D.P.; Griffith, M.; Aten, A.; Chattopadhyay, S.K.; Smith, S.C.; Habarta, N.; Goetzel, R.Z.; et al. A systematic review of selected interventions for worksite health promotion. The assessment of health risks with feedback. *Am. J. Prev. Med.* **2010**, *38*, S237–S262. [CrossRef] [PubMed]
7. Baicker, K.; Cutler, D.; Song, Z. Workplace wellness programs can generate savings. *Health Aff. Proj. Hope* **2010**, *29*, 304–311. [CrossRef] [PubMed]

8. Goetzel, R.Z.; Ozminkowski, R.J. The health and cost benefits of work site health-promotion programs. *Annu. Rev. Public Health* **2008**, *29*, 303–323. [CrossRef] [PubMed]
9. Pelletier, K.R. A review and analysis of the clinical and cost-effectiveness studies of comprehensive health promotion and disease management programs at the worksite: update VIII 2008 to 2010. *J. Occup. Environ. Med.* **2011**, *53*, 1310–1331. [CrossRef] [PubMed]
10. Ortman, J.; Velkoff, V.; Hogan, H. *An Aging Nation: The Older Population in the United States*; Current Population Reports; U.S. Census Bureau: Washington, DC, USA, 2014; p. 28.
11. Anderko, L.; Roffenbender, J.S.; Goetzel, R.Z.; Howard, J.; Millard, F.; Wildenhaus, K.; Desantis, C.; Novelli, W. Promoting prevention through the affordable care act: Workplace wellness. *Prev. Chronic. Dis.* **2012**, *9*, E175. [CrossRef] [PubMed]
12. Goetzel, R.Z.; Pei, X.; Tabrizi, M.J.; Henke, R.M.; Kowlessar, N.; Nelson, C.F.; Metz, R.D. Ten modifiable health risk factors are linked to more than one-fifth of employer-employee health care spending. *Health Aff. Proj. Hope* **2012**, *31*, 2474–2484. [CrossRef]
13. Koh, H.K.; Sebelius, K.G. Promoting prevention through the Affordable Care Act. *N. Engl. J. Med.* **2010**, *363*, 1296–1299. [CrossRef]
14. McCoy, K.; Stinson, K.; Scott, K.; Tenney, L.; Newman, L.S. Health promotion in small business: A systematic review of factors influencing adoption and effectiveness of worksite wellness programs. *J. Occup. Environ. Med.* **2014**, *56*, 579–587. [CrossRef]
15. Mattke, S.; Liu, H.H.; Caloyeras, J.P.; Huang, C.Y.; Van Busum, K.R.; Khodyakov, D.; Shier, V. *Workplace Wellness Programs Study: Final Report*; RAND Corporation: Santa Monica, CA, USA, 2013.
16. Goetzel, R.Z.; Henke, R.M.; Tabrizi, M.; Pelletier, K.R.; Loeppke, R.; Ballard, D.W.; Grossmeier, J.; Anderson, D.R.; Yach, D.; Kelly, R.K.; et al. Do workplace health promotion (wellness) programs work? *J. Occup. Environ. Med.* **2014**, *56*, 927–934. [CrossRef] [PubMed]
17. Centers for Disease Control and Prevention. Workplace Health Promotion: Planning/Workplace Governance. Available online: https://www.cdc.gov/workplacehealthpromotion/planning/index.html (accessed on 30 January 2019).
18. McLellan, D.L.; Cabán-Martinez, A.J.; Nelson, C.C.; Pronk, N.P.; Katz, J.N.; Allen, J.D.; Davis, K.L.; Wagner, G.R.; Sorensen, G. Organizational characteristics influence implementation of worksite health protection and promotion programs: Evidence from smaller businesses. *J. Occup. Environ. Med. Am. Coll. Occup. Environ. Med.* **2015**, *57*, 1009–1016. [CrossRef] [PubMed]
19. Centers for Disease Control and Prevention. *CDC Worksite Health ScoreCard Manual: An Assessment Tool to Promote Employee Health and Well-Being*; U.S. Department of Health and Human Services: Atlanta, GA, USA, 2019.
20. Tamers, S.L.; Chosewood, L.C.; Childress, A.; Hudson, H.; Nigam, J.; Chang, C.-C. Total worker health 2014–2018: The novel approach to worker safety, health, and well-being evolves. *Int. J. Environ. Res. Public. Health* **2019**, *16*, E321. [CrossRef] [PubMed]
21. NIOSH. *Fundamentals of Total Worker Health Approaches: Essential Elements for Advancing Worker Safety, Health, and Well-Being*; U.S. Department of Health and Human Services, Public Health Service, Centers for Disease Control and Prevention, National Institute for Occupational Safety and Health: Cincinnati, OH, USA, 2016.
22. Kish, L. Weighting for unequal pi. *J. Off. Stat.* **1992**, 183–200.
23. Pronk, N. Best practice design principles of worksite health and wellness programs. *ACSMs Health Fit. J.* **2014**, *18*, 42–46. [CrossRef]
24. Payne, J.; Cluff, L.; Lang, J.; Matson-Koffman, D.; Morgan-Lopez, A. Elements of a workplace culture of health, perceived organizational support for health, and lifestyle risk. *Am. J. Health Promot. AJHP* **2018**, *32*, 1555–1567. [CrossRef]
25. Linnan, L.; Bowling, M.; Childress, J.; Lindsay, G.; Blakey, C.; Pronk, S.; Wieker, S.; Royall, P. Results of the 2004 national worksite health promotion survey. *Am. J. Public Health* **2008**, *98*, 1503–1509. [CrossRef]
26. Cooklin, A.; Joss, N.; Husser, E.; Oldenburg, B. Integrated approaches to occupational health and safety: A systematic review. *Am. J. Health Promot. AJHP* **2017**, *31*, 401–412. [CrossRef]
27. Haberkorn, J. Health policy brief: The prevention and public health fund. *Health Aff. (Millwood)* **2012**. [CrossRef]
28. Chait, N.; Glied, S. Promoting prevention under the affordable care act. *Annu. Rev. Public Health* **2018**, *39*, 507–524. [CrossRef]

29. Hannon, P.A.; Garson, G.; Harris, J.R.; Hammerback, K.; Sopher, C.J.; Clegg-Thorp, C. Workplace health promotion implementation, readiness, and capacity among mid-sized employers in low-wage industries: A national survey. *J. Occup. Environ. Med. Am. Coll. Occup. Environ. Med.* **2012**, *54*, 1337–1343. [CrossRef] [PubMed]
30. Glasgow, R.E.; McCaul, K.D.; Fisher, K.J. Participation in worksite health promotion: A critique of the literature and recommendations for future practice. *Health Educ. Q.* **1993**, *20*, 391–408. [CrossRef] [PubMed]
31. Stiehl, E.; Shivaprakash, N.; Thatcher, E.; Ornelas, I.J.; Kneipp, S.; Baron, S.L.; Muramatsu, N. Worksite health promotion for low-wage workers: A scoping literature review. *Am. J. Health Promot. AJHP* **2018**, *32*, 359–373. [CrossRef] [PubMed]
32. Merchant, J.A.; Lind, D.P.; Kelly, K.M.; Hall, J.L. An employee total health management-based survey of Iowa employers. *J. Occup. Environ. Med. Am. Coll. Occup. Environ. Med.* **2013**, *55*, S73–S77. [CrossRef] [PubMed]
33. Gomaa, A.E.; Tapp, L.C.; Luckhaupt, S.E.; Vanoli, K.; Sarmiento, R.F.; Raudabaugh, W.M.; Nowlin, S.; Sprigg, S.M. Occupational traumatic injuries among workers in health care facilities—United States, 2012–2014. *MMWR Morb. Mortal. Wkly. Rep.* **2015**, *64*, 405–410. [PubMed]
34. Helmkamp, J.C.; Lincoln, J.E.; Sestito, J.; Wood, E.; Birdsey, J.; Kiefer, M. Risk factors, health behaviors, and injury among adults employed in the transportation, warehousing, and utilities Super SECTOR. *Am. J. Ind. Med.* **2013**, *56*, 556–568. [CrossRef]
35. Sieber, W.K.; Robinson, C.F.; Birdsey, J.; Chen, G.X.; Hitchcock, E.M.; Lincoln, J.E.; Nakata, A.; Sweeney, M.H. Obesity and other risk factors: The national survey of U.S. long-haul truck driver health and injury. *Am. J. Ind. Med.* **2014**, *57*, 615–626. [CrossRef]
36. Marcum, J.L.; Chin, B.; Anderson, N.J.; Bonauto, D.K. Self-reported work-related injury or illness—Washington, 2011–2014. *MMWR Morb. Mortal. Wkly. Rep.* **2017**, *66*, 302–306. [CrossRef]
37. Luckhaupt, S.E.; Calvert, G.M. Prevalence of coronary heart disease or stroke among workers aged <55 Years—United States, 2008–2012. *MMWR Morb. Mortal. Wkly. Rep.* **2014**, *63*, 645–649.
38. Dong, X.S.; Wang, X.; Largay, J.A. Occupational and non-occupational factors associated with work-related injuries among construction workers in the USA. *Int. J. Occup. Environ. Health* **2015**, *21*, 142–150. [CrossRef]
39. U.S. Bureau of Labor Statistics. 2017 Survey of Occupational Injuries & Illnesses Charts Package. Available online: https://www.bls.gov/iif/osch0062.pdf (accessed on 30 January 2019).
40. Apostolopoulos, Y.; Sönmez, S.; Mona, S.; Haldeman, L.; Strack, R.; Jones, V. Barriers to truck drivers' healthy eating: Environmental influences and health promotion strategies. *J. Workplace Behav. Health* **2011**, *26*, 122–143. [CrossRef]
41. Lemke, M.; Apostolopoulos, Y. Health and wellness programs for commercial motor-vehicle drivers: Organizational assessment and new research directions. *Workplace Health Saf.* **2015**, *63*, 71–80. [CrossRef]
42. Anderson, N.J.; Smith, C.K.; Byrd, J.L. Work-related injury factors and safety climate perception in truck drivers. *Am. J. Ind. Med.* **2017**, *60*, 711–723. [CrossRef]
43. Pronk, N.P. Integrated worker health protection and promotion programs: Overview and perspectives on health and economic outcomes. *J. Occup. Environ. Med. Am. Coll. Occup. Environ. Med.* **2013**, *55*, S30–S37. [CrossRef]
44. Sorensen, G.; McLellan, D.; Dennerlein, J.T.; Pronk, N.P.; Allen, J.D.; Boden, L.I.; Okechukwu, C.A.; Hashimoto, D.; Stoddard, A.; Wagner, G.R. Integration of health protection and health promotion: Rationale, indicators, and metrics. *J. Occup. Environ. Med. Am. Coll. Occup. Environ. Med.* **2013**, *55*, S12–S18. [CrossRef]
45. Loeppke, R.R.; Schill, A.L.; Chosewood, L.C.; Grosch, J.W.; Allweiss, P.; Burton, W.N.; Barnes-Farrell, J.L.; Goetzel, R.Z.; Heinen, L.; Hudson, T.W.; et al. Advancing workplace health protection and promotion for an aging workforce. *J. Occup. Environ. Med.* **2013**, *55*, 500–506. [CrossRef]
46. Anger, W.K.; Kyler-Yano, J.; Vaughn, K.; Wipfli, B.; Olson, R.; Blanco, M. Total worker health intervention for construction workers alters safety, health, well-being measures. *J. Occup. Environ. Med.* **2018**, *60*, 700–709. [CrossRef]
47. Peters, S.E.; Grant, M.P.; Rodgers, J.; Manjourides, J.; Okechukwu, C.A.; Dennerlein, J.T. A cluster randomized controlled trial of a Total Worker Health® intervention on commercial construction sites. *Int. J. Environ. Res. Public. Health* **2018**, *15*, E2354. [CrossRef]
48. Anger, W.K.; Elliot, D.L.; Bodner, T.; Olson, R.; Rohlman, D.S.; Truxillo, D.M.; Kuehl, K.S.; Hammer, L.B.; Montgomery, D. Effectiveness of total worker health interventions. *J. Occup. Health Psychol.* **2015**, *20*, 226–247. [CrossRef]

49. Carr, L.J.; Leonhard, C.; Tucker, S.; Fethke, N.; Benzo, R.; Gerr, F. Total worker health Intervention increases activity of sedentary workers. *Am. J. Prev. Med.* **2016**, *50*, 9–17. [CrossRef]
50. Bradley, C.J.; Grossman, D.C.; Hubbard, R.A.; Ortega, A.N.; Curry, S.J. Integrated interventions for improving total worker health: A panel report from the National Institutes of Health pathways to prevention workshop: Total worker health—What's work got to do with it? *Ann. Intern. Med.* **2016**, *165*, 279–283. [CrossRef]
51. Fishta, A.; Backé, E.-M. Psychosocial stress at work and cardiovascular diseases: An overview of systematic reviews. *Int. Arch. Occup. Environ. Health* **2015**, *88*, 997–1014. [CrossRef]
52. Chandola, T.; Brunner, E.; Marmot, M. Chronic stress at work and the metabolic syndrome: Prospective study. *BMJ* **2006**, *332*, 521–525. [CrossRef]
53. Kubo, J.; Goldstein, B.A.; Cantley, L.F.; Tessier-Sherman, B.; Galusha, D.; Slade, M.D.; Chu, I.M.; Cullen, M.R. Contribution of health status and prevalent chronic disease to individual risk for workplace injury in the manufacturing environment. *Occup. Environ. Med.* **2014**, *71*, 159–166. [CrossRef]
54. Thiese, M.S.; Hanowski, R.J.; Kales, S.N.; Porter, R.J.; Moffitt, G.; Hu, N.; Hegmann, K.T. Multiple conditions increase preventable crash risks among truck drivers in a cohort study. *J. Occup. Environ. Med.* **2017**, *59*, 205–211. [CrossRef]
55. Schulte, P.A.; Pandalai, S.; Wulsin, V.; Chun, H. Interaction of occupational and personal risk factors in workforce health and safety. *Am. J. Public Health* **2012**, *102*, 434–448. [CrossRef]
56. Taylor, A.W.; Pilkington, R.; Montgomerie, A.; Feist, H. The role of business size in assessing the uptake of health promoting workplace initiatives in Australia. *BMC Public Health* **2016**, *16*, 353. [CrossRef]
57. Grosch, J.W.; Alterman, T.; Petersen, M.R.; Murphy, L.R. Worksite health promotion programs in the U.S.: Factors associated with availability and participation. *Am. J. Health Promot. AJHP* **1998**, *13*, 36–45. [CrossRef]

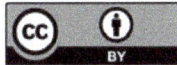

© 2019 by the authors. Licensee MDPI, Basel, Switzerland. This article is an open access article distributed under the terms and conditions of the Creative Commons Attribution (CC BY) license (http://creativecommons.org/licenses/by/4.0/).

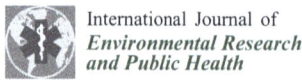

Article

Effect of a Job Demand-Control-Social Support Model on Accounting Professionals' Health Perception

José Joaquín Del Pozo-Antúnez [1], Antonio Ariza-Montes [2,3,*], Francisco Fernández-Navarro [4] and Horacio Molina-Sánchez [1]

1. Financial Economic and Accounting Department, Universidad Loyola Andalucía, 14004 Córdoba, Spain; jjpozo@uloyola.es (J.J.D.P.-A.); hmolina@uloyola.es (H.M.-S.)
2. Management Department, Universidad Loyola Andalucía, 14004 Córdoba, Spain
3. Department of Business Administration, Universidad Autónoma de Chile, 7500912 Santiago, Chile
4. Quantitative Methods Department, Universidad Loyola Andalucía, 14004 Córdoba, Spain; fafernandez@uloyola.es
* Correspondence: ariza@uloyola.es

Received: 23 September 2018; Accepted: 27 October 2018; Published: 1 November 2018

Abstract: The Job Demand-Control and Job Demand-Control-Support (JDCS) models constitute the theoretical approaches used to analyze the relationship between the characteristics of labor and occupational health. Few studies have investigated the main effects and multiplicative model in relation to the perceived occupational health of professional accountants. Accountants are subject to various types of pressure in performing their work; this pressure influences their health and, ultimately, their ability to perform a job well. The objective of this study is to investigate the effects of job demands on the occupational health of 739 accountants, as well as the role of the moderator that internal resources (locus of control) and external resources (social support) have in occupational health. The proposed hypotheses are tested by applying different models of neural networks using the algorithm of the Extreme Learning Machine. The results confirm the relationship between certain stress factors that affect the health of the accountants, as well as the direct effect that the recognition of superiors in occupational health has. Additionally, the results highlight the moderating effect of professional development and the support of superiors on the job's demands.

Keywords: Perceived Occupational Health (POH); Job Demands-Control-Social Support (JD-R) model; professional accountants

1. Introduction

As indicated by Reference [1], workplace health management is crucial for improvements in psychosocial working conditions and health. Promoting healthy work environments is a matter of ethics as well as business interest, since the most competitive companies are those with mentally and physically healthy workers due to policies supporting and protecting their health [2]. There is no doubt that work is part of the social dimension of health. The National Institute for Occupational Safety and Health (NIOSH) recognizes the importance of the well-being of workers, their families and communities through a series of factors linked to the employment relationship, such as wages, hours of work, workload and stress levels, interactions with co-workers and supervisors, access to paid leave, and health-promoting workplaces [3]. Therefore, Total Worker Health promotes an integral intervention in health where measures aimed at the protection of the health of employees are combined with others supportive of well-being. From this perspective, Total Worker Health integrates the individual dimension of health with the organizational dimension and the environment [4]. The Job Demand-Control (JDC) model [5] and the Job Demand-Control-Support (JDCS) model [6,7] constitute the most widely used theoretical approaches to understanding and interpreting the relationships between the characteristics of health, work and well-being [8]. In fact, according to Reference [9], the occupational stress literature is dominated by these models.

Undoubtedly, every effort to improve the integral health of workers translates into greater working efficiency, as shown by the meta-analysis by Reference [10]. The JDCS model warns that the greatest risks to physical and mental health are manifested among workers who experience a high isolation-strain (iso-strain) job—that is, those that are subject to high job demands in a context of low control or decision latitude and low social support (iso-strain hypothesis). However, empirical evidence of this three-way interaction effect is still limited, primarily by the variety that exists in terms of the characteristics and conditions of labor between different jobs and occupations. Many authors, such as Reference [11], indicate that the samples used to test the JDCS model should be as homogeneous as possible, although they are heterogeneous with respect to the level of exposure of workers to the labor environment variables. This circumstance suggests the need to carry out research in occupations with similar characteristics. In addition, not all professions are subject to the same degree of strain, but some occupations tend to combine certain conditions that make workers in those jobs more vulnerable in terms of their physical and mental health [12].

Accountants play an important role in the financial market because they provide accurate information for decision making. Expert judgement and mental equilibrium are required for sound decisions. Despite this, an important gap of research exists in relation to pressures on accountants and its effects. Recently, a professional publication has shown how leading firms of accountants have taken steps to improve their health at work: Training the team leaders on issues of occupational health, creating spaces for healthier work practices, knowledge of such risks, sharing experiences among team members, etc. [13].

A profession as important as accounting is subject to heavy job demands that may affect one's perceived occupational health (POH). Occupational health is the result of the confluence of a number of stress factors and mechanism moderators in organizations. The effect of stressors on accountants has been studied in terms of different effects: For example, dysfunctional behaviour [14–16], personal well-being [17,18], labor satisfaction [17], performance [17] or turnover intention [17,19–22]. This research used theoretical frameworks compatible with those that explain the effect of the job demands in occupational health deterioration and, in particular, one of its major manifestations: Burnout [17,19–26]. Thus, the literature on the accountancy profession has identified several main categories of stressors, which highlight role overload, role conflict and role ambiguity [23]. The Job Demand-Job Control-Social Support (JDCS) model provides a holistic framework to investigate the direct effects and moderators of these stressors on occupational health. To our knowledge, this model has not has been tested on a group of accountants, so this paper covers an important gap in the literature.

This paper tries to cover gaps in the research on this topic in the European context. Thus, the objective of this study is to investigate the effects of job demands on the occupational health of the accountants, as well as the role of the moderator that internal resources (locus of control) and external resources (social support) have in occupational health. To meet the objectives of this research, Section 2 presents the theoretical framework and hypotheses that are derived from the framework. Section 3 describes the empirical study design and methodology used, which are based mainly on the analysis of neural networks. Section 4 displays the main results. The article ends with a discussion of the results (Section 5) and the main limitations of the study and future lines of research (Section 6).

2. Theoretical Framework and Hypothesis Development

This work deals with the study of the health of accountants based on a theoretical framework that uses the Job Demand-Control-Support (JDCS) model formulated by References [5–7]. Different authors have used this model to explain the effect of the job demands on occupational health [27–29].

The general formulation of the JDCS model states that job demands cause a strain. However, it may moderate (or intensify) depending on the degree of control that the employee has on their work and the social support available (see Figure 1).

Job control involves the employees' ability to organize their work and adopt their own initiatives. This perspective would have to be considered a double dimension of the work. On the one hand, the axis of the strain warns that jobs with high demands and low autonomy generate more strain, as opposed to jobs with low demands and high control, where the level of strain would be small. On the other hand, the axis of learning suggests that there is a type of challenging job with a favorable environment for career development when demands are high but also has a high degree of autonomy and implementation of their skills, as is possibly the case of this research.

The model proposed by Reference [5] originally contains two hypotheses. First, the strain hypothesis suggests that demanding activities with low control increase the risk of worker well-being, which is the effect of an additive and multiplicative character. Second, the buffer hypothesis emphasizes a character moderator that exerts job control on the relationship of job demand-strain. According to Reference [30], the two scenarios are not alternatives but are complementary, resulting in an extension of the hypothesis of the voltage buffer hypothesis.

As indicated above, in an extension of the original model, Reference [6] incorporated a second buffer factor of the job demands: Social support for both co-workers and supervisors. Given that the nature of the work of the accountants is based on teamwork, the dimension of social support in this context is a particularly relevant research framework.

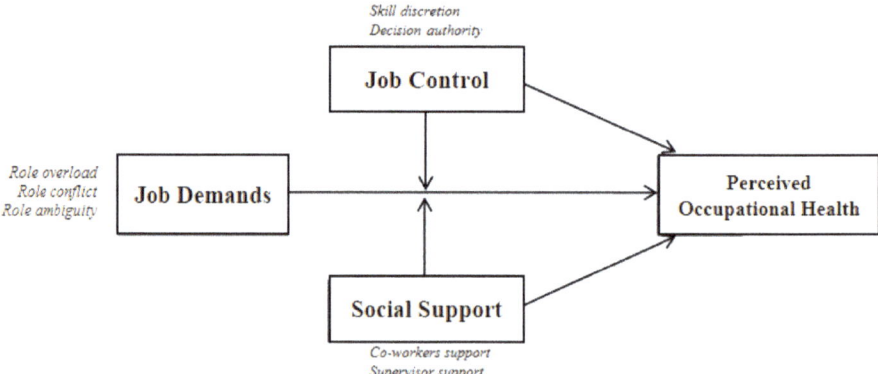

Figure 1. Model of Job Demand-Control-Support (JDCS) applied to the work of accountants.

2.1. Job Demands of Accountants

Accountancy firms are hierarchical and competitive entities to the point that several authors, such as Reference [31], believed that stress is a tool used intentionally by managers to achieve the maximum effectiveness from their subordinates in accounting firms. For example, the pressure of time improves the effectiveness of professional accountants, as Reference [32] observes, especially in the decision-making process, since it causes them to focus only on relevant information. However, work overload and time pressures, far from improving the performance of the professionals, endanger the quality of the work. The duality of effects, positive and negative, that the scientific literature has identified in relation to work overload is explained with the approach of the Arousal Theory, for which the relationship between stress and performance is U-shaped inverted, as pointed out in Reference [33]. As Reference [34] points out, the elimination of stress in accounting is a utopia, given the characteristics of this type of activity—for instance, seasonality linked to compliance with trade regulations, tight deadlines (so that customers can give timely information to the markets), tight time and monetary budgets by the increased competitiveness of the sector, the complexity of some decisions of the audit, manipulation of information by customers. However, scientific research can provide useful tools that contribute to coping and managing stress better.

The Stress Diagnosis Survey (SDS) of Reference [35] is one of the most used tools to analyze the demands that cause greater stress to the accountants. The SDS considers two categories of stressors: Individual and organizational. Individual stress includes role conflict, role ambiguity, quantitative and qualitative overload, time pressures, responsibility, professional careers and the scope of the work. Organizational factors include internal policy, development of human resources, compensation policy, participation, underutilization, style of supervision and organizational structure [36–38].

The model of Reference [23] is a reference for some work done later in the accounting field [17,21,24]. Nevertheless, as is noted above, perhaps the theoretical framework that is more accepted to explain the influence of the employment context in the well-being of employees is the JDCS model. However, in the specific field of audit accounting, its use has been much more limited. Thus, the relationship between stressors and the quality of the work of audit under this framework is explained by Reference [39], noting that the quality of the audit work is not affected by stressful situations if it remains under control. These authors warn that the buffering effect does not occur in the first year in which a client is audited. This will manifest in successive years as experience is acquired with the customer since personal competencies are enhanced to address work that translates into less stress.

This research uses the classification of the job demands that Reference [23] discusses around three broad categories of stressors: Work overload, role conflict and role ambiguity.

2.1.1. Work Overload

Work overload is observed the factor that most influences the deterioration of occupational health [38]. This is produced by taking on a large number of engagements, the tight time allowance to carry out the work or by the imposition of overly tight deadlines. If the prestige of the accountant increases, the demand for their services increases too, resulting in the paradox that excess demand on actual capacity may harm the work quality [40].

Another troubling circumstance is that increasing competition forces price adjustment and reduces the budgets of the implementation of the engagements. This can lead to two dysfunctional practices: Reduce the scope of procedures, again compromising the quality of the work; or underreporting time [41–43]. Time pressure inversely affects the quality of work. Performing audit judgements that entail a high level of subjectivity means that the professional accountant may be tempted to relieve pressure by skewing his own judgement. In this way, professional accountants who work with more time pressure assessed a lower risk of significant error in the audited financial statements, which leads them to decrease the intensity of the procedures and the workload [16,44]. In addition, reporting less than the actual number of hours worked (time underreporting) produces a double negative effect. On the one hand, planning future engagements considers the budget timetable of the previous year, thus conditioning the planning of future work. On the other hand, the evaluation of a professional's performance is distorted and is expected within an unrealistic time frame. Underreporting time is considered a more ethical strategy than devoting fewer hours than necessary when the budget is too tight [45].

Work overload also occurs when deadlines are so tight that they cause negative consequences for the quality of the work [46,47]. For example, professional accountants tended to consider less important errors detected on tight deadlines, especially when these deadlines have been established by the own professional accountants [48]. The obligation to comply with the rule of law creates peaks and concentration of work, which result in work overload and higher role conflict, which leads to emotional exhaustion among professional accountants, as References [25,26] have shown.

2.1.2. Role Conflict

Economic effects arising from the financial information prepared by accountants can sometimes lead to conflicts of an ethical nature. For example, the auditors attempt to preserve relations with customers. Therefore, using findings that may have a negative influence on the client, their judgements tend to be more relaxed, especially if the work contains a high level of subjectivity (for example, judgements on the materiality of the deviations identified in the internal control [48]). Thus, as the client portfolio of the professional accountant expands, the independence level increases, thus reducing the role conflict but increasing the workload [49].

Role conflict is more likely to occur at lower levels of a professional career due to the pressure from superiors (managers and partners) on these individuals, which has come to be called "pressure by obedience". This pressure may cause less-skilled team members to violate professional standards to meet the demands of their superiors [50].

All of the above issues translate into greater role conflict, which, according to Reference [34], cause greater stress and lower job satisfaction, thus affecting the health of the accountants.

2.1.3. Role Ambiguity

Another factor that can affect the quality of the work of professional accountants is the lack of understanding of the tasks to be carried out [15]. As indicated by Reference [31], the risk of significant errors during the performance of work creates a sense of fear among professional accountants. This sensation may have both positive (e.g., stimulates professional diligence) and negative effects (since it can induce the adoption of defensive strategies). What does appear clear is that the accountants experience less comfort to perform more complex tasks than when they perform more routine tasks [51].

Undoubtedly, as Reference [34] proposed, all these elements of role ambiguity have a negative influence on satisfaction and perception of performance.

2.2. Job Control

The negative effects that generate the high job demands can be buffered or intensified depending on the degree of control that the accountant has on the activity. This control is highlighted mainly by two factors: The possibility of applying one's own skills (skill discretion) and the level of autonomy over decisions that affect you (decision authority) [5]. In a recent study, professionals with greater competence and autonomy experienced less role ambiguity [52]. This circumstance occurs because higher levels of competition allowed attention to the complexity associated with the tasks of the profession with less pressure. At the same time, these authors found that less autonomy reduced access to information, which resulted in greater ambiguity.

There is evidence that shows that the degree of job autonomy in decision-making, such as the ability to decide one's workload, moderates some variables related to occupational health, such as stress [53]. Although the work overload may cause adverse effects on the quality of the work, the fact is that accountancy firms are impregnated with an organizational culture that accepts, encourages and imposes high standards of work that translate into levels of high demand. Despite this, there is empirical evidence showing that if the accountant chooses the workload voluntarily, harmful effects on the quality of the work are not produced.

Job autonomy in the field of auditing can cause dysfunctional behaviours; in fact, in a sample of Chinese professional accountants, the dysfunctional behaviour increased because the professional had greater autonomy [54]. In a positive sense, these authors also noted that accountants perceived job autonomy as a sign of support from the organization, which resulted in greater job satisfaction.

The pressure caused by tight time budgets also leads to dysfunctional behaviours. However, these vary at different hierarchical levels and are more likely in positions requiring less experience—for example, in roles with less autonomy in the activity planning [46]. In addition, these authors observed that the perception of a greater degree of involvement in time programming has a positive influence on the achievement of the budgetary targets.

On the other hand, control over the activity also manifests itself when accountants can fully display their abilities. This situation makes work exciting and encourages accountants to do their best work rather than adopting dysfunctional behaviours [47]. In this way, because the content of the tasks corresponds to the level of professional development, stressors are cushioned by the incentive that involves applying one's own professional competencies. Professional judgement develops as experience is gained. In the early professional stages, tasks are more structured and require a level of minor professional judgement. Over time, the responsibility of professional accountants on more complex decisions leads to higher ambiguity. Without a doubt, the experience provides greater comfort in complex decision-making, in keeping with the principles of Social Cognitive Theory. The experience leads to better assessments of the risk of significant errors [44,55], which determines greater control of the activities and leads to highly stimulating work when personal skills are applied to help solve complex situations. Finally, because experience is gained when a customer increases knowledge about such situations [56,57], improving control over activities and diluting the negative effects of work overload may result in the quality of the work of the professional accountant [58].

2.3. Social Support

Several authors believe that quality relations between the accountancy firms and their professionals develop more intensely when they perceived a fair deal and when they feel supported by the organization, which reduces burnout and intention to leave the organization [19,22].

Collectivism exerts a positive influence on the level of well-being of professional accountants, which is measured by its three components: Job satisfaction, work-life balance and life satisfaction [18]. For these authors, as the engagements become more complex, professional accountants develop a feeling of belonging to the work and a spirit of team-oriented organization. In this context, the behaviour of superiors is influential, since they create an organizational culture, which defines what practices are encouraged and desired by the firm. Thus, if superiors expressly and honestly reject the practices that generate stress (such as the underreporting the hours spent in completing work), subordinates feel that their stress levels are alleviated.

In this sense, there is a negative relationship between job autonomy and counterproductive behaviours, an effect that is compensated for and reversed by a set of factors, among which perceived organizational support stands out [54]. This circumstance suggests that the negative consequences associated with job autonomy are mitigated in organizations that promote positive attitudes among their employees. In addition, firms that promote values and ethical behaviour increase the level of socialization of its professionals, significantly reducing dysfunctional practices that could arise from time pressures [45].

Social support depends greatly on one's superiors. The style of leadership of these superiors has a direct effect on the performance of teams and in superior-subordinate relations, even in relations between the members of the team. Team performance improves when superiors stimulate innovation, serve the personal needs of team members, offer positive reinforcement and conform to the budgets schedules [59]. More recently, in an investigation on accountants, leaders who promote a strong team culture achieve smoother communication and greater cohesion among members [60].

Feelings emerge in opposite directions when subordinates do not feel supported by their immediate supervisor. This is something that happens all too often in accountancy firms due to the feeling of fear that is cultivated more or less informally with the intention of stimulating monitoring, promoting self-improvement, mitigating the anaesthetizing effect of habit and maintaining reputation [31]. This feeling is more unusual because auditors are accountable in more instances and when more complex tasks become especially intense [51].

2.4. Hypothesis Development

Figure 2 shows the theoretical model on which this work is based, as well as the hypotheses that seek to demonstrate the purpose of this investigation. These are divided into two groups: The direct effects of three model factors and moderator effects.

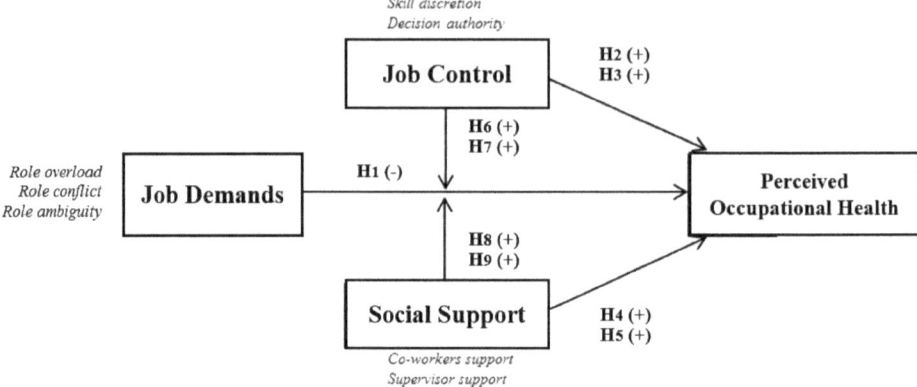

Figure 2. Model hypotheses.

2.4.1. Direct Effects

Hypothesis 1 (H1). *As the job demands become more demanding, perceived occupational health of professional accountants decreases.*

Hypothesis 2 (H2). *As accountants have greater autonomy in the implementation of their professional skills, perceived occupational health increases.*

Hypothesis 3 (H3). *As the accountant has higher degree of autonomy in decision-making, perceived health increases.*

Hypothesis 4 (H4). *As the accountant has more support from his superiors, perceived occupational health increases.*

Hypothesis 5 (H5). *As the accountant has greater support from peers, perceived occupational health increases.*

2.4.2. Moderating Effects

Hypothesis 6 (H6). *Autonomy in the implementation of professional competences buffers the relationship between job demands and perceived occupational health.*

Hypothesis 7 (H7). *Autonomy in decision-making buffers the relationship between job demands and perceived occupational health.*

Hypothesis 8 (H8). *Support from one's superiors serves as a moderator of the relationship between the demands of the job role in perceived occupational health.*

Hypothesis 9 (H9). *Peer support serves as a moderator of the relationship between the demands of work on perceived occupational health.*

3. Design of the Empirical Research

3.1. Sample

The data used for the development of this research were obtained from the sixth European Working Conditions Survey, which was developed by the European Foundation for the Improvement of the Conditions of Life and Work in 2015 [61]. This survey analyzes the working conditions in the 27 countries of the European Union, providing valuable information on different aspects of the working conditions in Europe: Attitudes, perceptions and behavior of employees. The population consists of all persons aged 15 or above who are employed or self-employed and whose usual place of residence is in one of the member states of the European Union. The field work was carried out in 2015 based on 43,850 valid surveys.

To achieve the objectives of the present research, a sub-sample of 739 professional accountants were extracted using codes 2411 (accountants) and 3313 (accounting associate professionals) of the International Standard Classification of Occupations.

Of the respondents, 75.2% are women, while the remaining 24.8% are men. The average age of the professional accountants is 43.9 years. Most respondents working in the private sector (82.5%) with a contract mainly have indefinite work contracts (88.8%) that are an average of 10.9 years old. With respect to the main variable of this research, it should be noted that 17.7% of respondents believe that the development of the work directly affects their health, compared to 82.3% who considered otherwise.

3.2. Measures

The dependent variable of this research is the perceived occupational health of professional accountants. A single item measures this variable: Whether the professionals perceive that their work directly affects their health. The respondents had three response options: No; yes, mainly positively; and yes, mainly negatively.

The job demands were measured using 7 items grouped into three categories: Role overload (e.g., "Does your job involve working with tight deadlines?"), role ambiguity (e.g., "Do you know what is expected of you at work?") and role conflict (e.g., "Does your job involve being in situations that are emotionally disturbing for you?").

The scale of job control integrates 4 items that measure skill discretion (e.g., "Does your job involve solving unforeseen problems on your own?") and 7 items that assess the decision authority (e.g., "Are you consulted before objectives are set for your work?" or "Do you have a say in the choice of your work colleagues?").

Finally, the scale of social support measures support from superiors with 7 items (e.g., "Your immediate supervisor provides useful feedback on your work" or "Your immediate boss encourages and supports your development"), while the support of co-workers is determined by a unique item that ask directly if "your colleagues help and support you."

3.3. Methodology

The methodology proposed in this research is developed in three phases: Preparation of the constructs of the first order from the application of a factor analysis, analysis of neural networks with the Extreme Learning Machine algorithm, and finally, interpretation of the resulting model using a sensitivity analysis.

A factor analysis was run with a rotation promax on the original data set. Promax rotation allows the factors obtained to be correlated (unlike the varimax rotation or orthogonal rotation). Following the recommendations of Reference [62], items that were not correlated with any specific factor were excluded from the analysis, while the loading used for other factor was 0.40. Variables that are grouped without any logical meaning according to the nature of the problem were also eliminated. The factor analysis revealed the existence of first-order factors for the constructs: Job Demands (JD),

Skill Discretion (SD), Decision Authority (DA) and Supervisor Support (SS). The construct Co-Worker Support (WS) was composed of a single item. Since the input variables were represented in different ranges, it was decided to standardize them to a [0, 1] scale linearly according to the function min (max).

The main analysis was carried out with artificial neural networks. This method has shown satisfactory results in solving complex problems and constitutes a useful tool in data analysis of different areas or disciplines: Medicine, economics, engineering, biology and psychology [63]. Increasingly, more authors appreciate their applicability with regard to models derived from classic statistics [64,65]. From a methodological perspective, the priority themes that apply neural networks deal with the classification of patterns (classification and prediction) and approximation of functions [63]. It is possible that the growing interest in neural networks lies in its capacity for the treatment of nonlinear problems [66], since better yields are achieved because there is independence from the fulfilment of the theoretical assumptions of traditional techniques. Neural networks have proven to be an effective tool for classifying cases under the non-linearity hypothesis. A neural network is a linear model in which the basis functions can be a sigmoid type. In the case that concerns us, the analysis was performed using a neural network in a single layer, which allows for modelling interactions of an order greater than two (and not only multiplicative); interactions will be key to analyzing the moderator effect of job control and social support. The parameters of the model have been estimated using the algorithm Extreme Learning Machine [67]. In this algorithm, the weights of the input layer to the hidden layer (which models the nonlinear part of the system) are initialized randomly. In addition, the parameters that bind the hidden layer with the layer's output are estimated analytically after solving a problem of least squares with regularization.

To finish the investigation, a sensitivity analysis was conducted. The main disadvantage of the models of neural networks is that they are considered a "black box" type, since they are effective at finding hidden relationships between inputs and outputs with a high capacity for approximation, but they do not provide information on how they have managed to do so. This limitation causes many academics to scrap the use of these models in their research. A sensitivity analysis is used to overcome this restriction. The present study uses a global sensitivity analysis inspired by a decomposition functional ANOVA [68]. This method makes it possible to decompose the nonlinear function on a set of elements associated with the parts of the independent variables, the interactions of the variable two by two, to the interactions between variables three to three and so on until all interactions of the input variables are analyzed. This methodology was already proposed for the classification problem and has been adapted ad hoc in this study for the case of regression [69]. To evaluate the stability of the method, an analysis with two subsamples that gave rise to two estimates of parameters of sensitivity (estimate 1 and 2 estimate) was performed.

4. Results

In the case of factor analysis, the construct Job Demands (JD) was reduced to a single component that explained 35.38% of total variance (the other elements presented eigenvalues below one). The construct Job Control (JC) was composed of two elements: Skill Discretion (SD) and Decision Authority (DA). These are summarized in two factors that explained 38.55% and 46.84% of variance, respectively. The construct Social Support (SS) was composed, as explained above, by two elements: Supervisor Support (SS) and Co-Worker Support (WS). The first is represented by a factor that explained 75.54% of variance, while the second was a construct consisting of a single item.

First, we analyze the mean square error (MSE) of the linear regression, including interactions considered in this research, compared to the model of the trained neural network according to Extreme Learning Machine. The classical model earned an MSE of 31.8862 and a neural network 11.4588 MSE, which justifies that the neural network model summarizes data more effectively than the classic model. The result of the regularization was cross-validated, resulting in a value of 10E3. In addition, the number of hidden layer neurons was fixed at 500.

After verifying that the non-linear model had greater precision than the linear model, its parameters were interpreted by applying the above sensitivity analysis. The first-order analysis qualifies the contribution to the output of the different input variables (job demands, skill discretion, decision authority, supervisor support and co-worker support) in a direct way without interactions. Table 1 presents the contribution to the variance of each of these variables and their signs (which were estimated empirically).

Table 1. Analysis of the first order. Contribution to the variance and sign.

	JD	SD	DA	SS	WS
Estimate 1	0.610426 (−)	0.0255825 (+)	0.0148224 (+)	0.283876 (+)	0.0231483 (+)
Estimate 2	0.560802 (−)	0.0019926 (+)	0.0151903 (+)	0.332172 (+)	0.0015737 (+)

JD (Job Demands), SD (Skill Discretion), DA (Decision Authority), SS (Social Support), WS (Co-Worker Support).

The variables that contribute most significantly to the explanation of perceived occupational health of accountants are job demands, with a negative sign, and supervisor support, with a positive sign. These results highlight, on the one hand, that an accountant's health deteriorates as job demands increase, while having the support of immediate superiors contributes positively to perceived occupational health. Since the results of estimation 1 and 2 are close (see Table 1), they can be considered robust. Table 1 also shows that the direct effect of the other variables (skill discretion, decision authority and co-worker support) is irrelevant in the perception of accountants' health.

Then, we analyzed the possible moderating effect of job control and social support in the relationship between job demands and perceived occupational health. This was solved by incorporating the contribution to the variance of the different interactions of the variable two by two.

The results of such interactions, all of them with positive signs, are presented in Table 2. The positive sign of the interactions when job demands had a negative relationship with perceived occupational health confirms the moderating effect that show both social support and job control. Focusing on Table 2, we can appreciate that the possibility of practicing skills as well as having the confidence in support from the top are the two variables that largely reduce the negative effect of job demands in perceived occupational health by the accountants.

Table 2. Analysis of the iterations of the variables. Contribution to the variance.

	JD	SD	DA	SS	WS
JD	-	0.0543336	0.0065206	0.0761218	0.0044644
SD	0.0847528	-	0.0097692	0.0191648	0.0254918
DA	0.0058920	0.0104552	-	0.0004655	0.0059129
SS	0.0800194	0.0189461	0.0009225	-	0.0007901
WS	0.0036139	0.0249092	0.0056966	0.0000172	-

JD (Job Demands), SD (Skill Discretion), DA (Decision Authority), SS (Social Support), WS (Co-Worker Support). Above, the axis values correspond to interactions in Scenario 1, while values below the axis correspond to Scenario 2. In bold, the highest values are highlighted.

5. Discussion

Accountants play an important role in market economies. Financial information reduces costs of transaction in agency relationship; therefore, accountants are an essential link in the relations between owners and managers [70]. In this context, professional accountants that audit give credibility to the system, constituting an effective signaling mechanism in corporate governance [71] and influence in credit decisions [72]. Likewise, Positive Accounting Theory has shown the influence of accounting figures in taxation, sectoral regulation and executive compensation plans [73].

The significance and relevance of this profession places stress on accountants, who are forced to contend with strong demands that can affect their health. The most significant include professionals who work with tight deadlines, with significant seasonality (since most companies issue financial reports at the same time, coinciding with the calendar year) and in an environment of extreme competition, which reduces prices and increases pressure on resource allocation.

In this context of strain, the accountant must "juggle" to put into practice the independence, judgement, and professional skepticism that international auditing agencies require. Therefore, any deterioration in the health of these professionals, which alter their emotional balance, will decisively affect the judgement of the professional accountant and the quality of their work.

The present paper is relevant in the European context and investigates the effects of job demands in occupational health perceived by the accountants, as well as the moderator role that job control exerts over work and the social support of colleagues and superiors. The results, after the application of a neural network model, confirm some of the hypotheses raised in this research, both with regard to the outcomes and the effects of the moderators.

On the one hand, in relation to the direct effects of the job demands, job control and social support on perceived occupational health (H1 to H5), it has been shown that job demands are the factor that best explains the deterioration of accountants' health, which is in line with the prior literature that has verified the existence of this relationship in other manifestations of loss of health, such as burnout [38]. The other variable that exerts an important influence on perceived occupational health is supervisor support—in this case, in a positive sense. This result is consistent with the model of an organization staffed by professional accountants and is based mainly on professional talent. The implementation of professional talent requires the support and trust of the organization. The results of this study highlight better occupational health among professionals who receive explicit support from their superiors. On the other hand, job control does not exert a significant direct effect on perceived occupational health, possibly because the work of the accountants is structured and formalized, leaving little room for individual initiative.

Otherwise, the JDCS model discusses a number of mechanisms that contribute to cushioning the pernicious effect of the job demands on perceived occupational health. The results derived from the neural network model suggest that these mechanisms indeed improve the perception of one's own occupational health—specifically, the implementation of vocational skills and perception of greater support of hierarchical superiors. Accounting firms are characterized by their high level of hierarchy and fierce pyramidal structure. This design requires a high degree of staff turnover, which allows the channels of promotion to be open [74]. Since accountants' immediate superiors evaluate them, support from superiors is one of the mechanisms for recognition with greater impact on the development of a healthy work environment [41]. In a qualitative study, the importance of superiors in the self-esteem of subordinates is underlined: "To hear my senior say I've done a good job is a real boost to my morale!". The comment of this assistant illustrates the process governing her approach to auditing: She was congratulated for her work, and she takes the compliment personally ("I'm doing a good job"), thus strengthening her identity, and this prospect is precisely what motivates her to do her best [31]. To fulfil their expectations in terms of self-achievement, some auditors go further. Undoubtedly, support of one's superiors and a feeling of justice decrease the feeling of burnout among accountants [19,22]. In addition, the confidence of being supported by the organization and its managers in a competitive environment where lawsuits are frequent contributes to a vital balance [18].

The other variable with a significant moderating effect in the relationship between job demand and perceived occupational health is the possibility of practicing personal skills (skill discretion). The analysis of this effect, which has much to do with the concept of hardiness, is especially relevant in the profession discussed in this research. People with hardy personalities perceive stimulating and challenging situations as stressful (commitment dimension), probably because they believe that stress factors are controllable thanks to their professional skills (skill discretion), thus transforming risk into an opportunity for personal growth (challenge dimension). Commitment and challenge show a significant relationship with exhaustion, one of the fundamental dimensions of burnout, as point out Reference [26]. This result offers the possibility of aligning the needs of firms to respond to a competitive market with the professional interests of the accountants to the point where many professionals consider joining these companies as a promising start to a career or as a highly stimulating professional activity [47].

In short (see Figure 3), the direct effects on perceived occupational health come primarily from job demands (Hypothesis 1) and the recognition of superiors (Hypothesis 4), while the incidence of the two dimensions of job control (Hypothesis 2 and 3) and co-worker support (Hypothesis 5) is not relevant. For the moderating effects, the relationship between job demand and perceived occupational health is reducing among professionals who can practice their professional skills (Hypothesis 6) and have the support of their superiors (Hypothesis 8). The rest of the moderator effects scarcely explain the variance of the model: Decision authority (Hypothesis 7) and co-worker support (Hypothesis 9).

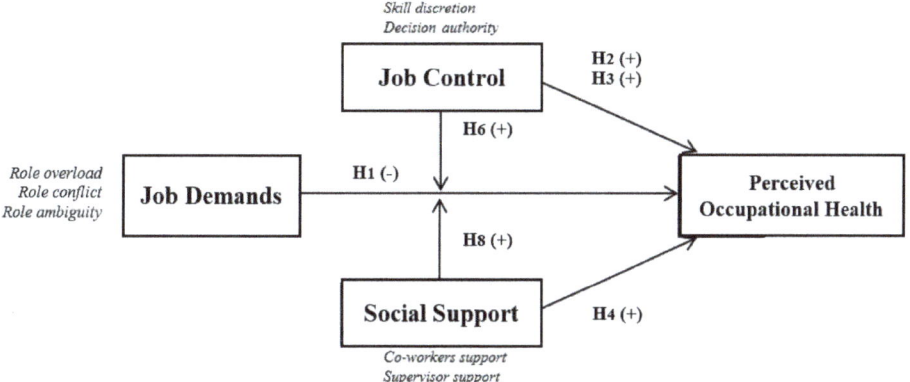

Figure 3. Model hypotheses confirmed.

Two important practical implications for organizations and their human resource managers can be drawn from this research. On the one hand, recruitment and selection processes should pay special attention to candidates with hardiness, i.e., those who are capable of transforming stressful situations into opportunities for growth. Professionals who have this competence profile better bear the pressure inherent in the work, and hardiness is especially valuable for developing professional careers with long spans, such as accountancy firms. On the other hand, in an environment that is as demanding as the object of this paper in which one is subjected to intense pressures of time and deadlines, superiors play a central role in the promotion of a healthy work environment. Therefore, superiors should receive practical training in managing people so that they are aware of and develop the skills needed to provide the social support that accounting professionals need and demand. Leading practices and training programmes implemented by large accountancy firms to support the mental health of employees are displayed by Reference [13].

As noted in the introduction to this research, Total Worker Health promotes integral intervention in health that considers both the individual perspective and the organizational context. In this sense, JDCS model is one of the theoretical approaches more suited to understanding and interpreting the relationships between work features and the health and well-being of employees [8]. As a conclusion, we can say that this research confirms the basic postulates of the JDCS model (professional development and supervisor support mainly constitute the basic mechanisms for moderating the high pressures of the accounting work), thus contributes to explaining the perceived occupational health of accounting profession from an original and novel theoretical framework on this field.

6. Limitations and Future Lines of Research

Finally, it is necessary to mention the major methodological limitations of this study. First, perceived occupational health was measured through individual self-perceptions. Second, the problem of social desirability is a setback of studies that ask about how labor conditions affect employees. Self-perception and the social desirability may cause bias in responses. Third, the relationship between the variables being investigated cannot be considered causally since we studied cross-sectional data, not experimental data. Finally, the study is limited to the scope of the European Union. Future studies should investigate the influence of the JDCS model in professional accountants who develop their activities in other cultural contexts.

7. Conclusions

Scarce studies have explored the main effects and multiplicative model in relation to the perceived occupational health of professional accountants. The Job Demand-Control and Job Demand-Control-Support (JDCS) models adopted in this article are an appropriate theoretical framework to analyze the relationship between the characteristics of labor and occupational health.

In conclusion, the obtained results confirm the relationship between certain stress factors that affect the health of the accountants, as well as the direct effect that has the recognition of superiors in occupational health. Additionally, the results highlight the moderating effect of professional development and the support of superiors on the job's demands.

The implications of these findings could assist human resource managers in facilitating, to some extent, good social relationships amongst accountants.

Author Contributions: For research articles with several authors, a short paragraph specifying their individual contributions must be provided. The following statements should be used "Conceptualization, H.M.-S., A.A.-M. and J.J.D.P.-A.; Methodology, F.F.-N.; Software, F.F.-N.; Validation, F.F.-N.; Formal Analysis, H.M.-S., A.A.-M.; Investigation, H.M.-S., A.A.-M. and J.J.D.P.-A.; Resources, H.M.-S. and J.J.D.P.-A.; Data Curation, A.A.-M. and J.J.D.P.-A. Writing-Original Draft Preparation, J.J.D.P.-A.; Writing-Review & Editing, H.M.-S. and A.A.-M.; Visualization, H.M.-S. and A.A.-M.; Supervision, H.M.-S. and A.A.-M. and F.F.-N.; Project Administration, A.A.-M.; Funding Acquisition, N/A", please turn to the CRediT taxonomy for the term explanation. Authorship must be limited to those who have contributed substantially to the work reported.

Funding: This research received no external funding.

Acknowledgments: We thank Eurofound for providing the data set for this research. Reference [60], European Working Conditions Survey Integrated Data File, 1991–2015, [data collection], UK Data Service. SN: 7363, https://doi.org/10.5255/UKDA-SN-7363-4.

Conflicts of Interest: The authors declare no conflict of interest.

References

1. Shain, M.; Kramer, D. Health promotion in the workplace: Framing the concept; reviewing the evidence. *Occup. Environ. Med.* **2004**, *61*, 643–648. [CrossRef] [PubMed]
2. World Health Organization (WHO). *Healthy Workplaces: A WHO Global Model for Action*; World Health Organization: Geneva, Switzerland, 2010; Available online: http://www.who.int/occupational_health/publications/healthy_workplaces_model_action.pdf (accessed on 12 September 2018).
3. NIOSH. *Fundamentals of Total Worker Health Approaches: Essential Elements for Advancing Worker Safety, Health, and Well-Being*; U.S. Publication No. 2017-112; Department of Health and Human Services, Centers for Disease Control and Prevention, National Institute for Occupational Safety and Health—DHHS (NIOSH): Cincinnati, OH, USA, 2016. Available online: https://www.cdc.gov/niosh/docs/2017-112/pdfs/2017_112.pdf?id=10.26616/NIOSHPUB2017112 (accessed on 12 September 2018).
4. Schulte, P.; Pandalai, S.; Wulsin, V.; HeeKyonung, C. Interaction of Occupational and Personal Risk Factors in Workforce Health and Safety. *Am. J. Public Health* **2012**, *102*, 434–448. [CrossRef] [PubMed]
5. Karasek, R. Job demands, job decision latitude, and mental strain: Implications for job redesign. *Adm. Sci. Quart.* **1979**, *24*, 285–308. [CrossRef]
6. Johnson, J.V.; Hall, E.M. Job strain, work place social support, and cardiovascular disease: A cross-sectional study of a random sample of the Swedish working population. *Am. J. Public Health* **1988**, *78*, 1336–1342. [CrossRef] [PubMed]
7. Karasek, R.A.; Theorell, T. *Healthy Work: Stress, Productivity and the Reconstruction of Working Life*; Basic Books: New York, NY, USA, 1990.

8. Ibrahim, R.Z.A.R.; Ohtsuka, K. Review of the job demand-control and job demand-control-support models: Elusive moderating predictor effects and cultural implications. *Southeast Asia Psychol. J.* **2014**, *1*, 10–21.
9. Haly, M.K. A review of contemporary research on the relationship between occupational stress and social support: Where are we now? *Aust. J. Organ. Psychol.* **2009**, *2*, 44–63. [CrossRef]
10. Ford, M.T.; Cerasoli, C.P.; Higgins, J.A.; Decesare, A.L. Relationships between psychological, physical, and behavioural health and work performance: A review and meta-analysis. *Work Stress* **2011**, *25*, 185–204. [CrossRef]
11. Janssen, P.P.; Bakker, A.B.; De Jong, A. A test and refinement of the Demand–Control–Support Model in the construction industry. *Int. J. Stress Manag.* **2001**, *8*, 315–332. [CrossRef]
12. Eurofound. Occupational Profiles in Working Conditions: Identification of Groups with Multiple Disadvantages. Available online: https://www.eurofound.europa.eu/publications/report/2014/working-conditions/occupational-profiles-in-working-conditions-identification-of-groups-with-multiple-disadvantages (accessed on 9 September 2018).
13. Skoulding, L. What Are the Big Four Doing to Support Mental Health in the Workplace. Accountancy Age. May 2018. Available online: https://www.accountancyage.com/2018/05/17/what-are-the-big-four-doing-to-support-mental-health-in-the-workplace/ (accessed on 29 October 2018).
14. Utary, A.R. Effect of Time Budget Pressure on Dysfunctional Audit and Audit Quality, Information technology as Moderator. *Int. J. Econ. Res.* **2014**, *11*, 689–698.
15. Svanström, T. Time Pressure, Training Activities and Dysfunctional Auditor Behaviour: Evidence from Small Audit Firms. *Int. J. Audit.* **2016**, *20*, 40–51. [CrossRef]
16. Broberg, P.; Tagesson, T.; Argento, D.; Gyllengham, N.; Mårtensson, O. Explaining the influence of time budget pressure on audit quality in Sweden. *J. Manag. Gov.* **2017**, *21*, 331–350. [CrossRef]
17. Jones, A.; Strand Norman, C.; Wier, B. Healthy Lifestyle as a Coping Mechanism for Role Stress in Public Accounting. *Behav. Res. Account.* **2010**, *22*, 21–41. [CrossRef]
18. Umans, T.; Broberg, T.; Schmidt, M.; Nilsson, P.; Olsson, E. Feeling well by being together: Study of Swedish auditors. *Work* **2016**, *54*, 79–86. [CrossRef] [PubMed]
19. Herda, D.N.; Lavelle, J.J. The Auditor-Audit Firm Relationship and Its Effect on Burnout and Turnover Intention. *Account. Horiz.* **2012**, *26*, 707–723. [CrossRef]
20. Pradana, A.; Salehudin, I. Work overload and turnover intention of junior auditors in Greater Jakarta, Indonesia. *South East Asian J. Manag.* **2015**, *9*, 108–124.
21. Chong, V.K.; Monroe, G.S. The impact of the antecedents and consequences of job burnout on junior accountants' turnover intentions: A structural equation modelling approach. *Account. Financ.* **2015**, *55*, 105–132. [CrossRef]
22. Cannon, N.H.; Herda, D.N. Auditors' Organizational Commitment, Burnout, and Turnover Intention: A Replication. *Behav. Res. Account.* **2016**, *28*, 69–74. [CrossRef]
23. Fogarty, T.J.; Singh, J.; Rhoads, G.K.; Moore, R.K. Antecedents and Consequences of Burnout in Accounting: Beyond the Role Stress Model. *Behav. Res. Account.* **2000**, *12*, 31–67.
24. Almer, E.D.; Kaplan, S.E. The Effects of Flexible Work Arrangements on Stressors, Burnout, and Behavioral Job Outcomes in Public Accounting. *Behav. Res. Account.* **2002**, *14*, 1–34. [CrossRef]
25. Sweeney, J.T.; Summers, S.L. The effect of busy season workload on public accountants' job burnout. *Behav. Res. Account.* **2002**, *14*, 223–245. [CrossRef]
26. Law, D.W.; Sweeney, J.T.; Summers, S.L. An Examination of the influences of contextual and individual variables on public accountants' exhaustation. *Adv. Account. Behav. Res.* **2016**, *11*, 129–153.
27. Rafferty, Y.; Friend, R.; Landsbergis, P.A. The association between job skill discretion, decision authority and burnout. *Work Stress* **2001**, *15*, 73–85. [CrossRef]
28. De Jonge, J.; Dollard, M.F.; Dormann, C.; Le Blanc, P.M.; Houtman, I.L.D. The Demand-Control Model: Specific demands, specific control, and well-defined groups. *Int. J. Stress Manag.* **2000**, *7*, 269–287. [CrossRef]
29. Brouwers, A.; Evers, W.J.G.; Tomic, W. Self-efficacy in eliciting social support and burnout among secondary-school teachers. *J. Appl. Soc. Psychol.* **2001**, *32*, 1474–1491. [CrossRef]
30. Hausser, J.A.; Mojzisch, A.; Niesel, M.; Schulz-Hardt, S. Ten years on: A review of recent research on the Job Demand-Control (-Support) model and psychological well-being. *Work Stress* **2010**, *24*, 1–35. [CrossRef]
31. Guénin-Paracini, H.; Marsch, B.; Marché Paillé, A. Fear and risk in the audit process. *Account. Organ. Soc.* **2014**, *39*, 264–288. [CrossRef]

32. Glover, S.M. The Influence of Time Pressure and Accountability on Auditors' Processing of Nondiagnostic Information. *J. Account. Res.* **1997**, *35*, 213–226. [CrossRef]
33. Pietsch, C.P.; Messier, W.F., Jr. The Effects of Time Pressure on Belief Revision in Accounting: A Review of Relevant Literature within a Pressure-Arousal-Effort-Performance Framework. *Behav. Res. Account.* **2017**, *29*, 51–71. [CrossRef]
34. Rebele, J.E.; Michaels, R.E. Independent Auditors' Role Stress: Antecedents, Outcome, and Moderating Variables. *Behav. Res. Account.* **1990**, *2*, 124–153.
35. Ivancevich, J.M.; Matteson, M.T. *Stress Diagnostic Survey*; University of Houston: Houston, TX, USA, 1983.
36. Collins, K.M. Stress and departures from the public accounting profession: A study of gender differences. *Account. Horiz.* **1993**, *7*, 29–38.
37. Larson, L.L.; Meier, H.H.; Poznanski, P.J.; Murff, E.J.T. Concepts and Consequences of Internal Auditor Job Stress. *J. Account. Financ. Res.* **2004**, *12*, 35–46.
38. Larson, L.L.; Tipton Murff, E.J. An Analysis of Job Stress Outcomes among Bank Internal Auditors. *Bank Account. Financ.* **2006**, *19*, 39–43.
39. Yan, H.; Xie, S. How does auditors' work stress affect audit quality? Empirical evidence from the Chinese stock market. *China J. Account. Res.* **2016**. [CrossRef]
40. Pritchard, A.C.; Ferris, S.P.; Jagannathan, J. Too Busy to Mind the Business? Monitoring by Directors with Multiple Board Appointments. *J. Financ.* **2003**, *58*, 1087–1111. [CrossRef]
41. Pierce, B.; Sweeney, B. Cost–Quality Conflict in Audit Firms: An Empirical Investigation. *Eur. Account. Rev.* **2004**, *13*, 415–441. [CrossRef]
42. Nehme, R.; Al Mutawa, A.; Jizi, M. Dysfunctional Behavior of External Auditors. The collision of time budget and time deadline. Evidence from developing country. *J. Dev. Areas* **2016**, *50*, 373–388. [CrossRef]
43. Baldacchino, P.J.; Tabone, N.; Agius, J.; Bezzina, F. Organizational Culture, Personnel Characteristics and Dysfunctional Audit Behavior. *IUP J. Account. Res. Audit Pract.* **2016**, *15*, 34–63.
44. Sayed Hussin, S.A.H.; Iskandar, T.M.; Saleh, N.M.; Jaffar, R. Professional Skepticism and Auditors' Assessment of Misstatement Risks: The Moderating Effects of Experience and Time Budget Pressure. *Econ. Sociol.* **2017**, *10*, 225–250. [CrossRef] [PubMed]
45. Espinosa-Pike, M.; Barrainkua, I. El efecto de los valores profesionales y la cultura organizativa en la respuesta de los auditores a las presiones de tiempo. *Span. J. Financ. Account.* **2017**, *46*, 507–534. [CrossRef]
46. McNamara, S.M.; Liyanatachchi, G.A. Time Budget pressure and auditor dysfunctional behaviour within an occupational stress model. *Account. Bus. Public Interest* **2008**, *7*, 1–43.
47. Umar, M.; Sitorus, S.M.; Surya, R.L.; Shauki, E.R.; Diyanti, V. Pressure, Dysfunctional Behavior, Fraud Detection and Role of Information Technology in the Audit Process. *Aust. Account. Bus. Financ. J.* **2017**, *11*, 102–115. [CrossRef]
48. Bennett, G.B.; Hartfield, R.C. Do Approaching Deadlines Influence Auditors' Materiality Assessments? *Audit. J. Pract. Theory* **2017**, *36*, 29–48. [CrossRef]
49. DeAngelo, L. Auditor size and audit quality. *J. Account. Econ.* **1981**, *3*, 189–199. [CrossRef]
50. DeZoort, F.T.; Lord, A.T. An Investigation of Obedience Pressure Effects in Auditor' Judgments. *Behav. Res. Account.* **1994**, *6*, 1–30.
51. Bagley, P.L. Negative Affect: A Consequence of Multiple Accountabilities in Auditing. *Audit. J. Pract. Theory* **2010**, *29*, 141–157. [CrossRef]
52. Fazli, S.; Muhammaddun, Z.; Ahmad, A. The Effects of Personal Organizational Factors on Role Ambiguity amongst Internal Auditors. *Int. J. Audit.* **2014**, *18*, 105–114. [CrossRef]
53. Goodwin, J.; Wu, D. What is the Relationship between Audit Partner Busyness and Audit Quality? *Contemp. Account. Res.* **2015**, *33*, 341–377. [CrossRef]
54. Brink, A.G.; Emerson, D.J.; Yang, L. Job Autonomy and Counterproductive Behaviors in Chinese Accountants: The Role of Job-Related Attitudes. *J. Int. Account. Res.* **2016**, *15*, 115–131. [CrossRef]
55. Knapp, C.A.; Knapp, M.C. The effects of experience and explicit fraud risk assessment in detecting fraud with analytical procedures. *Account. Organ. Soc.* **2001**, *26*, 25–37. [CrossRef]
56. Chen, C.-Y.; Lin, C.-J.; Lin, Y.-C. Audit Partner Tenure, Audit Firm Tenure, and Discretionary Accruals: Does Long Auditor Tenure Impair Earnings Quality? *Contemp. Account. Res.* **2008**, *25*, 415–445. [CrossRef]
57. Gul, F.A.; Fung, S.; Jaggi, B. Earnings quality: Some evidence on the role of auditor tenure and auditors' industry expertise. *J. Account. Econ.* **2009**, *47*, 265–287. [CrossRef]

58. Gul, F.A.; Ma, S.; Lai, K. Busy Auditors, Partner-Client Tenure, and Audit Quality. Evidence from an Emerging Market. *J. Int. Account. Res.* **2017**, *16*, 83–105. [CrossRef]
59. Pratt, J.; Jiambalvo, J. Relationships between leader behavior and audit team performance. *Account. Organ. Soc.* **1981**, *6*, 133–142. [CrossRef]
60. Nelson, M.W.; Proell, C.A.; Randel, A.E. Team-Oriented Leadership and Auditors' Willingness to Raise Audit Issues. *Account. Rev.* **2016**, *91*, 1781–1805. [CrossRef]
61. Eurofound. *European Working Conditions Survey Integrated Data File, 1991–2015, [Data Collection]*; SN: 7363; UK Data Service: Colchester, UK, 2017. [CrossRef]
62. Laher, S. Using exploratory factor analysis in personality research: Best-practice recommendations. *SA J. Ind. Psychol.* **2010**, *36*, 1–7. [CrossRef]
63. Cajal, B.; Jiménez, R.; Losilla, J.M.; Montaño, J.J.; Navarro, J.B.; Palmer, A.; Pitarque, A.; Portell, M.I.; Rodrigo, M.F.; Ruíz, J.C.; et al. Las redes neuronales artificiales en psicología: Un estudio bibliométrico. *Metodología de las Ciencias del Comportamiento* **2001**, *3*, 53–64.
64. Bonilla, M.; Puertas, R. *Análisis de las Redes Neuronales: Aplicación a Problemas de Predicción y Clasificación Financiera*; Servei de Publicacions, Universitat de València: Valencia, Spain, 1997.
65. West, P.; Brockett, P.; Golden, L. A comparative analysis of neural networks and statistical methods for predicting consumer choice. *Mark. Sci.* **1997**, *16*, 370–391. [CrossRef]
66. Pitarque, A.; Ruiz, J.C.; Roy, J.F. Las redes neuronales como herramientas estadísticas no paramétricas de clasificación. *Psicothema* **2000**, *12*, 459–463.
67. Huang, G.B.; Zhu, Q.Y.; Siew, C.K. Extreme Learning Machine: Theory and Applications. *Neurocomputing* **2006**, *70*, 489–501. [CrossRef]
68. Sobol, I.M. Global sensitivity indices for nonlinear mathematical models and their monte carlo estimates. *Math. Comput. Simul.* **2001**, *55*, 271–280. [CrossRef]
69. Fernandez Navarro, F.; Carbonero, M.; Becerra, D.; Torres, M. Global Sensitivity Estimates for Neural networks classifiers. *IEEE Trans. Neural Netw. Learn. Syst.* **2017**, *28*, 2592–2604. [CrossRef] [PubMed]
70. Jensen, M.C.; Meckling, W.H. Theory of the firm: Managerial behavior, agency costs and ownership structure. *J. Financ. Econ.* **1976**, *3*, 305–360. [CrossRef]
71. Ashbaugh, H.; Warfield, T.D. Audits as a Corporate Governance Mechanism: Evidence from the German Market. *J. Int. Account. Res.* **2003**, *2*, 1–21. [CrossRef]
72. Durendez Gómez-Guillamón, A. The usefulness of the audit report in investment and financing decisions. *Manag. Audit. J.* **2003**, *18*, 549–559. [CrossRef]
73. Watts, R.L.; Zimmerman, J.L. Towards a Positive Theory of the Determination of Accounting Standards. *Account. Rev.* **1978**, *53*, 112–134.
74. Collins, K.M.; Killough, L.N. An Empirical Examination of Stress in Public Accounting. *Account. Organ. Soc.* **1992**, *17*, 535–547. [CrossRef]

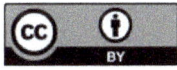

© 2018 by the authors. Licensee MDPI, Basel, Switzerland. This article is an open access article distributed under the terms and conditions of the Creative Commons Attribution (CC BY) license (http://creativecommons.org/licenses/by/4.0/).

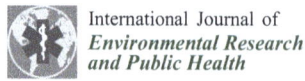

Article

Challenging Cognitive Demands at Work, Related Working Conditions, and Employee Well-Being

Sophie-Charlotte Meyer * and Lena Hünefeld

German Federal Institute for Occupational Safety and Health, D-44149 Dortmund, Germany; Huenefeld.Lena@baua.bund.de
* Correspondence: meyer.sophie-charlotte@baua.bund.de; Tel.: +49-(0)-231-9071-2709

Received: 8 October 2018; Accepted: 11 December 2018; Published: 19 December 2018

Abstract: In times of digitalized workplaces the extent of challenging cognitive demands at work is rising and employees increasingly have to manage new and unlearned tasks. Yet, these work characteristics have received little attention on how they relate to the worker's well-being. Thus, we analyze associations between cognitive work demands—also in interaction with other job characteristics—and indicators of employee well-being. The analyses are based on the BIBB/BAuA Employment Survey 2018, a cross-section that is representative for the German working population and covers approximately 20,000 employed individuals. Ordinary least squares (OLS) regressions suggest that cognitive demands are associated with a higher probability of feeling fatigued. In contrast, the results with respect to the employees' self-rated health status and job satisfaction are ambiguous, depending on which cognitive demand is considered. Overall, the findings indicate that cognitive demands might be related to both resource and demand, depending on the individual resources of employees.

Keywords: cognitive demands; occupational health; employee well-being; working conditions

1. Introduction

The world of work is undergoing permanent changes, which imply new challenges for organizations and individuals [1]. In globalized markets, organizations need to be more flexible, less hierarchical, and continually reorganizing to maintain competitiveness and prosperity. Furthermore, changes in the world of work are enabled and accelerated by digitization processes [2–4]. On the one hand, new technologies—such as information and communication technologies—are introduced as a strategy for adapting to constant market pressure. On the other hand, new technologies are again the basis for fundamental reorganization within organizations [5]. This results in a cycle of changes and the developments occur at an increased speed [3,4]. Overall, the world of work becomes more flexible, more unpredictable, and changes at an accelerated pace.

All these phenomena involve altered job demands for employees and lead to changes in job quality. Besides an intensification of work effort [6–8], as well as planning and decision-making demands [9–11], increases in cognitive and learning demands at work are discussed as outcomes of change in the working world [2,12,13]. Generating new knowledge, as well as problem solving, has become an integral part of employees' work tasks [14,15]. Furthermore, employees have to acquire new skills constantly in order to adapt to rapidly changing demands at work [12]. Therefore, maintaining one's skills has become more difficult due to increasing skill variety in recent years [11] and employees are more frequently confronted with tasks they have not learned or they are not familiar with. Coping with the new requirements and tasks is becoming increasingly relevant, not only for everyday working life but also for personal development, regarding competencies and skills learned in order to maintain employability [16–18].

In the past decades, research on the quality of work has often focused on work intensification and autonomy [19], showing that an appropriate balance between work requirements and autonomy is particularly important for a good quality of work, and in turn for employee well-being [20–27]. However, empirical studies on learning and cognitive demands are scarce and so far little is known about how these demands relate to the well-being of employees. The existing studies predominantly focus on learning demands and point to an ambivalent picture regarding the relationship between these demands and employee well-being [13,28]. Moreover, the studies are based on non-representative survey data with small sample sizes, rendering it difficult to generalize the findings for the entire working population. There is also no distinct definition between learning or cognitive demands and both terms are largely used interchangeably. While both refer to confrontation with new tasks at work and the requirement to acquire new knowledge, learning demands can be understood as a superordinate term that includes cognitive demands [29]. In general, learning demands can be defined as demands which "require employees to acquire knowledge and skills that are necessary to perform their jobs effectively" [13]. Cognitive demands involve confrontation with new tasks, unpredictable developments, and solving routine problems [28]. Using this definition, it remains unclear whether an individual learning process is achieved or not and which demands contribute to the cognitive development of the employees [30].

In this study, we add to the existing literature and empirically explore the relationship between cognitive demands and employee well-being. The analyses are based on the German BIBB/BAuA Employment Survey 2018, a large representative cross-section providing recent data on the work and health situation of the working population in Germany (approximately 20,000 respondents). In a first step, we explore the determinants of cognitive demands in order to identify groups frequently facing cognitive demands at work. To measure cognitive demands, we considere three different variables: facing new tasks, improving work, and doing unlearned things. Analyzing the status quo is crucial in order to identify groups of workers with an increased need for additional training or assistance to cope with new requirements. This is of particular relevance as cognitive demands will likely become more prominent in the future and will gradually affect the whole working population. In a second step, we analyze the relationship between cognitive demands—also in interaction with other work demands—and employee well-being. We consider indicator variables for fatigue, self-rated health, and job satisfaction to measure employee well-being.

2. Work–Stress Theories and the Role of Cognitive Demands

Researchers developed different theoretical models to describe the relationship between different working conditions and employee health (e.g., Job Demands Control Model (JDC) [25], Job Demands-Resources Model (JD-R) [31], or Action Regulation Theory (ART) [32]. While these models consider various working conditions, only a few explicitly include cognitive demands. In the context of our study, two models are of particular importance. Firstly, we rely on the integrated model of psychosocial work characteristics and the consequences of job strain introduced by Glaser et al. [28]. Based on various theories and models [33–35] on the impact of working conditions on attitudes and health, the authors [28] developed a model embedding learning demands, work-related resources, and job stressors in order to predict processes of learning, performance, and health impairment. An important assumption of this model—in line with Karasek [25]—is that not all working conditions should be defined as job demands, regardless of their impact on employee well-being. When cognitive demands are predisposed as working conditions that trigger effort-driven processes and are thus associated with physical and psychological costs, the potential positive effects of cognitive demands for skill acquisition and performance are neglected. The absence of cognitive demands at work could also be negatively related to employee well-being and motivation [28]. Therefore, the authors combine the assumptions of different work-stress theories, including the challenge–hindrance framework that distinguishes between challenge and hindrance demands [36]. Hindrance demands are supposed to reduce personal growth and promote strain and health impairments [36,37]. Challenge demands also trigger strain, but they are also supposed to have a motivating effect and enable employees to learn and to further develop their own personality. The classification of job demands as challenge or hindrance demands depends on the individual assessment of employees. Therefore, the cognitive appraisals (challenge and hindrance appraisal) of individuals are the important explanatory mechanisms behind the positive and negative effects of job demands on a workers well-being [13,38–40]. In line with this framework, Glaser et al. [28] distinguish between beneficial learning (e.g., task variety and cognitive demands), work-related resources (e.g., autonomy and social support), and stressors or adverse conditions (e.g., overload and conflicts). The proposed model predicts a positive effect of learning demands on personality development and a negative effect of stressors or adverse conditions on health. Empirical analyses exploring this model indicate that problem solving and learning requirements are crucial for creativity and motivation. Other studies confirm these results. For instance, Prem et al. [13] find a significant relationship between learning demands and personal development. Personal development was in turn positively associated with vitality in this study. Furthermore, Crawford et al. [41] show that the correlation between work demands and engagement strongly depends on the specific type of work demand. Demands that were appraised by workers as hindrance were negatively associated with engagement and demands that were appraised by workers as challenges were positively associated with engagement. However, the study of Glaser et al. [28] also showed that learning requirements may be detrimental to health if accompanied by work overload. The authors thus demonstrate—in line with other studies [30,42]—the importance of the interaction of cognitive demands with other working conditions for employee well-being. Based on the model of Glaser et al. [28], we assume that cognitive demands might be both positively and negatively related to the personal development of employees, and in turn also to their attitudes and health. Furthermore, we assume that autonomy and work intensification moderate the effect of cognitive demands on employee well-being.

Secondly, person–environment fit theories (P–E fit) are crucial to explain why cognitive demands at work could have different consequences for different groups of employees. All P–E fit theories assume that the extent to which people fit their work environments has significant consequences (e.g., with respect to their satisfaction, performance, stress, productivity, or turnover). A better fit is associated with better outcomes [43–45]. Moreover, Kristof-Brown and Guay [46] showed that stress is a consequence of a poor person–environment fit. The fit of the individual and the environment is determined by the fulfilment of needs resulting in favorable attitudes, such as job satisfaction or organizational commitment [47,48]. In addition, P–E fit is a reciprocal and ongoing process whereby individuals shape their environments and environments shape individuals [49]. Work environments are associated with cognitive demands to varying degrees. Furthermore, individuals also differ in terms of their needs at work and require different conditions in order to achieve favorable attitudes. In line with the P–E fit theories, we suppose that cognitive demands at work do not equally meet the needs of different employment groups. Consequently, we expect that the probability of perceiving cognitive demands at work as stressful varies across different groups of employees (e.g., with respect to different socio-demographic groups, such as gender or educational level).

3. Data and Methods

The analyses are based on the BIBB/BAuA Employment Survey 2018, a representative cross-sectional survey covering approximately 20,000 employed individuals in Germany who work at least 10 h per week and are at least 15 years old [50] (see Table A1 for an overview). The BIBB/BAuA Employment Survey is representative for the German labor force, including employed as well as self-employed individuals, and covers various occupational groups. For the analyses, we exclude individuals above the age of 65, as working individuals above that age (age 65 ≈ statutory retirement age in Germany) are a selective and highly heterogeneous group (e.g., self-employed, as well as individuals depending on additional income to increase their pension). Further, the analyses are restricted to individuals with valid data for the included variables. The analysis sample amounts to 18,554 individuals, although the number of observations varies slightly according to the analyses performed. The sample consists of 54.5% men and 45.5% women, with the majority (51.2%) being aged between 35–54 years (see Table A2 in Appendix A). Before the BIBB/BAuA Employment Survey 2018 has been carried out, it has been inspected and received a positive vote of the ethics commission.

3.1. Variables

The BIBB/BAuA Employment Survey 2018 includes three different variables indicating cognitive demands: facing new tasks, improving work, and doing unlearned things. We consider all of the three items in order to cover different dimensions of cognitive demands. Although the wording of the questions on cognitive demands is not identical, the indicators are still comparable to those used in previous studies [13,28]. The respondents were asked how often they face these demands during their work and the response scale was frequently, sometimes, rarely, never (see Table 1). In order to keep the analyses simple and reduce complexity, we recode the variables into indicator variables. For new tasks and improving work, these dichotomous variables equal 1 if someone reports to experience a cognitive demand frequently and 0 otherwise. As comparatively few individuals report doing unlearned things frequently, we collapse sometimes and frequently into one category for this variable.

Table 1. Distribution of cognitive demands.

	How Frequently Does It Happen during Your Work ...	Frequently	Sometimes	Rarely	Never	N	Stressful? (If Frequently)
New tasks	... that you are faced with new tasks that you have to try to understand and become familiar with?	40.2	39.9	15.0	5.0	19,509	18.3
Improve work	... that you improve previous procedures or try out something new?	29.2	44.8	17.6	8.4	19,485	n.a.
Unlearned things	... that you are required to do things that you have not learned or do not have a mastery of?	8.2	28.6	29.2	34.0	19,489	42.16

Source: Own calculations based on the BIBB/BAuA Employment Survey 2018, weighted results.

A special feature of the BIBB/BAuA Employment Survey is that individuals who report frequently facing a specific job demand are subsequently asked whether or not they perceive this job demand as stressful. This allows us to take the individual assessment whether the specific cognitive demand is perceived as a resource or rather as a demand into account. For the variable "improve work", the question whether it is stressful or not was not asked, as this question was not defined as a stressor due to its rather positive meaning.

Employee well-being is operationalized by three different outcomes. Work-related fatigue (yes = 1, no = 0) is based on the question of whether the respondent has frequently suffered from emotional exhaustion in the last 12 months during work, on working days, or both. A comparable dichotomous measure of fatigue is collected within the European Working Conditions Survey (EWCS) and has been previously used to study work-related differences in well-being [51]. Moreover, respondents were asked about their general state of health, which was recoded into an indicator variable for self-rated good health (excellent/very good/good = 1, not so good/poor = 0). Self-rated health has been a widely used measure and it was found that it likely considers chronic and acute illnesses [52,53]. Finally, we consider overall job satisfaction (by asking the question: "And now, all things considered, how satisfied are you with your work on the whole?"), recoded into an indicator variable (very satisfied/satisfied = 1, less satisfied/not satisfied = 0), as a measure for overall well-being. Single-item measures of global job satisfaction have been found to be as reliable as multiple-item measures [54].

As additional working conditions, we consider a measure for work intensity (by asking the question: "How frequently does it happen during your work that you have to work under great time pressure or pressure to perform?"), as well as an indicator for the respondent's autonomy at work (by asking the question: "How frequently does it occur that you can plan and arrange your own work yourself?"). These variables equal 1 if the individuals report frequently facing the working conditions, and 0 otherwise (sometimes/rarely/never).

As control variables, we include gender, three age groups (15–34, 35–54, 55–65), three dummies for schooling (low, intermediate, high), four dummies for the occupational status, as well as five sector dummies (see Table A2 in Appendix A).

3.2. Methods

For ease of interpretation, we performed Ordinary Least Squares (OLS) regression analyses with robust standard errors. We thus applied linear probability models, given that the cognitive demands, as well as the health outcome measures, were coded as indicator variables. Coefficients may thus be interpreted as differences in the probability of the outcome variable—in this case facing a specific cognitive demand or a certain health condition. Given that linear and logistic models often render very similar results, we preferred this model, as this interpretation is much more intuitive and fits the research questions studied somewhat better compared to the interpretation of other methods (e.g., odds ratios derived from logistic regressions) [55]. In order to adjust for the violation of homoscedasticity, heteroscedasticity-consistent standard errors were applied.

In a first step, we explored the determinants of cognitive demands by regressing the cognitive demands on the control variables to get an idea of the groups frequently facing cognitive demands at work. Second, we explored whether, and to what extent, cognitive demands are related to employee well-being. We additionally exploited the information on whether or not the specific cognitive demand is perceived as stressful by restricting the analyses to those reporting to be frequently facing new tasks or doing unlearned things. In doing so, we aimed to make an effort in testing the P–E fit (see Section 2) and assess whether the cognitive demands are related to health or whether it depends on the individual's characteristics. Moreover, these analyses enabled us to estimate the relationship between cognitive demands and health at the intensive margin, and thus mitigate the potential bias resulting from selection into the extent of facing cognitive demands. Previous studies suggest that cognitive demands might be harmful if they co-occur with work overload [28]. Therefore, in the final analyses we included interaction terms between one specific cognitive demand (i.e., doing unlearned things) and two working conditions (work intensity and autonomy) in the regressions of well-being. As a result, we were able to assess whether or not facing high work intensity or autonomy moderates the relationship between this cognitive demand and employee well-being. We focused on this cognitive demand as our analyses revealed that it is strongly related to adverse health or well-being, and, therefore, can be interpreted as a stressor. Work intensity and job autonomy were chosen, as according to common work–stress theories, their importance for employee well-being is well explored and widely accepted. Both the measures for cognitive demands and working conditions were operationalized as indicator variables, and thus the interaction terms between these two variables can be interpreted as follows: a positive interaction suggests that the working condition strengthens the association between the specific cognitive demand and employee well-being, while a negative interaction term mitigates the association.

4. Results

4.1. Distribution of Cognitive Demands

Table 1 summarizes the variables for cognitive demands studied in this paper. A vast majority reported to facing new tasks sometimes (39.9%) or even frequently (40.2%). Similarly, about three quarters of the respondents stated they were either sometimes or frequently required to improve procedures or try out something new. Doing unlearned things during work was less common; only 8.2% reported that their job frequently required doing things they had not learned or were not able to perform. With respect to facing new tasks at work, this applied to 18.3%. Among those doing unlearned things frequently, 42.16% perceived it as stressful.

4.2. Heterogeneity in Cognitive Demands Across Groups

As a first step, we explored the determinants of workers facing the three different types of cognitive demands at work by regressing the cognitive demands on socio-demographic characteristics (Table 2, Columns 1–3). Table 2 shows the results and each column presents the estimates of a separate regression model taking the different measures of cognitive demands as dependent variables. In general, women faced cognitive demands at work significantly less often as compared to male employees. For instance, the probability of facing new tasks at work is 7 percentage points lower for women. With respect to age, we found that middle-aged and older workers were significantly less likely to perform any of the cognitive tasks explored as compared to younger workers. High-educated individuals faced cognitive demands more often than low-educated, whereas the estimate for intermediate-educated individuals turns out to be significant for facing new tasks only. For new tasks, the educational differences in cognitive demands were most pronounced; high-educated individuals had a 19 percentage point higher probability to face new tasks at work compared to low-educated individuals. Regarding occupational status, white-collar employees, civil servants, and self-employed individuals are significantly more likely to experience cognitive demands at work as compared to blue-collar workers. Moreover, the results indicate that cognitive demands are most common within the manufacture sector, while they are less common in the service sector.

Table 2. Determinants of Cognitive Demands (OLS Regression).

	New Tasks	Improve Work	Unlearned Things	Demand is Stressful [A]	
				New Tasks	Unlearned Things
Gender					
Men	Reference	Reference	Reference	Reference	Reference
Women	−0.0761 ***	−0.0427 ***	−0.0248 ***	0.0442 ***	0.0966 ***
	(0.0075)	(0.0071)	(0.0075)	(0.0090)	(0.0267)
Age					
15–34	Reference	Reference	Reference	Reference	Reference
35–54	−0.0225 *	−0.0207 *	−0.0276 **	0.0340 **	−0.023
	(0.0100)	(0.0096)	(0.0100)	(0.0104)	(0.0314)
55–65	−0.0521 ***	−0.0634 ***	−0.0684 ***	0.0988 ***	0.0901 *
	(0.0110)	(0.0104)	(0.0110)	(0.0127)	(0.0371)
Schooling					
Low	Reference	Reference	Reference	Reference	Reference
Intermediate	0.0565 ***	0.0153	0.0221	−0.0282	−0.0214
	(0.0114)	(0.0102)	(0.0115)	(0.0181)	(0.0427)
High	0.1924 ***	0.1154 ***	0.0714 ***	−0.0713 ***	−0.0916 *
	(0.0115)	(0.0104)	(0.0116)	(0.0176)	(0.0421)
Occupational status					
Blue-collar	Reference	Reference	Reference	Reference	Reference
White-collar	0.1193 ***	0.0985 ***	0.0551 ***	−0.0334	−0.047
	(0.0117)	(0.0102)	(0.0119)	(0.0186)	(0.0437)
Civil sevant	0.1847 ***	0.1498 ***	0.1793 ***	0.0385	0.0376
	(0.0181)	(0.0166)	(0.0181)	(0.0254)	(0.0610)
Self-employed	0.2003 ***	0.2207 ***	0.0273	−0.0706 **	−0.1430 *
	(0.0178)	(0.0167)	(0.0176)	(0.0222)	(0.0620)
Sector					
Public sector	Reference	Reference	Reference	Reference	Reference
Manufacture	0.0690 ***	0.0622 ***	0.0374 **	−0.0663 ***	−0.1013 *
	(0.0115)	(0.0110)	(0.0116)	(0.0135)	(0.0412)
Craft	−0.0033	−0.0444 ***	0.0336 *	−0.0964 ***	−0.1455 **
	(0.0151)	(0.0134)	(0.0151)	(0.0185)	(0.0526)
Service	−0.0332 ***	−0.0329 ***	−0.0180	−0.0710 ***	−0.0783 *
	(0.0099)	(0.0091)	(0.0098)	(0.0126)	(0.0375)
Other	−0.0352 **	−0.0085	0.0103	−0.0335	−0.0827
	(0.0135)	(0.0126)	(0.0135)	(0.0175)	(0.0478)
Constant	0.2719 ***	0.1964 ***	0.3209 ***	0.2486 ***	0.5362 ***
	(0.0173)	(0.0159)	(0.0175)	(0.0254)	(0.0627)
Adj. R^2	0.0538	0.0388	0.0170	0.0345	0.0460
N	18,554	18,532	18,535	8235	1561

[A] Corresponds to the subgroup of individuals who reported frequently facing the specific cognitive demand; Note: * $p < 0.05$, ** $p < 0.01$, *** $p < 0.001$; Robust standard errors in parentheses. Source: Own calculations based on the BIBB/BAuA Employment Survey 2018, unweighted results.

Interestingly, the results were opposed (Table 2, Columns 4 and 5) when we focused on the subjective perception of cognitive demands with respect to the question on whether it is stressful or not (given the respondent faced the specific cognitive demand frequently).; the probability of perceiving new tasks or doing unlearned things at work as stressful was significantly higher for women and older people as well as low-educated individuals.

4.3. Cognitive Demands and Well-Being

In the next step, we assessed whether cognitive demands were related to indicators of well-being (Table 3, Columns 1–3). Again, each column reports the estimates of separate regressions taking the different indicators of well-being as dependent variables. Overall the estimates revealed that cognitive demands played an important role for employee well-being—independent from their socio-demographic characteristics. With respect to fatigue, it turned out that all cognitive demands considered were associated with a higher probability of feeling fatigued. For instance, doing unlearned things sometimes or frequently was associated with a 10.6 percentage point higher probability of suffering from fatigue during work or on working days. Regarding overall health, the results varied across the different cognitive demands. While the probability of reporting to be in good health was not significantly related to facing new tasks at work, it was positively correlated with improving work. In contrast, doing unlearned things was associated with a reduced probability of reporting good health. Regarding job satisfaction, it turned out that on average, individuals facing new tasks and improving work frequently were more likely to be satisfied with their job. On the contrary, doing unlearned things was often associated with lower job satisfaction. The results indicate that cognitive demands might be related to both resource and demand.

Table 3. Cognitive Demands and Well-Being (OLS Regression).

	Fatigue	Overall Health	Satisfaction	Demand is Stressful [A]		
				Fatigue	Overall Health	Satisfaction
Cognitive demands						
New tasks	0.0289 ***	−0.0038	0.0138 **	0.1665 ***	−0.0867 **	−0.0826 **
	(0.0073)	(0.0056)	(0.0046)	(0.0383)	(0.0334)	(0.0299)
Improve work	0.0184 *	0.0147 **	0.0252 ***			
	(0.0077)	(0.0056)	(0.0045)			
Unlearned things	0.1064 ***	−0.0454 ***	−0.0510 ***	0.2227 ***	−0.1065 ***	−0.1312 ***
	(0.0071)	(0.0055)	(0.0046)	(0.0356)	(0.0287)	(0.0255)
Adj. R^2	0.0339	0.0396	0.0149	0.1256	0.1282	0.0591
N	18,453	18,462	18,475	1146	1151	1151

[A] Corresponds to the subgroup of individuals who reported frequently facing the specific cognitive demand; Note: * $p < 0.05$, ** $p < 0.01$, *** $p < 0.001$; Robust standard errors in parentheses; control variables included gender as well as dummies for age group, schooling, occupational status, and sector (see Table 2). Source: Own calculations based on the BIBB/BAuA Employment Survey 2018, unweighted results.

The relationship between cognitive demands and well-being might be (partly) driven by whether or not individuals perceive the respective cognitive demand as stressful. For that reason, we now focus on individuals facing cognitive demands frequently and compare those perceiving it as stressful to those who do not regard it as a stressor (Table 3, Columns 4–6). As expected, the estimates became much larger. Perceiving it stressful to face new tasks or to do unlearned things at work was significantly associated with adverse health, e.g., with a higher probability of feeling fatigued but also with a lower probability of being satisfied with the job.

4.4. Cognitive Demands, Interactions with Other Working Conditions, and Well-Being

Table 4 reports the results of the interaction models with each column presenting the results of a separate regression. The models presented in Table 4 differ from the model estimated in Table 3, as the other cognitive demands (new tasks and improve work) are not included. For this reason, we also report the results for the relationship between unlearned things and the indicators for well-being where work intensity and autonomy have not been included (Table 4, Column 1, 3, 5). However, the estimates are quantitatively and qualitatively comparable to those presented in Table 4.

Table 4. Cognitive Demands, Interactions with Work Intensity and Autonomy, and Well-Being (OLS Regression).

	Fatigue	Fatigue	Overall Health	Overall Health	Satisfaction	Satisfaction
Cognitive demands						
Unlearned things	0.1148 ***	0.1234 ***	−0.0449 ***	−0.0578 ***	−0.0450 ***	−0.0649 ***
	(0.0069)	(0.0153)	(0.0053)	(0.0128)	(0.0045)	(0.0114)
Other working conditions						
Work intensity		0.1561 ***		−0.0713 ***		−0.0557 ***
		(0.0081)		(0.0064)		(0.0050)
Autonomy		−0.0282 **		0.0414 ***		0.0682 ***
		(0.0091)		(0.0077)		(0.0064)
Interactions						
Unlearned things × work intensity		0.0077		−0.0049		0.0031
		(0.0138)		(0.0106)		(0.0088)
Unlearned things × autonomy		−0.0437 **		0.0314 *		0.0310 **
		(0.0158)		(0.0133)		(0.0119)
Adj. R^2	0.0324	0.0654	0.0397	0.0550	0.0123	0.0380
N	18,491	17,839	18,499	17,845	18,513	17,861

Note: * $p < 0.05$, ** $p < 0.01$, *** $p < 0.001$; Robust standard errors in parentheses; control variables included gender as well as dummies for age group, schooling, occupational status, and sector (see Table 2). Source: Own calculations based on the BIBB/BAuA Employment Survey 2018, unweighted results.

The interaction terms (Table 4, Column 2, 4, 6) revealed that work autonomy likely buffers the adverse relationship between cognitive demands (i.e., doing unlearned things) and employee well-being to some extent. While doing unlearned things was related to a 12.3 percentage point higher probability of feeling fatigued for those employees experiencing little autonomy at work, the association was reduced by 4.4 percentage points for those individuals reporting a high level of job autonomy. The same was also true with respect to overall health and job satisfaction. For instance, while doing unlearned things was related to a 5.8 percentage point lower probability of being in good health for individuals with a low level of job autonomy, the negative association was about half as strong for employees with a high level of autonomy. Regarding work intensity, the interactions turned out to be insignificant and quantitatively negligible.

5. Discussion and Conclusions

Cognitive Demands are an integral part of work environments nowadays. However, these demands have received little attention on how they relate to employee well-being. Based on the integrated model of psychosocial work characteristics and consequences of strain [28], we assumed that cognitive demands might be both positively and negatively related to the employees' attitudes and health. Furthermore, based on P–E fit theories, we expected that the perception of whether cognitive demands are stressful or not would largely depend on socio-demographic and work-related characteristics.

The theoretical assumptions were largely supported and the main result of our study is that cognitive demands play an important role in the workers' well-being. Our analyses suggest that all cognitive demands considered are associated with a higher probability of feeling fatigued. However, with respect to self-rated overall health status and job satisfaction, the results are ambiguous, depending on the specific cognitive demand considered. On the one hand, improving work is positively related to good health and job satisfaction, while doing unlearned things is negatively associated with these outcomes. Therefore, the results indicate that cognitive demands might be related to both resource and demand—depending on the specific type of cognitive demand. These findings emphasize the immanent assumption of Glaser et al.'s [28] model that a fine-grained distinction of job demands is needed to analyze the associations between working conditions and the employees' attitudes and health. Furthermore, the results strengthen the theoretical challenge–hindrance framework. Cognitive demands trigger strain, but they can also have a satisfying effect. That is because cognitive demands often involve task variation or learning, which likely improves the employees' personal development and might thus be health-enhancing in the long run [19]. However, how the cognitive demands are designed seems to be crucial, and whether or not these demands co-occur with other job demands and if employees assess cognitive demands as stressful. While facing new tasks and improving work are to some extent positively related to well-being, doing unlearned things is consistently negatively related to employee well-being. In addition, perception of stress in relation to facing new tasks or to doing unlearned things at work is significantly associated with a higher probability of feeling fatigued, but also with a lower probability of being satisfied with the job. This result strengthens the importance of the challenge and hindrance appraisal as an explanatory mechanism for the relationship between cognitive demands and well-being. The challenge appraisal thus reflects the perception of situations enabling personal development. In contrast, the hindrance appraisal is related to individual frustration due to the prevention of the fulfilment of self-relevant goals [13,38,40]. The interaction analyses further reveal that autonomy might mitigate the negative association between doing unlearned things and well-being to some extent. In line with previous studies and theories, this finding further emphasizes the role of autonomy as an important resource to buffer stressors at work [34,56]. Overall, our findings support the idea that specific working conditions might be related to both demand and resource and that more research based on integrated models of different working conditions, including cognitive demands, are needed.

Moreover, our analyses on the determinants of cognitive demands reveal that different groups of employees face cognitive demands at work to varying degrees. A vast majority reported facing new tasks at work, while doing unlearned things during work was less common. This might partly be attributable to the relatively negative wording of this question (see Table 1). Moreover, the three variables are also different from a theoretical perspective; performing new tasks and improving procedures at work also refer to task variation, which might be interpreted as a resource, not only as a stressor. The analyses also indicate that the extent to which individuals perceive cognitive demands as stressful varies across different groups of employees. High-educated employees most frequently report facing cognitive demands as compared to low-educated employees. As expected, this suggests that knowledge-intensive occupations in particular are exposed to cognitive demands. In contrast, the probability of perceiving cognitive demands at work as stressful is significantly higher for low-educated individuals. This is in accordance with the assumptions derived from the P–E fit theories. Cognitive demands are an integral part of the work of high-educated employees and thus probably also a significant part of the satisfaction of needs. It can also be assumed that highly educated individuals are more likely to actively ask for new tasks to reach job satisfaction of needs. In addition, high-educated employees often dispose of more resources at work, such as a higher level of autonomy, as compared to low-educated employees [57]. Our findings emphasize that the match of individual needs and requirements in the workplace is crucial. Future research should focus on this in more depth in order to investigate the impact of different cognitive demands with regard to content and varying degrees of difficulty on the attitudes and health of different employment groups.

5.1. Limitations

Although this study is the first examining the relationship between cognitive demands and employee well-being based on a large data set representative for the German working population, there are some limitations that have to be acknowledged. First, the interpretation is limited due to the cross-sectional nature of the study. Thus, the analyses allow alternative explanations as we are not able to account for reverse causality or unobserved heterogeneity. Consequently, future research should elaborate on this, for example by replicating the analyses within a longitudinal study design.

Second, all measures were based on self-reports from participants, raising the risk of overestimated results due to common method biases [58]. However, various authors point out that subjective views are certainly an important indicator of objective health-related outcomes [59]. Self-reports may not be too problematic when investigating interaction effects: Common method effects are likely attenuating rather than strengthening interactions [60]. Third, we used single items to measure cognitive demands. Although single item measures are found to be valid [55,61], studies and theories presented at the beginning of the paper suggest that cognitive demands might be a multi-dimensional concept on which future research should focus on. Finally, our analyses are based on the whole working population rendering knowledge on the relationship between cognitive demands and employee well-being in a general sense, which can be interpreted as a first step in discovering this issue. In order to better understand this relationship, future research should elaborate on the heterogeneity across groups, for example by performing subgroup analyses with respect to gender, age groups, and educational level, but also occupations. This is crucial in order to derive concrete recommendations for action.

5.2. Practical Implications

This study adds to the limited research on the relationship between cognitive demands and employee well-being. Our results indicate that cognitive demands are both stressors and resources. Considering the rise of new (communication) technologies [62], cognitive demands at work seem to be an important but widely neglected topic in modern societies. On the one hand, the results underline the beneficial effects of cognitive demands at work. Cognitive demands should be included in work tasks, giving employees the opportunity to improve their personal development. However, the cognitive demands should not over-strain employees. Organizations have the responsibility to design workplaces according to the needs of their employees. To ensure that the employer is informed about the cognitive demands of their employees, cognitive demands should also be included in the risk assessment and be a part of employee appraisals. Furthermore, organizations could create competence teams in which employees could exchange information on new challenges and learn from each other. Finally, organizations should offer additional training in order to support employees in developing individual coping strategies by considering the needs of different groups of employees.

Author Contributions: Conceptualization, S.-C.M. and L.H.; data curation, S.-C.M.; methodology, S.-C.M.; writing—original draft, S.-C.M. and L.H.

Funding: This research received no external funding.

Acknowledgments: We would like to thank three anonymous referees for their valuable comments which helped to improve earlier versions of this paper.

Conflicts of Interest: The authors declare no conflict of interest.

Appendix A

Table A1. Overview of BIBB/BAuA Employment Survey.

	BIBB/BAuA Employment Survey
Data owner	German Federal Institute for Vocational Education and Training (BIBB) and the German Federal Institute for Occupational Safety and Health (BAuA)
Survey	Repeated cross-section, conducted every six years (comparable since 2006); Latest survey carried out in 2018
Interview	Telephone interviews (CATI) since 2006
Sample	Approximately 20.000 employees

Table A1. *Cont.*

	BIBB/BAuA Employment Survey
Target population	Representative for the German working population; Includes individuals belonging to the labor force (having a paid work), aged 15 and over, with a regular work time of at least 10 h per week. Apprentices are excluded.
Purpose of Data Collection	Research according to the research programs of BIBB and BAuA; Aim to provide differentiated and representative information regarding the working population and jobs in Germany for quantitative employment and qualification research as well as for occupational health and safety reporting.
Subjects	Among others: Working conditions, work load, work-related health, main fields of responsibility, level of requirements, knowledge requirements, work requirements, need for advanced training, school education, vocational and advanced training, professional career, employment that is adequate to the vocational training, career changes, applicability of professional qualifications
Further information	https://www.bibb.de/en/12138.php

Table A2. Sample Statistics.

Variables	%
Cognitive Demands	
New tasks (frequently)	40.2
Improve work (frequently)	29.2
Unlearned things (frequently/sometimes)	36.8
Gender	
Men	54.5
Women	45.5
Age	
15–34	27.2
35–54	51.2
55–65	21.7
Schooling	
Low	22.4
Intermediate	38.1
High	39.6
Occupational status	
Blue-collar	18.7
White-collar	68.4
Civil sevant	5.4
Self-employed	7.5
Sector	
Public sector	25.0
Manufacture	20.6
Craft	11.7
Service	32.3
Other	10.4
Work intensity (frequently)	
Time pressure/pressure to perform	48.2
Autonomy (frequently)	
Arranging own work	65.4

Source: Own calculations based on the BIBB/BAuA employment survey 2018, weighted results.

References

1. Cascio, W.F. The changing world of work. In *Oxford Handbook of Positive Psychology and Work*; Linley, P.A., Harrington, S., Garcea, N., Eds.; Oxford University Press: Oxford, UK, 2010; pp. 13–14.
2. Korunka, C.; Kubicek, B. Job Demands in a Changing World of Work. In *Job Demands in a Changing World of Work*; Springer: Berlin, Germany, 2017; pp. 1–5.
3. Rosa, H. *Alienation and Acceleration: Towards a Critical Theory of Late-Modern Temporality*; NSU Press: Malmö, Sweden, 2010.
4. Rosa, H. *High-Speed Society: Social Acceleration, Power, and Modernity*; Penn State Press: University Park, PA, USA, 2010.
5. Castells, M. *The Rise of the Network Society*; John Wiley & Sons: Oxford, UK, 2011.
6. Burchell, B.; Ladipo, D.; Wilkinson, F. *Job Insecurity and Work Intensification*; Routledge: Abingdon, UK, 2005.
7. Green, F. Work intensification, discretion, and the decline in well-being at work. *East. Econ. J.* **2004**, *30*, 615–625.
8. Green, F.; McIntosh, S. The intensification of work in Europe. *Labour Econ.* **2001**, *8*, 291–308. [CrossRef]
9. Allvin, M.; Aronsson, G.; Hagström, T.; Johansson, G.; Lundberg, U. *Work Without Boundaries: Psychological Perspectives on the New Working Life*; John Wiley & Sons: Hoboken, NJ, USA, 2011.
10. Flecker, J.; Fibich, T.; Kraemer, K. Socio-economic changes and the reorganization of work. In *Job Demands in a Changing World of Work*; Springer: Berlin, Germany, 2017; pp. 7–24.
11. Wood, L.A. *The Changing Nature of Jobs: A Meta-Analysis Examining Changes in Job Characterisitcs Over Time*; University of Georgia Athens: Athens, GA, USA, 2011.
12. Loon, M.; Casimir, G. Job-demand for learning and job-related learning: The moderating effect of need for achievement. *J. Manag. Psychol.* **2008**, *23*, 89–102. [CrossRef]
13. Prem, R.; Ohly, S.; Kubicek, B.; Korunka, C. Thriving on challenge stressors? Exploring time pressure and learning demands as antecedents of thriving at work. *J. Organ. Behav.* **2017**, *38*, 108–123. [CrossRef] [PubMed]
14. Paulsson, K.; Sundin, L. Learning at work-a combination of experience based learning and theoretical education. *Behav. Inf. Technol.* **2000**, *19*, 181–188. [CrossRef]
15. Shalley, C.E.; Gilson, L.L.; Blum, T.C. Interactive effects of growth need strength, work context, and job complexity on self-reported creative performance. *Acad. Manag. J.* **2009**, *52*, 489–505. [CrossRef]
16. Kubicek, B.; Paškvan, M.; Korunka, C. Development and validation of an instrument for assessing job demands arising from accelerated change: The intensification of job demands scale (IDS). *Eur. J. Work Organ. Psychol.* **2015**, *24*, 898–913. [CrossRef]
17. Obschonka, M.; Silbereisen, R.K.; Wasilewski, J. Constellations of new demands concerning careers and jobs: Results from a two-country study on social and economic change. *J. Vocat. Behav.* **2012**, *80*, 211–223. [CrossRef]
18. Nijhof, W.J. Lifelong learning as a European skill formation policy. *Hum. Resour. Dev. Rev.* **2005**, *4*, 401–417. [CrossRef]
19. Rau, R.; Buyken, D. Current Status of Knowledge About Health Risk From Mental Workload: Evidence Based on a Systematic Review of Reviews. *Zeitschrift für Arbeits-und Organisationspsychologie* **2015**, *59*, 113–129.
20. Bonde, J.P.E. Psychosocial factors at work and risk of depression: A systematic review of the epidemiological evidence. *Occup. Environ. Med.* **2008**, *65*, 438–445. [CrossRef] [PubMed]
21. Demerouti, E.; Bakker, A.B.; de Jonge, J.; Janssen, P.P.; Schaufeli, W.B. Burnout and engagement at work as a function of demands and control. *Scand. J. Work Environ. Health* **2001**, *27*, 279–286. [CrossRef]
22. Kivimäki, M.; Nyberg, S.T.; Batty, G.D.; Fransson, E.I.; Heikkilä, K.; Alfredsson, L.; Bjorner, J.B.; Borritz, M.; Burr, H.; Casini, A.; et al. Job strain as a risk factor for coronary heart disease: A collaborative meta-analysis of individual participant data. *Lancet* **2012**, *380*, 1491–1497. [CrossRef]
23. Kivimäki, M.; Virtanen, M.; Elovainio, M.; Kouvonen, A.; Väänänen, A.; Vahtera, J. Work stress in the etiology of coronary heart disease—A meta-analysis. *Scand. J. Work Environ. Health* **2006**, *32*, 431–442. [CrossRef] [PubMed]
24. Landsbergis, P.A.; Dobson, M.; Koutsouras, G.; Schnall, P. Job strain and ambulatory blood pressure: A meta-analysis and systematic review. *Am. J. Public Health* **2013**, *103*, e61–e71. [CrossRef] [PubMed]

25. Karasek, R. Job demands, job decision latitude, and mental strain: Implications for job redesign. *Adm. Sci. Q.* **1979**, *24*, 285–308. [CrossRef]
26. Karasek, R. Demand/Control model: A social-emotional, and psychological approach to stress risk and active behavior development. In *ILO Encyclopedia of Occupational Health and Safety*; ILO: Geneva, Switzerland, 1998.
27. Steptoe, A.; Kivimäki, M. Stress and cardiovascular disease: An update on current knowledge. *Annu. Rev. Public Health* **2013**, *34*, 337–354. [CrossRef] [PubMed]
28. Glaser, J.; Seubert, C.; Hornung, S.; Herbig, B. The impact of learning demands, work-related resources, and job stressors on creative performance and health. *J. Pers. Psychol.* **2015**, *14*, 37–48. [CrossRef]
29. Büssing, A.; Glaser, J. *Das Tätigkeits-und Arbeitsanalyseverfahren für das Krankenhaus-Selbstbeobachtungsversion (TAA-KH-S)*; Hogrefe: Göttingen, Germany, 2002.
30. Layer, J.K.; Karwowski, W.; Furr, A. The effect of cognitive demands and perceived quality of work life on human performance in manufacturing environments. *Int. J. Ind. Ergon.* **2009**, *39*, 413–421. [CrossRef]
31. Bakker, A.B.; Demerouti, E. The job demands-resources model: State of the art. *J. Manag. Psychol.* **2007**, *22*, 309–328. [CrossRef]
32. Hacker, W. Action regulation theory: A practical tool for the design of modern work processes? *Eur. J. Work Organ. Psychol.* **2003**, *12*, 105–130. [CrossRef]
33. Hackman, J.R.; Oldham, G.R. Motivation through the design of work: Test of a theory. *Organ. Behav. Hum. Perform.* **1976**, *16*, 250–279. [CrossRef]
34. Richter, P.; Hacker, W. *Belastung und Beanspruchung: Streß, Ermüdung und Burnout im Arbeitsleben [Workload and Strain: Stress, Fatigue, and Burnout in Working Life]*; Asanger: Heidelberg, Germany, 1998.
35. Karasek, R.A.; Theorell, T. *Health Work*; Basic Book: New York, NY, USA, 1990.
36. Cavanaugh, M.A.; Boswell, W.R.; Roehling, M.V.; Boudreau, J.W. An empirical examination of self-reported work stress among US managers. *J. Appl. Psychol.* **2000**, *85*, 65–74. [CrossRef] [PubMed]
37. Podsakoff, N.P.; LePine, J.A.; LePine, M.A. Differential challenge stressor-hindrance stressor relationships with job attitudes, turnover intentions, turnover, and withdrawal behavior: A meta-analysis. *J. Appl. Psychol.* **2007**, *92*, 438–454. [CrossRef]
38. Folkman, S.; Lazarus, R.S. If it changes it must be a process: Study of emotion and coping during three stages of a college examination. *J. Pers. Soc. Psychol.* **1985**, *48*, 150–170. [CrossRef]
39. LePine, J.A.; Podsakoff, N.P.; LePine, M.A. A meta-analytic test of the challenge stressor–hindrance stressor framework: An explanation for inconsistent relationships among stressors and performance. *Acad. Manag. J.* **2005**, *48*, 764–775. [CrossRef]
40. Searle, B.J.; Auton, J.C. The merits of measuring challenge and hindrance appraisals. *Anxiety Stress Coping* **2015**, *28*, 121–143. [CrossRef]
41. Crawford, E.R.; LePine, J.A.; Rich, B.L. Linking job demands and resources to employee engagement and burnout: A theoretical extension and meta-analytic test. *J. Appl. Psychol.* **2010**, *95*, 834–848. [CrossRef]
42. Jinnett, K.; Schwatka, N.; Tenney, L.; Brockbank, C.V.; Newman, L.S. Chronic conditions, workplace safety, and job demands contribute to absenteeism and job performance. *Health Aff.* **2017**, *36*, 237–244. [CrossRef]
43. Kristof-Brown, A.L.; Zimmerman, R.D.; Johnson, E.C. Consequences of individualis' fit at work: A meta-analysis of person-job, person-organization, person-group, and person-supervisor fit. *Pers. Psychol.* **2005**, *58*, 281–342. [CrossRef]
44. Caplan, R.D. Person-environment fit theory and organizations: Commensurate dimensions, time perspectives, and mechanisms. *J. Vocat. Behav.* **1987**, *31*, 248–267. [CrossRef]
45. Su, R.; Murdock, C.; Rounds, J. Person-environment fit. In *APA Handbook of Career Intervention*; Hartung, P.J., Savickas, M.L., Wals, W.B., Eds.; American Psychological Association: Washington, DC, USA, 2015; pp. 81–98.
46. Kristof-Brown, A.L.; Guay, R.P. Person–environment fit. In *PA Handbooks in Psychology. APA Handbook of Industrial and Organizational Psychology*; Zedeck, S., Ed.; American Psychological Association: Washington, DC, USA, 2011.
47. Arthur, W., Jr.; Bell, S.T.; Villado, A.J.; Doverspike, D. The use of person-organization fit in employment decision making: An assessment of its criterion-related validity. *J. Appl. Psychol.* **2006**, *91*, 786–801. [CrossRef]
48. Greguras, G.J.; Diefendorff, J.M. Different fits satisfy different needs: Linking person-environment fit to employee commitment and performance using self-determination theory. *J. Appl. Psychol.* **2009**, *94*, 465–477. [CrossRef] [PubMed]

49. Rounds, J.B.; Tracey, T.J. *From Trait-and-Factor to Person-Environment Fit Counseling: Theory and Process*; Lawrence Erlbaum Associates, Inc.: Hillsdale, NJ, USA, 1990.
50. Rohrbach-Schmidt, D.; Hall, A. *BIBB/BAuA Employment Survey 2012*; BIBB-FDZ Data and Methodological Report; Bundesinstitut für Berufsbildung (BIBB): Bonn, Germany, 2013.
51. Benach, J.; Gimeno, D.; Benavides, F.G.; Martínez, J.M.; Torné Mdel, M. Types of employment and health in the European Union: Changes from 1995 to 2000. *Eur. J. Public Health* **2004**, *14*, 314–321. [CrossRef] [PubMed]
52. Simon, J.; De Boer, J.B.; Joung, I.M.; Bosma, H.; Mackenbach, J.P. How is your health in general? A qualitative study on self-assessed health. *Eur. J. Public Health* **2005**, *15*, 200–208. [CrossRef]
53. Idler, E.L.; Benyamini, Y. Self-rated health and mortality: A review of twenty-seven community studies. *J. Health Soc. Behav.* **1997**, *38*, 21–37. [CrossRef] [PubMed]
54. Wanous, J.P.; Reichers, A.E.; Hudy, M.J. Overall job satisfaction: How good are single-item measures? *J. Appl. Psychol.* **1997**, *82*, 247–252. [CrossRef]
55. Hellevik, O. Linear versus logistic regression when the dependent variable is a dichotomy. *Qual. Quant.* **2009**, *43*, 59–74. [CrossRef]
56. Bakker, A.B.; Demerouti, E.; Euwema, M.C. Job resources buffer the impact of job demands on burnout. *J. Occup. Health Psychol.* **2005**, *10*, 170–180. [CrossRef]
57. Ross, C.E.; Wu, C.-L. Education, age, and the cumulative advantage in health. *J. Health Soc. Behav.* **1996**, *37*, 104–120. [CrossRef]
58. Podsakoff, P.M.; MacKenzie, S.B.; Lee, J.Y.; Podsakoff, N.P. Common method biases in behavioral research: A critical review of the literature and recommended remedies. *J. Appl. Psychol.* **2003**, *88*, 879–903. [CrossRef] [PubMed]
59. Marmot, M.G.; Fuhrer, R.; Ettner, S.L.; Marks, N.F.; Bumpass, L.L.; Ryff, C.D. Contribution of psychosocial factors to socioeconomic differences in health. *Milbank Q.* **1998**, *76*, 403–448. [CrossRef] [PubMed]
60. Conway, N.; Briner, R.B. Full-time versus part-time employees: Understanding the links between work status, the psychological contract, and attitudes. *J. Vocat. Behav.* **2002**, *61*, 279–301. [CrossRef]
61. DeSalvo, K.B.; Bloser, N.; Reynolds, K.; He, J.; Muntner, P. Mortality prediction with a single general self-rated health question. *J. Gen. Intern. Med.* **2006**, *21*, 267–275. [CrossRef] [PubMed]
62. Kompier, M.A. New systems of work organization and workers' health. *Scand. J. Work Environ. Health* **2006**, *32*, 421–430. [CrossRef] [PubMed]

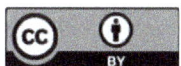

© 2018 by the authors. Licensee MDPI, Basel, Switzerland. This article is an open access article distributed under the terms and conditions of the Creative Commons Attribution (CC BY) license (http://creativecommons.org/licenses/by/4.0/).

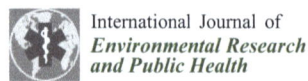

Article

Larger Workplaces, People-Oriented Culture, and Specific Industry Sectors Are Associated with Co-Occurring Health Protection and Wellness Activities

Aviroop Biswas [1,*], Colette N. Severin [1], Peter M. Smith [1,2,3], Ivan A. Steenstra [1,4], Lynda S. Robson [1] and Benjamin C. Amick III [1,5]

1. Institute for Work & Health, Toronto, ON M5G 2E9, Canada; cseverin@iwh.on.ca (C.N.S.); psmith@iwh.on.ca (P.M.S.); isteenstra@morneaushepell.com (I.A.S.); lrobson@iwh.on.ca (L.S.R.); bamickii@fiu.edu (B.C.A.)
2. Dalla Lana School of Public Health, University of Toronto, Toronto, ON M5T 3M7, Canada
3. Centre of Occupational and Environmental Health, Monash University, Melbourne, VIC 3004, Australia
4. Morneau Shepell, Toronto, ON M5S 3A9, Canada
5. Florida International University, Miami, FL 33199, USA
* Correspondence: abiswas@iwh.on.ca; Tel.: +1-416-927-2027 (ext. 2290)

Received: 29 October 2018; Accepted: 28 November 2018; Published: 4 December 2018

Abstract: Employers are increasingly interested in offering workplace wellness programs in addition to occupational health and safety (OHS) activities to promote worker health, wellbeing, and productivity. Yet, there is a dearth of research on workplace factors that enable the implementation of OHS and wellness to inform the future integration of these activities in Canadian workplaces. This study explored workplace demographic factors associated with the co-implementation of OHS and wellness activities in a heterogenous sample of Canadian workplaces. Using a cross-sectional survey of 1285 workplaces from 2011 to 2014, latent profiles of co-occurrent OHS and wellness activities were identified, and multinomial logistic regression was used to assess associations between workplace demographic factors and the profiles. Most workplaces (84%) demonstrated little co-occurrence of OHS and wellness activities. Highest co-occurrence was associated with large workplaces (odds ratio (OR) = 3.22, 95% confidence interval (CI) = 1.15–5.89), in the electrical and utilities sector (OR = 5.57, 95% CI = 2.24–8.35), and a high people-oriented culture (OR = 4.70, 95% CI = 1.59–5.26). Promoting integrated OHS and wellness approaches in medium to large workplaces, in select industries, and emphasizing a people-oriented culture were found to be important factors for implementing OHS and wellness in Canadian organizations. Informed by these findings, future studies should understand the mechanisms to facilitate the integration of OHS and wellness in workplaces.

Keywords: workforce demographics; health promotion; injury prevention; occupational health

1. Introduction

The workplace is a social determinant of health, with employment and working conditions linked to a range of health, functioning, and quality-of-life outcomes [1,2]. Work-related injuries and illnesses are associated with morbidity and substantial financial and social costs, and health hazards from work can also impact people's personal lives and lifestyle [3,4]. Studies also show that lifestyle risk factors (e.g., being a smoker, stressful lives outside of work, being obese, and heavy alcohol use) can increase the likelihood of sustaining workplace injuries more so than among those without such risk factors [5,6]. North American employers are required to provide occupational health and safety (OHS) activities that minimize negative health effect due to worker exposures to job-related risks and hazards.

In comparison, workplace health promotion or wellness activities are voluntarily provided by some employers to improve worker wellbeing through health behavior changes and are shown to have short and long-term health and productivity benefits [7,8].

There has been a shift in thinking about how workplaces can better integrate safety into the overall wellbeing of their workforce [9]. Wellness and OHS programs share the goal of protecting and improving worker health and given these overlaps it makes sense to integrate both. Integrating OHS and wellness activities is expected to have greater effects on health, safety, and wellbeing than if the activities operated separately from each other [10,11]. This approach, commonly referred to as Total Worker Health® in the US, is widely endorsed by international health and labor agencies [12–14] with the consensus that it will lead to improvements in the long-term well-being of workers and their families, and reduce pressures on healthcare and social security systems [13,14].

Several studies have demonstrated links between the characteristics of workplaces (workplace demographic factors) and the implementation and integration of OHS and wellness activities. For example, the manufacturing sector reports a higher number of OHS and wellness activities than other sectors [15,16], and smaller workplaces are likely to offer fewer OHS and wellness programs than larger organizations [15,17,18]. Examining workplaces in the US Midwest, McLellan et al. found leadership support and having an OHS committee to be important contributors to implementing integrated approaches [19]. Tremblay et al. examined Massachusetts employers and found a high degree of coordinated activities among unionized workplaces and in construction, healthcare, manufacturing, and entertainment industries [18]. These and other studies are limited in their focus on small workplaces [17,19] and sampled few larger workplaces [18]. A greater focus on medium to large in addition to smaller workplaces can further uncover factors enabling integrated activities as larger workplaces are likely to have more resources to support these activities [20]. Furthermore, much of the research examining relationships between workplace factors and the implementation of OHS and wellness have focused on US workplaces and little is known about the extent that these activities co-occur in Canadian workplaces. To inform research and policy recommendations towards the widespread adoption of integrated worker health approaches in Canada, research evidence is needed to understand the extent that OHS and wellness activities co-occur as a necessary first step towards identifying the current status quo and the workplace factors that can be amenable targets for integrated approaches in the future.

The objective of this study was to explore the workplace demographic factors associated with the concurrent implementation of OHS and wellness activities in Canadian workplaces. The study has two research questions (RQ): RQ1—"What is the extent that OHS and wellness activities co-occur in workplaces?" RQ2—"Are there associations between workplace demographic characteristics and the co-occurrence of OHS and wellness activities?" These questions were explored in a cross-section of a large, heterogenous sample of small, medium, and large workplaces in Ontario, Canada. Informed by evidence from US studies, we hypothesized that large and unionized workplaces in specific industry sectors have a higher co-occurrence of OHS and wellness activities than workplaces with other demographic characteristics.

2. Materials and Methods

2.1. Data Sources

This study analyzed data from the Ontario Leading Indicators Project (OLIP), a cross-sectional survey conducted by researchers at the Institute for Work & Health from 2011 to 2014 in partnership with health and safety associations in Ontario, Canada. The aim of the OLIP study was to identify leading indicator measures for workplaces to improve their health and safety performance before injuries and illnesses occur. Study details are available elsewhere [21]. Briefly, OHS and wellness data were collected in collaboration with four OHS associations representing employers from most labor sectors in Ontario. The target population consisted of organizations registered with the

Workplace Safety & Insurance Board (WSIB), an organization responsible for workers' compensation to approximately 62.5% of Ontario's workforce [22]. Workplace Safety & Insurance Board compensation coverage is optional for certain workers such as independent contractors, sole proprietors, and partners in partnerships. Organizations included in the study analysis had at least one full-time employee in the following industries: education, electrical and utilities, agriculture, manufacturing, municipal, healthcare, service, pulp and paper, forestry, and mining. Other industries were not examined.

2.2. Sampling and Recruitment

Workplaces were identified by random stratified sampling based on the following variables: industrial sector, geographic region, and size. Study recruitment took place from 15 March 2011, to 27 August 2012, which began with the OLIP study's health and safety association partners making initial contact with organizations to solicit their interest. If an organization consented to take part in the study, the person most knowledgeable about health and safety at their organization completed an online English-language questionnaire. Respondents were also given the option to complete the questionnaire by mail or phone. Questionnaires were administered to each respondent in a random sequence. Three to ten follow-up e-mails or phone calls were sent to remind participants to complete questionnaires. The study was approved by the University of Toronto's research ethics board (protocol 25363).

2.3. Measures

2.3.1. Independent Variables: Workplace Demographic Characteristics

The independent variables used in the analysis were workplace demographic characteristics chosen a priori from the available literature as they were found to be linked to the co-occurrence of OHS and wellness activities. The following variables were examined, workplace size (four categories; small and without a Joint Health and Safety Committee, JHSC (reference category)), union status (unionized, non-unionized (reference category), don't know), industry sector (eight sectors; manufacturing sector (reference category)). Workplace culture factors previously found to be associated with OHS and wellness implementation [19,23] were examined using a measure of workplace health and safety leadership (lowest = 1 (reference category), highest = 4), and a measure of people-oriented culture (lowest = 1 (reference category), highest = 4) (Supplementary Table S1).

Union status (i.e., at least part of the workforce is represented by a union) was self-reported in the OLIP questionnaire. Questionnaire responses were linked to corresponding 2009 WSIB administrative records to obtain additional information on a workplace's industry sector classification. Workplace size was self-reported and categorized according to Statistics Canada classifications [24] as follows, small workplaces had 1 to 99 employees, medium workplaces had 100 to 499 employees, and large workplaces had ≥500 employees. Workplace size was a proxy of OHS infrastructure and accordingly, small workplaces were further classified by whether they reported having a JHSC (consists of labor and management representatives regularly meet to deal with health and safety issues). This categorization was based on the mandatory Ontario labor requirement that workplaces with >20 employees must have a JHSC. An organization's leadership support and culture were examined using two subscales selected a priori from the Organizational Policies and Practices questionnaire [25,26]: Health and Safety Leadership (six items) and People-Oriented Culture (four items). Participants rated the extent their organization achieved these subscales on a five-point scale from 0% (never) to 100% (always). Each subscale item was averaged to a score ranging from 0 (low) to 4 (high).

2.3.2. Occupational Health and Safety and Wellness Activities

A workplace's OHS activities were measured by the availability of factors related to safe and effective OHS performance as an alternative measure to the number of OHS activities offered by workplaces as these can vary by working conditions and industry sector. For example, workplaces in high hazard industries are likely to overrepresent higher OHS activities than other workplaces.

Occupational health and safety performance was measured using the Institute for Work & Health's Organizational Performance Metric (IWH-OPM) tool, which has been shown to be predictive (i.e., valid and reliable) of future injury and illness rates [27,28]. The eight-item IWH-OPM tool was developed by a consensus process among a team of researchers and health and safety professionals [28]. For each IWH-OPM item, respondents rated the percent of time that certain practices occurred in their workplace, from 1 (0–20%) to 5 (80–100%). Scores for each item were summed to estimate a total OHS performance score, with a highest score of 40 (a score of 5 for all items) indicating that all eight OHS practices took place most to all the time in a workplace.

A workplace's wellness activities were assessed by dichotomous ("yes" or "no") responses to the question: "during the last 12 months, did your company offer any of the following programs to employees and/or their families?" The range of wellness activities were selected from the literature and the Centers for Disease Control and Prevention's Workplace Health Model [29,30]. Wellness programs included screenings (blood pressure, diabetes, cholesterol, and cancer), smoking cessation classes, physical activity and/or fitness classes, and educational resources. Wellness policies included flexible work hours to engage in wellness activities, encouraging fitness breaks, and healthy food choices. Supportive environments for wellness activities included providing shower facilities, signage to encourage stair use, and on-site fitness facilities or walking trails. The total number of wellness activities was derived from a total score of 25 possible options.

2.3.3. Outcome Variable: Co-Occurrence of Occupational Health and Safety and Wellness Activities

Occupational health and safety performance and wellness activities were examined as continuous variables and categorized into profiles based on similar response probability patterns for the total scores of each activity.

2.4. Analyses

Statistical analyses were conducted using commercially-available statistical software, SAS v. 9.4 (SAS Institute Inc., Cary, NC, USA) [31] and Mplus v. 8.0 (Muthén & Muthén, Los Angeles, CA, USA) [32], and tests were two-sided with significance set at $p = 0.05$. Workplaces represented by OLIP questionnaire responses were statistically weighted to permit inferences from the sample to a comparable population of Ontario organizations based on strata of workplace size, region, and industry sector. For RQ1, mean values of OHS and wellness activities were compared separately according to workplace size, union status, industry sector, health and safety leadership, and people-oriented culture. Analysis of variance was used to examine differences in the mean OHS and wellness activities scores. Workplaces were assigned to 'profiles' based on the probability that they had similar numbers of OHS and wellness activities to other workplaces using Mplus's latent profile analysis function. The latent profile analysis statistical technique aims to recover hidden groups from observed data, similar to clustering techniques, but is more flexible because the approach is based on an explicit model of the data, and accounts for the fact that recovered groups are uncertain [33]. Data on OHS performance scores and number of wellness activities were transferred from SAS to Mplus and analyzed as continuous variables in a mixture model with sample weights. Several models were fit with increasing numbers of profiles (one profile, two profiles, three profiles etc.). A decision on the most suitable number of profiles fitting the data was made by inspecting model-fit statistics for the Lo–Mendell–Rubin adjusted likelihood ratio test. The Lo–Mendell–Rubin test had a p-value of 0.58 when comparing four profiles to three profiles, suggesting that three profiles sufficiently modelled the data. For RQ2, associations between the latent profile groups and workplace demographic characteristics (independent variables) were estimated using multinomial logistic regression by transferring latent profile probability data generated from Mplus back into SAS and matching them to corresponding data from individual survey respondents. The odds of a co-occurrence profile associated with a workplace characteristic of interest compared to the odds of the lowest co-occurrence profile and a reference workplace characteristic (e.g., a small workplace without a JHSC) were described as odds ratios (OR) and 95% confidence intervals (CIs).

3. Results

3.1. Descriptive Statistics

Representatives from 1692 organizations responded to the OLIP survey from 7285 approached (23.2% response rate). Excluded from the analysis were respondents with missing data for the variables of interest or if respondents did not indicate "none of the above" if indicating the absence of wellness activities rather than overlooking the question, to leave a final analytical sample of 1285 responses. Most respondents were managers (36%) and had >5 years of experience at their organization (70%). Table 1 describes the workplace demographic characteristics. Most workplaces were classified as small and without a JHSC (53%), non-unionized (90%), and in the manufacturing (30%) or service (54%) sectors. The most frequently reported wellness programs were employee assistance programs (EAPs) (15%), physical activity and/or fitness programs (14%), and stress reduction programs (13%), while different health screening and education programs were reported the least. The most frequent wellness policy was flexible hours (40%) followed by working from home (14%). Onsite shower facilities (15%) was the most frequently reported environmental support.

Table 1. Characteristics of surveyed workplaces (n = 1285). Statistically-weighted values described.

Characteristic	n	% or M	SD
Workplace size			
Small (<100 employees) without a JHSC	171	53.2	4.1
Small (<100 employees) with a JHSC	511	28.3	3.3
Medium (100 to 499 employees)	267	8.0	1.8
Large (>500 employees)	81	1.9	0.8
Union status			
Non-unionized	964	90.1	1.9
Unionized	304	5.9	0.9
Don't know	10	4.1	4.2
Industry sector			
Manufacturing	440	30.4	1.4
Service	412	53.6	2.9
Healthcare	197	4.4	0.6
Agriculture	161	10.2	1.4
Education	81	0.8	0.1
Municipal	62	0.4	0.1
Pulp and paper	24	0.1	<0.1
Electrical and utilities	13	0.1	<0.1
Occupational health & safety performance (IWH-OPM, range: 1 to 5)			
Formal safety audits at regular intervals		3.3	15.3
Organization values ongoing safety improvement		4.3	9.4
Safety as important as work production and quality		4.4	9.5
Workers and supervisors have information to work safely		4.5	8.5
Employees always involved in health and safety decisions		4.3	9.3
Those in charge of safety have authority to make necessary changes		4.5	9.1
Positive recognition for those who act safely		4.0	11.9
Everyone has the tools and/or equipment to complete work safely		4.6	7.9

Table 1. Cont.

Characteristic	n	% or M	SD
Workplace wellness activities			
Flexible work hours for wellness	484	39.8	2.2
Have onsite shower facilities	365	15.0	2.2
Employee assistance programs	394	14.6	2.5
Physical activity and/or fitness programs	272	14.2	2.4
Programs to prevent/reduce stress	226	12.6	2.4
Self-care books/tools	210	11.9	2.1
Nutrition education	221	11.7	2.4
Education on balancing work and family	164	11.4	2.2
Provide or encourage fitness breaks	158	8.1	1.7
Have fitness or walking trails on site	133	6.4	1.5
Health risk assessment	87	5.8	1.9
Smoking cessation classes/counselling	184	5.7	1.5
Weight management classes/counselling	115	5.2	1.9
Screenings for high blood pressure	83	5.2	1.6
Alcohol or drug abuse support programs	173	4.3	0.9
Cholesterol reduction education	68	4.1	1.4
Screenings for cholesterol level	35	3.2	1.6
Screening for diabetes	30	2.4	1.3
Chronic disease management programs	66	2.3	0.9
Promotions/discounts to encourage health food choices	158	2.2	0.9
Label health food choices in cafeteria	76	2.2	1.0
Nurse advice line	41	1.9	0.8
Screenings for any form of cancer	24	1.7	0.9
Have signage to encourage people to use the stairs	41	1.7	0.9
HIV/AIDS education	22	0.4	0.1

M, Mean; SD, Standard Deviation; JHSC, Joint Health and Safety Committee; IWH-OPM, Institute for Work & Health-Organizational Performance Metric tool; HIV/AIDS, Human Immunodeficiency Virus/Acquired Immune Deficiency Syndrome.

3.2. Co-Occurrence of Occupational Health and Safety and Wellness Activities

The number of OHS and wellness activities were found to be poorly correlated (Pearson's $r = 0.14$) indicating that the co-occurrence of both was low among the surveyed workplaces. Figure 1 shows common profiles of co-occurrent OHS and wellness activities according to latent profile analysis. Three distinct profiles of workplace OHS and wellness activities were identified. Profile 1 indicated the group of workplaces with the lowest occurrence of OHS and wellness activities (84% of responses), with a mean of 33 OHS activities and no wellness activities. Profile 2 indicated the group of workplaces with the highest occurrence of OHS and wellness activities (4% of responses), with a mean of 37 OHS activities and 10 wellness activities. Profile 3 indicated the group of workplaces with a moderate co-occurrence of OHS and wellness activities (13% of responses), with a mean of 34 OHS activities and four wellness activities.

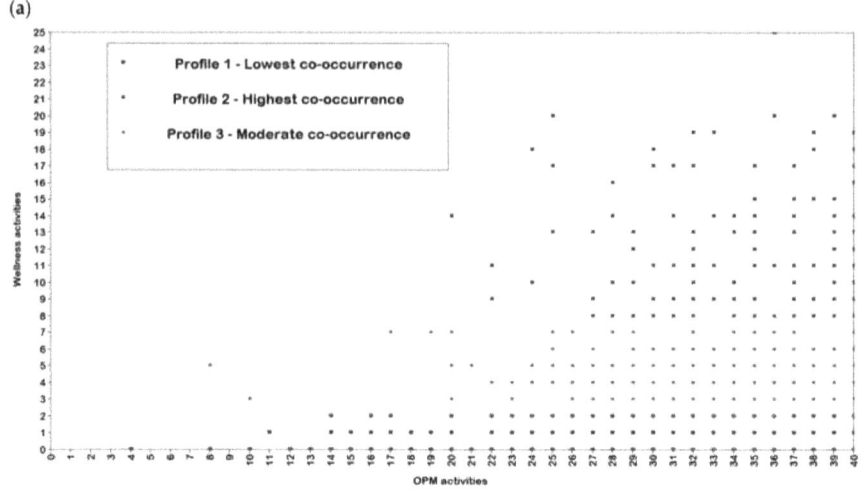

Figure 1. Co-occurrence of workplace occupational health and safety (OHS) and wellness activities based on workplaces with similar profiles. (**a**) Co-occurrence profiles (lowest co-occurrence (red circle), moderate co-occurrence (orange diamond), highest co-occurrence (green cross)) and (**b**) descriptive characteristics of the profiles. SE, Standard Error.

3.3. Asociations between Workplace Demographic Characteristics and the Co-Occurrence of Occupational Health and Safety and Wellness Activities

Table 2 shows associations between workplace demographic characteristics and the co-occurrence profiles of OHS and wellness activities. Increasing workplace size was associated with greater odds of a workplace being classified in the highest (profile 2) and moderate (profile 3) co-occurrence profiles compared to small workplaces without a JHSC. Large workplaces were estimated to have the greatest odds of being in the highest co-occurrence profile compared to small, non-JHSC workplaces (OR = 3.22, 95% CI = 1.15–5.89). Compared to small, non-JHSC workplaces, medium workplaces were most likely to be classified in the moderate co-occurrence profile (profile 3) (OR = 4.71, 95% CI = 1.42–8.74), followed by large workplaces (OR = 2.22, 95% CI = 1.05–4.52). Unionized workplaces were more likely to be a member of the highest co-occurrence profile (profile 2) (OR = 1.52, 95% CI = 0.48–4.88) or moderate co-occurrence profile (OR = 1.03, 95% CI = 0.33–3.27) compared to non-unionized workplaces, although these estimates were not statistically significant. Workplaces in the electrical and utilities (OR = 5.57, 95% CI = 2.24–8.35) and municipal (OR = 5.52, 95% CI = 0.91–8.43) industry sectors were most likely to be classified as a highest occurrence profile compared to the manufacturing sector, although the association with the municipal sector was not statistically significant. Workplaces in the electrical and utilities (OR = 7.67, 95% CI = 2.46–10.50) and municipal sectors (OR = 6.97, 95% CI = 1.80–9.06) were also most likely to be classified in the moderate co-occurrence profile. No statistically significant associations were found between scores for health and safety leadership and the likelihood of highest and moderate co-occurrence profiles. Workplaces rated highest for people-oriented culture were likely to be classified in the highest co-occurrence profile (OR = 4.70, 95% CI = 1.59–5.26) compared to lowest-rated workplaces. No statistically significant associations were found between people-oriented culture ratings and the moderate co-occurrence profile.

Table 2. Associations between workplace demographic characteristics and the co-occurrence of occupational health and safety and wellness activities (n = 1285) [1].

Characteristic	Profile 2 Highest Co-Occurrence	Profile 3 Moderate Co-Occurrence
	OR (95% CI)	
Workplace size		
Small (<100 employees) without a JHSC	Reference	Reference
Small (<100 employees) with a JHSC	0.32 (0.05–2.19)	1.48 (1.15–4.25)
Medium (100 to 499 employees)	2.76 (0.43–3.59)	4.71 (1.42–8.74)
Large (>500 employees)	3.22 (1.15–5.89)	2.22 (1.05–4.52)
Union status		
Non-unionized	Reference	Reference
Unionized	1.52 (0.48–4.88)	1.03 (0.33–3.27)
Industry sector		
Manufacturing	Reference	Reference
Agriculture	1.00 (0.11–9.20)	0.78 (0.46–1.50)
Pulp and paper	0.50 (0.11–2.21)	0.51 (0.10–2.70)
Education	0.74 (0.15–3.67)	4.90 (0.28–8.77)
Electrical and utilities	5.57 (2.24–8.35)	7.97 (2.46–10.50)
Municipal	5.52 (0.91–8.43)	6.97 (1.80–9.06)
Healthcare	1.76 (0.68–4.56)	2.12 (0.72–6.28)
Service	0.13 (0.03–0.59)	1.87 (0.73–4.80)
Health and safety leadership		
1 (low)	Reference	Reference
2	1.77 (0.25–2.66)	0.52 (0.12–2.24)
3	5.19 (0.95–7.52)	0.50 (0.15–1.69)
4 (high)	4.77 (0.73–5.99)	0.60 (0.21–1.74)
People-oriented culture		
1 (low)	Reference	Reference
2	1.63 (0.96–2.40)	3.59 (0.77–6.88)
3	1.73 (2.20–4.41)	4.63 (0.93–6.02)
4 (high)	4.70 (1.59–5.26)	2.77 (0.62–5.42)

[1] Reference profile category: Profile 1 (lowest co-occurrence). Reference, OR = 1.00; OR, odds ratio; CI, confidence interval; JHSC, Joint Health and Safety Committee.

4. Discussion

This study surveyed a large and diverse sample of workplaces to examine the extent that OHS and wellness activities co-occur and identified the workplace characteristics most likely to be associated with the co-occurrence of the activities. Most workplaces surveyed reported having few OHS and wellness activities. Large workplaces, those in the electrical and utilities sector, and with a high rating for people-oriented culture were factors most associated with a high co-occurrence of OHS and wellness activities. Large and medium-size workplaces, those in the electrical and utilities, and municipal sectors were associated with a moderate co-occurrence of activities.

This study found a fewer number of wellness activities in Ontario workplaces compared to US studies where at least three-quarters of workplaces reported one or more wellness activity [17,18]. This difference may be due to the fewer incentives for Canadian employers to invest in wellness activities as most medically-necessary services are covered by Canada's public healthcare system. Furthermore, employer contributions to healthcare costs are comparatively modest. The higher number of EAPs compared to other wellness activities is unsurprising as small workplaces represented the highest proportion of respondents in the study. The outsourcing of resources to EAPs can represent a better investment for small workplaces compared to more costly investments in onsite wellness activities [20]. Small organizations also experience several obstacles to implementing wellness activities such as constraints in assigning resources and dedicated staff for wellness initiatives, perceiving a lack of employee interest in participating in wellness activities, or have poor access to health promotion resources and wellness providers [20]. While stress management, physical activity promotion, and flexible hours were reported frequently, others such as healthy food choices and shower facilities were less frequently reported. This suggests that workplaces might be primarily focusing on encouraging their workers to change their own behaviors. Yet only focusing on changing individual behaviors is unlikely to lead to meaningful worker health improvements since a small percentage of workers participate in wellness activities without workplace policies and environmental supports also in place [3].

A small proportion of workplaces indicated a moderate or high co-occurrence of OHS and wellness activities, and similar findings have also been reported elsewhere [17,18]. Medium and large organizations were more likely to provide moderate to high co-occurrence of OHS and wellness activities compared to small workplaces, while having a JHSC did not show meaningful differences in wellness activities among small workplaces. This suggests that medium- to large-size workplaces are more likely than small workplaces to have the resources and supports in place to promote these efforts concurrently. Workplaces in the service, agriculture, and pulp and paper sectors were least likely to report co-occurring activities, while the electrical and utilities and municipal sectors were most likely. These differ from findings previously reported among employers in Massachusetts [18]. Whether the differences in our study reflect true differences in the employer population in Ontario compared to Massachusetts or reflects selection bias between the two studies, requires closer inspection. Further research is also needed to examine the workplace practices in sectors pertaining to low and high OHS and wellness activities to better understand the reasons for the implementation differences in Canada. Our findings also suggest that a people-oriented culture can at the very least support a higher implementation of wellness activities. Employer efforts to create a workplace culture of trust and respect might enhance workers' receptivity and openness to messages and programs designed to change behaviors and improve health [34,35].

Some limitations need to also be acknowledged when interpreting these findings. First, this was a cross-sectional study and causal relationships cannot be directly inferred. Second, the response rate was low, although the study's large initial sample size can facilitate the detection of more robust and reproducible statistical relationships than previous research with smaller sample sizes. We also reduced nonresponse bias by statistically weighting all modelling estimates to infer responses from a population of comparable organizations in the Ontario labor market. Third, our findings are only generalizable to the industry sectors we sampled and future studies need to examine how our findings relate to other industries such as the finance, information, professional, and entertainment sectors. Fourth, our use of a self-reported survey is prone to recall and social desirability biases. Differential measurement error is also possible across OHS and wellness activities. Respondents to the survey were selected based on their knowledge of OHS activities in the workplace, not on wellness activities. As such, it is possible that respondents could estimate OHS activities more accurately than wellness activities. Fifth, it is possible that some wellness activities were counted more than once if they were also provided as part of an EAP service (e.g., education, risk management tools, and self-care materials). Nonetheless, we conducted a sensitivity analysis and found that co-occurrence profiles did not meaningfully change when wellness activities that might be part of an EAP were removed. Lastly, the OLIP survey was not designed to collect detailed wellness information or the extent that these are integrated and coordinated with OHS activities.

Integrated OHS and wellness activities are widely promoted as an effective approach to chronic disease prevention [36]. This is partly explained by the emergence of evidence supporting the idea that workplace factors contribute to adverse health outcomes traditionally considered to be unrelated to work (such as stress, heart disease, and mental health) [10,11,37]. While distinguishing workplaces by their implementation of OHS and wellness activities may not reflect a truly integrated worker health approach [23], our findings provide a better understanding of the workplace factors associated with having suitable resources to support an integrated approach in the Canadian labor market. In 2016, a panel report from the National Institute of Health Pathways to Prevention Workshop identified small workplaces as a priority area for supporting integrated approaches through Total Worker Health® [38]. However, as our study and others have shown [15–18], there is a lack of demonstrated effectiveness in smaller workplaces in the concurrent adoption of health protection and wellness programming. Smaller workplaces might not integrate their OHS and wellness resources not because of a lack of support or motivation per se, but because of a lack of resources, including personnel, which might make it challenging to just perform traditional OHS hazard control alone [39]. Findings show that larger workplaces, with a people-oriented culture, and in the electrical and utilities, and municipal sectors are associated with more health protection and wellness resources that can be streamlined into integrated approaches. The next logical step is to examine intermediate and long-term health and productivity changes for these workplaces expected to benefit the most from co-occurring and integrated OHS and wellness activities. Subsequent findings can inform studies that are extended or scaled to other industries and smaller workplaces. Actionable recommendations whereby Canadian workplaces can integrate their existing OHS and wellness activities and ingrain these within a workplace's culture is also an area of research that needs to be explored further. Integration can also be enabled by an integrated safety and wellness committee, shared budgets and resources, and incentivizing employees in health protection and health promotion efforts [23].

5. Conclusions

This study provides valuable information on the co-occurrence of OHS and wellness activities and identifies workplace demographic factors most associated with their implementation in Canadian workplaces. Large workplaces, those in the electrical and utilities sector, and with a high rating for people-oriented culture are factors strongly related to the implementation of both OHS and wellness and might benefit most from integrated worker health activities. Future research needs to understand how to facilitate the uptake of OHS and wellness activities in workplaces with fewer concomitant organizational resources to increase OHS and wellness implementation. Furthermore, our findings need to be verified in other workplace contexts that were not explored in this study, and the factors that influence organizational change and worker participation need also to be better understood. Finally, it will be important to understand how to streamline OHS and wellness activities in workplaces for an integrated worker health approach.

Supplementary Materials: The following are available online at http://www.mdpi.com/1660-4601/15/12/2739/s1, Table S1: Ontario Leading Indicators Project (OLIP): survey variable names.

Author Contributions: Conceptualization, A.B. and B.C.A.III; Methodology, A.B.; Software, A.B.; Validation, A.B. and B.C.A.III; Formal Analysis, A.B.; Investigation, A.B.; Resources, A.B., P.M.S., and B.C.A.III; Data Curation, C.N.S. and B.C.A.III; Writing—Original draft preparation, A.B.; Writing—Review and editing, C.N.S., P.M.S., L.S.R., I.A.S., and B.C.A.III; Visualization, A.B.; Supervision, B.C.A.III; Project Administration, C.N.S.; Funding Acquisition, C.N.S., P.M.S., L.S.R., I.A.S., and B.C.A.III.

Funding: This research was supported by a grant from the Workplace Safety and Insurance Board's Research Advisory Council (#09032) and the Province of Ontario, Canada.

Acknowledgments: The authors thank the other members of the 'Ontario Leading Indicators Project' research team: Sheilah Hogg-Johnson, Cameron Mustard, Michael Swift, Selahadin Ibrahim, and Sara Macdonald. The authors also provide a special thank you to our health and safety association partners in Ontario who helped us recruit workplaces, and to the workplaces themselves for participating.

Conflicts of Interest: The authors declare no conflicts of interest. The funders had no role in the design of the study; in the collection, analyses, or interpretation of data; in the writing of the manuscript, or in the decision to publish the results.

References

1. Raphael, D. *Social Determinants of Health: Canadian Perspectives*; Canadian Scholars' Press and Women's Press: Toronto, ON, Canada, 2009; pp. 150–191.
2. Solar, O.; Irwin, A. A conceptual framework for action on the social determinants of health. In *Social Determinants of Health Discussion Paper 2 (Policy and Practice)*; WHO Press: Geneva, Switzerland, 2010; pp. 32–33.
3. Schulte, P.A.; Pandalai, S.; Wulsin, V.; Chun, H. Interaction of occupational and personal risk factors in workforce health and safety. *Am. J. Public Health* **2012**, *102*, 434–448. [CrossRef] [PubMed]
4. Ljungblad, C.; Granström, F.; Dellve, L.; Åkerlind, I. Workplace health promotion and working conditions as determinants of employee health. *Int. J. Workplace Health Manag.* **2014**, *7*, 89–104. [CrossRef]
5. Musich, S.; Napier, D.; Edington, D.W. The association of health risks with workers' compensation costs. *J. Occup. Environ. Med.* **2001**, *43*, 534–541. [CrossRef] [PubMed]
6. Trogdon, J.; Finkelstein, E.; Hylands, T.; Dellea, P.; Kamal-Bahl, S. Indirect costs of obesity: A review of the current literature. *Obes. Rev.* **2008**, *9*, 489–500. [CrossRef] [PubMed]
7. Conn, V.S.; Hafdahl, A.R.; Cooper, P.S.; Brown, L.M.; Lusk, S.L. Meta-analysis of workplace physical activity interventions. *Am. J. Prev. Med.* **2009**, *37*, 330–339. [CrossRef] [PubMed]
8. Noblet, A.; LaMontagne, A.D. The role of workplace health promotion in addressing job stress. *Health Promot. Int.* **2006**, *21*, 346–353. [CrossRef]
9. Hymel, P.A.; Loeppke, R.R.; Baase, C.M.; Burton, W.N.; Hartenbaum, N.P.; Hudson, T.W.; McLellan, R.K.; Mueller, K.L.; Roberts, M.A.; Yarborough, C.M. Workplace health protection and promotion: A new pathway for a healthier—And safer—Workforce. *J. Occup. Environ. Med.* **2011**, *53*, 695–702. [CrossRef] [PubMed]
10. Sorensen, G.; Stoddard, A.M.; LaMontagne, A.D.; Emmons, K.; Hunt, M.K.; Youngstrom, R.; McLellan, D.; Christiani, D.C. A comprehensive worksite cancer prevention intervention: Behavior change results from a randomized controlled trial (United States). *Cancer Causes Control* **2002**, *13*, 493–502. [CrossRef]
11. Cooklin, A.; Joss, N.; Husser, E.; Oldenburg, B. Integrated approaches to occupational health and safety: A systematic review. *Am. J. Health Promot.* **2017**, *31*, 401–412. [CrossRef]
12. World Health Organization. *Healthy Workplaces: A WHO Global Model for Action. For Employers, Workers, Policy-Makers and Practitioners*; World Health Organization: Geneva, Switzerland, 2010.
13. International Labour Organization. The SOLVE Training Package: Integrating Health Promotion into Workplace OSH Policies. Available online: http://www.ilo.org/safework/info/instr/WCMS_178438/lang--en/index.htm (accessed on 21 November 2018).
14. Schill, A.L.; Chosewood, L.C. The NIOSH Total Worker Health™ program: An overview. *J. Occup. Environ. Med.* **2013**, *55*, S8–S11. [CrossRef] [PubMed]
15. Hannon, P.A.; Garson, G.; Harris, J.R.; Hammerback, K.; Sopher, C.J.; Clegg-Thorp, C. Workplace health promotion implementation, readiness, and capacity among mid-sized employers in low-wage industries: A national survey. *J. Occup. Environ. Med.* **2012**, *54*, 1337–1343. [CrossRef]
16. Sinclair, R.C.; Cunningham, T.R. Safety activities in small businesses. *Saf. Sci.* **2014**, *64*, 32–38. [CrossRef] [PubMed]
17. McLellan, D.L.; Cabán-Martinez, A.J.; Nelson, C.C.; Pronk, N.P.; Katz, J.N.; Allen, J.D.; Davis, K.L.; Wagner, G.R.; Sorensen, G. Organizational characteristics influence implementation of worksite health protection and promotion programs: Evidence from smaller businesses. *J. Occup. Environ. Med.* **2015**, *57*, 1009–1016. [CrossRef] [PubMed]
18. Tremblay, P.A.; Nobrega, S.; Davis, L.; Erck, E.; Punnett, L. Healthy workplaces? A survey of Massachusetts employers. *Am. J. Health Promot.* **2013**, *27*, 390–400. [CrossRef] [PubMed]
19. McLellan, D.L.; Williams, J.A.; Katz, J.N.; Pronk, N.P.; Wagner, G.R.; Cabán-Martinez, A.J.; Nelson, C.C.; Sorensen, G. Key organizational characteristics for integrated approaches to protect and promote worker health in smaller enterprises. *J. Occup. Environ. Med.* **2017**, *59*, 289–294. [CrossRef]
20. McCoy, M.K.; Stinson, M.K.; Scott, M.K.; Tenney, M.L.; Newman, L.S. Health promotion in small business: A systematic review of factors influencing adoption and effectiveness of worksite wellness programs. *J. Occup. Environ. Med.* **2014**, *56*, 579–587. [CrossRef] [PubMed]

21. Institute for Work & Health. Measures in the Ontario Leading Indicators Project (OLIP) Survey. Available online: https://www.iwh.on.ca/sites/iwh/files/iwh/reports/iwh_project_olip_about_the_measures_august_2013.pdf (accessed on 21 November 2018).
22. Workplace Safety and Insurance Board of Ontario. 2017 Highlights: By the Numbers. Available online: http://www.wsibstatistics.ca/S2/Workplaces%20%20WSIB%20By%20The%20Numbers_P.php (accessed on 21 November 2018).
23. Sorensen, G.; McLellan, D.; Dennerlein, J.T.; Pronk, N.P.; Allen, J.D.; Boden, L.I.; Okechukwu, C.A.; Hashimoto, D.; Stoddard, A.; Wagner, G.R. Integration of health protection and health promotion: Rationale, indicators, and metrics. *J. Occup. Environ. Med.* **2013**, *55*, S12. [CrossRef]
24. Leung, D.; Rispoli, L.; Chan, R. Small, Medium-Sized, and Large Businesses in the Canadian Economy: Measuring Their Contribution to Gross Domestic Product from 2001 to 2008. Available online: https://www150.statcan.gc.ca/n1/en/pub/11f0027m/11f0027m2012082-eng.pdf (accessed on 21 November 2018).
25. Amick, B.C.; Habeck, R.V.; Hunt, A.; Fossel, A.H.; Chapin, A.; Keller, R.B.; Katz, J.N. Measuring the impact of organizational behaviors on work disability prevention and management. *J. Occup. Rehabil.* **2000**, *10*, 21–38. [CrossRef]
26. Hunt, H.A.; Habeck, R.V.; VanTol, B.; Scully, S.M. *Disability Prevention among Michigan Employers, 1988–1993*; Report No. 93-004; W.E. Upjohn Institute for Employment Research: Kalamazoo, MI, USA, 1993.
27. Shea, T.; De Cieri, H.; Donohue, R.; Cooper, B.; Sheehan, C. Leading indicators of occupational health and safety: An employee and workplace level validation study. *Saf. Sci.* **2016**, *85*, 293–304. [CrossRef]
28. Institute for Work & Health. Benchmarking Organizational Leading Indicators for the Prevention and Management of Injuries and Illnesses: Final Report. Available online: https://www.iwh.on.ca/sites/iwh/files/iwh/reports/iwh_report_benchmarking_organizational_leading_indicators_2011.pdf (accessed on 21 November 2018).
29. Centers for Disease Control and Prevention. Workplace Health Model. Available online: https://www.cdc.gov/workplacehealthpromotion/pdf/WorkplaceHealth-model-update.pdf (accessed on 21 November 2018).
30. Goetzel, R.Z.; Henke, R.M.; Tabrizi, M.; Pelletier, K.R.; Loeppke, R.; Ballard, D.W.; Grossmeier, J.; Anderson, D.R.; Yach, D.; Kelly, R.K. Do workplace health promotion (wellness) programs work? *J. Occup. Environ. Med.* **2014**, *56*, 927–934. [CrossRef]
31. SAS Institute. *Base SAS 9.4 Procedures Guide*; SAS Institute: Cary, NC, USA, 2015.
32. Muthén, L.K.; Muthén, B.O. *Mplus User's Guide*, 7th ed.; Muthén & Muthén: Los Angeles, CA, USA, 2012.
33. Oberski, D. Mixture models: Latent profile and latent class analysis. In *Modern Statistical Methods for Human-Computer Interaction*; Springer: Geneva, Switzerland, 2016; pp. 275–287.
34. Aldana, S.G.; Anderson, D.R.; Adams, T.B.; Whitmer, R.W.; Merrill, R.M.; George, V.; Noyce, J. A review of the knowledge base on healthy worksite culture. *J. Occup. Environ. Med.* **2012**, *54*, 414–419. [CrossRef] [PubMed]
35. Pronk, N.; Allen, C. Chapter 26: A culture of health: Creating and sustaining supportive organizational environments for *health*. In *ACSM's Worksite Health Handbook. A Guide to Building Healthy and Productive Companies*, 2nd ed.; Pronk, N., Ed.; Human Kinetics Publishers: Champaign, IL, USA, 2009; pp. 224–230.
36. Feltner, C.; Peterson, K.; Weber, R.P.; Cluff, L.; Coker-Schwimmer, E.; Viswanathan, M.; Lohr, K.N. The effectiveness of Total Worker Health interventions: A systematic review for a National Institutes of Health Pathways to Prevention Workshop. *Ann. Intern. Med.* **2016**, *165*, 262–269. [CrossRef] [PubMed]
37. Anger, W.K.; Elliot, D.L.; Bodner, T.; Olson, R.; Rohlman, D.S.; Truxillo, D.M.; Kuehl, K.S.; Hammer, L.B.; Montgomery, D. Effectiveness of Total Worker Health interventions. *J. Occup. Health Psychol.* **2015**, *20*, 226–247. [CrossRef] [PubMed]

38. Bradley, C.J.; Grossman, D.C.; Hubbard, R.A.; Ortega, A.N.; Curry, S.J. Integrated interventions for improving Total Worker Health: A panel report from the National Institutes of Health Pathways to Prevention Workshop: Total Worker Health—What's Work Got to Do with It? *Ann. Intern. Med.* **2016**, *165*, 279–283. [CrossRef] [PubMed]
39. Rohlman, D.S.; Campo, S.; Hall, J.; Robinson, E.L.; Kelly, K.M. What could Total Worker Health® look like in small enterprises? *Ann. Work Expo. Health* **2018**, *62*, S34–S41. [CrossRef] [PubMed]

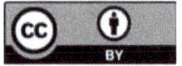

© 2018 by the authors. Licensee MDPI, Basel, Switzerland. This article is an open access article distributed under the terms and conditions of the Creative Commons Attribution (CC BY) license (http://creativecommons.org/licenses/by/4.0/).

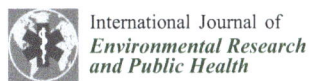

Article

New Burnout Evaluation Model Based on the Brief Burnout Questionnaire: Psychometric Properties for Nursing

María del Carmen Pérez-Fuentes [1,*], María del Mar Molero Jurado [1], África Martos Martínez [1] and José Jesús Gázquez Linares [1,2]

[1] Department of Psychology, Faculty of Psychology, University of Almería, 04120 Almería, Spain; mmj130@ual.es (M.d.M.M.J.); amm521@ual.es (Á.M.M.); jlinares@ual.es (J.J.G.L.)
[2] Department of Psychology, Universidad Autónoma de Chile, Región Metropolitana, Providencia 7500000, Chile
* Correspondence: mpf421@ual.es; Tel.: +34-950-015-598

Received: 19 November 2018; Accepted: 30 November 2018; Published: 2 December 2018

Abstract: Health care personnel are considered one of the worker sectors most exposed to heavier workloads and work stress. One of the consequences associated with the exposure to chronic stress is the development of burnout syndrome. Given that evaluating this syndrome requires addressing the context in which they are to be used, the purpose of this work was to analyze the psychometric properties and structure of the Burnout Brief Questionnaire (CBB), and to propose a more suitable version for its application to health professionals, and more specifically nurses. The final study sample was made up of 1236 working nursing professionals. An exploratory factorial analysis was carried out and a new model was proposed through a confirmatory factorial analysis. Thus, validation of the CBB questionnaire for nursing health care personnel showed an adequate discrimination of the items and a high internal consistency of the scale. With respect to the factorial analysis, four factors were extracted from the revised model. Specifically, these new factors, called job dissatisfaction, social climate, personal impact, and motivational abandonment, showed an adequate index of adjustment. Thus, the Brief Burnout Questionnaire Revised for nursing staff has favorable psychometric properties, and this model can be applied to all health care professionals.

Keywords: burnout; psychometric properties; nursing

1. Introduction

The number of health care workers in Spain increases year after year, as the number of official association members testifies, in fields such as medicine, which in 2015 increased by 1.9%. The number of nurses rose by 3.4% [1] to nearly 300,000 registered nurses according to the latest data from the National Statistics Institute [2]. Furthermore, the role of nursing personnel is more and more important, and the emotional skills and stressful work climate of nurses must be taken into account, but not only for them, as there are now studies analyzing these factors even in students of physiotherapy, for example [3]. Therefore, nurses are gradually facing situations and settings with more pressure and heavier workloads [4], which produce scenarios filled with strain and job stress [5].

According to the Encyclopedia of Mental Health, burnout syndrome is a type of response to chronic emotional and interpersonal stress factors at work, which is recognized as a serious occupational hazard [6]. The presence of stressors at work maintained over long periods of time can cause burnout in workers, especially those who maintain a constant direct care relationship with service users, as is the case of health care personnel [7], although this syndrome may also be discussed in other areas [8–10].

The presence of burnout syndrome in workers leads to physical, occupational, and psychological consequences, in particular, cardiovascular problems, pain, depressive symptoms, sleep problems, alcohol abuse, absenteeism, and job dissatisfaction [11]. Its appearance has also been associated with a multitude of individual and psychosocial variables [12,13].

One of the behaviors associated with this syndrome is demotivation [5,14]. Specifically, the deterioration of professional motivation, which affects almost half of nursing personnel [15], is a process derived from the perception of absence of reward and culminates in the individual's depersonalization [16]. Motivation, which refers to choices of ends and means, depends in large part on an individual's beliefs and values at the time a situation is evaluated. Motivation generates feelings that lead to action on the job, while demotivation creates limits and promotes expressions of displeasure and distress [17]. According to a study by Achour et al. [18], lack of recognition and motivation are two challenges that health care personnel must face as heavier workloads are assigned and measurements of performance become stricter. This directly affects their performance and job satisfaction [19]. So nursing professionals with the most intrinsic motivation (that is, motivated by their own enjoyment of performing the task for humanitarian reasons) and extrinsic motivation (associated with economic characteristics and scheduling flexibility) show higher levels of job satisfaction and less burnout [20].

Job satisfaction specifically refers to the enjoyment individuals find in their job [21]. Lack of satisfaction in health care jobs has been associated with the presence of burnout in workers, and also with the intention of quitting the profession and diminishing quality of the care given [22,23]. According to Farnaz et al. [24], job satisfaction in nursing is associated mainly with environmental factors, in detriment to sociodemographic and individual factors, so improving satisfaction in job positions involves enriching the characteristics of the organizations nurses work in.

The workplaces with the highest quality, with regard to both setting and structure, are associated with greater well-being and lower levels of burnout among health care personnel [25,26]. Therefore, it is of vital importance that healthy work environments, where the psychological health of nursing staff is given attention, be promoted [27]. In turn, study of the prevention, treatment, and measurement of severe widespread problems in this population, such as burnout syndrome, must continue to progress [28].

The most widely used instrument for the evaluation of burnout is the Maslach Burnout Inventory (MBI) [29]. This instrument was designed for evaluating professionals, such as nurses, who perform their job while interacting with users of their service [30], and has been extensively described and validated internationally [31]. Its manual describes burnout as occurring at high levels of emotional exhaustion and depersonalization, in combination with low scores in personal accomplishment. However, other studies [32] make use of alternative proposals to determine the presence of burnout, such as the definition by Poncet et al. [33], who estimated that this syndrome is present among professionals with a cumulative score over −9 on the MBI.

Although there are studies confirming the Maslach Burnout Inventory questionnaire's three dimensions [34–36], other studies have found factor structures based on two [37,38] and five dimensions [39,40]. Densten [39], after confirmatory analysis of the instrument, found that the structure based on five scales was more strongly supported than the model of three, or even four. Thus, while the depersonalization factor was maintained in this new division of factors, emotional exhaustion was divided into "somatic strain" and "psychological strain," while personal accomplishment was broken down into "self-accomplishment" and "working with others."

Another alternative instrument to the MBI for evaluating burnout is the Brief Burnout Questionnaire (CBB) [41]. The CBB comprises 21 items that evaluate not only the syndrome itself, but also its antecedents and consequences. That is, it understands burnout as a process [42]. The instrument was validated in teaching professionals, showing adequate convergent validity with the MBI on the total burnout scale (but not, however, on all the syndrome factors), so the authors recommended it for evaluating some elements present in the burnout process (specifically antecedents, burnout, and consequences), but not for direct evaluation of its specific components. Few studies have used this questionnaire [43–45], as shown in the review by Ahola et al. [46], who indicated that they were unaware of the existence of the questionnaire's validation. It has also been adapted for use with housewives [47], in which a three-factor structure similar to the one found in the original questionnaire was found. However, this instrument has received some criticism. For example, in the validation done in a sample of teachers in Aragon Province, Spain [48], no significant differences were found on some of the scales between men and women, which might be due to the inappropriateness of the items in showing the behavior associated on each scale. The results have also shown low reliability, and it was concluded that its use has generated little validity, mainly because of its factor division [49].

According to Domínguez-Lara [50], the multifactor internal structure of burnout evaluation instruments must be analyzed considering the context where they are going to be used, since even though the construct may have a good theoretical basis, the configuration of its structure may vary when used in real environments. Therefore, the purpose of this study is to show that the CBB is a valid model for different cultures and societies, as this scale has awakened great interest in recent years. In addition to analyzing its psychometric properties and structure, this study proposes the best version or model for its application to health care professionals, and nurses in particular.

2. Materials and Methods

2.1. Participants

The sample was made up of 1352 nurses selected at random from several health centers, and therefore actively employed at the time data were collected. Subjects who did not complete the questionnaire or who gave random answers (detected by control questions) were eliminated from the study. The final sample consisted of a total of 1236 participants, of whom 69.3% ($n = 857$) were working under temporary contracts and the other 30.7% ($n = 379$) had permanent contracts.

The mean participant age was 31.50 years ($SD = 6.18$), in a range of 21 to 57 years. Of the whole sample, 84.5% ($n = 1044$) were women and 15.5% ($n = 192$) were men, with a mean age of 31.65 years ($SD = 6.23$) and 30.71 years ($SD = 6.17$), respectively. Their marital status was 55% ($n = 680$) single, 42.1% ($n = 520$) married or in a stable relationship, 2.8% ($n = 34$) divorced or separated, and 0.2% ($n = 2$) widowed. In addition, 68.9% ($n = 852$) of the participants had no children, 14.5% ($n = 179$) had 1 child, 13.2% ($n = 163$) had 2 children, and the remaining 3.3% ($n = 41$) had 3 or more.

Their distribution by area of work was 32% ($n = 396$) staff nurse and 21.9% ($n = 271$) on emergency teams, while 11.4% ($n = 141$) were working in the ICU, 10.7% ($n = 132$) in surgery, 2.3% ($n = 28$) in outpatient care, and 4% ($n = 50$) in the mental health unit. The remaining 17.6% ($n = 218$) were working in other areas.

2.2. Instruments

An ad hoc questionnaire was prepared to collect sociodemographic data (age, sex, marital status, and degree) and to compile information on their profession and work experience: years of experience, employment situation (permanent or temporary), work shifts (rotating, 12 h or more, nights only, and morning/afternoon), and number of patients attended to in a workday.

The CBB [41] was used to evaluate burnout syndrome in the professionals. This instrument consists of 21 items in three blocks corresponding to antecedents of burnout and its elements and consequences. Even though the purpose of the questionnaire is to evaluate the professional burnout process, it includes factors proposed in the Maslach and Jackson model [29] and components that precede and support it. The answer format is a 5-point Likert-type scale. Items 2, 4, 8, 9, and 16 must be inverted and recoded after inversion to find the corresponding overall subscale scores.

2.3. Procedure

Before the data were collected, compliance with participant information standards, confidentiality, and ethics in data processing was guaranteed. Questionnaires were implemented on a Web platform, which enabled participants to fill them out online. A series of control questions were included to detect chance or incongruent answers, and any such cases were discarded from the study sample.

2.4. Data Analysis

The descriptive and confirmatory data analyses were done following the steps by Pérez-Fuentes et al. [51]; in addition, validation was performed in two stages following the steps by Álvarez-García et al. [52]. The first stage was intended to study the structure of the CBB. To approach this objective, the sample was first randomly divided into two independent homogeneous subsamples. The first (n = 605) was used as a calibration sample for confirmatory factor analysis (CFA) of the burnout model proposed (Figure 1). Then CFA was done for the proposed model, taking the following fit indices as measures: χ^2/gl, comparative fit index (CFI), Tucker–Lewis index (TLI), root mean square error of approximation (RMSEA), with the confidence interval (CI) at 90%. The index χ^2/gl was used considering values below 5 acceptable [53], Comparative Fit Index (CFI) and Incremental Fit Index (IFI) over or near 0.95, and RMSEA below or very near 0.06 [54]. As a general rule, good fit of the model would be found when ratio 2/GL (degrees of freedom)$\leq$ 3; Goodness-of-fit index (GFI), adjusted goodness of fit index (AGFI), and TLI > 0.90; CFI > 0.95; and RMSEA $\leq$ 0.05. The advisable respecifications were made to the proposed model, which showed good fit indices, considering theoretical and statistical criteria (modification indices, estimation errors, standardized errors of measurement). The Akaike information criterion [55] was used for model selection based on the second subsample (n = 635), which was used as the validation sample to validate the respecified model. Cronbach's alpha [56] and split halves were used for the reliability analysis of the new scale.

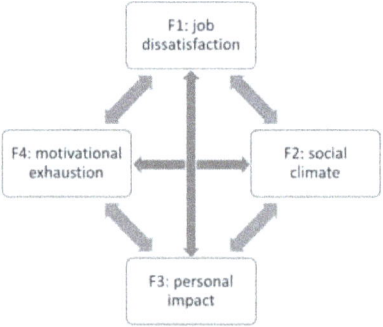

Figure 1. Proposed Burnout model.

In the second stage, an analysis was done to support the proposed invariant factor structure across type of contract (permanent or temporary) and gender (male/female). First, both subsamples were checked to see the goodness of fit of these structures (model M0a, Permanent-Male, and model M0b, Temporary-Female). The four resulting nested models were evaluated: (a) Model 1. Both subsamples were considered simultaneously with free parameter estimation. (b) Model 2. Metric invariance was demonstrated. (c) Model 3. Scalar invariance was demonstrated. (d) Model 4. Strict invariance. There was no consensus criterion to determine the criteria to be used to evaluate the difference in fit of the nested models [57]. This study used ΔCFI to evaluate its fit. ΔCFI interprets the model as fully invariant if the value found is below 0.01 [58]. The analyses were performed using the SPSS version 23.0 Statistical Package for Windows (IBM, Armonk, NY, USA) and the AMOS 22 program (IBM, Armonk, NY, USA).

3. Results

3.1. Preliminary Analyses

In the first place, the data show that the CBB items have a normal distribution according to the criterion of Finney and DiStefano [59], who give 2 and 7 as the maximum permissible for skew and kurtosis, respectively. In our study, the maximum was 1.24 and 2.15, respectively. In the exploratory factor analysis, principal component extraction was used with direct oblimin rotation (KMO = 0.85), which allows correlation between factors. Based on the exploratory analysis and various previous studies on validation of the questionnaire itself, other versions, and previous research, a new model is proposed.

3.2. Exploratory Factor Analysis of the Original CBB Model

The principal component analysis (chosen since the determinant of $p = 0.086$ showed intercorrelation of the variables, required for this method) revealed the existence of two components with eigenvalues over 1 in the first block, that is, the general antecedents scale. Thus, the scree test indicated the advisability of rotation with two factors with eigenvalues of 3.56 and 1.37, since they were clearly distanced from the third, with a score of 0.86.

After factor analysis, the items with factor saturations over 0.40 were selected from the direct oblimin rotation matrix of rotated components. As seen in Table 1, factor 1 corresponds to the items that make up the scale's organization factor. Factor 1 comprises four items, all with loadings over 0.60, which explain 38.18% of the variance. Factor 2 is made up of five items and forms part of the task component, and explains 15.22% of the variance.

Table 1. Factor structure, communalities (h2), eigenvalues, Cronbach's alpha, and percentage of explained variance ($n = 1236$). Extraction method: principal component analysis.

Principal component analysis	F1	F2	h^2
Item 2	0.56	0.63	0.53
Item 4	0.65		0.42
Item 6		0.79	0.63
Item 8	0.81		0.66
Item 9	0.79		0.62
Item 10		0.55	0.31
Item 14		0.68	0.48
Item 16	0.78		0.63
Item 20		0.80	0.64
Eigenvalue	3.56	1.37	
Percentage explained variance	39.51	15.22	54.73
Kaiser–Meyer–Olkin		0.85	
Barlett's sphericity	$\chi^2_{(36)} = 3019.35, p < 0.000$		
Cronbach's alpha	0.75	0.73	0.79

Note: Items are listed in decreasing order by saturation. Visualization coefficient > 0.40. F1: organization; F2: task.

In the second block of the burnout syndrome scale, principal component analysis (determinant $p = 0.124$ shows intercorrelation of the variables) revealed the existence of one component with an eigenvalue over 1. As the theoretical structure of the construct was three factors, we used principal axis factoring to force the presence of three factors with varimax rotation. The scree test shows the adequacy of rotation with one factor with a value of 3.38, and the following two are scarcely below 1, with values of 0.98 and 0.96, although they are at a distance from the quartile score of 0.84.

After the factor analysis, we selected the items with the highest factor saturations from the matrix of rotated components (varimax rotation). Table 2 shows how factor 1 corresponds to the items that make up the scale's emotional exhaustion factor. This factor comprises three items, all with loadings over 0.60, explaining 31.93% of the variance. The original questionnaire did not include item 3 in this factor, which saturated highest in factor 3. Factor 2 comprises four items, which form the lack of accomplishment component, explaining 4.99% of the variance. Item 18 is included in this factor, but not in the original version, where it was in factor 3. Finally, it should be mentioned that factor 3, which is formed by the depersonalization component, is composed of two items, and that item 3 is in this factor, unlike the original questionnaire.

Table 2. Factor structure, communalities (h^2), eigenvalues, Cronbach's alpha, and percentage of explained variance ($n = 1236$). Extraction method: principal component analysis.

Principal component analysis	F1	F2	F3	h^2
Item 1	0.76			0.68
Item 3			0.72	0.58
Item 5		0.49		0.27
Item 7	0.60			0.48
Item 11			0.44	0.37
Item 12		0.50		0.33
Item 15	0.72			0.66
Item 18		0.28		0.11
Item 19		0.30		0.17
Eigenvalue	3.38	0.98	0.96	
Percentage explained variance	31.93	4.99	3.74	40.66
Kaiser–Meyer–Olkin		0.84		
Barlett's sphericity		$\chi^2_{(36)} = 2569.33, p < 0.000$		
Cronbach's alpha	0.81	0.49	0.57	0.76

Note: Items are listed order by saturation in decreasing. Visualization coefficient >0.40. F1: emotional exhaustion; F2: lack of accomplishment; F3: depersonalization.

Table 3. Factor structure, communalities (h^2), eigenvalues, Cronbach's alpha, and percentage of explained variance ($n = 1236$). Extraction method: principal component analysis.

Principal component analysis	F1	F2	F3	F4	h^2
Item 1	0.56	0.41	0.65		0.61
Item 2	0.59	0.58			0.55
Item 3			0.62	0.45	0.49
Item 4		0.65			0.43
Item 5	0.43			0.57	0.41
Item 6	0.70			0.56	0.64
Item 7	0.44		0.62		0.51
Item 8		0.80			0.66
Item 9		0.78			0.62
Item 10				0.61	0.38
Item 11			0.40	0.67	0.51
Item 12	0.44			0.62	0.47
Item 13			0.78		0.62
Item 14	0.56		0.41		0.40
Item 15	0.56		0.70		0.66
Item 16		0.77	0.41		0.64
Item 17			0.66		0.47
Item 18				0.53	0.30
Item 19	0.66				0.44
Item 20	0.76				0.64
Item 21			0.62		0.46
Eigenvalue	6.67	1.76	1.39	1.06	
Percentage explained variance	31.77	8.41	6.64	5.05	51.86
Kaiser–Meyer–Olkin		0.92			
Barlett's sphericity		$\chi^2_{(210)} = 8449.54, p < 0.000$			
Cronbach's alpha	0.74	0.75	0.82	0.59	0.88

Note: Items are listed in decreasing order by saturation. Visualization coefficient >0.40. F1: job dissatisfaction; F2: social climate; F3: personal impact; F4: motivational exhaustion.

The third part of the scale corresponds to the consequences of burnout, and analysis of principal components revealed the existence of one component with eigenvalues over 1. It comprises three items (13, 17, and 21), all with loadings over 0.75 (.79, 0.79, and 0.76, respectively), which explain 60.53% of the variance (KMO = 0.66; $\chi^2_{(3)}$ = 560.17, $p < 0.000$; Cronbach's alpha = 0.67).

3.3. Exploratory Factor Analysis of Revised CBB Model (CBB-R)

Principal component analysis (chosen because the determinant of $p = 0.001$ shows intercorrelation of the variables, required by this method) revealed the existence of four components with eigenvalues over 1. The scree plot recommends rotating with four factors, with eigenvalues of 3.56 and 1.37, respectively, as they are at a clear distance from the third with a score of 0.86.

After factor analysis, we selected the items with factor saturations over 0.40 from the direct oblimin rotation matrix of rotated components. As seen in Table 3, factor 1 corresponds to the items that make up the scale's job dissatisfaction factor. This factor comprises five items, all with loadings over 0.55, explaining 31.77% of the variance. Factor 2 has four items that form the social climate component, explaining 8.41% of the variance. Factor 3 has seven items, which make up the personal impact component and explain 5.05% of the variance. Finally, factor 4 (five items) is related to motivational exhaustion.

3.4. Confirmatory Factor Analysis of CBB Model and CBB-R Model

Table 4 analyzes the fit of the various models of the questionnaire by the original CBB model, the unidimensional CBB model, the proposed four-factor CBB model, and the revision of that model first proposed (CBB-R). The original model and the unidimensional model show values that are not very adequate. The proposed four-factor CBB model, which corresponds to what was found in the exploratory analysis, is better, but while it showed good fit indices, the advisable respecifications were made considering theoretical and statistical criteria (modification indices, errors of estimation, standardized errors of measurement), which led to elimination of items 2, 16, 3, 13, 17, and 11. The revised model showed much better fit with the calibration sample. The difference between the AIC default model value (248.497) and the AIC saturated model value (240.000) is also very small, showing that this is probably the best of the models according to the Akaike model selection criteria.

Fit indices for the proposed CBB-R model with the validation sample ($n = 635$) are shown in Figure 2. Confirmatory factor analysis for the proposed model was done, taking the following fit indices as measures: $\chi^2/gl = 2.241$, CFI = 0.961, TLI = 0.951, RMSEA = 0.044 (0.036–0.053).

Table 4. Fit indices for the models proposed (calibration sample; $n = 605$).

Model	χ^2 (df)	χ^2/df	CFI	TLI	RMR	Est.	RMSEA CI 90% Bel.	RMSEA CI 90% Abv.
Original CBB model	931.446 (179)	5.204	0.822	0.791	0.042	0.083	0.078	0.089
Unidimensional CBB model	1305.043 (189)	6.904	0.735	0.706	0.059	0.099	0.094	0.104
Proposed CBB model	664.676 (183)	3.632	0.886	0.869	0.044	0.066	0.061	0.071
Proposed CBB-R model	176.497 (84)	2.101	0.965	0.956	0.027	0.043	0.034	0.052

Note: CFI, comparative fit index; TLI, Tucker–Lewis index; RMSEA, root mean square error of approximation; CI, confidence interval; df, degrees of freedom; Est., estimation; Bel., below; Abv., above. CBB: CBB-R (Revised CBB Model).

The reliability of the model was analyzed using Cronbach's alpha, where $\alpha = 0.89$ for the total sample; for factor 1 (job dissatisfaction), comprising four items, $\alpha = 0.697$; for factor 2 (social climate), made up of three items, $\alpha = 0.666$; for factor 3 (personal impact), made up of four items, $\alpha = 0.808$; and for factor 4 (motivational exhaustion), comprising four items, $\alpha = 0.529$. Furthermore, the data found by split halves also showed both equal-length (Spearman–Brown coefficient = 0.818) and unequal-length (Spearman–Brown coefficient = 0.819) consistency of the scales.

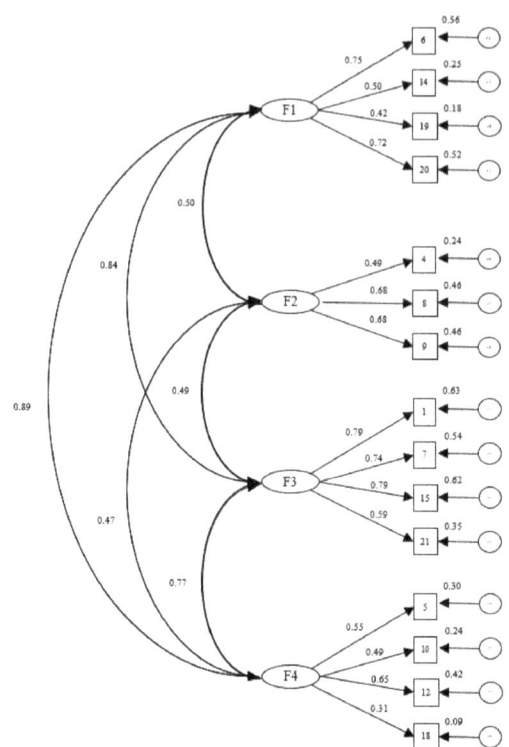

Figure 2. Proposed CBB-R model (validation sample $n = 635$). Note: F1: job dissatisfaction; F2: social climate; F3: personal impact; F4: motivational exhaustion.

Table 5 shows the values for all six models. It can be seen how ΔCFI is over 0.01 for models 3 and 4, accepting the configural and metric invariance. Specifically, ΔCFI between model 1 (configural and metric base model) and models 3 and 4 is 0.024, so scalar and strict invariance cannot be accepted. In the analysis of variance by gender, in all cases ΔCFI is under 0.01, so the configural, metric, scalar, and strict invariances are accepted.

Table 5. Multigroup analysis of variance by type of contract (permanent/temporary) and gender (male/female).

Model	x^2	gl	x^2/gl	Δx^2	CFI	ΔCFI	IFI	RMSEA (CI 90%)
M0a (permanent)	376.265 ($p = 0.000$)	168	2.239		0.960		0.961	0.032 (0.027–0.036)
M0b (temporary)	417.761 ($p = 0.000$)	179	2.333		0.955		0.955	0.033 (0.029–0.037)
M1 (base model set)	505.309 ($p = 0.000$)	194	2.604		0.941		0.941	0.036 (0.032–0.040)
M2 (FS)	544.696 ($p = 0.000$)	209	2.606	39.387	0.936	0.005	0.936	0.036 (0.032–0.040)
M3 (FS + Int)	376.265 ($p = 0.000$)	168	2.239	129.044	0.960	0.024	0.961	0.032 (0.027–0.036)
M4 (FS + Int + Err)	376.265 ($p = 0.000$)	168	2.239	129.044	0.960	0.024	0.961	0.032 (0.027–0.036)
M0a (male)	383.819 ($p = 0.000$)	168	2.284		0.959		0.960	0.032 (0.028–0.037)
M0b (female)	407.567 ($p = 0.000$)	179	2.276		0.957		0.957	0.032 (0.028–0.036)
M1 (base model set)	446.771 ($p = 0.000$)	194	2.302		0.952		0.953	0.032 (0.029–0.036)
M2 (FS)	474.727 ($p = 0.000$)	209	2.271	27.956	0.950	0.002	0.950	0.032 (0.028–0.036)
M3 (FS + Int)	383.819 ($p = 0.000$)	168	2.284	62.952	0.959	0.009	0.960	0.032 (0.028–0.037)
M4 (FS + Int + Err)	376.265 ($p = 0.000$)	168	2.284	62.952	0.959	0.009	0.960	0.032 (0.028–0.037)

Nota FS = factor saturation; Int = intercepts; Err = error.

4. Discussion

The validation of the CBB questionnaire for health care personnel in nursing shows adequate discrimination of items. Cronbach's alpha for this scale was 0.089, which shows its high internal consistency.

With respect to the factor analysis, four factors were extracted from the revised model, which differed from the original structure of the Brief Burnout Questionnaire [41]. This model was proven to generate better fit of the data than the original. The percentage explained by this model was 51.86%, emphasizing the first factor, where all the items loaded over 0.55 and explained 31.77% of the variance. This factor, called job dissatisfaction, clusters indicators in two dimensions, burnout factors and burnout syndrome. This factor compiles items that refer to the balance between job expectations and reality, and how much enjoyment the individual finds in the job [21]. This coincides with the proposal made by Moreno et al. [35], in their questionnaire for evaluating professional burnout in doctors, where a factor referring to the loss of job expectations was included. Similarly, the second factor, made up of four items, groups indicators corresponding to the relationship the worker establishes with fellow workers and superiors at work. This factor, which is called social climate, responds to a cluster that may be due to the importance in developing burnout of chronic stressful interpersonal situations in the workplace [6]. The third factor grouped seven items, which in the original questionnaire were in the burnout syndrome scale, except for one, which was on the consequences scale. The cluster of these items is called the personal impact factor and refers to the direct consequences exhaustion has on different areas of an employee's life.

Finally, the fourth factor, called motivational exhaustion, combines five items that in the original model were part of the burnout syndrome scale. The questions grouped under this factor of motivational exhaustion refer to the absence of job growth and stimulation for development in the job position. These are aspects that promote work demotivation, generate distress [17], and are among the challenges health care personnel face most frequently [18].

Although this four-factor model showed adequate fit, after making the corresponding respecifications according to theoretical and statistical criteria, items 2, 16, 3, 13, 17, and 11 were eliminated, so all 21 items in the original questionnaire were not retained. The items that were finally kept in each of the factors in the Brief Burnout Questionnaire Revised were items 6, 14, 19, and 20 for job dissatisfaction; 4, 8, and 9 in the social climate factor; 1, 7, 15, and 21 in personal impact; and 5, 10, 12, and 18 in the motivational exhaustion factor.

The model fit improved considerably this way, and also showed consistency in the validation sample. Configural and metric invariance of the model across the type of job (permanent/temporary) is also assumed, and invariance in all cases (configural, metric, scalar, and strict) across gender. Given the divergence found when clustering items, inquiry into the adequacy of the structure reported by the CBB-R for nursing personnel will have to continue. The multifactorial construct of burnout shown here, which differs from the one reported by the authors of the original study, shows the need for further study of the internal structure of the evaluation instruments in this construct in the population studied [50]. In the process of adapting and validating instruments for certain populations, it must be known whether the factor structure coincides or not with the terms of the original version, as the job characteristics of each sample partly moderate the conditions where burnout appears. The proposed model also includes an analysis of all the burnout risk and protection factors now known as found in the theoretical review.

5. Conclusions

The Brief Burnout Questionnaire Revised for health care personnel in nursing has favorable psychometric properties. The internal consistency of the total scale and each of the factors is adequate, therefore the general fit is acceptable. However, it is recommended that goodness and fit of the model continue to be analyzed to test the psychometric properties of the instrument in other groups, since this model of burnout can be applied to all care professionals.

This new evaluation model based on the CBB questionnaire adapted as an instrument for evaluation of the syndrome in health care personnel is intended to approach even closer to knowledge of burnout, exploring the different facets that comprise it. Thus, the purpose of validating the instrument was to approach burnout's present reality. As a syndrome linked to the work environment of individuals, burnout will continue to evolve with it, accumulating new factors workers must cope with that may also lead to burnout.

Author Contributions: M.d.M.M.J., Á.M.M., and M.d.C.P.-F. contributed to the conception and design of the review. J.J.G.L. applied the search strategy. All authors applied the selection criteria. All authors completed the assessment of risk of bias. All authors analyzed the data and interpreted data. M.d.M.M.J., M.d.C.P.-F., and Á.M.M. wrote this manuscript. M.d.C.P.-F. and J.J.G.L. edited this manuscript. M.d.C.P.F. is responsible for the overall project.

Funding: This research received no external funding.

Acknowledgments: The present study was undertaken in collaboration with the Excma. Diputación Provincial de Almería. Part of this work has been developed thanks to the financing of the 2018 Own Research Plan of the University of Almería, for the help for the hiring of research personnel in predoctoral training, granted to África Martos Martínez.

Conflicts of Interest: The authors declare no conflict of interest.

References

1. National Statistics Institute. *España en Cifras*; INE: Madrid, Spain, 2017.
2. Profesionales Sanitarios Colegiados 2016. Available online: http://www.ine.es/jaxi/Datos.htm?path=/t15/p416/a2016/l0/&file=s08004.px (accessed on 15 August 2018).
3. González-Cabanach, R.; Souto-Gestal, A.; Fernández-Cervantes, R. Emotion regulation profiles and academic stress in Physiotherapy students. *Eur. J. Educ. Psychol.* **2017**, *10*, 57–67. [CrossRef]
4. Zhou, J.; Yang, Y.; Qiu, X.; Pan, H.; Ban, B.; Qiao, Z.; Wang, L.; Wang, W. Serial multiple mediation of organizational commitment and job burnout in the relationship between psychological capital and anxiety in Chinese female nurses: A cross-sectional questionnaire survey. *Int. J. Nurs. Stud.* **2018**, *83*, 75–82. [CrossRef] [PubMed]
5. García-Camapayo, J.; Puebla-Guedea, M.; Herrera-Mercadal, P.; Daudén, E. Burnout Syndrome and Demotivation among Health Care Personnel. Managing Stressful Situations: The Importance of Teamwork. *Actas Dermosifiliogr.* **2016**, *107*, 400–406. [CrossRef]
6. Maslach, C. Burnout. In *Encyclopedia of Mental Health*, 2nd ed.; Friedman, H., Ed.; Elsevier: Oxford, UK, 2016; pp. 222–227. ISBN 978-0-12-397045-9.
7. Gómez, L.; Estrella, D. Síndrome de *Burnout*: Una revisión breve. *Ciencia Humanismo Salud* **2015**, *2*, 116–122.
8. De Francisco, C.; Arce, C.; Vílchez, M.P.; Vales, A. Antecedents and consequences of burnout in athletes: Perceived stress and depression. *Int. J. Clin. Health Psychol.* **2016**, *16*, 221–314. [CrossRef]
9. Pérez-Fuentes, M.C.; Gázquez, J.J.; Ruiz, M.D.; Molero, M.M. Inventory of Overburden in Alzheimer's Patient Family Caregivers with no Specialized Training. *Int. J. Clin. Health Psychol.* **2017**, *17*, 56–64. [CrossRef] [PubMed]
10. Martos, Á.; Pérez-Fuentes, M.C.; Molero, M.M.; Gázquez, J.J.; Simón, M.M.; Barragán, A.B. Burnout y engagement en estudiantes de Ciencias de la Salud. *Eur. J Investig.* **2018**, *8*, 23–36. [CrossRef]
11. Jodas, D.A.; Nesello, F.; Eumann, A.; Durán, A.; Lopez, F.; de Andrade, S.M. Physical, psychological and occupational consequences of job burnout: A systematic review of prospective studies. *PLoS ONE* **2017**, *12*, e0185781. [CrossRef]
12. Iorga, M.; Socolov, V.; Muraru, D.; Dirtu, C.; Soponaru, C.; Ilea, C.; Socolov, D.G. Factors Influencing Burnout Syndrome in Obstetrics and Gynecology Physicians. *BioMed Res. Int.* **2017**, *2017*, 1–10. [CrossRef]
13. Schneider, A.; Weigl, M. Associations between psychosocial work factors and provider mental well-being in emergency departments: A systematic review. *PLoS ONE* **2018**, *13*, e0197375. [CrossRef]
14. Frenet, C.; Trépanier, S.G.; Demers, M.; Austin, S. Motivational pathways of occupational and organizational turnover intention among newly registered nurses in Canada. *Nurs. Outlook* **2017**, *65*, 444–454. [CrossRef]
15. Obradovic, Z.; Obradovic, A.; Cesir-Skoro, I. Nurses and burnout síndrome. *J. Health Biol.* **2013**, *3*, 60–64.

16. Basinska, B.A.; Wilczek-Ruzyczka, E. The role of rewards and demansd in burnout among surgical nurses. *Int. J. Occup. Med. Environ. Health* **2013**, *26*, 593–604. [CrossRef]
17. Pucheu, A. ¿Existen diferencias en la motivación de distintas generaciones en enfermería? *Rev. Méd. Clín. Las Condes* **2018**, *29*, 336–342. [CrossRef]
18. Achour, N.; Munokaran, S.; Barker, F.; Soetanto, R. Staff Stress: The Sleeping Cell of Healthcare Failure. *Procedia Eng.* **2018**, *212*, 459–466. [CrossRef]
19. Contreras, F.; Espinal, L.; Pachón, A.M.; González, J. Burnout, liderazgo y satisfacción laboral en el personal asistencial de un hospital de tercer nivel en Bogotá. *Perspect. Psicol.* **2013**, *9*, 65–80. [CrossRef]
20. Dill, J.; Erickson, R.J.; Diefendorff, J.M. Motivation in caring labor: Implications for the well-being and employment outcomes of nurses. *Soc. Sci. Med.* **2016**, *167*, 99–106. [CrossRef]
21. Kabir, M.N.; Parvin, M.M. Factors affecting employee job satisfaction of pharmaceutical sector. *Aust. J. Bus. Manag. Res.* **2011**, *1*, 113–123.
22. Elbarazi, I.; Loney, T.; Yousef, S.; Elias, A. Prevalence of and factors associated with burnout among health care professionals in Arab countries: A systematic review. *BMC Health Serv. Res.* **2017**, *17*, 1–10. [CrossRef]
23. Van Bogaert, P.; Van Heusden, D.; Verspuy, M.; Wouters, K.; Slootmans, S.; Van der Straeten, J.; Aken, V.; White, M. The Productive Ward Program™: A Two-Year Implementation Impact Review Using a Longitudinal Multilevel Study. *Can. J. Nurs. Res.* **2017**, *49*, 28–38. [CrossRef]
24. Farnaz, R.; Kalateh, A.; Hemmati, S.; Ebrahimzade, N.; Sarikhani, Y.; Heydari, S.T.; Lankarani, K.B. The impact of environmental and demographic factors on nursing job satisfaction. *Electron. Phys.* **2018**, *10*, 6712–6717. [CrossRef]
25. Molero, M.M.; Pérez-Fuentes, M.C.; Gázquez, J.J.; Simón, M.M.; Martos, Á. Burnout Risk and Protection Factors in Certified Nursing Aides. *Int. J. Environ. Res. Public Health* **2018**, *15*, 1116. [CrossRef] [PubMed]
26. Mudallal, R.H.; Othman, W.M.; Al Hassan, N.F. Nurses' Burnout: The Influence of Leader Empowering Behaviors, Work Conditions, and Demographic Traits. *Inquiry* **2017**, *54*, 1–10. [CrossRef] [PubMed]
27. Wei, H.; Sewell, K.A.; Woody, G.; Rose, M.A. The state of the science of nurse work environments in the United States: A systematic review. *Int. J. Nurs. Sci.* **2018**, *5*, 1–14. [CrossRef]
28. Pérez-Fuentes, M.C.; Molero, M.M.; Gázquez, J.J.; Oropesa, N.F. The Role of Emotional Intelligence in Engagement in Nurses. *Int. J. Environ. Res. Public Health* **2018**, *15*, 1915. [CrossRef]
29. Maslach, C.; Jackson, S.E. *Maslach Burnout Inventory*; Consulting Psychologists Press: Palo Alto, CA, USA, 1981.
30. Squieres, A.; Finlayson, C.; Gerchow, L.; Cimiotti, J.P.; Matthews, A.; Schwendimann, R.; Griffiths, P.; Busse, R.; Heinen, M.; Brzostek, T.; et al. Methodological considerations when translating "burnout". *Burn Res.* **2014**, *1*, 59–68. [CrossRef] [PubMed]
31. Martins, S.; Teixera, C.M.; Carvalho, A.S.; Hernández-Marrero, P. Compared to Palliative Care, Working in Intensive Care More than Doubles the Chances of Burnout: Results from a Nationwide Comparative Study. *PLoS ONE* **2016**, *11*, e0162340. [CrossRef]
32. Merlani, P.; Verdon, M.; Businger, A.; Domenighetti, G.; Pargger, H.; Ricou, B. Burnout in ICU Caregivers: A Multicenter Study of Factors Associated to Centers. *Am. J. Respir. Crit.* **2011**, *184*, 1140–1146. [CrossRef]
33. Poncet, M.C.; Toullic, P.; Papazian, L.; Barnes, N.K.; Timsit, J.F.; Pochard, F.; Chevret, S.; Schlemmer, B.; Azoulay, E. Burnout Syndrome in Critical Care Nursing Staff. *Am. J. Respir. Crit.* **2007**, *175*, 698–704. [CrossRef]
34. Guerra, C.; Mújica, A.; Nahmias, A.; Rojas, N. Análisis psicométrico de la escala de conductas de autocuidado para psicólogos clínicos. *Rev. Latinoam. Psicol.* **2011**, *43*, 319–328. [CrossRef]
35. Moreno, B.; Gálvez, M.; Garrosa, E.; Mingote, J.C. Nuevos planteamientos en la evaluación del *burnout*. La evaluación específica del desgaste profesional médico. *Aten Prim.* **2006**, *38*, 544–549. [CrossRef]
36. Pisanti, R.; Lombardo, C.; Lucidi, F.; Violani, C.; Lazzari, D. Psychometric properties of the Maslach Burnout Inventory for Human Services among Italian nurses: A test of alternative models. *J. Adv. Nurs.* **2013**, *69*, 697–707. [CrossRef] [PubMed]
37. Kalliath, T.J.; O'Driscoll, M.P.; Gillespie, D.F.; Bluedorn, A.C. A test of the Maslach Burnout Inventory in three samples of healthcare professionals. *Work Stress* **2000**, *14*, 35–50. [CrossRef]
38. Kim, H.; Ji, J. Factor structure and longitudinal invariance of the Maslach Burnout Inventory. *Res. Soc. Work Pract.* **2009**, *19*, 325–339. [CrossRef]
39. Densten, I.L. Re-thinking burnout. *J. Organ. Behav.* **2001**, *22*, 833–847. [CrossRef]

40. García, J.M.; Herrero, S.; León, J.L. Validez factorial del Maslach Burnout Inventory (MBI) en una muestra de trabajadores del Hospital Psiquiátrico Penitenciario de Sevilla. *Apuntes Psicol.* **2007**, *25*, 157–174.
41. Moreno-Jiménez, B.; Bustos, R.; Matallana, A.; Miralles, T. La evaluación del burnout. Problemas y alternativas. El CBB como evaluación de los elementos del proceso. *Rev. Psicol. Trabajo Organ.* **1997**, *13*, 185–207.
42. Mingote, J.C.; Moreno, B.; Gálvez, M. Desgaste profesional y salud de los profesionales médicos: Revisión y propuestas de prevención. *Med. Clínica* **2004**, *123*, 265–270. [CrossRef]
43. Blanco-Álvarez, T.M.; Thoen, M.A. Factores asociados al estrés laboral en policías penitenciarios costarricenses. *Rev. Costarric. Psicol.* **2017**, *36*, 45–59. [CrossRef]
44. Correa-Correa, Z.; Muñoz-Zambrano, I.; Chaparro, A.F. Síndrome de Burnout en docentes de dos universidades de Popayán, Colombia. *Rev. Salud Pública* **2010**, *12*, 589–598. [CrossRef]
45. Roger, M.C.; Abalo, J.G.; Pérez, C.M.; Ochoa, I.I.; Abalo, R.G.; Abalo, Y. El control of burnout syndrome de desgaste professional o burnout en enfermeria oncológica: Una experiencia de intervención. *Terapia Psicol.* **2006**, *24*, 39–53.
46. Ahola, K.; Toppinen-Tanner, S.; Seppänen, J. Interventions to alleviate burnout symptoms and to support return to work among employees with burnout: Systematic review and meta-analysis. *Burn Res.* **2017**, *4*, 1–11. [CrossRef]
47. González-Ramírez, M.T.; Landero, R.; Moral de la Rubia, J.M. Cuestionario de Burnout para amas de casa (CUBAC): Evaluación de sus propiedades psicométricas y del Modelo Secuencial de Burnout. *Univ. Psychol.* **2009**, *8*, 533–544.
48. Montero, J.; García-Campayo, J.; Andrés, E. Validez factorial de la estructura del Cuestionario Breve de Burnout (CBB) en una muestra de docentes en Aragón. *Rev. Psicopatol. Psicol. Clin.* **2009**, *14*, 123–132. [CrossRef]
49. Domínguez-Lara, S.; Fernández-Arata, M. Cuestionario breve de Burnout, ¿una elección adecuada? *Enferm Clín.* **2018**, *28*, 214–215. [CrossRef] [PubMed]
50. Domínguez-Lara, S.A. Análisis factorial y confiabilidad del Burnout Screening Inventory. *Educ. Méd.* **2017**, *19*, 125–130. [CrossRef]
51. Pérez-Fuentes, M.C.; Molero, M.M.; Martos, A.; Barragán, A.B.; Gázquez, J.J.; Sánchez-Marchán, C. Spanish analysis and validation of Peer Conflict Scale. *Eur. J. Educ. Psychol.* **2016**, *9*, 56–62. [CrossRef]
52. Álvarez-García, D.; Barreiro-Collazo, A.; Núñez, J.C.; Dobarro, A. Validity and reliability of the Cyber-aggression Questionnaire for Adolescents (CYBA). *Eur. J. Psychol. Appl. Legal Context* **2017**, *8*, 69–77. [CrossRef]
53. Bentler, P.M. *EQS Structural Equations Program Manual*; BMDP Statistical Software: Los Angeles, CA, USA, 1989.
54. Hair, J.F.; Black, W.C.; Babin, B.J.; Anderson, R.E.; Tatham, R.L. *Multivariate Data Analysis*, 7th ed.; Pearson Prentice Hall: Upper Saddle River, NJ, USA, 2006.
55. Akaike, H. A new look at the statistical model identification. *IEEE Trans. Autom. Control* **1974**, *19*, 716–723. [CrossRef]
56. Cronbach, L.J. Coefficient alpha and the internal structure of tests. *Psychometrika* **1951**, *16*, 297–334. [CrossRef]
57. Byrne, B.M.; Stewart, S.M. The MACS approach to testing for multigroup invariance of a second-order structure: A walk through the process. *Struct. Equ. Models* **2006**, *13*, 287–321. [CrossRef]
58. Cheung, G.W.; Rensvold, R.B. Evaluating goodness-of-fit indexes for testing measurement invariance. *Struct. Equ. Models* **2002**, *9*, 233–255. [CrossRef]
59. Finney, S.J.; DiStefano, C. Non-normal and categorical data in structural equation modeling. In *Structural Equation Modeling: A Second Course*; Hancock, G.R., Mueller, R.O., Eds.; Information Age: Greenwich, CT, USA, 2006; pp. 269–314.

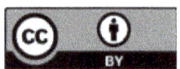

© 2018 by the authors. Licensee MDPI, Basel, Switzerland. This article is an open access article distributed under the terms and conditions of the Creative Commons Attribution (CC BY) license (http://creativecommons.org/licenses/by/4.0/).

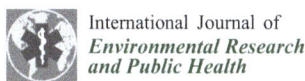

Article

Employee Stress, Reduced Productivity, and Interest in a Workplace Health Program: A Case Study from the Australian Mining Industry

Tamara D. Street *, Sarah J. Lacey and Klaire Somoray

Wesley Medical Research, Brisbane, QLD 4066, Australia; slacey@wesleyresearch.com.au (S.J.L.); KSomoray@wesleyresearch.com.au (K.S.)
* Correspondence: tstreet@wesleyresearch.com.au; Tel.: +61-7-3271-1706

Received: 15 October 2018; Accepted: 23 December 2018; Published: 31 December 2018

Abstract: The Australian mining sector has an elevated industry prevalence of stress and high stress related productivity impairment costs. This study surveyed 897 employees from an Australian mining company to identify characteristics associated with: (a) high stress related productivity impairment costs; and (b) likelihood of stressed employees wanting stress management assistance at work. Groups associated with average annual productivity impairment costs in excess of $50,000 per employee included: permanent day shift employees; employees who reported being stressed at work most of the time; employees who reported being stress at work all of the time; and employees who were contemplating better managing their stress in the next 6 months. Overall, 52% of employees who identified as being in the contemplation stage of change for stress management and 52% of employees who experienced stress most of the time reported wanting stress assistance with stress. However, only 33% of stressed permanent day shift employees and 36% of employees who experienced stress all the time reported wanting stress assistance. To achieve a high return on investment when implementing workplace stress management programs in the mining industry, practitioners need to strategically target health promotion to engage stressed employees with high productivity impairment costs and low desire for stress management assistance.

Keywords: work stress; productivity; impairment cost; stress management; employee characteristics; workplace health promotion; health and safety

1. Introduction

Stress management refers to the act of engaging in deliberate strategies to control ones level of stress, particularly chronic stress. Managing employee stress is a priority for advancing worker health in the global mining industry. An elevated industry prevalence of stress and the high associated personal and organisational costs of stress indicates a need for workplace health and safety risk management action. In Australia where this study was conducted, research has identified that psychological distress is significantly more prevalent in Australian mining workforces than in the general Australian population [1,2]. More specifically, in an adult Australia population sample, 11.7% of respondents had Kessler Psychological Distress Scale (K10) scores that indicated high/very high psychological distress [3]. Comparatively, 28% of employees from mine sites in South Australia and Western Australia [1], and 12.7% of employees from mine sites in New South Wales and Queensland [2] had K10 scores indicating high/very high psychological distress.

High economic costs of stress related absenteeism and presenteeism have been reported in the Australian mining sector. For example, in a Queensland mining company work-related stress accounted for the highest financial burden (compared across 25 medical conditions) [4]. Employees who reported experiencing stress at work were 19% less productive than employees who did not report experiencing stress [4]. Furthermore, based on productive time lost calculations from Queensland and New South Wales mines it has been estimated that psychological distress has an annual economic cost of $153.8 million to the Australian coal mining industry, representing almost 9% of pre-tax operating profit [5].

Work-related stress has been linked to detrimental employee health outcomes. For example, a longitudinal study spanning 14 years found that higher levels of workplace stress were associated with an increased risk of metabolic syndrome, a precursor of coronary heart disease [6]. Workplace stress has also been indirectly linked to employees' health through the experience of stress being associated with greater engagement in negative health behaviours such as tobacco smoking, inadequate diet, insufficient physical activity, and alcohol use [7,8]. It has been speculated that conditions associated with mining employment including long work rosters and remote work locations may increase the risk of miners experiencing stress [9]. Concerns for miners' health have been raised with several recent public enquires into work practices associated with the Australian mining industry, such as fly-in fly-out (FIFO) or drive-in drive-out (DIDO) arrangements, and impacts on mental health and suicide [10,11]. Some studies have found that Australian FIFO miners report work-life balance difficulties and relationship stress [12] and family stress associated with frequent miner absence from home [13]. McPhedran and De Leo [9] recommend caution when interpreting associations between mining employment and stress noting that work practices, rather than employment industry, had a direct relationship with some stress measures. In their comparison of male miners to males in other occupations, they identified that mine employees on average worked longer hours than employees in other occupations and working longer hours was independently associated with perceived lower quality family relationships and higher levels of relationship stress [9].

There are many workplace risk management strategies with research evidence of effectiveness [14,15]. Effective stress management has also been linked to improvements in other health behaviours. For instance, Lipschitz et al. [16] demonstrated that individuals who improved their stress management also increased their likelihood of exercising and managing their depression over a period of six months. A key challenge for health and safety practitioners is engaging stressed employees to proactively seek stress management assistance. This is particularly important given that low help seeking behaviours have been associated with the male-dominated mining industry [17].

Historically, studies have researched stress management strategies for adults assuming that anyone who requires assistance with stress management is ready to change their behaviour, with limited consideration to the actual readiness of the individual [18]. Although existing workplace based stress management studies have not specified the percentage of stressed employees who are prepared to adopt stress management practices, a population based study including 1085 adults recruited from national market research directories identified that at baseline measurement, over 80% of the sample were not ready to adopt stress management practices [18]. These individuals were not practicing effective stress management behaviours, including physical activity, regular relaxation, taking time for social activities, and/or talking with others, and not intending to start practing stress management strategies in the immediate future. Applying the Stages of Change Model of behaviour change, these adults were classified as being in a pre-contemplation or contemplation stage of change for stress management [18]. The randomised clinical trial study found that adults who participated in a Stages of Change Model stage-matched stress management intervention, as compared longitudinally to a control group, had significantly greater progress towards stress management action and maintenance behaviours, significantly lower stress levels, and were significantly more likely to be practicing healthy stress management and avoiding unhealthy stress management behaviours [18].

Within a mining workforce, research has identified that stage of readiness was not associated with likelihood of wanting assistance with reducing or quitting smoking [19], but was associated with wanting assistance with healthy weight management [20]. It was found that employees who were in the contemplative, preparation, and action stages for improving their eating habits were more likely to desire assistance for healthy weight programs compared to employees in the pre-contemplative stage. Employees in the action and maintenance stages for improving their physical activity habits were also more likely to desire assistance for healthy weight programs compared to employees in the pre-contemplative stage [20]. Research is needed within a mining workforce to identify the prevalence of employees ready to adopt stress management assistance and to explore whether stage of readiness is associated with stress impairment productivity costs and likelihood of seeking stress management assistance.

Although companies need to equitably provide health support for all employees, to maximize return on program investment targeted program promotion is critical to engage employees at risk of stress related health issues. In addition to understanding the employee characteristics associated with stress and readiness to change, practitioners would benefit from understanding if employee characteristics (including socio-demographic and work characteristic variables, e.g., age and job role) are associated with stress productivity costs and likelihood of seeking stress management assistance.

Research within the Australian mining sector suggests that certain employee demographic and work characteristics are associated with greater risk for psychological distress [1,2]. More specifically, Bowers et al. [1] found that mining employees aged 25 to 35 years and shift-work employees (rostered as two weeks on, one week off) were more likely to report psychological distress. However, it is unclear from the available literature which employee characteristics are associated with high stress-related productivity impairment costs. Similarly, empirical research indicates that females and middle-aged persons [21–23] are significantly more likely to access professional services to address stress management and other mental health concerns. Previous studies using a mining workforce also indicate that gender and age influence preference for health promotion programs [19]. For example, females and employees aged 24 years and under have been found to be more likely to want assistance for smoking cessation [19].

The limited available research to date suggests that employee characteristics and employee readiness for change may be associated with preference for health promotion programs such as those that target stress management. The aim of this study was two-fold: (a) To investigate, within employees' who reported high levels of stress, the relationship between employee characteristics, stage of change for stress management, and productivity impairment costs; and (b) The relationship between employee characteristics, stage of change for stress management, and desire for assistance with stress management through a workplace health promotion program. Although this case study focuses on the Australian mining workforce, it is likely that the findings will have practical application for the development of stress management strategies in the global mining industry.

2. Materials and Methods

2.1. Participants

A sample of 897 employees from an Australian mining company were recruited to participate in the study. Participants were aged between 17 and 73 years. Consistent with the organizations workforce characteristics, the majority of participants (74%) were male. It was not possible to calculate a response rate due to the recruitment process, however the mining organisation confirmed that the sample was representative of the workforce demographic characteristics. Furthermore, variance in survey responses indicated that participants included a range of employees. Participant employment characteristics are detailed in Table 1. Reported percentages exclude missing data and are, therefore, calculated from different sample sizes as a few participants chose not to report some of their demographic and work information.

Of the 893 employees who responded to the stress item ($n = 4$ were missing data), 375 employees reported experiencing stress while at work 'some of the time' to 'all of the time' (refer Table 2). The majority of these stressed employees reported that they were not ready to adopt stress management practices, with 34.0% ($n = 106$) in the pre-contemplation stage and 22.8% ($n = 71$) in the contemplation stage. Of the stressed employees who were ready to adopt stress management behaviours, 6.4% ($n = 20$)

were in the preparation stage, 27.2% (n = 85) in the action stage. The remaining 9.6% (n = 30) were in the maintenance stage, reporting that they were attempting to continue managing their stress. The sample of stressed employees was analysed to identify employee characteristics and stress management stages of change associated with (a) high productivity impairment costs and (b) desire for assistance with stress management.

Table 1. Participant employment characteristics.

Characteristic		n	%
Roster (n = 892)	Permanent day Shift	456	50.9
	Rotating/alternating shift	440	49.1
Employment Status (n = 888)	Permanent contract	777	87.5
	Contractor	111	12.5
Living arrangement (n = 889)	Resident	693	78.0
	FIFO/DIDO	196	22.0

Notes. n = 897; FIFO/DIDO = Fly-in, Fly-out/Drive-in, Drive-out.

Table 2. Group differences on work impairment percentage and annual productivity cost per person.

		Work Impairment (%)		Productivity Cost ($)		t-Value	p-Value
	n	M	SD	M	SD		
Gender							
Male	265	33.1	23.0	$44,549.93	$31,023.54	68	0.499
Female	110	34.8	22.1	$46,904.83	$29,822.75		
Roster							
Permanent day shift	206	37.6	23.5	$50,915.48	$31,501.24	3.86	<0.001
Rotating shift	169	28.7	20.9	$38,624.79	$28,134.91		
Contract							
Permanent employee	324	34.6	22.7	$46,700.16	$30,578.24	2.65	0.008
Contractor	48	25.4	21.1	$34,285.68	$28,446.86		
Residency status							
Resident	282	35.4	23.1	$47,776.63	$31,173.21	2.82	0.005
FIFO/DIDO	88	27.7	20.6	$37,295.35	$27,811.39		

Notes. n = 375; FIFO/DIDO = Fly-in, Fly-out/Drive-in, Drive-out; Differences in group sample size (n) is due to missing data on employee characteristics.

2.2. Design

This study was approved by the by the Uniting Care Health Human Research Ethics Committee (#2013.03.74). The study utilized a cross-sectional design. Voluntary informed consent was obtained from each participant.

2.3. Procedure

The research team visited two Australian mining sites and a corresponding residential mine village. Due to safety regulations the team was prohibited from entering some work site areas. Company managers nominated working units with the goal of obtaining a representative sample of employees. In these work units, participant information sheets were displayed in common gathering areas and announcements were made by mangers at daily work group meetings. All employees of the selected work units who were sighted by the researchers during the data collection period were invited by the researchers to participate in the health survey. The survey was provided in hard copy (on paper) and once complete returned to the research team. All data were entered and analysed in IBM SPSS version 21 (IBM, Armonk, NY, USA). Participants included a mixture of operational, managerial, and administrative roles. Managers were not informed of which employees participated in the research.

2.4. Measures

Demographic and employment characteristic measures replicated government survey and corporate health survey items [4,24]. Consistent with previous research [4], stress was measured by the item "How much of the time in the past four weeks did you feel stressed while at work?" Response options included: none of the time; a little of the time; some of the time; a good bit of the time; most of the time; and all of the time. Participants were classified as stressed if they selected: some of the time; a good bit of the time; most of the time; or all of the time. Participants were classified as low risk of stress and excluded from stress analyses if they responded: none of the time; or a little of the time.

Consistent with previous research measuring miners' readiness to change healthy behaviours using the Stages of Change Model [25], participants were asked to select one of five statements in response to the following question. 'How would you describe your approach to stress management?' Response option statements were amended from previously published nutrition and physical activity focused statements [25] to focus on stress management and were based on the traditional Stages of Change Model of behaviour change stage descriptions [26]. More specifically, stress management stage of change was measured by the selection of one of the following statements: pre-contemplative "As far as I'm concerned my stress management habits don't need changing"; contemplative "I'm seriously intending to better manage my stress in the next 6 months"; preparation "I have definite plans to better manage my stress in the next month"; action "I am doing something to better manage my stress"; and maintenance "I took action more than six months ago to better manage my stress and I'm working hard to maintain this change".

The Worker Productivity and Activity Impairment—General Health (WPAI:GH) questionnaire [27] items including hours worked, work absenteeism (i.e., work time missed due to health), and work presenteeism (i.e., impairment while working due to health) were replicated with minor amendments. Consistent with previous research using a shift work mining sample [4], the original seven-day measurement period was extended to a four-week period to minimize the impact of acute illnesses and shift work rosters to read, "During the past four weeks, how many days did you miss from work because of your health problems?"

Based on established World Health Organization and government survey items [24,28] the following outcome item "Would you like assistance with stress management?" was asked in the workplace health program survey section to measure employees' preference for assistance.

2.5. Analyses

All analyses were conducted using the IBM software package SPSS version 21. Consistent with previous research [4], the current study followed the protocol outlined by Lenneman et al. [29]. However, it was not necessary to calculate 'excess costs' as the study was limited to a subset of employees who reported experiencing stress at work ($n = 375$). As presented by previous research [4], productivity impairment was calculated based on a modified version of the WPAI:GH. Specifically, productivity impairment was calculated for each employee who reported experiencing stress at work using the sum of days absent from work multiplied by 5 (which represents five days of work during a working week), and rate of presenteeism expressed as an overall impairment percentage. The following formula was used in calculating the work impairment percentage (1).

Formula:

$$\text{Absenteeism impairment} = \text{days off work} \times 5$$
$$\text{Presenteeism impairment} = \text{presenteeism score} \times (20 - \text{days off work}) \quad (1)$$
$$\text{Work impairment percentage} = \text{absenteeism impairment} \times \text{presenteeism impairment}$$

Productivity costs were calculated by multiplying the overall work impairment percentage by the average Australian mining annual salary of $134,784 [30]. Finally, independent sample t-tests and a one-way ANOVAs were performed to examine the differences in productivity costs depending on employee characteristics and stage of change.

3. Results

3.1. Stress-Related Productivity Impairment Costs

Of the 375 employees who reported experiencing stress at work, 23.4% ($n = 82$) reported at least one day of absence from work due to personal health problems in the past four weeks. Twenty-five employees (6.7%) also stated a high degree of presenteeism, reporting that they had trouble concentrating at work or doing their best due to personal health problems 'most of the time' or 'all of the time' in the past four weeks. Overall, stressed employees were associated with an average of 33.6% work impairment and $45,240.70 (SD = 30,655.26) in productivity costs per employee.

Independent sample t-tests and a one-way ANOVA were performed to examine the differences in productivity costs depending on employee characteristics (see Tables 2 and 3). Significant differences were identified between roster type, contract, and residency status. As seen in Table 2, employees on permanent day shifts were more likely to be associated with higher productivity costs compared to employees on rotating/alternating shifts, Cohen's $D = 0.41$. Permanent employees were significantly more likely to report higher work impairment which was associated with higher productivity costs compared to contractors, Cohen's $D = 0.42$. Employees who resided in the mining towns were also more likely to be associated with higher productivity costs compared to FIFO/DIDO employees, Cohen's $D = 0.35$. Based on Cohen's D conventions, these differences were considered small to medium. Productivity costs did not significantly differ between males and females and among the different age groups.

Table 3. Group differences based on work impairment percentage and annual productivity cost.

	n	Work Impairment (%)		Productivity Cost ($)		F-Ratio	p-Value
		M	SD	M	SD		
Age (years)							
Under 18 to 24	41	30.3	21.2	$40,895.44	$28,529.37		
25–34	131	35.5	22.8	$47,915.20	$30,745.12		
35–44	75	34.0	22.0	$45,862.50	$29,635.07	0.74	0.565
45–54	64	33.0	22.0	$44,478.72	$29,591.15		
55 and over	27	29.2	25.1	$39,336.96	$33,828.53		
Stress level							
Some of the time	212	27.3	18.4	$36,830.36	$24,793.38		
A good bit of the time	100	36.2	22.5	$48,764.85	$30,300.98	20.61	<0.001
Most of the time	44	48.0	22.7	$64,757.59	$30,594.89		
All of the time	19	55.9	35.2	$75,337.16	$47,379.12		

Notes. $n = 375$; FIFO/DIDO = Fly-in, Fly-out/Drive-in, Drive-out; Differences in group sample size (n) is due to missing data on employee characteristics.

Productivity costs also significantly differed between self-reported levels of stress at work (see Table 3). A trend is observed in Table 3 with increased frequency of experiencing stress at work being associated with increased productivity costs. Employees who reported feeling stressed 'all of the time' in the previous four week period reported the highest productivity costs ($M = $75,337.16; SD = $47,379.12). Post-hoc analysis using Games-Howell test were performed due to the unequal variances and sample sizes between the groups. Employees who reported experiencing stress 'all of the time' showed significantly higher costs compared to employees who reported only feeling stressed 'some of the time', $p = 0.012$ and the difference showed a large effect, Cohen's $D = 1.02$. Employees who reported feeling stressed 'most of the time' were also associated with significantly higher productivity costs compared to those who only experienced stress 'some of the time', $p < 0.001$, Cohen's $D = 1.00$ and 'a good bit of the time', $p = 0.024$, Cohen's $D = 0.53$. The effect sizes were large and medium, respectively. Employees who reported feeling stressed 'a good bit of the time' were also associated with higher productivity costs compared to employees who only felt stressed 'some of the time' at work, $p = 0.004$, and the effect was small to medium size, Cohen's $D = 0.43$.

Differences in productivity costs depending on stage of change for stress management were examined. Table 4 reveals that, on average, the highest productivity impairment costs were associated with employees classified in the contemplation stage of change for stress management while employees in the pre-contemplation stage were associated with the lowest average productivity impairment cost. A one-way ANOVA was conducted to assess the differences in productivity costs based on employees' readiness to change their stress management behaviours. An overall significant difference was found, $F (4, 307) = 6.78$, $p < 0.001$. Post hoc analysis using Games-Howell test suggest that, contemplation employees were associated with significantly higher productivity costs compared to pre-contemplation employees, $p < 0.001$ and the difference had a medium to large effect, Cohen's $D = 0.77$. Employees in the action stage were also associated with significantly higher productivity costs compared to pre-contemplation employees, $p = 0.015$. However, the effect size was only small to medium, Cohen's $D = 0.46$. No other significant differences were found between the other groups.

Table 4. Work impairment percentage and annual productivity cost per person based on stage of change.

Stage of Change		Work Impairment (%)		Productivity Cost ($)	
	n	M	SD	M	SD
Pre-contemplation—As far as I'm concerned my stress management habits do not need changing	106	24.0	21.4	$32,284.58	$28,803.25
Contemplation—I'm seriously intending to better manage my stress in the next 6 months	71	39.9	19.9	$53,761.73	$26,829.95
Preparation—I have definite plans to better manage my stress in the next month	20	34.7	19.1	$46,702.66	$25,708.73
Action—I am doing something to better manage my stress	85	33.3	19.4	$44,922.71	$26,106.93
Maintenance—I took action more than 6 months ago to better manage my stress and I'm working hard to maintain it	30	33.9	24.8	$45,691.78	$33,484.98

Notes. $n = 375$.

3.2. Desire for Assistance with Stress Management

Of the 375 employees who reported experiencing stress at work, only 28% ($n = 105$) reported wanting assistance to manage their stress. A hierarchical logistic regression was performed to predict the likelihood for wanting assistance with stress management. Participants' employee characteristics and reported levels of stress at work were included in Step 1 to partial out their effect in the regression model. The stage of change for stress management variable was included in Step 2. Step 1 was significant, $\chi^2(8) = 39.76$, $p < 0.001$, explaining 19.4% of the total variance (Nagelkerke $r^2 = 0.19$) and correctly classified 76.4% of the cases. The model's sensitivity was 37.7 and specificity was 91.4. As shown in Table 5, being female and having higher levels of stress were significant predictors of desiring stress management assistance. Female employees were twice as likely to want stress management assistance compared to male employees. Employees who reported experiencing stress more frequently were significantly more likely to report desiring stress management assistance compared to employees who reported experiencing stress less frequently. Age, shift work rotation, employment status, and current work arrangement were not significant predictors within the Step 1 of the model.

Table 5. Logistic regression predicting the likelihood of desiring assistance with stress management.

		Do Not Want Assistance (n = 270; 72%)	Want Assistance (n = 105; 28%)				
	n	% or M (SD)	% or M (SD)	OR	95% C.I. (OR)		p-Value
Step 1—Employee and work characteristics							
Gender							
Male †	265	76.6%	23.4%	-	-	-	
Female	110	60.9%	39.1%	2.27	1.27	4.08	0.006
Age	338	36.66 (11.74)	36.44 (9.99)	1.01	0.98	1.03	0.697
Roster Type							
Permanent Day Shift †	206	66.5%	33.5%	-	-	-	
Rotating/Alternating	169	78.7%	21.3%	0.81	0.43	1.54	0.515
Contract Type							
Employee †	324	69.4%	30.6%	-	-	-	
Contractor	48	87.5%	12.5%	0.41	0.13	1.35	0.139
Residency Status							
Resident †	282	69.9%	30.1%	-	-	-	
FIFO/DIDO	88	78.4%	21.6%	1.10	0.50	2.30	0.809
Stress Levels							
Some of the time	212	83.5%	16.5%	-	-	-	
A good bit of the time	100	60.0%	40.0%	3.18	1.66	6.08	<0.001
Most of the time	44	47.7%	52.3%	6.47	2.78	15.03	<0.001
All of the time	19	63.2%	36.8%	4.45	1.21	16.37	0.025
Step 2—Stage of Change							
Pre-contemplation †	106	86.8%	13.2%	-	-	-	
Contemplation	71	47.9%	52.1%	11.05	4.26	28.70	<0.001
Preparation	20	60.0%	40.0%	7.13	1.97	25.87	0.003
Action	85	77.6%	22.4%	2.85	1.07	7.62	0.037
Maintenance	30	66.7%	33.3%	5.22	1.60	16.99	0.006

Notes. n = 375; Differences in group sample size (n) is due to missing data on employee characteristics; logistic regression sample included in analysis N = 275 due to missing values; FIFO/DIDO = fly-in, fly-out/DRIVE-in, drive-out; OR = odds ratio; CI = confidence intervals; † Reference.

When the stages of readiness to change were added in the model, the second block was significant, $\chi^2(4) = 32.65$, $p < 0.001$, explaining an additional 13.9% of the total variance. Overall, the model was significant, $\chi^2(12) = 72.42$, $p < 0.001$ and explained 33.3% of the total variance (Nagelkerke $r^2 = 0.33$) and accurately classified 78.2% of the cases. The model's sensitivity was 49.4 and specificity was 89.4. Pre-contemplation employees were the reference category for the readiness to change one's approach to stress management. As shown in Table 5, employees in all readiness stages were significantly more likely to desire stress management assistance than stressed employees who reported that their stress management habits do not need changing. However, it is important to note that the odds ratio's lower confidence intervals for employees in the action stage nearly encompasses 1, indicating that being in the action stage may not necessarily increase the employees' likelihood to desire assistance for their stress. The odds ratio of the action group in desiring assistance is also small (OR = 2.85) compared to employees in the pre-contemplation stage. Examination of the other groups revealed that employees in the contemplation stage showed the highest odds ratio, indicating that this group were 11.05 times more likely to want assistance for stress management compared to the pre-contemplation group. Furthermore, compared to the pre-contemplative employees, preparation employees were 7.13 times and maintenance employees were 5.22 times more likely to desire assistance for stress management.

4. Discussion

Within a mining workforce sample, this study identified employee characteristics and stress management stages of change associated with high stress-related productivity impairment costs and desire for assistance with stress management. Of the employees who reported experiencing stress at work, employee groups associated with significantly higher productivity impairment costs included: day shift workers; permanent contract employees; employees who reside within the mining towns; frequently stressed employees; employees intending to better manage their stress in the next six months; and employees who are actively managing their stress. Although previous research has reported that FIFO miners were at risk of stress due to their work arrangements [12,13] in the current study they had lower stress impairment costs than permanent day shift employees.

The lower productivity impairment costs associated with alternating rosters, contractors and FIFO/DIDO employment may be related to the roles and responsibilities associated with the different types of employees appointed to permanent day shifts versus alternating contracts. To protect participant anonymity the current study did not gather data regarding job position, however, the researchers are aware that within the current sample, employees working permanent day shifts included managers, professionals, administrative, and operational staff. Comparatively, employees with alternating rosters, FIFO/DIDO employment, and contractual work were more likely to be appointed to operational mining roles. A study by Ling et al. [5] showed that managers within the coal mining industry had higher average lost productivity time costs compared to machine operators and trade workers. Managers were also associated with higher psychological distress [2].

In this mining workforce sample, employees in the contemplation stage for stress management had the highest average annual stress-related productivity impairment cost ($53,761 per employee). Although individuals who are classified as contemplative intend to improve their behaviour in the next six months, they are considered not ready to self-initiate immediate changes [18]. Research has shown in a national population based sample that a stage-matched stress management intervention was effective in achieving rapid progression through the stages of effective stress management strategy adoption [18]. Given that the contemplation group for stress management in this study had high impairment costs, savings could be achieved by assisting these employees to manage or remove stress that is impacting on their work productivity. Future research should be conducted to identify if implementation of a stage of change matched stress management intervention could achieve similar results in a mining workforce as achieved in the population based sample.

Consistent with previous research that found females were more likely to exhibit help-seeking behaviours and access professional stress management or mental health support services [21–23], the current study found that females were significantly more likely to report wanting assistance with stress management. Although males and females had similar average impairment costs, the higher proportion of males in the mining workforce and the lower likelihood of males to want assistance suggests that practitioners need to ensure that stress management promotion is appropriate for engaging males. Male employees appear to be unlikely to initiate help seeking behaviours despite experiencing stress at work. Given that this study found that higher frequency of experiencing stress at work was associated with higher impairment costs, it was encouraging to identify that higher stress frequency was also associated with greater desire for assistance with stress management. This suggests that workplace provided stress management assistance will likely appeal to high productivity impairment cost employees that were frequently experiencing stress at work.

Similarly, stage of change for adoption of effective stress management behaviours analyses revealed that employees in the contemplation stage had the both the highest cost impairment and highest likelihood to report wanting assistance. By contrast, employees in the pre-contemplation stage who believed their stress management habits did not need changing, were found to have both the lowest cost impairment and lowest likelihood to report wanting assistance. This again indicates that workplace provided stress management assistance will likely appeal to high productivity impairment cost employees that were intending to improve their stress management in the next six months.

4.1. Limitations and Future Resarch

Limitations include the recruitment process, use of self-report data, and generalizability of results. Specifically, the recruitment of participants was restricted due to the operational demands to those whom attended the work site on the day and the researchers were unable to record the number of employees who were present but declined to participate. Therefore, it was not possible to accurately evaluate the extent to which the sample reflected the wider workforce of approximately 8000 employees or response rate. Furthermore, it is not possible based on this case study to determine the extent to which the results outlined herein are reflective of employees within the broader mining industry both in Australia and globally. Additional studies are needed to longitudinally examine if demographic and work characteristics and employees' readiness to change is associated with actual participation in workplace stress management programs. The voluntary recruitment of participants could also have exposed this study to a selection bias, with research participants potentially being more likely than the average employee to engage in healthy lifestyle behaviours.

4.2. Practical Implications

From a research perspective, future studies should explore whether permanent day shift and local employment are significantly associated with higher productivity impairment costs after controlling for the potential contribution of job role related responsibilities, job demands, and salaries. However, from a practical point of view, regardless of whether role or work arrangement is directly related to productivity cost impairment, based on the current findings stress management strategies should be available to all employees with a particular focus on engaging employee groups with high impairment costs. Employee groups associated with average annual productivity impairment costs in excess of $50,000 per employee included: permanent day shift employees; employees who experienced stress at work most of the time; employees who experienced stress at work all of the time; and employees who were contemplating better managing their stress in the next 6 months. To guide effective stress management in the Australian mining industry, future research should be conducted to identify whether implementation of a stage-matched stress management intervention achieves similar results in a mining workforce as achieved in a population-based sample [18].

5. Conclusions

To effectively design and tailor stress management strategies for a mining workforce that will deliver a high return on investment, practitioners must identify high cost employee groups and those receptive of participation in a workplace health promotion program. This study makes a novel contribution to the workplace health literature by identifying characteristics in a mining workforce associated with: (a) high stress related productivity impairment costs; and (b) characteristics of stressed employees who desire assistance with stress management in an Australian mining company.

Overall, it is likely that the observed high productivity impairment costs associated with roster and residential status (i.e., permanent day workers and local residents) is reflective of employee job roles within these groups which may include persons who reside locally and are employed in supervisory or management roles. Therefore, a targeted workplace stress management program aimed at employees in such roles may result in the greatest return on investment.

Stage of change for stress management reflects an individuals' readiness to change and desire for assistance with stress management. According to the Stages of Change Model, individuals in the precontemplation and contemplation stages are not attempting to manage their stress. Only 13.2% of employees in the precontemplation stage and 52.1% of employees in the contemplation stage reported wanting assistance with stress management. Therefore, workplace health promotion programs targeting stress management must, in the first instance, convince employees of the value and benefit of participation in order to ensure high levels of enrolment that would result in the greatest benefit for employees and return on investment for the organisation.

Overall, these findings suggest that, within the organisation presented in this study, workplace provided stress management assistance will likely appeal to over a third of the high the productivity impairment cost employees. Furthermore, strategically targeted health promotion will be required to engage the remainder of the stressed employees with high productivity impairment costs and low desire for stress management assistance.

Author Contributions: T.D.S. and S.J.L. contributed equally to the project design and data collection. T.D.S., S.J.L., and K.S. contributed equally to the data analysis and manuscript preparation. All authors contributed substantially to the work reported, and have read and approved the final manuscript.

Funding: This research received no external grant funding.

Acknowledgments: The authors acknowledge the corporate and community supporters who donated to Wesley Medical Research to advance health and medical research.

Conflicts of Interest: The authors declare no conflict of interest.

References

1. Bowers, J.; Lo, J.; Miller, P.; Mawren, D.; Jones, B. Psychological distress in remote mining and construction workers in Australia. *Med. J. Aust.* **2018**, *208*, 391–397. [CrossRef] [PubMed]
2. Considine, R.; Tynan, R.; James, C.; Wiggers, J.; Lewin, T.; Inder, K.; Perkins, D.; Handley, T.; Kelly, B. The contribution of individual, social and work characteristics to employee mental health in a coal mining industry population. *PLoS ONE* **2017**, *12*, e0168445. [CrossRef] [PubMed]
3. Australian Bureau of Statistics. National Health Survey: First Results, 2014e15; Table 7 Psychological Distress—Australia. Available online: http://www.abs.gov.au/AUSSTATS/abs@.nsf/DetailsPage/4364.0.55.0012014-15?OpenDocument (accessed on 15 September 2018).
4. Street, T.D.; Lacey, S.J. Accounting for Employee Health: The Productivity Cost of Leading Health Risks. *Health Promot. J. Aust.* **2018**. [CrossRef] [PubMed]
5. Ling, R.; Kelly, B.; Considine, R.; Tynan, R.; Searles, A.; Doran, C.M. The economic impact of psychological distress in the Australian coal mining industry. *J. Occup. Environ. Med.* **2016**, *58*, e171–e176. [CrossRef]
6. Chandola, T.; Brunner, E.; Marmot, M. Chronic stress at work and the metabolic syndrome: Prospective study. *BMJ* **2006**, *332*, 521–525. [CrossRef]
7. Eakin, J.M. Work-related determinants of health behavior. In *Handbook of Health Behavior Research I: Personal and Social Determinants*; Gochman, D., Ed.; Plenum Press: New York, NY, USA, 1997; pp. 337–357.
8. Siegrist, J.; Rodel, A. Work stress and health risk behavior. *Scand. J. Work Environ. Health* **2006**, *32*, 473–481. [CrossRef]

9. McPhedran, S.; De Leo, D. Relationship quality, work-family stress, and mental health among Australian male mining industry employees. *J. Relationsh. Res.* **2014**, *5*, 1–9. [CrossRef]
10. House of Representatives Committee. Cancer of the Bush or Salvation for Our Cities? Fly-In, Fly-Out and Drive-In, Drive-Out Workforce Practices in Regional Australia. Available online: https://www.aph.gov.au/Parliamentary_Business/Committees/House_of_Representatives_Committees?url=ra/fifodido/report/fullreport.pdf (accessed on 15 September 2018).
11. Education Health Standing Committee the Impact of FIFO Work Practices on Mental Health: Final Report. Available online: http://www.parliament.wa.gov.au/Parliament/commit.nsf/(Report+Lookup+by+Com+ID)/2E970A7A4934026448257E67002BF9D1/$file/20150617%20-%20Final%20Report%20w%20signature%20for%20website.htaccess (accessed on 15 September 2018).
12. Torkington, A.M.; Larkins, S.; Gupta, T.S. The psychosocial impacts of fly-in fly-out and drive-in drive-out mining on mining employees: A qualitative study. *Aust. J. Rural Health* **2011**, *19*, 135–141. [CrossRef]
13. Kaczmarek, E.; Sibbel, A.; Cowie, C. Australian military and Fly-In/Fly-Out (FIFO) mining families: A comparative study. *Aust. J. Psychol.* **2003**, *55*, 187–188.
14. Harvey, S.B.; Joyce, S.; Tan, L.; Johnson, A.; Nguyen, H.; Modini, M.; Groth, M. Developing a Mentally Healthy Workplace: A Review of the Literature. 2014. Available online: https://www.headsup.org.au/docs/default-source/resources/developing-a-mentally-healthy-workplace_final-november-2014.pdf?sfvrsn=8 (accessed on 24 September 2018).
15. Richardson, K.M.; Rothstein, H.R. Effects of occupational stress management intervention programs: A meta-analysis. *J. Occup. Health psychol.* **2008**, *13*, 69. [CrossRef]
16. Lipschitz, J.M.; Paiva, A.L.; Redding, C.A.; Butterworth, S.; Prochaska, J.O. Co-occurrence and coaction of stress management with other health risk behaviors. *J. Health Psychol.* **2015**, *20*, 1002–1012. [CrossRef] [PubMed]
17. Tynan, R.J.; Considine, R.; Rich, J.L.; Skehan, J.; Wiggers, J.; Lewin, T.J.; James, C.; Inder, K.; Baker, A.L.; Kay-Lambkin, F. Help-seeking for mental health problems by employees in the Australian Mining Industry. *BMC Health Serv. Res.* **2016**, *16*, 498. [CrossRef] [PubMed]
18. Evers, K.E.; Prochaska, J.O.; Johnson, J.L.; Mauriello, L.M.; Padula, J.A.; Prochaska, J.M. A randomized clinical trial of a population-and transtheoretical model-based stress-management intervention. *Health Psychol.* **2006**, *25*, 521. [CrossRef] [PubMed]
19. Street, T.D.; Lacey, S.J. Employee characteristics and health belief variables related to smoking cessation engagement attitudes. *Work* **2018**, *60*, 75–83. [CrossRef] [PubMed]
20. Street, T.D.; Thomas, D.L. Beating obesity: Factors associated with interest in workplace weight management assistance in the mining industry. *Saf. Health Work* **2017**, *8*, 89–93. [CrossRef] [PubMed]
21. Wang, P.S.; Aguilar-Gaxiola, S.; Alonso, J.; Angermeyer, M.C.; Borges, G.; Bromet, E.J.; Bruffaerts, R.; De Girolamo, G.; De Graaf, R.; Gureje, O. Use of mental health services for anxiety, mood, and substance disorders in 17 countries in the WHO world mental health surveys. *Lancet* **2007**, *370*, 841–850. [CrossRef]
22. Burgess, P.M.; Pirkis, J.E.; Slade, T.N.; Johnston, A.K.; Meadows, G.N.; Gunn, J.M. Service use for mental health problems: Findings from the 2007 National Survey of Mental Health and Wellbeing. *Aust. N. Z. J. Psychiatry* **2009**, *43*, 615–623. [CrossRef] [PubMed]
23. Olesen, S.C.; Butterworth, P.; Leach, L.S.; Kelaher, M.; Pirkis, J. Mental health affects future employment as job loss affects mental health: Findings from a longitudinal population study. *BMC Psychiatry* **2013**, *13*, 144. [CrossRef]
24. Australian Bureau of Statistics. Australian Health Survey: Users Guide, 2011–2013 (No. 4363.0.55.001). Available online: http://www.abs.gov.au (accessed on 14 September 2018).
25. Lacey, S.J.; Street, T.D. Measuring healthy behaviours using the stages of change model: An investigation into the physical activity and nutrition behaviours of Australian miners. *BioPsychoSocial Med.* **2017**, *11*, 30. [CrossRef]
26. Prochaska, J.O.; Butterworth, S.; Redding, C.A.; Burden, V.; Perrin, N.; Leo, M.; Flaherty-Robb, M.; Prochaska, J.M. Initial efficacy of MI, TTM tailoring and HRI's with multiple behaviors for employee health promotion. *Prev. Med.* **2008**, *46*, 226–231. [CrossRef]
27. Reilly, M.C.; Zbrozek, A.S.; Dukes, E.M. The validity and reproducibility of a work productivity and activity impairment instrument. *Pharmacoeconomics* **1993**, *4*, 353–365. [CrossRef] [PubMed]

28. World Health Organization Regional. Guidelines for the Development of Healthy Workplaces. Available online: http://www.who.int/occupationalhealth/publications/wproguidelines/en/ (accessed on 15 September 2018).
29. Lenneman, J.; Schwartz, S.; Giuseffi, D.L.; Wang, C. Productivity and health: An application of three perspectives to measuring productivity. *J. Occup. Environ. Med.* **2011**, *53*, 55–61. [CrossRef] [PubMed]
30. Australian Bureau of Statistics. Employee Earnings and Hours, Australia. Available online: http://www.abs.gov.au/ausstats/abs@.nsf/mf/6306.0/ (accessed on 15 September 2018).

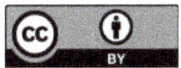
© 2018 by the authors. Licensee MDPI, Basel, Switzerland. This article is an open access article distributed under the terms and conditions of the Creative Commons Attribution (CC BY) license (http://creativecommons.org/licenses/by/4.0/).

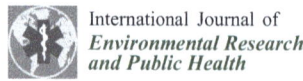

Article

Association between Occupational Injury and Subsequent Employment Termination among Newly Hired Manufacturing Workers

Nathan C. Huizinga [1], Jonathan A. Davis [1,2], Fred Gerr [1] and Nathan B. Fethke [1,3,*]

[1] Department of Occupational and Environmental Health, University of Iowa, Iowa City, IA 52242, USA; nhuizi6@gmail.com (N.C.H.); jonathan-a-davis@uiowa.edu (J.A.D.); fred-gerr@uiowa.edu (F.G.)
[2] University of Iowa Injury Prevention Research Center, University of Iowa, Iowa City, IA 52242, USA
[3] Healthier Workforce Center of the Midwest, University of Iowa, Iowa City, IA 52242, USA
* Correspondence: nathan-fethke@uiowa.edu

Received: 14 December 2018; Accepted: 31 January 2019; Published: 2 February 2019

Abstract: Few longitudinal studies have examined occupational injury as a predictor of employment termination, particularly during the earliest stages of employment when the risk of occupational injury may be greatest. Human resources (HR) records were used to establish a cohort of 3752 hourly employees newly hired by a large manufacturing facility from 2 January 2012, through 25 November 2016. The HR records were linked with records of employee visits to an on-site occupational health center (OHC) for reasons consistent with occupational injury. Cox regression methods were then used to estimate the risk of employment termination following a first-time visit to the OHC, with time to termination as the dependent variable. Analyses were restricted to the time period ending 60 calendar days from the date of hire. Of the 3752 employees, 1172 (31.2%) terminated employment prior to 60 days from date of hire. Of these, 345 terminated voluntarily and 793 were terminated involuntarily. The risk of termination for any reason was greater among those who visited the OHC during the first 60 days of employment than among those who did not visit the OHC during the first 60 days of employment (adjusted hazard ratio = 2.58, 95% CI = 2.12–3.15). The magnitude of effect was similar regardless of the nature of the injury or the body area affected, and the risk of involuntary termination was generally greater than the risk of voluntary termination. The results support activities to manage workplace safety and health hazards in an effort to reduce employee turnover rates.

Keywords: turnover; employment duration; occupational injury; manufacturing; newly-hired workers

1. Introduction

In certain occupational contexts, such as knowledge-based work, some level of employee turnover is considered potentially healthy for an organization (e.g., by providing opportunities to replace poor performers) [1,2]. More broadly, however, it is widely believed that a high level of turnover is a marker for one or more undesirable characteristics of the employment circumstance, including safety and health hazards [3–5]. Increased levels of employee turnover are also commonly associated with decreased organizational performance and profitability [3,5,6]. Thus, understanding and mitigating factors leading to employee turnover is an important business management strategy.

An increased risk of occupational injury during the earliest periods of employment has been observed in numerous studies spanning many decades [7,8]. Examinations of early data compiled by the US Bureau of Labor Statistics observed that both the proportion and incidence rates of occupational injuries were greatest during the first three months of employment [9,10]. Many subsequent studies also observed greater injury frequencies, prevalence, or incidence rates among employees with the lowest job tenure. For example, from 1995 to 2004, 28% of >86,000 injuries among mining workers occurred among those in the first year of employment, while 33% occurred among those employed 1–5 years [11]. Among logging workers, the rate of workers' compensation claims (from 1999 to 2003) was more than double among those with two or fewer months of job tenure (vs. those with >2 months of job tenure) [12]. In addition, substantially greater incidence rates and relative risks of first-time workers' compensation claims involving lost work days were observed among those employed (across a range of industrial sectors) for less than one month (vs. those employed for at least 13 months) [13]. This effect was consistent across injury event classifications, including those typical of acute, traumatic injuries (e.g., contact with objects/equipment and falls) and those typical of more chronic, musculoskeletal outcomes (e.g., repetitive motion). Recent meta-analyses also suggest that negative impacts of turnover on safety outcomes (e.g., occupational injury rates) are among the strongest drivers of reduced organizational financial performance [14]. Thus, if turnover levels are high, then an employer will find itself continuously (i) replenishing its workforce with new employees at greatest risk of injury and associated costs (e.g., workers' compensation) and (ii) incurring potentially avoidable costs associated with hiring and training new employees.

While employment duration or worker experience has frequently been examined as a risk factor for occupational injury, occupational injury has less often been examined as a risk factor for employment duration (or termination). The relationship between occupational injury and employee turnover, if any, is likely complex. Cree and Kelloway [15] suggested a model whereby employees' turnover intentions are influenced by the perception of risk associated with the work, which itself is a function of (i) employees' "accident history," either direct (i.e., actual injury experience) or indirect (i.e., knowledge of others' injury experiences) and (ii) the attitudes of coworkers, supervisors, and management regarding workplace safety and health. In this context, it is important to note that turnover intentions relate to voluntary employment termination, which is also influenced by factors not directly related to workplace safety and health, such the availability of alternative employment options [16]. Associations between occupational injury and subsequent employment termination (both voluntary and involuntary) have been recently observed among health care workers [17,18]. It is not known, however, if the associations observed among health care workers also apply to manufacturing settings, in which entry into the workforce may not require specific knowledge and skills, and in which workers may not be afforded the same level of autonomy [19].

The objective of this study was to estimate the association between occupational injury and subsequent employment termination among newly hired manufacturing workers. Specifically, we merged human resources information with information from an on-site occupational health center to create a time history for each worker in relation to both occupational injury events and employment duration (and/or termination). We also restricted our analyses to the first 60 days from the date of hire, and hypothesized that those experiencing an occupational injury during this time were more likely to terminate employment (for both voluntary and involuntary reasons) prior to 60 days from the date of hire.

2. Materials and Methods

2.1. Study Overview

A cohort of all hourly employees newly hired from 2 January 2012 through 25 November 2016 by a large manufacturing facility in the US Midwest was established using the employer's human resources records database. We did not include employees newly hired into administrative, managerial, or other salaried positions (e.g., engineering). Occupational injury data from the same time period were extracted from a separate database maintained by the facility's on-site occupational health center. The two datasets were linked using an identification number assigned to each employee. The employer redacted all personal identifiers from the merged dataset prior to delivery to the research team. Written approval was obtained from the employer for use of the merged (de-identified) dataset, and the University of Iowa Institutional Review Board determined that the study did not meet the regulatory definition of human subjects' research.

2.2. Study Facility and Setting

The study facility produces consumer-grade household appliances. At any given time during the study period, the facility employed approximately 2300 hourly workers and occupied approximately 232,000 m^2 of production space. Production employees were organized by a labor union. Production output during the study period was roughly 5000 completed products per day across three main product assembly lines and one premium product line. Human resources onboarding and basic safety training for new hires occurred during the first four hours of each of the first two days of employment. The facility also has a dedicated training area used to orient new hires to the materials, equipment (e.g., machinery and tools), and processes that are common throughout the production areas. New hires practice simulated production tasks in the training area, gaining proficiency while learning expectations for compliance with safety policies in a hands-on manner. During the second four hours of each of the first two days of employment, new hires shadowed a current employee to learn the production processes required of the jobs to which they were assigned. Transition from shadowing to full-time production activities was expected by the third day of employment.

2.3. Probationary Period

Based on the collective bargaining agreement between workers and management, each new hourly employee was considered "probationary" for a period of 60 calendar days from the date of hire. During the probationary period, new employees (i) were not under the jurisdiction of the collective bargaining agreement, (ii) had limited access to overtime work, and (iii) were unable to request job reassignment within the facility. After 60 calendar days from the date of hire, each employee was considered a "regular" employee subject to all collective bargaining provisions regardless of formal affiliation with the labor organization.

The 60-day probationary period is also consistent with estimates of the time required to recover costs associated with hiring and training unskilled workers [20]. Facility management estimated that the hiring and training costs associated with each new hire were $5500 (on average). New hires at the study facility earn an average initial wage of approximately 15.00 $/h. Assuming the value of labor is equivalent to the pay rate, hiring and training costs would be recovered after 367 work hours, or just over 45 8-hour work days. Generally, 45 8-hour work days will occur within 60 calendar days from the date of hire.

2.4. Study Sample

The human resources database included records on 3834 employees hired during the observation period. For employees hired multiple times during the observation period, only the first instance was included in the final dataset (resulting in exclusion of 13 records). Employees hired between 26 September 2016 and 25 November 2016, were also excluded (69 records) in order to ensure all employees in the final dataset had the potential to work the full 60-day probationary period. Therefore, the final study sample included 3752 employees.

2.5. Employment Termination

The primary outcome event was any termination of employment during the 60-day probationary period, dichotomized as "yes" or "no." Outcome variables were created using information available in the human resources records database. Information was also available regarding the reason for termination, as recorded by the employer. We classified the following reasons as involuntary terminations: termination without pay, violation of workplace violence policy, absenteeism, unsatisfactory performance, and safety violation. We classified the following reasons as voluntary terminations: personal reasons, return to school, relocation, another job, and "3-day no call/no show."

The "3-day no call/no show" reason refers to an employer policy stating that an employee will be terminated if he/she is absent for three consecutive work days and does not communicate an explanation for the absence. We considered such a circumstance a voluntary termination, in contrast to absenteeism, which was related to the number of absent days regardless of communication between the employee and the employer (which we considered an involuntary termination). Terminations also occurred for other reasons for which neither involuntary nor voluntary could be assigned, including: promotion from hourly to salaried employment, catastrophic injury outside of work that removed the employee from the workforce, and unspecified circumstances.

2.6. Occupational Health Center Visits

The primary predictor variable was the occurrence of any first-time visit to the on-site occupational health center (OHC) within 60 calendar days from the date of hire (i.e., early OHC visit, dichotomized as yes/no), regardless of the nature of injury/event or the body part/area affected. Secondary predictor variables were created by classifying early OHC visits according to (i) the "nature of injury," recorded in the OHC database as repetitive strain, acute sprain/strain, struck/caught/injured by, cut/puncture/scrape, slip/trip/fall, temperature extreme, and a variety of other descriptors (e.g., chemical burns, allergic reactions, and foreign objects in eye, among others), and (ii) the "body part/area affected," recorded in the OHC database as abdominal area, chest area, a variety of lower extremity areas (hips, knees, ankles, feet, thighs, and calves), head/eye, low back, shoulder/arm, wrist/hand, upper back/neck, and other (e.g., heat-related). To manage small cell sizes for analysis purposes, the nature of injury categories were collapsed to repetitive strain, acute sprain/strain, and general occupational injuries (i.e., all others). Collapsing the nature of injury categories also separated injuries that typically result from exposure to physical risk factors for musculoskeletal outcomes from injuries that typically result from exposure to other hazards. The body part/area affected categories were also collapsed to low back, shoulder/arm, wrist/hand, and other (i.e., all other body parts/areas) to manage small sizes.

Primary and secondary predictor variables were created from information available in the OHC database. Employer policy required the immediate reporting of acute occupational injuries as well as signs and symptoms consistent with non-acute adverse musculoskeletal health outcomes to OHC nursing staff. Nursing staff were required to document all OHC visits, including the employee number, the date of the visit, the nature of the injury/event which brought the employee to the center, as well as the body part/area affected. The OHC database did not contain information regarding other, personal health concerns for which an employee might seek care.

2.7. Demographic Variables

Demographic variables available for each new hire included gender, age, and race/ethnicity. Age was analyzed as a continuous variable. Race/ethnicity was categorized as White/Caucasian, Black/African-American, Hispanic/Latino(a) and other (including Asian/Pacific islanders, Alaskan natives and American Indians).

2.8. Job Characteristics

The human resources records database included information about the work shift to which each new hire was assigned, categorized as First (7:00 a.m.–3:30 p.m., Monday–Friday), Second (3:30 p.m.–11:30 p.m., Monday–Friday), Third (11:30 p.m.–7:00 a.m., Monday–Friday), and Premium (5:00 a.m.–3:30 p.m., Monday–Thursday). In addition, information was available for job classification and assigned department. At the study facility, a department is an organizational unit consisting of a group of production tasks under the supervision of one or more production team leaders. We used the job classification and department information to assign a "nature of work" to each new hire, categorized as assembly, fabrication, inspection, material handling, or maintenance.

Assembly work was machine-paced and cyclic. Workers in the assembly classification performed one or more production tasks according to a standard sequence of steps, with a cycle time typically on the order of 35 seconds. Assembly work involved a range of hand-intensive activities, including manual manipulation and installation of parts and the use of both manual and powered hand tools. Fabrication work involved the operation of in-house machinery and fabrication equipment (e.g., presses, vacuum forming machines, and foam injection machines, among many others). Fabrication work was often cyclic, but self-paced rather than machine-paced (in contrast to assembly work). Fabrication areas received daily orders for parts to support the assembly lines and workers would feed raw material into the equipment and either manipulate manual controls or operate digital interfaces. Inspection work involved visual inspection of the completed products or sub-assemblies. Inspection work was distributed throughout the assembly lines but, in contrast to assembly work, was not always cyclic and involved less biomechanically demanding activity (e.g., placing/scanning bar code labels and completing paperwork). Material handling generally involved the use of powered industrial vehicles and manual push/pull carts to transport parts and completed products throughout the facility. Finally, maintenance work involved electrical work, powered industrial vehicle repair, tool and die maintenance, as well as repair of assembly and fabrication equipment.

2.9. Statistical Analyses

The duration of employment was dichotomized as ≤60 days (i.e., termination of employment during the probationary period) and >60 days (i.e., working at least to end of the probationary period). The demographic variables (gender, age, race/ethnicity) and job characteristic variables (shift, and nature of work) were then stratified and summarized by duration of employment for descriptive purposes. Age was reported using the mean and standard deviation; all other variables were reported using observation frequencies and proportions.

We calculated incidence rates of OHC visits to provide additional context to the analysis. Specifically, incidence rates were calculated as the number of first-time OHC visits divided by the total person-time at risk of visiting the OHC across the full duration of the study period (i.e., 2 January 2012 to 25 November 2016). For employees with an OHC visit, person-time at risk was censored on the date of the first OHC visit recorded in the OHC database. For employees with no OHC visit, person-time was censored on either (i) the date at which employment was terminated or (ii) the end of the study period. In addition, we calculated incidence rates of first-time OHC visits that occurred during the 60-day probationary period (i.e., early OHC visits). The same censoring criteria were used for these calculations, although each employee contributed a maximum of 60 days of person-time at risk of visiting the OHC.

Hazard ratios (HRs) of the crude associations between early OHC visits and time to termination during the 60-day probationary period were estimated using Cox regression methods [21,22]. Nine models were constructed, each representing one of the combinations of one OHC visit definition (any early OHC visit, nature of injury, or body part/area affected) and one time to termination definition (any, involuntary, or voluntary). In all models, the referent category was limited to those employees without an early OHC visit. Time-varying measures of the three OHC visit variables (listed immediately above) were created to capture person-time both before and following an OHC visit [23]. Specifically, among those with an early OHC visit, the number of days from the date of hire to the date of the early OHC visit was analyzed as unexposed time (but time while still at risk of employment termination), while the number of days from the date of the early OHC visit to the date on which person-time was censored was analyzed as exposed time. Among those without an early OHC visit, all person-time of observation was analyzed as unexposed time. Also, in models with involuntary termination as the outcome event, we included person-time accumulated among those with voluntary or other terminations because these employees were still at risk of involuntary termination prior to the time of voluntary or other termination. Similarly, in models with voluntary termination as the outcome event, we included person-time accumulated among those with involuntary or other terminations because these employees were still at risk of voluntary termination prior to the time of involuntary or other termination.

For all crude analyses, the proportional hazards assumption was tested by including interaction terms between each predictor variable and time; no statistically significant interaction terms were observed, indicating that the proportional hazards assumption was not violated. Cox regression methods were also used to estimate crude associations between each demographic and job characteristic variable and time to each of the termination types (any, involuntary, and voluntary).

Adjusted associations between early OHC visits and time to termination were also estimated using Cox regression. As in the crude analyses, models were constructed for each combination of one OHC visit definition and one time to termination definition (i.e., nine total models). Demographic and job characteristic variables crudely associated with the risk of employment termination (with $p < 0.10$) were included in all multivariable models. No further model specification criteria were applied (e.g., backward elimination) given the small number of available demographic and job characteristic variables relative to the sample size.

To assess bias of the adjusted hazard ratios between early OHC visits and time to involuntary termination potentially introduced by retaining in the analyses person-time accumulated among those with voluntary or other termination (and vice versa), additional analyses were conducted with datasets (i) restricted only to those with involuntary or no termination (i.e., excluding those with voluntary or other termination) and (ii) restricted only to those with voluntary or no termination (i.e., excluding those with involuntary or other termination). All statistical procedures were performed using SAS (version 9.4, SAS Institute, Inc., Cary, NC, USA).

3. Results

A summary of demographic and job characteristic variables is provided in Table 1. The mean age of the 3752 employees was 33.9 ± 10.9 years, and 68.0% were male. 58.4% of the employees identified as white/Caucasian, 39.1% as black/African-American, 2.7% as Hispanic/Latino, and 3.4% as other racial/ethnic designations. Larger proportions of new hires were placed into the first (34.6%) and second (43.7%) shifts compared to third (18.7%) and premium (3.0%) shifts. A substantial majority (87.2%) was assigned to assembly work.

1172 (31.2%) of the new hires were employed 60 days or less. Of these, 793 (67.7%) were terminated for involuntary reasons, 345 (20.4%) for voluntary reasons, and 34 (2.9%) for other reasons (Table 1). Differences in the distributions of demographic and job characteristic variables between employment duration strata (i.e., employed >60 days vs. employed ≤60 days) were generally small. However, those employed ≤60 days were less frequently male, more frequently white/Caucasian, and more frequently assigned to assembly work. In addition, a smaller proportion of those employed ≤60 days was assigned to the premium product line, although the number of new hires in this category was relatively small.

Employees contributed a total of 856,845 person-days (2348 person-years (PY)) of observation during the study period (2 January 2012–25 November 2016). During this time, a total of 1090 first-time OHC visits were recorded, yielding an overall incidence rate (IR) of 46.4/100PY. Of the 1090 first-time visits, 453 (41.6%) were classified as general occupational injuries (IR = 19.3/100PY), 429 (39.3%) as repetitive strain (IR = 18.3/100PY), and 208 (19.1%) as acute sprain/strain (IR = 8.9/100PY). The body part/area affected most commonly was the wrist/hand (29.3%), followed by the shoulder/arm (25.2%) and the low back (10.9%), with other body parts/areas accounting for the remainder (34.6%).

Table 1. Demographic and job characteristic variables.

Variable	Full Sample (n = 3572)		Employed > 60 days (n = 2580)		Employed ≤ 60 days							
					All (n = 1172)		Involuntary (n = 793)		Voluntary (n = 345)		Other (n = 34)	
	N	(%)	N	(%)	N	(%)	N	(%)	N	(%)	N	(%)
Demographics												
Age [1]	33.9	(10.9)	34.0	(10.7)	33.7	(11.3)	34.0	(11.1)	32.9	(11.7)	34.1	(11.3)
Male gender	2550	(68.0)	1808	(70.0)	742	(63.3)	501	(63.2)	221	(64.1)	20	(58.8)
Race/ethnicity												
White/Caucasian	2057	(54.8)	1360	(52.7)	697	(59.5)	446	(56.2)	238	(69.0)	13	(38.2)
African-American	1467	(39.1)	1064	(41.2)	403	(34.4)	285	(35.9)	100	(29.0)	18	(52.9)
Hispanic/Latino(a)	102	(2.7)	61	(2.4)	41	(3.5)	36	(4.5)	5	(1.4)	0	(0.0)
Other [2]	126	(3.4)	95	(3.7)	31	(2.7)	26	(3.3)	2	(0.6)	3	(8.8)
Job characteristics												
Shift assignment												
First	1297	(34.6)	885	(34.3)	412	(35.2)	316	(39.9)	88	(25.5)	8	(23.5)
Second	1639	(43.7)	1120	(43.4)	519	(44.3)	295	(37.2)	199	(57.7)	25	(73.5)
Third	702	(18.7)	472	(18.3)	230	(19.6)	177	(22.3)	52	(15.1)	1	(2.9)
Premium [3]	114	(3.0)	103	(4.0)	11	(0.9)	5	(0.6)	6	(1.7)	0	(0.0)
Nature of work												
Non-assembly	480	(12.8)	428	(16.6)	52	(4.4)	42	(5.3)	9	(2.6)	1	(2.9)
Fabrication	203	(5.4)	181	(7.0)	22	(1.9)	16	(2.0)	5	(1.4)	0	(0.0)
Inspection	75	(2.0)	61	(2.4)	14	(1.2)	12	(1.5)	2	(0.6)	0	(0.0)
Material handling	142	(3.8)	128	(5.0)	14	(1.2)	13	(1.6)	1	(0.3)	0	(0.0)
Maintenance	60	(1.6)	58	(2.3)	2	(0.2)	1	(0.1)	1	(0.3)	1	(2.9)
Assembly	3272	(87.2)	2152	(83.4)	1120	(95.6)	751	(94.7)	336	(97.4)	33	(97.1)

Notes: [1] Age reported as mean(sd); [2] includes Asian/Pacific Islanders, Alaska natives, and American Indians; [3] employees assigned to the premium product line worked four, 10-hr shifts per week.

Of the 1090 first-time OHC visits, 339 (31.1%) occurred during the 60-day probationary period (i.e., early OHC visits). The median number of calendar days from the date of hire to the date of any early OHC visit was 20 (interquartile range: 10–32 days), with a range zero days (i.e., employee reported to the OHC on the first day of employment) to 60 days. Employees contributed a total of 173,816 probationary days (476 PY) of observation, resulting in an incidence rate for early OHC visits of 71.2/100PY. Of the 339 early OHC visits, 142 (41.9%) were classified as general occupational injuries (IR = 29.8/100PY), 129 (38.1%) as repetitive strain (IR = 27.1/100PY), and 68 (20.0%) as acute sprain/strain (IR = 14.3/100PY). The body part/area affected most commonly was the wrist/hand (28.3%), followed by the shoulder/arm (24.5%) and the low back (12.1%), with other body parts/areas accounting for the remainder (35.1%).

Crude estimates of association between the demographic and job characteristic variables and time to termination are provided in Table 2. Statistically significant reductions in the risk of any employment termination were observed among (i) males (HR = 0.79, 95% CI = 0.70–0.89), (ii) those identifying as black/African-American (HR = 0.77, 95% CI = 0.68–0.87) and other racial/ethnic categories (HR = 0.70, 95% CI = 0.49–1.00), and (iii) those assigned to the premium shift (HR = 0.26, 95% CI = 0.14–0.48). In contrast, the risk of any employment termination during the probationary period was elevated among those assigned to assembly positions (HR = 3.69, 95% CI = 2.79–4.87). This pattern was consistent for involuntary and voluntary terminations. However the precision of many HR estimates was reduced as a consequence of small cell sizes. For example, the risk of voluntary terminations among those assigned to assembly positions was highly elevated (HR = 7.0, 95% CI = 3.60–13.56), but the referent category (i.e., those assigned to non-assembly positions) included only nine (2.6%) of the 345 voluntary terminations. A few differences were observed when examining the associations among those with involuntary and voluntary employment termination. Most notably, among those assigned to second shift, the risk of involuntary employment termination was reduced (HR = 0.77, 95% CI = 0.66–0.90) while the risk of voluntary employment termination was elevated (HR = 1.72, 95% CI = 1.72–2.21).

Table 2. Crude associations between demographic and job characteristic variables and employment termination within the 60-day probationary period.

Variable	Any Termination		Involuntary Termination		Voluntary Termination	
	HR	[95% CI]	HR	[95% CI]	HR	[95% CI]
Demographics						
Age	1.00	[0.99, 1.01]	1.00	[0.99, 1.01]	0.99	[0.98, 1.00]
Male gender	0.79	[0.70, 0.89]	0.77	[0.67, 0.89]	0.77	[0.62, 0.96]
Race/ethnicity						
White/Caucasian		-REF-		-REF-		-REF-
African-American	0.77	[0.68, 0.87]	0.84	[0.72, 0.97]	0.55	[0.44, 0.70]
Hispanic/Latino	1.25	[0.91, 1.71]	1.67	[1.19, 2.35]	0.48	[0.20, 1.17]
Other [1]	0.70	[0.49, 1.00]	0.87	[0.59, 1.29]	0.13	[0.03, 0.52]
Job characteristics						
Shift						
First		-REF-		-REF-		-REF-
Second	1.00	[0.88, 1.14]	0.77	[0.66, 0.90]	1.72	[1.34, 2.21]
Third	1.04	[0.88, 1.22]	1.05	[0.88, 1.27]	1.10	[0.78, 1.55]
Premium [2]	0.26	[0.14, 0.48]	0.16	[0.16, 0.38]	0.59	[0.26, 1.35]
Nature of work						
Non-assembly		-REF-		-REF-		-REF-
Assembly	3.69	[2.79, 4.87]	3.20	[2.35, 4.37]	7.00	[3.60, 13.56]

Notes: [1] includes Asian/Pacific Islanders, Alaska natives, and American Indians; [2] employees assigned to the premium product line worked four, 10-h shifts per week.

Crude and adjusted estimates of association between early OHC visits and employment termination during the probationary period are provided in Table 3. Any instance of an early OHC was associated with a statistically significant increase in risk of any employment termination prior to the end of the probationary period (adjusted HR = 2.58, 95% CI = 2.12–3.15). The effect magnitude was similar when analyzing OHC visits by the nature of the injury, with statistically significant adjusted HRs of 2.38 for repetitive strain, 2.61 for acute sprain/strain, and 2.78 for general occupational injuries. Associations were also statistically significant when analyzing early OHC visits by the body part/area affected, although of somewhat greater magnitude for the shoulder/arm (adjusted HR = 3.58) and low back (adjusted HR = 3.12) than for the wrist/hand (adjusted HR = 1.95) and other body parts/areas (adjusted HR = 2.26). The magnitude of effect was generally greater for involuntary termination than for voluntary termination, but substantial overlap of the 95% confidence intervals around the HR estimates suggests minimal statistical difference (if any).

Table 3. Crude and adjusted [1] associations between occupational health center (OHC) visits and employment termination within the 60-day probationary period. [2]

	Any Termination		Involuntary Termination		Voluntary Termination	
	Crude	Adjusted	Crude	Adjusted	Crude	Adjusted
	HR [95% CI]	HR [95% CI]	HR [95% CI]	HR [95% CI]	HR [95% CI]	HR [95% CI]
Any early OHC visit	2.35 [1.93, 2.85]	2.58 [2.12, 3.15]	2.54 [2.02, 3.20]	2.74 [2.17, 3.45]	2.06 [1.37, 3.09]	2.29 [1.52, 3.45]
Nature of injury						
Repetitive strain	2.25 [1.65, 3.07]	2.38 [1.74, 3.25]	2.48 [1.73, 3.54]	2.55 [1.78, 3.65]	1.68 [0.86, 3.26]	1.87 [0.96, 3.66]
Acute sprain/strain	2.40 [1.62, 3.54]	2.61 [1.77, 3.87]	2.26 [1.40, 3.67]	2.50 [1.54, 4.07]	2.24 [1.06, 4.75]	2.33 [1.09, 4.96]
General occup.	2.40 [1.79, 3.21]	2.78 [2.07, 3.72]	2.53 [1.80, 3.56]	2.89 [2.05, 4.07]	1.73 [0.92, 3.26]	2.04 [1.08, 3.85]
Body part/area affected						
Low back	2.45 [1.47, 4.08]	3.12 [1.87, 5.22]	2.83 [1.60, 5.01]	3.52 [1.98, 6.26]	1.69 [0.54, 5.29]	2.29 [0.73, 7.20]
Shoulder/arm	3.40 [2.46, 4.68]	3.58 [2.59, 4.94]	3.65 [2.51, 5.30]	3.84 [2.64, 5.58]	2.70 [1.39, 5.25]	2.82 [1.44, 5.51]
Wrist/hand	1.79 [1.20, 2.66]	1.95 [1.31, 2.91]	1.96 [1.24, 3.09]	2.09 [1.32, 3.31]	1.00 [0.37, 2.68]	1.13 [0.42, 3.05]
Other	2.06 [1.48, 2.87]	2.26 [1.62, 3.15]	1.94 [1.29, 2.91]	2.10 [1.39, 3.17]	1.93 [1.03, 3.64]	2.13 [1.13, 4.03]

Notes: [1] All models adjusted for gender, race/ethnicity, shift, and nature of work based on associations with $p < 0.10$ in crude analyses; [2] referent category in all models includes those with no OHC visit and no termination of the specified type within the 60-day probationary period.

Results of the additional analyses with restricted datasets showed minimal change in the adjusted HRs. Specifically, HRs in the additional analyses were, on average, 6% greater than those presented in Table 3. In no case was a HR reported in Table 3 greater than the analogous HR estimated in the analysis of the restricted dataset.

4. Discussion

The results of this study show a strong association between visiting an on-site occupational health center and subsequent termination of employment within 60 days from the date of hire among a large sample of newly hired manufacturing workers. Specifically, the risk of termination was more than double among those who visited the on-site occupational health center compared to those who did not. The magnitudes and precisions of the risk estimates were also consistent across different injury classifications and mostly consistent across different body parts/areas affected. Associations were also elevated regardless of the reason for termination, although of somewhat greater magnitude among those with terminations classified as involuntary compared to those with terminations classified as voluntary.

Few longitudinal studies are available to which the results of the current study can be compared. Most recently, Okechukwu et al. [18] examined the association between self-reported occupational injury and both involuntary and voluntary "job loss" among a sample of 1331 nursing home workers. Injury data were collected at the time of enrollment and again after six and 12 months of follow-up, and then linked to employers' administrative records to identify those with job loss occurring in the subsequent six months. Overall, 24.2% of the sample experienced job loss within the 18 months of observation, which is much lower than the frequency of employment termination observed in the current study (in the current study, 31.2% of new hires were employed fewer than 60 days from the date of hire). Similar to the current study, statistically significant associations were observed between occupational injury and both voluntary and involuntary job loss, and the magnitude of the association was also greater for involuntary job loss. However, important differences in the study sample (nursing home workers with an average of 6.3 years of experience at the time of enrollment vs. newly hired manufacturing workers) and differences in the nature of work between the cohorts limit comparisons between the results of our study and those reported in Okechukwu et al. [18].

The incidence rates of early OHC visits were approximately 50–60% greater than the incidence rates observed across the full study period, suggesting an increase in the risk of occupational injury during the earliest stages of employment. Gerr et al. [24] reported results from a prospective study of physical risk factors and upper extremity musculoskeletal outcomes among 386 workers at the same facility as that of the current study. In contrast to the current study, Gerr et al. [24] ascertained incident musculoskeletal symptoms with a weekly self-reported survey and incident musculoskeletal disorders via clinical evaluation (following a self-report of symptoms). Compared to the employees included in the current study, participants of Gerr et al. [24] were experienced (average of 15.8 years at the facility at the time of entry vs. all new hires), older (mean age 43.1 years vs. 33.9 years), and less frequently male (48.1% vs. 68.0%). Incidence rates were reported as 58/100PY for hand/arm symptoms, 19/100PY for hand/arm disorders, 54/100PY for neck/shoulder symptoms, and 14/100PY for neck shoulder disorders. Analogous incidences rates in the current study (by combining the nature of injury categories with the body part/area affected categories) were 8.5/100PY for OHC visits classified as either acute sprain/strain or repetitive strain and affecting the wrist/hand and 8.4/100PY for injuries classified as either acute sprain/strain or repetitive strain and affecting the neck/shoulder. The difference in incidence rates might appear to contradict the evidence suggesting that the risk of occupational injury is greatest during the earliest stages of employment. However, the active case-finding approach used by Gerr et al. [24] is expected to result in greater observed incidence rates than the use of passive surveillance sources, such as the OHC database used in the current study [25]. It is possible that only those experiencing the greatest levels of musculoskeletal discomfort reported to the OHC. In addition, it is possible that some employees, upon experiencing musculoskeletal discomfort, elected to terminate employment but did not report to the OHC.

Error in the ascertainment of dates of employment termination (of any type) was unlikely given the use of human resources data and inclusion of all newly hired employees in the study sample. While it is possible that some terminations were recorded one or more business days following the actual event, we have no way of validating the accuracy of the termination dates. Regardless, any error was unlikely to have differed systematically between those who visited the OHC and those who did not. However, the classification of each termination as involuntary or voluntary relied on our interpretation of the information included in the human resources database. We discussed our termination classification strategy with the employer prior to analyses. The only heterogeneity of opinion occurred for the "3-day no-call/no-show" reason for termination ($n = 216$), which we classified as voluntary. Ultimately, we believe our choice was appropriate since the employee made an active decision both to not report to work and to not communicate an explanation for the absence.

Errors in the ascertainment of exposure may have occurred. First, it is possible that some employees experienced an occupational injury and did not report to the OHC (despite employer policy). If employment termination during the probationary period were more likely as a result of the unreported occupational injury, then the observed hazard ratios would have been attenuated. We believe it is likely that the dates of events classified as general occupational injuries (e.g., chemical exposures and foreign objects in the eye) were captured accurately given their acute nature and the policy requiring employees to immediately report to the OHC. However, the date of an event classified as "acute sprain/strain" or "repetitive strain" does not necessarily reflect the date of symptom onset. Any lag between the onset of symptoms and the OHC visit date would increase the number of unexposed days and decrease the time to termination following the OHC visit date, and therefore inflate the observed hazard ratios. However, we have no reason to believe that the frequency or duration of reporting lags were of sufficient magnitude to cause meaningful bias of the estimated hazard ratios. Finally, the OHC was staffed by multiple occupational health nurses and so some (inter-observer) misclassification may have occurred of the nature of the injury/event which brought the employee to the center and/or the body part/area affected.

5. Conclusions

In summary, newly hired manufacturing workers who visited an on-site occupational health center for reasons consistent with an occupational injury experienced increased risk employment termination within 60 days from the date of hire. In addition, the incidence rate of occupational health center visits within 60 days from the date of hire was substantially greater than that observed over longer time frames. Together, these results suggest that management of workplace safety and health hazards to prevent the occurrence of occupational injury may reduce turnover rates.

Finally, the end of the study observation period (November 2016) corresponds approximately with a major shift in strategic production management practices at the study facility. Specifically, starting in early 2017, the facility has adopted the "world-class manufacturing (WCM)" model attributed most commonly to Hayes and Wheelwright [26], reformulated by Schonberger [27], and further refined and formalized by large, multi-national manufacturing enterprises such as Fiat Chrysler Automobiles. A key component of WCM is an organizational commitment to safety, such that "WCM cannot be implemented when the company is not assuring a robust safety system" [28] (p. 600). We hope to revisit the analyses described in this manuscript after complete roll-out and maturation of the WCM systems and procedures in order to evaluate the effect of WCM on occupational injury rates and employee turnover.

Author Contributions: Conceptualization, N.C.H. and N.B.F.; Methodology, N.C.H., N.B.F., J.A.D. and F.G.; Formal analysis, N.C.H., N.B.F. and F.G.; Investigation, N.C.H. and N.B.F.; Resources, N.B.F.; Data curation, N.C.H., N.B.F. and J.A.D.; Writing—original draft preparation, N.C.H. and N.B.F.; Writing—review and editing, N.C.H., N.B.F., J.A.D. and F.G.; Visualization, N.C.H. and N.B.F.; Project administration, N.B.F.; Funding acquisition, N.B.F.

Funding: This research was supported by a grant from the National Institute for Occupational Safety and Health (NIOSH) for the Heartland Center for Occupational Health and Safety at the University of Iowa, grant number T42OH008491. Additional support was provided by the NIOSH-funded Healthier Workforce Center of the Midwest at the University of Iowa, grant number U19OH008868.

Acknowledgments: The authors wish to thank the workers and management at the study facility for their support of this project.

Conflicts of Interest: The authors declare no conflict of interest. The funders had no role in the design of the study; in the collection, analyses, or interpretation of data; in the writing of the manuscript, or in the decision to publish the results.

References

1. Meier, K.J.; Hicklin, A. Employee turnover and organizational performance: Testing a hypothesis from classical public administration. *J. Publ. Adm. Res. Theor.* **2007**, *18*, 573–590. [CrossRef]
2. Wynen, J.; Van Dooren, W.; Mattijs, J.; Deschamps, C. Linking turnover to organizational performance: The role of process conformance. *Public Manag. Rev.* **2018**. [CrossRef]
3. Heavey, A.L.; Holwerda, J.A.; Hausknecht, J.P. Causes and consequences of collective turnover: A meta-analytic review. *J. Appl. Psychol.* **2013**, *98*, 412–453. [CrossRef] [PubMed]
4. Glebbeek, A.C.; Bax, E.H. Is high employee turnover really harmful? An empirical test using company records. *Acad. Manag. J.* **2004**, *47*, 277–286.
5. Hausknecht, J.P.; Trevor, C.O. Collective turnover at the group, unit, and organizational levels: Evidence, issues, and implications. *J. Manag.* **2011**, *37*, 352–388. [CrossRef]
6. Park, T.-Y.; Shaw, J.D. Turnover rates and organizational performance: A meta-analysis. *J. Appl. Psychol.* **2013**, *98*, 268–309. [CrossRef]

7. Burt, C.D. *New Employee Safety: Risk Factors and Management Strategies*; Springer: Cham, Switzerland, 2016.
8. Hom, P.W.; Lee, T.W.; Shaw, J.D.; Hausknecht, J.P. One hundred years of employee turnover theory and research. *J. Appl. Psychol.* **2017**, *102*, 530–545. [CrossRef]
9. Root, N.; Hoefer, M. The first work-injury data available from new BLS study. *Mon. Lab. Rev.* **1979**, *102*, 76–80.
10. Siskind, F. Another look at the link between work injuries and job experience. *Mon. Lab. Rev.* **1982**, *105*, 38–40.
11. Groves, W.; Kecojevic, V.; Komljenovic, D. Analysis of fatalities and injuries involving mining equipment. *J. Saf. Res.* **2007**, *38*, 461–470. [CrossRef]
12. Bell, J.L.; Grushecky, S.T. Evaluating the effectiveness of a logger safety training program. *J. Saf. Res.* **2006**, *37*, 53–61. [CrossRef] [PubMed]
13. Breslin, F.C.; Smith, P. Trial by fire: A multivariate examination of the relation between job tenure and work injuries. *Occup. Environ. Med.* **2006**, *63*, 27–32. [CrossRef] [PubMed]
14. Hancock, J.I.; Allen, D.G.; Bosco, F.A.; McDaniel, K.R.; Pierce, C.A. Meta-analytic review of employee turnover as a predictor of firm performance. *J. Manag.* **2013**, *39*, 573–603. [CrossRef]
15. Cree, T.; Kelloway, E.K. Responses to occupational hazards: Exit and participation. *J. Occup. Health Psychol.* **1997**, *2*, 304. [CrossRef] [PubMed]
16. Griffeth, R.W.; Hom, P.W.; Gaertner, S. A meta-analysis of antecedents and correlates of employee turnover: Update, moderator tests, and research implications for the next millennium. *J. Manag.* **2000**, *26*, 463–488. [CrossRef]
17. Brewer, C.S.; Kovner, C.T.; Greene, W.; Tukov-Shuser, M.; Djukic, M. Predictors of actual turnover in a national sample of newly licensed registered nurses employed in hospitals. *J. Adv. Nurs.* **2012**, *68*, 521–538. [CrossRef] [PubMed]
18. Okechukwu, C.A.; Bacic, J.; Velasquez, E.; Hammer, L.B. Marginal structural modelling of associations of occupational injuries with voluntary and involuntary job loss among nursing home workers. *Occup. Environ. Med.* **2016**, *73*, 175–182. [CrossRef] [PubMed]
19. Young, A.E. Return to work following disabling occupational injury-facilitators of employment continuation. *Scand. J. Work Environ. Health* **2010**, 473–483. [CrossRef]
20. Hinkin, T.R.; Tracey, J.B. The cost of turnover: Putting a price on the learning curve. *Cornell Hotel Restaur. Adm. Q.* **2000**, *41*, 14–21. [CrossRef]
21. Cox, D.R.; Oakes, D. *Analysis of Survival Data*; Chapman and Hall: London, UK, 1984.
22. Kalbfleisch, J.D.; Prentice, R.L. *The Statistical Analysis of Failure Time Data*; John Wiley and Sons: New York, NY, USA, 1980.
23. Fisher, L.D.; Lin, D.Y. Time-dependent covariates in the Cox proportional-hazards regression model. *Annu. Rev. Public Health* **1999**, *20*, 145–157. [CrossRef]
24. Gerr, F.; Fethke, N.B.; Merlino, L.; Anton, D.; Rosecrance, J.; Jones, M.P.; Marcus, M.; Meyers, A.R. A prospective study of musculoskeletal outcomes among manufacturing workers: I. Effects of physical risk factors. *Hum. Factors* **2014**, *56*, 112–130. [CrossRef] [PubMed]
25. Silverstein, B.A.; Stetson, D.S.; Keyserling, W.M.; Fine, L.J. Work-related musculoskeletal disorders: Comparison of data sources for surveillance. *Am. J. Ind. Med.* **1997**, *31*, 600–608. [CrossRef]
26. Hayes, R.H.; Wheelwright, S.C. *Restoring Our Competitive Edge: Competing Through Manufacturing*; Wiley: New York, NY, USA, 1984; Volume 30.
27. Schonberger, R.J. *World Class Manufacturing*; Simon and Schuster: New York, NY, USA, 2008.
28. Chiarini, A.; Vagnoni, E. World-class manufacturing by Fiat. Comparison with Toyota Production System from a Strategic Management, Management Accounting, Operations Management and Performance Measurement dimension. *Int. J. Prod. Res.* **2015**, *53*, 590–606. [CrossRef]

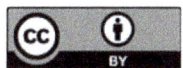

© 2019 by the authors. Licensee MDPI, Basel, Switzerland. This article is an open access article distributed under the terms and conditions of the Creative Commons Attribution (CC BY) license (http://creativecommons.org/licenses/by/4.0/).

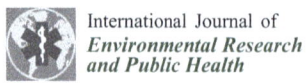

Article

It Doesn't End There: Workplace Bullying, Work-to-Family Conflict, and Employee Well-Being in Korea

Gyesook Yoo [1] and Soomi Lee [2,*]

[1] Department of Child and Family Studies, Kyung Hee University, Seoul 02447, Korea; dongrazi@khu.ac.kr
[2] Department of Biobehavioral Health, Pennsylvania State University, State College, PA 16802, USA
* Correspondence: soomilee1104@gmail.com

Received: 7 June 2018; Accepted: 20 July 2018; Published: 22 July 2018

Abstract: Workplace bullying entails negative consequences on workers' life. Yet, there is lack of research on workplace bullying in an Asian context. Moreover, less is known about the potential mechanisms linking workplace bullying and employee well-being. This study examined the associations between workplace bullying and Korean employees' well-being (quality of life, occupational health) and whether the associations were mediated by work-to-family conflict. Cross-sectional data came from 307 workers in South Korea who were employed in healthcare, education, and banking industries. Analyses adjusted for industry, age, gender, education, marital status, and work hours. Employees who had more exposure to workplace bullying reported lower levels of quality of life and occupational health. These associations were mediated by work-to-family conflict, such that more exposure to workplace bullying was associated with greater work-to-family conflict, which, in turn, was associated with lower levels of quality of life and occupational health. These mediating pathways were consistent across the three industries. Korean employees who experience more workplace bullying may bring unfinished work stress to the home (thus greater work-to-family conflict), which impairs their well-being. Future research may need to consider the role of work-to-family conflict when targeting to reduce the negative consequences of workplace bullying.

Keywords: workplace bullying; quality of life; occupational health; work-to-family conflict; Korean workplaces

1. Introduction

Workplace bullying entails negative consequences on workers' life, by exposing workers to negative acts of co-workers, supervisors or subordinates [1,2]. The prevalence of workplace bullying is high across nations [3] and it is becoming an increasingly serious issue in South Korea (Korea, hereafter) in recent years. The vast majority of Korean employees (87%) report they have experienced some form of bullying within the previous six months [4]. The rate of workplace bullying experiences is even higher among employees who work long hours and non-regular employees who may have job insecurity [5]. Workplace bullying may impair employees' mental and physical health. However, there is lack of empirical research focusing on workplace bullying in Korea and its associations with Korean employees' well-being. Moreover, less is known about potential mediating mechanisms linking workplace bullying and employee well-being [6].

Work-to-family conflict is a possible mediator between workplace bullying and employee well-being. Work-to-family conflict refers to time-based, strain-based, and behavior-based interrole conflict between mutually incompatible demands from work and family domains in some respect [7]. According to the work-family interface model [7–9], negative experiences and stressors from workplaces often spill over into employees' personal and family life via work-to-family conflict [10–13]. Work-to-family conflict, in turn, is associated with employees' negative health and well-being outcomes [14–19].

Based on the work-family interface model, previous studies have paid much attention to the negative work-to-family spillover effects of employees' emotional labor, abusive supervision, and social ostracism at workplaces [10–13,20–23]. However, there has been lack of research examining the negative work-to-family spillover effects originate from workplace bullying. To address this gap in occupational literature, this study examines the potential mediating role of work-to-family conflict in the link between workplace bullying and employee well-being outcomes assessed by quality of life and occupational health. Most of existing studies on workplace bullying have been based on Western samples, lacking in consideration of different cultural values on interpersonal relationships or organizational hierarchies and cultures in non-Western countries [6,23,24]. Findings from the Korean employee sample may enrich our understanding of the mechanism in which workplace bullying impairs employee well-being in a cultural context where employees are particularly vulnerable to experiencing workplace bullying and work-to-family conflict.

1.1. Theoretical and Empirical Background Linking Workplace Bullying to Employee Well-Being

Workplace bullying is generally defined as situations where an employee is exposed to negative actions on the part of co-workers, supervisors or subordinates repeatedly and over a period of time [25]. It is different from workplace violence [26] or occupational stalking [27] in its nature of repetition, persistency, hostile intentionality of negative acts, and power imbalance. Some forms of workplace bullying behaviors include wrong or unjust judgement about a bullied employee's work performance, criticizing one's personal life, restricting expression of personal opinion, assigning meaningless tasks, and backbiting. Such negative actions are unwanted and resented by the victim employees and may cause humiliation and distress in victims and also potentially in observers [28].

Previous research has observed the negative consequences of workplace bullying on employees' health and well-being, including deterioration of psychological well-being, complaints about physical and somatic symptoms, and poor quality of life [29–32]. Both the victims of bullying and the observers report more general stress and mental stress than those without bullying experiences [33]. There may also be a long-term health consequences of workplace bullying. A 3-wave follow-up study from Danish employees in a period of four years has shown that negative health problems caused by workplace bullying (e.g., poor self-rated health, sick-leave, depressive disorders, and sleep problems) last over several years even after bullying was discontinued [34].

1.2. Work-to-Family Conflict as a Mediating Mechanism

Work-family conflict refers to *"a form of interrole conflict in which the role pressures from work and family domains are mutually incompatible in some respect"* ([7], p. 77), which includes time-based, strain-based, and behavior-based conflict. The work-family interface model [7–9] suggests that negative experiences from work often spill over into employees' non-work domains and interfere with family and personal activities (i.e., work-to-family conflict) that are critical for employee well-being. The emotional and strain-based work demands can threaten employees' psychological resources including needs for autonomy, competence, and relatedness and hamper their involvement to meet role requirements in family and personal domains [35–39]. Through this work-to-family conflict mechanism, employees may transmit their negative emotions toward and come into conflict with family members, thereby their family roles, relationships, and family time may be negatively influenced [23,40]. Previous studies found the effects of work-to-family conflict on employee's psychological distress [17,19], somatic symptoms and health complaints [14–16], and occupational well-being [18].

Many studies have examined work-to-family conflict consequences associated with employees' emotional labor, non-supportive or abusive supervision, psychopathic leadership, and ostracism in workplaces [10–13,20–23]. Scant empirical research has been done on the work-to-family conflict effect on the link between workplace bullying and employee well-being outcomes such as quality of life and occupational health. Employees who are frequently exposed to workplace bullying may experience considerable strain at work in trying to defend and protect themselves. This consumption of victims' physical and psychological resources might negatively spill over into their family and personal domains, which could impair well-being. One of the rare studies of this kind was recently performed by Sanz-Vergel and Rodríguez-Muñoz [41], who examined the mediating effect of work-to-family conflict on the relationship between workplace bullying and employees' health problems in the telecommunications sector in Spain. They found that work-to-family conflict partially mediated the positive association between employee's workplace bullying experiences and health problems including somatic symptoms, anxiety, and insomnia. Thus, based on the work-family interface model [7–9], we could propose that more exposure to workplace bullying is associated with lower well-being outcomes, mediated by higher work-to-family conflict.

1.3. Extent of Workplace Bullying in Korean Workplaces

Contextual characteristics in a certain culture and nation may influence on the people's work and family life [42]. According to the well-known Hofstede's cultural dimensions, Korea is considered to be a society with high levels of power distance, uncertainty avoidance, collectivism, Confucianism, and restraint [43,44]. In this culture, Korean workplaces have tended to have strong hierarchy of top-down organizational culture with the hard work ethic for long hours and let the group interests take precedence over the individual rights of employees [42,45,46], which is more likely to be a breeding ground for workplace bullying acts and behaviors [47]. For example, abusive supervisors or colleagues might exploit the victim's work-oriented attitude by top-down leadership or collectivistic peer pressure.

According to Seo's survey in 2010, 4% of Korean employees working in healthcare, manufacturing, service, and financial industries were the victims of workplace bullying and only 13.4% reported that they had never experienced any forms of workplace bullying during the past six months [4]. Among a number of Korean industries, employees working in education, banking, and healthcare industries seem more vulnerable; about 25% of education industry workers were the victims of workplace bullying and banking industry workers reported average 34 exposure to workplace bullying per month [5]. The most frequent negative acts experienced by the respondents were 'being urged to resign', 'ideas or opinions being ignored', and 'being humiliated'. Especially, employees in education, banking, and healthcare sectors came under pressure to resign once a week. Employees who worked long hours or non-regular workers reported more exposure to workplace bullying [5].

Although workplace bullying is one of the major social problems in Korea and the media is paying attention to the recent suicide cases of employees due to severe stress from workplace bullying [48], this topic has received little scholarly attention. There has been lack of knowledge about the prevalence, antecedents, consequences, and mechanisms of bullying in Korean workplaces. To examine the associations between workplace bullying, work-to-family conflict, and employee well-being, the current study used data collected from employees in education, banking, and healthcare industries in Korea, where workplace bullying is a particular concern.

1.4. Present Study

Building on the work-family interface model [7–9], we examined the cross-sectional associations between workplace bullying, work-to-family conflict, and employees' well-being outcomes. Using data collected from three service industries (i.e., healthcare, education, and banking) in Korea, we tested the mediating role of work-to-family conflict in the associations of workplace bullying with quality of life and occupational health, two outcomes reflecting employees' overall well-being. Our hypotheses are as follows, with specific paths are illustrated in Figure 1.

Hypotheses 1. *More exposure to workplace bullying will be associated with higher work-to-family conflict ("a" path).*

Hypotheses 2. *Higher work-to-family conflict will be associated with lower well-being, assessed by quality of life and occupational health ("b" path).*

Hypotheses 3. *More exposure to workplace bullying will be indirectly associated with lower well-being, mediated by higher work-to-family conflict ("a × b").*

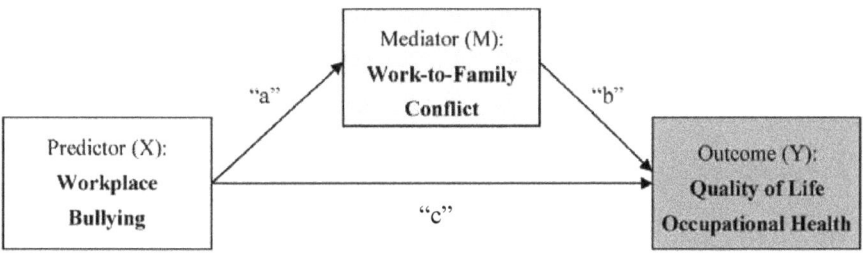

Figure 1. Conceptual model examining the effect of workplace bullying on employees' well-being outcomes mediated by work-to-family conflict. **Note**: "a × b" indicates the indirect effect of X on Y through M. "c" indicates the total effect of X on Y.

2. Materials and Methods

2.1. Participants and Procedure

Employees working in healthcare, education, and banking industries in South Korea participated in this study. Participants were recruited across multiple worksites within each industry from July to September 2014. Those worksites included 4 clinics and hospitals ("healthcare" industry), 6 elementary, middle and high schools ("education" industry), and 12 banks, insurance companies, and other financial institutions ("banking" industry). All worksites were located in Seoul and Gyeonggi-do, the capital city and the province area surrounding the capital city, respectively. Only regular employees (full-time, permanent employees, not temporary) and middle managers and below level (not high-level and executives) were invited to participate in the study.

A paper-pencil questionnaire measuring respondent's exposure to workplace bullying, work-to-family conflict, quality of life, occupational health, and demographic variables was administrated for about twenty minutes in the employee lounges, cafeterias, and lobbies at each workplace. Participants were briefed about the research purpose and requirements of this study, and then informed that their participation would be voluntary and anonymous, guaranteeing confidentiality. After they agreed to participate and provided consent, 444 questionnaires were distributed and 410 employees completed the survey, resulting in a high response rate of 92.3%. One of our main variables asked about the extent to which work experiences interfere with family and personal life (i.e., work-to-family conflict). Thus, we restricted our sample to those who were in heterosexual married/partnered status, because homosexual relationship is socially unacceptable and against the law in South Korea. Out of 410 employees who completed the questionnaire, 307 employees were heterosexual married/partnered, regular employees, and middle managers and below level at the time of survey, thus the final analytic sample of the current study. Their demographic information is provided in Table 1.

Table 1. Descriptive statistics of variables by sub-industry.

	Total (N = 307)		Healthcare (n = 105)		Education (n = 88)		Banking (n = 114)		Difference Test
	M or %	(SD)	M or %	(SD)	M or %	(SD)	M or %	(SD)	χ^2 or F-test
Sociodemographic characteristics									
Age	42.85	(8.01)	41.28$_b$	(7.99)	43.07$_{ab}$	(8.52)	44.14$_a$	(7.41)	3.60 *
Gender (%)									15.41 ***
Male	38.76		46.67		21.59		44.74		
Female	61.24		53.33		78.41		55.26		
Education (%)									31.59 ***
College graduate or higher	70.03		69.52		90.91		54.39		
Under college graduate	29.97		30.48		9.09		45.61		
Work hours (per week)	43.83	(6.22)	43.34$_b$	(4.44)	41.89$_b$	(4.00)	45.78$_a$	(8.20)	10.89 ***
Main variables									
Workplace bullying	5.30	(5.33)	6.00$_a$	(5.56)	3.64$_b$	(3.95)	5.95$_a$	(5.77)	6.25 **
Work-to-family conflict	2.97	(0.79)	2.88	(0.86)	2.94	(0.76)	3.07	(0.73)	1.58
Quality of life	3.62	(0.61)	3.58	(0.60)	3.74	(0.61)	3.55	(0.61)	2.70
Occupational health	3.19	(0.88)	3.16$_{ab}$	(0.94)	3.44$_a$	(0.79)	3.03$_b$	(0.84)	5.89 **

Note: N = 307 Korean employees. Differing subscripts of a, b, and c indicate the results of post hoc analyses where a is higher than b (ab is not significantly different from a or b). Means and percentages with no subscripts do not significantly differ. * $p < 0.05$, ** $p < 0.01$, *** $p < 0.001$.

2.2. Measures

2.2.1. Workplace Bullying

Exposure to workplace bullying was measured by twenty-two items of the Negative Acts Questionnaire (NAQ-Revised) [49]. Employees were asked to report the extent to which they had been exposed to specific negative behaviors at their workplace within the previous six months. Sample items include "Someone withholding information which affects your performance", "Being ordered to do work below your level of competence", and "Having your opinions and views ignored". Each item was rated on a 5-point scale such as 0 = *never*, 1 = *now and then*, 2 = *monthly*, 3 = *every week*, and 4 = *daily*. Some previous studies considered a frequency of roughly weekly exposure over about 6 months as severe cases of workplace bullying [1]. To capture the effect of any exposure to workplace bullying in this study, we considered responses 1 or higher as *having exposure to workplace bullying* (=1 vs. 0 = *no exposure to workplace bullying*). Then we summed the binary indicators across 22 items to create total workplace bullying exposure variable; higher scores representing more exposure to workplace bullying. The Cronbach's alpha for the 22 items was 0.92.

2.2.2. Work-to-Family Conflict

Work-to-family conflict was measured with four items of the Work to Family Conflict Scale [50], in which employees were asked to report the extent to which they had experienced work conflicts with family in the past year. Each item was rated on a 5-point scale from 1 = *never* to 5 = *all of the time*. Sample items include "Your job reduces the effort you can give to activities at home", "Stress at work makes you irritable at home", and "Your job makes you feel tired to do the things that need attention at home". The mean of the 4 items was calculated, with higher scores representing greater work-to-family conflict. The Cronbach's alpha for the 4 items was 0.82.

2.2.3. Quality of Life

Employees' perceptions of their quality of life were assessed via six items excerpted from the Quality of Life Scale-Parent Form [51]. Respondents rated their satisfaction in family life, time for work, family and leisure, and financial well-being on a 5-point Likert scale from 1 = *very dissatisfied* to 5 = *very satisfied*. Example items read, "How satisfied are you with your family life?", "How satisfied are you with your time?", and "How satisfied are you with your financial well-being?" The mean of the 6 items was calculated, with higher scores representing higher quality of life. The Cronbach's alpha for the 6 items was 0.81.

2.2.4. Occupational Health

To assess employees' overall perceived health affected by their occupation, we used two items adapted from Zoller's [52] interview question in terms of physical and psychological aspects. The items read, "How does your job affect your physical health?" and "How does your job affect your mental health?" Responses were coded as 1 = *very negatively*, 2 = *negatively*, 3 = *neither negatively nor positively*, 4 = *positively*, 5 = *very positively*. The mean of the two items was calculated, such that higher scores reflected greater occupational health.

2.2.5. Covariates

We controlled for employees' sociodemographic and work characteristics as covariates, including age, gender, education level, and work hours. Age and work hours as continuous variables were self-reported in years and hours, respectively. Gender (0 = *male*, 1 = *female*) and education level (0 = *under college graduate*, 1 = *college graduate or higher*) were dummy coded. In addition, we considered potential differences by industry. In our sample, the banking industry had the largest number of employees (see Table 1) and thus served as the reference group (1 = healthcare, 2 = education, 3 = banking; reference group).

2.3. Analytic Strategy

We used multiple mediation analyses with bootstrapping method using the SAS PROCESS macro [53]. This method allows for the estimation of the indirect effect, based on the product (×) of the effect of a predictor on a mediator and the effect of the mediator on an outcome. The indirect effect reflects "a × b" in Figure 1. The bootstrapping method also produces a bias-corrected confidence interval for the indirect effect [53]. In all models, we set the number of bootstrap samples to 10,000.

3. Results

Table 1 shows descriptive results of our variables and comparisons by industry. Beginning with sociodemographic characteristics, the average age of our sample was 42.85 years (SD = 8.01) and banking industry employees were older than healthcare industry employees (no difference with education industry employees). Sixty-one percent were women, with a higher proportion of women in the education industry (78%). The majority of the employees (70%) were college graduates or had higher education; this trend was more apparent in the education industry (91%) than in the banking industry (54%). The mean work hours was 43.83 h per week (SD = 6.22) and banking industry employees worked significantly longer hours than those in the other two industries.

In terms of our main variables, the mean exposure to workplace bullying for an average employee was not so high (M = 5.30 on a 0–22 range scale); yet, there was a great variability between employees (SD = 5.33). More than half of employees (54%) endorsed one particular item, "Someone withholding information which affects your performance." Employees in the healthcare and banking industries reported significantly more exposure to workplace bullying than those in the education industry (with no difference between healthcare and banking). Our sample of employees reported a moderate level of work-to-family conflict (M = 2.97 on a 5 point scale) and a high level of quality of life (M = 3.62 on a 5 point scale), on average, with no differences by industry. The mean level of occupational health was moderate (M = 3.19 on a 5 point scale), and it was higher for education industry employees than for banking industry employees.

Table 2 shows results of the mediation model examining the effect of workplace bullying on quality of life through work-to-family conflict. The first column presents the results of "a" path, the association of workplace bullying with work-to-family conflict adjusting for covariates. Employees in the healthcare and education industries reported lower work-to-family conflict than those in the banking industry. Women (vs. men), employees with college or higher education (vs. not), and those with longer work hours reported higher work-to-family conflict. After controlling for these effects, there was a significant association of workplace bullying with work-to-family conflict, such that more exposure to workplace bullying was associated with higher work-to-family conflict. Moreover, higher work-to-family conflict was associated with lower quality of life ("b" path, second column). Before including work-to-family conflict, there was a significant negative association of workplace bullying with quality of life ("c" path; B = −0.034, SE = 0.007, p < 0.001); this association was slightly reduced after including work-to-family conflict ("c'" path; B = −0.027, SE = 0.007, p < 0.001). The association was found after adjusting for industry, sociodemographic characteristics, and work hours (none of them were significant). On the whole, then, the model revealed a significant indirect effect of workplace bullying on quality of life mediated by work-to-family conflict. Twenty percent of the total effect of workplace bullying on quality of life was explained by the indirect effect through work-to-family conflict.

Table 3 shows results of the mediation model examining the effect of workplace bullying on occupational health through work-to-family conflict. Consistent with the previous model (Table 2), more exposure to workplace bullying was associated with higher work-to-family conflict ("a" path). Further, higher work-to-family conflict was associated with lower occupational health ("b" path).

This link was independent of the significant associations of education industry (vs. banking) and older age with higher occupational health. The total effect of workplace bullying on occupational health was also significant ("c" path; $B = -0.031$, $SE = 0.009$, $p < .01$). However, after including work-to-family conflict, the direct association of workplace bullying with occupational health was reduced ("c'" path; $B = -0.018$, $SE = 0.009$, $p < 0.05$). Overall, the model revealed a significant indirect effect of workplace bullying on occupational health mediated by work-to-family conflict. Forty-one percent of the total effect of workplace bullying on occupational health was due to the indirect effect through work-to-family conflict.

Table 2. The effect of workplace bullying on quality of life, mediated by work-to-family conflict.

	M: Work-to-Family Conflict				Y: Quality of Life			
	B			(SE)	B			(SE)
Intercept	−0.45	***		(0.10)	3.55	***		(0.08)
X: Workplace bullying	0.03	***		(0.01)	−0.03	***		(0.01)
M: Work-to-family conflict	−			−	−0.19	***		(0.05)
Industry, Healthcare (vs. Banking)	−0.22	*		(0.10)	−0.02			(0.08)
Industry, Education (vs. Banking)	−0.26	*		(0.11)	0.08			(0.09)
Age	−0.01			(0.01)	0.00			(0.00)
Women (vs. Men)	0.54	***		(0.09)	0.01			(0.07)
College graduates or higher (vs. Not)	0.38	***		(0.10)	0.07			(0.08)
Work hours (per week)	0.01	*		(0.01)	0.00			(0.01)
	$R^2 = 0.2285$				$R^2 = 0.1553$			
	$F(7299) = 12.65$ ***				$F(8298) = 6.85$ ***			
	Indirect Effect of X on Y: $B = -0.01$ **, $SE = 0.002$							
	95% CI = −0.0121 to −0.0129							

Note: $N = 307$ Korean employees. X refers to predictor; M refers to mediator; Y refers to outcome. * $p < 0.05$, *** $p < 0.001$.

Table 3. The effect of workplace bullying on occupational health, mediated by work-to-family.

	M: Work-to-Family Conflict				Y: Occupational Health			
	B			(SE)	B			(SE)
Intercept	−0.45	***		(0.10)	3.04	***		(0.12)
X: Workplace bullying	0.03	***		(0.01)	−0.02	*		(0.01)
M: Work-to-family conflict	−			−	−0.37	***		(0.07)
Industry, Healthcare (vs. Banking)	−0.22	*		(0.10)	0.13			(0.11)
Industry, Education (vs. Banking)	−0.26	*		(0.11)	0.36	**		(0.13)
Age	−0.01			(0.01)	0.02	**		(0.01)
Women (vs. Men)	0.54	***		(0.09)	0.03			(0.10)
College graduates or higher (vs. Not)	0.38	***		(0.10)	−0.03			(0.11)
Work hours (per week)	0.01	*		(0.01)	0.00			(0.01)
	$R^2 = 0.2285$				$R^2 = 0.2035$			
	$F(7299) = 12.65$ ***				$F(8298) = 9.52$ ***			
	Indirect Effect of X on Y: $B = -0.01$***, $SE = 0.004$							
	95% CI = −0.0214 to −0.0064							

Note: $N = 307$ Korean employees. * $p < 0.05$, ** $p < 0.01$, *** $p < 0.001$.

Figure 2 summarizes our results showing the mediating effects of work-to-family conflict on the links between workplace bullying and two well-being outcomes. More exposure to workplace bullying was associated with higher work-to-family conflict (i.e., H1 supported), which was, in turn, associated with lower levels of quality of life and occupational health (i.e., H2 supported). Work-to-family conflict was a significant mediator in the association between workplace bullying and well-being (i.e., H3 supported).

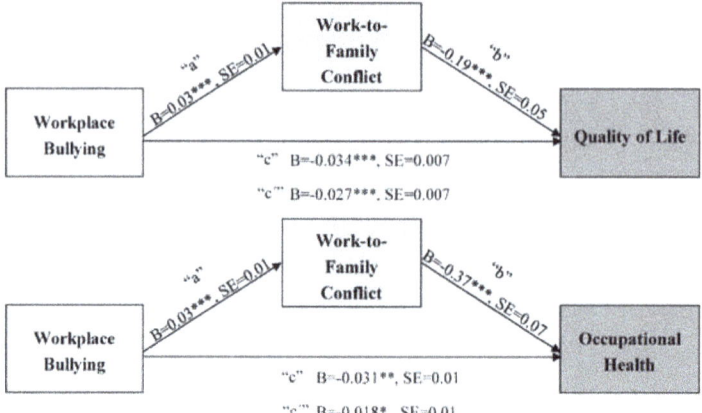

Figure 2. The mediating effects of work-to-family conflict on the links between workplace bullying on well-being outcomes. **Note:** Analyses adjusted for industry, age, gender, education, and work hours. "a × b" indicates the indirect effect of X on Y through M. "c" indicates the total effect of X on Y. "c'" indicates the direct effect of X on Y after controlling for the effect of M on Y.

4. Discussion

Guided by the work-family interface model [7–9], we examined the mediating role of work-to-family conflict in the associations between workplace bullying and well-being outcomes among Korean employees. Consistent with our hypotheses, results revealed that more exposure to workplace bullying was associated with greater work-to-family conflict, and greater work-to-family conflict was further associated with lower quality of life and occupational health. We have found no other studies that report the consequences and mechanisms of workplace bullying in Korean employees. Given that workplace bullying is a serious issue in many countries [3], our findings may add regional empirical evidence to the literature on workplace bullying.

We found that Korean employees who had more exposure to workplace bullying reported experiencing greater work-to-family conflict. This finding supports the work-family interface model [7–9] which suggests that stressful work experiences such as workplace bullying may spill over into employees' non-work domains and interfere with family and personal activities. Specifically, stress from workplace bullying experiences might have threatened employees' psychological resources and thus reduce their ability to be involved in family and personal roles and responsibilities [35–39]. Note that the mean levels of workplace bullying exposure and work-to-family conflict experiences were not high in our sample, but the two variables were positively covaried. It may also be important to mention differences in the levels of workplace bullying and work-to-family conflict by industry. We observed that Korean employees in the healthcare and banking industries reported significantly more exposure to workplace bullying than those in the education industry (see Table 1). Moreover, Korean employees in the healthcare and education industries reported higher work-to-family conflict than those in the banking industry after adjusting for sociodemographic characteristics and work hours (see Table 2). However, the positive association between workplace bullying and work-to-family conflict was found across the three industries, which may suggest the strong link between them.

Our results also revealed that greater work-to-family conflict was associated with lower levels of quality of life and occupational health. This is in line with previous studies that report the negative consequences of work-to-family conflict on employee health and well-being [14–19]. Korean employees work long hours and work in hierarchical culture [42,45,46], all of which may be risk factors for work-to-family conflict and degraded well-being. Given that happier employees are more productive at work [54], Korean employers should make more efforts to reduce work-to-family conflict and thereby improve their employees' well-being. For example, a workplace intervention designed to increase supervisor support may reduce work-to-family conflict [55], and by doing so, improve employee health and well-being [14,56].

Combining these results, this study observed that workplace bullying was associated with employee well-being (i.e., quality of life, occupational health), and this association was partially mediated by work-to-family conflict. Before adding work-to-family conflict in our analytic models, workplace bullying was significantly associated with quality of life and occupational health. However, these associations became weaker after including work-to-family conflict. Although not fully mediated, considerable proportions in the total effects of workplace bullying on quality of life (24%) and occupational health (41%) were explained by work-to-family conflict. This study contributes to understanding the mechanisms in which workplace bullying is linked to Korean employees' well-being. Future research may need to consider other potential mechanisms linking workplace bullying and employee well-being, as we found that work-to-family conflict did not fully mediate the association.

4.1. Practical Implications

Korea currently has no legal definition and laws on workplace bullying. This study urges that it's about time to develop rules to reduce workplace bullying incidences in Korea as well as to protect Korean workers from its negative consequences. Most of European countries and parts of Canada and Australia have established laws and regulations against workplace bullying [57,58]. Their practices and success stories may guide Korean government's legislation. In addition, work and life balance rather than achieving goals and career success is a continuously important topic among Korean employees because many Korean workplaces are highly competitive and demand individual sacrifice for the larger organization. The mediating effects of work-to-family conflict on the negative associations between workplace bullying and employee well-being found in this study suggest that each workplace needs to implement work-life balance policies and establish ethical standards and infrastructure [59] for the prevention and handling of workplace bullying. Workplace bullying may also involve substantial costs for the community due to degraded health as well as for the employers in terms of lost productivity. In order to legislate against workplace bullying in Korea, a business case needs to be made. Findings from this study may also provide broader implications for other countries who have similar issues of work and family life with Korea and want to improve their own workplace practices.

4.2. Limitations and Future Directions

Several of this study's limitations provide useful directions for future research. First, we used self-reports of workplace bullying, work-to-family conflict, quality of life, and occupational health that may pose a risk for common-method bias [60]. For example, an employee who experienced more workplace bullying might have responded negatively to the items of quality of life and occupational health. Future research may benefit from incorporating objective measures of well-being, such as clinical health measures or biomarkers of stress. Second, our sample was purposely selected from multiple worksites in three industries (healthcare, education, and banking) in South Korea, and thus it is not representative of Korean employees. In the future, it is necessary to include workplace bullying items in a national survey so that we can draw national-level inference about the negative influence of workplace bullying. It may also be that our measure of workplace bullying may not fully capture the real phenomenon of workplace bullying. According to Seo [5], only about 38% of victim employees in Korea report the incidents of bullying, because of their perception that some extent of bullying is unavoidable in Korean workplace culture. As such, we may underestimate the extent of workplace bullying. Future research may need to improve the validity of workplace bullying measure by cultural and occupational contexts. More specific measurements about workplace bullying are also needed. For example, there may be differences between men and women in the experience of workplace bullying consequences of it [61]. Moreover, more regional analyses are needed to see whether findings from our study are replicated in other settings. Finally, our cross-sectional analyses cannot determine the direction of effect. Although our analytic models imply that workplace bullying is a predictor, work-to-family conflict is a mediator, and quality of life and occupational health are outcomes, there is no temporal order between the variables and causality can operate in other directions. Future research should include multiple time points to identify the direction of effect.

5. Conclusions

Findings from this study highlight that workplace bullying is an important work-derived stressor associated with Korean employees' work-to-family conflict and well-being outcomes. All of our research hypotheses were supported: More exposure to workplace bullying was associated with lower levels of quality of life and occupational health among Korean employees; specifically, the negative associations were mediated by greater work-to-family conflict. At the most basic level, both workplace bullying and work-to-family conflict are societal concerns, and thus future research should continue to focus on this topic by examining multiple pathways linking workplace bullying to well-being outcomes in diverse employee samples across countries. A more harmonious workplace may improve the employees' well-being, which may ultimately enhance productivity and health at the larger society.

Author Contributions: Conceptualization, G.Y. & S.L.; Data Collection, G.Y.; Methodology and Formal Analysis, S.L.; Writing–Original Draft Preparation, Review & Editing, G.Y. & S.L.

Funding: This research received no external funding.

Conflicts of Interest: The authors declared no potential conflicts of interest with respect to the research, authorship, and/or publication of this article.

References

1. Einarsen, S.; Hoel, H.; Zapf, D.; Cooper, C.L. The concept of bullying and harassment at work: The European tradition. In *Bullying and Harassment in the Workplace: Developments in Theory, Research, and Practice*; Einarsen, S., Ed.; Taylor and Francis: Boca Raton, FL, USA, 2011; pp. 3–40.
2. Leymann, H. The content and development of mobbing at work. *Eur. J. Work Organ. Psychol.* **1996**, *5*, 165–184. [CrossRef]
3. Samnani, A.K.; Singh, P. 20 Years of workplace bullying research: A review of the antecedents and consequences of bullying in the workplace. *Aggress. Violent Behav.* **2012**, *17*, 581–589. [CrossRef]
4. Seo, Y. Workplace bullying in Korea. *KRIVET Issue Br.* **2013**, *20*, 1–4.
5. Seo, Y. The state of workplace bullying by job sector in Korea. *KRIVET Issue Br.* **2015**, *77*, 1–4.
6. Rai, A.; Agarwal, U. Workplace bullying: A review and future research directions. *South Asian J. Manag.* **2016**, *23*, 27–56.
7. Greenhaus, J.H.; Beutell, N.J. Sources of conflict between work and family roles. *Acad. Manag. Rev.* **1985**, *10*, 76–88. [CrossRef]
8. Grzywacz, J.G.; Marks, N.F. Reconceptualizing the work-family interface: An ecological perspective on the correlates of positive and negative spillover between work and family. *J. Occup. Health Psychol.* **2000**, *5*, 111–126. [CrossRef] [PubMed]
9. Greenhaus, J.H.; Parasuraman, S. A work-nonwork interactive perspective of stress and its consequences. *J. Organ. Behav. Manag.* **1987**, *8*, 37–60. [CrossRef]
10. Hoobler, J.M.; Brass, D.J. Abusive supervision and family undermining as displaced aggression. *J. Appl. Psychol.* **2006**, *91*, 1125–1133. [CrossRef] [PubMed]
11. Carlson, D.; Ferguson, M.; Hunter, E.; Whitten, D. Abusive supervision and work-family conflict: The path through emotional labor and burnout. *Leadersh. Q.* **2012**, *23*, 849–859. [CrossRef]
12. Carlson, D.; Ferguson, M.; Perrewe, P.L.; Whitten, D. The fallout from abusive supervision: An examiniation of subordinates and their partners. *Pers. Psychol.* **2011**, *64*, 937–961. [CrossRef]
13. Tepper, B.J. Consequences of abusive supervision. *Acad. Manag. J.* **2000**, *43*, 178–190.
14. Buxton, O.M.; Lee, S.; Beverly, C.; Berkman, L.F.; Moen, P.; Kelly, E.L.; Hammer, L.B.; Almeida, D.M. Work-family conflict and employee sleep: Evidence from IT workers in the Work, Family and Health Study. *Sleep* **2016**, *39*, 1871–1882. [CrossRef] [PubMed]

15. Geurts, S.; Rutte, C.; Peeters, M. Antecedents and consequences of work–home interference among medical residents. *Soc. Sci. Med.* **1999**, *48*, 1135–1148. [CrossRef]
16. Kinnunen, U.; Geurts, S.; Mauno, S. Work-to-family conflict and its relationship with satisfaction and well-being: A one-year longitudinal study on gender differences. *Work Stress* **2004**, *18*, 1–22. [CrossRef]
17. De Lange, A.H.; Taris, T.W.; Kompier, M.A.J.; Houtman, I.L.D.; Bongers, P.M. "The very best of the millennium": Longitudinal research and the demand-control-(support) model. *J. Occup. Health Psychol.* **2003**, *8*, 282–305. [CrossRef] [PubMed]
18. Lee, S.; Davis, K.D.; Neuendorf, C.; Grandey, A.; Lam, C.B.; Almeida, D.M. Individual- and organization-level work-to-family spillover are uniquely associated with hotel managers' work exhaustion and satisfaction. *Front. Psychol.* **2016**, *7*. [CrossRef] [PubMed]
19. Simon, M.; Kümmerling, A.; Hasselhorn, H.M. Work-home conflict in the European nursing profession. *Int. J. Occup. Environ. Health* **2004**, *10*, 384–391. [CrossRef] [PubMed]
20. Thomas, L.T.; Ganster, D.C. Impact of family-supportive work variables on work-family conflict and strain: A control perspective. *J. Appl. Psychol.* **1995**, *80*, 6–15. [CrossRef]
21. Wagner, D.T.; Barnes, C.M.; Scott, B.A. Driving it home: How workplace emotional labor harms employee home life. *Pers. Psychol.* **2014**, *67*, 487–516. [CrossRef]
22. Frye, N.K.; Breaugh, J.A. Family-friendly policies, supervisor support, work-family conflict, family-work conflict, and satisfaction: A test of a conceptual model. *J. Bus. Psychol.* **2004**, *19*, 197–220. [CrossRef]
23. Liu, J.; Kwan, H.K.; Lee, C.; Hui, C. Work-to-family spillover effects of workplace ostracism: The role of work-home segmentation preferences. *Hum. Resour. Manag.* **2013**, *52*, 75–93. [CrossRef]
24. Zhu, Y.; Li, D. Negative spillover impact of perceptions of organizational politics on work-family conflict in China. *Soc. Behav. Pers.* **2015**, *43*, 705–714. [CrossRef]
25. Einarsen, S. Harassment and bullying at work: A review of the Scandinavian approach. *Aggress. Violent Behav.* **2000**, *5*, 379–401. [CrossRef]
26. Acquadro Maran, D.; Varetto, A.; Zedda, M.; Magnavita, N. Workplace violence toward hospital staff and volunteers: A survey of an Italian sample. *J. Aggress. Maltreat. Trauma* **2018**, *27*, 76–95. [CrossRef]
27. Acquadro Maran, D.; Varetto, A.; Zedda, M.; Franscini, M. Health care professionals as victims of stalking: Characteristics of the stalking campaign, consequences, and motivation in Italy. *J. Interpers. Violence* **2017**, *32*, 2605–2625. [CrossRef] [PubMed]
28. Hauge, L.J.; Skogstad, A.; Einarsen, S. Relationships between stressful work environments and bullying: Results of a large representative study. *Work Stress* **2007**, *21*, 220–242. [CrossRef]
29. Arenas, A.; Giorgi, G.; Montani, F.; Mancuso, S.; Perez, J.F.; Mucci, N.; Arcangeli, G. Workplace bullying in a sample of italian and spanish employees and its relationship with job satisfaction, and psychological well-being. *Front. Psychol.* **2015**, *6*, 1–10. [CrossRef] [PubMed]
30. Casimir, G.; McCormack, D.; Djurkovic, N.; Nsubuga-Kyobe, A. Psychosomatic model of workplace bullying: Australian and Ugandan schoolteachers. *Empl. Relat.* **2012**, *34*, 411–428. [CrossRef]
31. Dehue, F.; Bolman, C.; Völlink, T.; Pouwelse, M. Coping with bullying at work and health related problems. *Int. J. Stress Manag.* **2012**, *19*, 175–197. [CrossRef]
32. Shahtahmasebi, S. Quality of life: A case report of bullying in the workplace. *Sci. World J.* **2004**, *4*, 118–123. [CrossRef] [PubMed]
33. Vartia, M.A.L. Consequences of workplace bullying with respect to the well-being of its targets and the observers of bullying. *Scand. J. Work Environ. Health* **2001**, *27*, 63–69. [CrossRef] [PubMed]
34. Bonde, J.P.; Gullander, M.; Hansen, Å.M.; Grynderup, M.; Persson, R.; Hogh, A.; Willert, M.V.; Kaerlev, L.; Rugulies, R.; Kolstad, H.A. Health correlates of workplace bullying: A 3-wave prospective follow-up study. *Scand. J. Work Environ. Health* **2016**, *42*, 17–25. [CrossRef] [PubMed]
35. Edwards, J.R.; Rothbard, N.P. Mechanisms linking work and family: Clarifying the relationship between work and family constructs. *Acad. Manag. Rev.* **2000**, *25*, 178–199. [CrossRef]
36. Frone, M.R.; Russell, M.; Cooper, M.L. Antecedents and outcomes of work-family conflict: Testing a model of the work-family interface. *J. Appl. Psychol.* **1992**, *77*, 65–78. [CrossRef] [PubMed]
37. Voydanoff, P. Toward a conceptualization of perceived work-family fit and balance: A demands and resources approach. *J. Marriage Fam.* **2005**, *67*, 822–836. [CrossRef]
38. Voydanoff, P. The effects of work demands and resources on work-to-family conflict and facilitation. *J. Marriage Fam.* **2004**, *66*, 398–412. [CrossRef]

39. Trépanier, S.G.; Fernet, C.; Austin, S. Workplace bullying and psychological health at work: The mediating role of satisfaction of needs for autonomy, competence and relatedness. *Work Stress* **2013**, *27*, 123–140. [CrossRef]
40. Jones, F.; Fletcher, B.C. An empirical study of occupational stress transmission in working couples. *Hum. Relat.* **1993**, *46*, 881–903. [CrossRef]
41. Sanz-Vergel, A.I.; Rodríguez-Muñoz, A. The effect of workplace bullying on health: The mediating role of work-family conflict. *Rev. Psicol. Trab. Organ.* **2011**, *27*, 93–102. [CrossRef]
42. Yoo, G. The effects of Confucian work views and gender role attitudes on job & family involvements and demands for family-friendly policies. *J. Fam. Relat.* **2010**, *14*, 91–108.
43. Kim, E.A. Hofstede's cultural dimensions: Comparison of South Korea and the United States. In Proceedings of the 2015 Cambridge Business & Economics Conference, Cambridge, UK, 1–2 July 2015.
44. Hofstede, G.; Bond, M.H. The Confucius connection: From cultural roots to economic growth. *Organ. Dyn.* **1988**, *16*, 5–21. [CrossRef]
45. Lee, S.; Duvander, A.-Z.; Zarit, S.H. How can family policies reconcile fertility and women's employment? Comparisons between South Korea and Sweden. *Asian J. Women's Stud.* **2016**, *22*. [CrossRef] [PubMed]
46. Lee, E. The influence of Confucian work value on the job involvement, job satisfaction, and organizational commitment. *Korean J. Ind. Organ. Psychol.* **2001**, *14*, 1–25.
47. Seo, Y.N.; Leather, P.; Coyne, I. South Korean culture and history: The implications for workplace bullying. *Aggress. Violent Behav.* **2012**, *17*, 419–422. [CrossRef]
48. Kim, H. Nurses Not Adequately Covered by the Psychological Counseling Service. Available online: http://news.donga.com/3/all/20180221/88765753/1 (accessed on 21 February 2018).
49. Einarsen, S.; Hoel, H. *Measuring Bullying and Harassment in the Workplace. Development and Validity of the Revised Negative Acts Questionnaire: A Manual*; University of Bergen: Bergen, Norway, 2006.
50. Grzywacz, J.G.; Bass, B.L. Work, family, and mental health: Testing different models of work-family fit. *J. Marriage Fam.* **2003**, *65*, 248–261. [CrossRef]
51. Olson, D.H.; Barnes, H.L. Quality of life. In *Family Social Science*; Olson, D.H., McCubbin, H.I., Barnes, H.L., Larsen, A.S., Muxen, M., Wilson, M., Eds.; University of Minnesota: St. Paul, MN, USA, 1985.
52. Zoller, H.M. Health on the line: Identity and disciplinary control in employee occupational health and safety discourse. *J. Appl. Commun. Res.* **2003**, *31*, 118–139. [CrossRef]
53. Hayes, A.F. *Introduction to Mediation, Moderation, and Conditional Process Analysis: A Regression-Based Approach*; Guilford Publications: New York, NY, USA, 2013.
54. Zelenski, J.M.; Murphy, S.A.; Jenkins, D.A. The happy-productive worker thesis revisited. *J. Happiness Stud.* **2008**, *9*, 521–537. [CrossRef]
55. Kelly, E.L.; Moen, P.; Oakes, J.M.; Fan, W.; Okechukwu, C.; Davis, K.D.; Hammer, L.B.; Kossek, E.E.; King, R.B.; Hanson, G.C.; et al. Changing work and work-family conflict: Evidence from the Work, Family, and Health Network. *Am. Sociol. Rev.* **2014**, *79*, 485–516. [CrossRef] [PubMed]
56. Almeida, D.M.; Lee, S.; Walter, K.N.; Lawson, K.M.; Kelly, E.L.; Buxton, O.M. The effects of a workplace intervention on employees' cortisol awakening response. *Community Work Fam.* **2018**, *21*, 151–167. [CrossRef]
57. Sanders, D.E.; Pattison, P.; Bible, J.D. Legislating "NICE": Analysis and assessment of proposed workplace bullying prohibitions. *South Law J.* **2012**, *22*, 1–36.
58. Squelch, J.; Guthrie, R. The Australian legal framework for workplace bullying. *Comp. Labor Law Policy J.* **2010**, *32*, 15–54.
59. Einarsen, K.; Mykletun, R.J.; Einarsen, S.V.; Skogstad, A.; Salin, D. Ethical infrastructure and successful handling of workplace bullying. *Nord. J. Work Life Stud.* **2017**, *7*. [CrossRef]
60. Podsakoff, P.M.; MacKenzie, S.B.; Lee, J.-Y.; Podsakoff, N.P. Common method variance in behavioral research: A critical review of the literature and recommended remedies. *J. Appl. Psychol.* **2003**, *88*, 879–903. [CrossRef] [PubMed]
61. Hoel, H.; Cooper, C.L.; Faragher, B. The experience of bullying in Great Britain: The impact of organizational status. *Eur. J. Work Organ. Psychol.* **2001**, *10*, 443–465. [CrossRef]

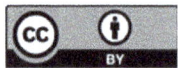

© 2018 by the authors. Licensee MDPI, Basel, Switzerland. This article is an open access article distributed under the terms and conditions of the Creative Commons Attribution (CC BY) license (http://creativecommons.org/licenses/by/4.0/).

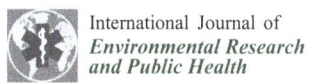

Article

Identifying Barriers and Supports to Breastfeeding in the Workplace Experienced by Mothers in the New Hampshire Special Supplemental Nutrition Program for Women, Infants, and Children Utilizing the Total Worker Health Framework

Eric A. Lauer [1,*], Karla Armenti [1], Margaret Henning [2] and Lissa Sirois [3]

[1] Institute on Disability, New Hampshire Occupational Health Surveillance Program, University of New Hampshire, College of Health and Human Services, Durham, NH 03824, USA; karla.armenti@unh.edu
[2] Department of Public Health, Keene State College, Keene, NH 03435, USA; mhenning@keene.edu
[3] State Director, Special Supplemental Nutrition Program for Women, Infants, and Children, New Hampshire Department of Health and Human Services, Concord, NH 03301, USA; lissa.sirois@dhhs.nh.gov
* Correspondence: eric.lauer@unh.edu

Received: 10 January 2019; Accepted: 11 February 2019; Published: 13 February 2019

Abstract: Variations in the barriers and contributors to breastfeeding across industries have not been well characterized for vulnerable populations such as mothers participating in the Special Supplemental Nutrition Program for Women, Infants, and Children (WIC). Our study used the Total Worker Health Framework to characterize workplace factors acting as barriers and/or contributors to breastfeeding among women participating in the New Hampshire WIC. Surveys were collected from WIC mothers ($n = 682$), which asked about employment, industry, and workplace accommodation and supports related to breastfeeding in the workplace. We found workplace policy factors supporting breastfeeding (i.e., having paid maternity leave, other maternity leave, and a breastfeeding policy) varied by industry. Women in specific service-oriented industries (i.e., accommodation and retail) reported the lowest rates of breastfeeding initiation and workplace supports for breastfeeding and pumping. Further, how a woman hoped to feed and having a private pumping space at work were significantly associated with industry, breastfeeding initiation, and breastfeeding duration. A substantial portion of women reported being not sure about their workplace environment, policies, and culture related to breastfeeding. Additional studies with larger sample sizes of women participating in WIC are needed to further characterize the barriers to breastfeeding associated with specific industries.

Keywords: total worker health; breastfeeding; industry; workplace accommodations; work environment; work culture; work policy; health promotion; occupational health surveillance

1. Introduction

Over the last two decades, the global public health community established that working outside the home was negatively associated with breastfeeding [1–4]. The World Health Organization has recently recognized the need for increased supports to improve breastfeeding duration and initiation rates, recommending women breastfeed for two years [5]. However, research in the United States (U.S.) found only 49% of women breastfeed for 6 months and breastfeeding initiation was impacted by working or planning to work postpartum [1,3,6,7]. Studies have found that breastfeeding incidence and duration were lower among employed, working-age women [1,3,8–10].

Moreover, women planning to work full-time postpartum were less likely to initiate breastfeeding than women who planned to work part-time and women were more likely to cease breastfeeding the first month prior or subsequent to returning to work [1,4]. Employment was also associated with breastfeeding less than two to three months postpartum [2]. Women who return to full-time employment six to twelve weeks postpartum were more than 50% less likely to meet their breastfeeding intentions, and women who return to full-time employment less than 6 weeks postpartum were more than twice as likely to not meet their breastfeeding intentions, compared to women who do not work [11].

Having identified this disparity, recent research has recognized the need to explore factors that influence breastfeeding cessation when returning to work [12]. Mothers themselves report multiple barriers to breastfeeding once returning to work, such as a lack of flexibility in the work schedule to allow for milk expression; lack of accommodations to express and/or store human milk; and concerns about support from supervisors and colleagues [13,14]. A woman's breastfeeding duration is also influenced by the existence and quality of maternity leave including its length, paid or unpaid status, and the attitudes, policies, and practices at her place of employment [15]. Among working women or women returning to work, research has found breastfeeding initiation and duration were lower for low-income women and women with less than a high school education [4,11]. However, this literature does not characterize specific, practical worksite factors that influence breastfeeding disparities among vulnerable populations.

1.1. Special Supplemental Nutrition Program for Women, Infants, and Children

Breastfeeding disparities experienced by low-income women due to individual, social, and environmental barriers are well documented [5,16]. Breastfeeding prevalence among low-income women, specifically women enrolled in the Special Supplemental Nutrition Program for Women, Infants, and Children (WIC), continues to be below national targets established in Healthy People 2020 [17]. Nationally, WIC mothers have lower rates of breastfeeding than non-participants, despite WIC's efforts to encourage breastfeeding through the Loving Support Makes Breastfeeding Work campaign and the WIC Peer Counseling Program [18–20]. Among WIC participants, barriers to breastfeeding include embarrassment toward breastfeeding in public, early return to work or school, infant behavior, lactation complications, lack of self-efficacy, low income, limited social support, less education, and unsupportive childcare [21–24].

The type of employment generally obtained by WIC eligible mothers further contributes to the disparities found in the U.S. WIC eligible mothers are more likely to have low-income jobs in childcare, home healthcare, or in one of the service industries [25]. These jobs are less likely to have flexible schedules or have paid-for breaks to express breast milk, both of which contribute to the mothers decision-making about continuing to breastfeed or early weaning [16]. These industries also usually lack workplace lactation policies and supports, which influence a woman's choice to continue breastfeeding upon returning to work [12].

The studies among WIC mothers identify a vulnerable population at risk of experiencing disparities in breastfeeding, which vary by employment type. However, employment supports and policies for breastfeeding are geographically and industry-dependent. For example, in New Hampshire (NH), according to the 2016 NH WIC Pediatric Nutrition Surveillance data, 76.8% of WIC mothers initiate breastfeeding after delivery, compared to 87.4% of all mothers in New Hampshire [26,27]. Further, previous studies have found that NH WIC mothers are less likely to have ever breastfed than other mothers in the U.S. or NH, and WIC mothers' breastfeeding duration was significantly related to employment status [21,28]. Additional state-specific research is needed to better understand and characterize breastfeeding disparities across employment types among WIC mothers.

1.2. The Total Worker Health Program and Benefits of Breastfeeding

The Total Worker Health (TWH) Program, created by the National Institute for Occupational Safety and Health (NIOSH) in 2012, supports protective and preventive efforts to improve the health and well-being of workers [29]. The TWH framework for worker well-being provides agreed-upon definitions and measures of worker well-being based on comprehensive, multidisciplinary literature reviews and expert panels consisting of occupational safety and health researchers [30]. The framework provides an opportunity to explore and characterize worksite factors that could improve breastfeeding behavior and supports for WIC mothers.

Breastfeeding-friendly worksites have been associated with benefits for both mothers and employers that include reduced employee absenteeism, increased employee retention, increased employee morale and loyalty, healthcare cost savings, and positive public relations and company image [31,32]. Although having space alone is not associated with increased duration of breastfeeding, women need the knowledge, support, encouragement, and environment to be successful in reaching their goals [33]. For every 1000 babies not breastfed, there are an extra 2033 physician visits, 212 days of hospitalization, and 609 prescriptions written [34].

1.3. Study Considerations

To the best of our knowledge there have been no studies exploring breastfeeding behavior across industries among WIC mothers. Using the TWH framework to characterize workplace factors for breastfeeding, this study examined the barriers and contributors to breastfeeding experienced by mothers in the NH WIC Program and focused on identifying workplace polices, supports, and practices that encourage or discourage breastfeeding after returning to work.

2. Methods

2.1. Study Design and Site Selection

This study used a cross-sectional design to survey women utilizing the WIC services in NH. In order to represent the entire state, all four local agencies providing WIC services in NH with catchment areas covering all ten counties in the state were utilized in the study.

2.2. Survey Development

As a first step towards designing this survey, a state-wide collaboration of multiple NH agencies, local coalitions, programs, and universities partnered to inform a questionnaire of breastfeeding in the workplace among NH WIC program participants. The team consisted of faculty and staff from the Institute on Disability, New Hampshire Occupational Health Surveillance Program in the University of New Hampshire's College of Health and Human Services, Keene State College Department of Public Health and Department of Health Science, New Hampshire Department of Health and Human Services' Division of Public Health Services, the Director of the New Hampshire WIC Nutrition Program, and a subcommittee of the New Hampshire Breastfeeding Taskforce. Based on a literature review of breastfeeding in the workplace and using focus groups, online feedback, and expert commentaries and reviews, a nine-page survey was iteratively developed to identify and measure person- and environment-level barriers and supports to breastfeeding initiation and continuation in the workplace.

Informed by prior breastfeeding studies of women using NH WIC services, survey questions were categorized into worker well-being domains operationalized by the NIOSH TWH Program [29]. The domains included in this study were (1) workplace physical environment and safety climate, (2) workplace policies and culture, (3) health status, and (4) work evaluation and experience [30]. The survey items used in this study identified concepts in the workplace related to the supports, knowledge/training, policies, physical space, and culture that encourage or discourage breastfeeding after returning to work.

Question content (i.e., concepts, topics, and phrasing) was based broadly on the existing literature and the state-wide partnership formed for this study. Survey questions were also included from (1) the Monadnock Region's Community Coalition for the Promotion of Breastfeeding Survey implemented in the Keene and Manchester NH WIC Programs, and (2) lactation support questions from the Centers for Disease Control and Prevention's Worksite Health ScoreCard [21,35]. Where possible, questions offered multiple choice responses similar to the 'Monadnock Region's Promotion of

Breastfeeding Survey, where the respondent could check more than one response [21]. This research, combined with the NH Breastfeeding Taskforce's experience and feedback, found breastfeeding to be a sensitive topic and recommended an anonymous survey with multiple choice responses to allow mothers to answer more honestly and in a fast, efficient manner.

When answering work questions, survey participants were instructed to reply for their current job, and if they were currently on maternity leave or recently left their job, they were asked to respond for their most recent job. Further, some survey items also included a step-wise, conditional design where participants were only asked to answer some secondary questions that were dependent on responses to the previous question in the survey. Topics with conditional questions included maternity leave, breastfeeding policies, break times for pumping at work, reactions to breastfeeding at work, and supports for breastfeeding longer at work.

The paper survey was pilot-tested for feasibility in the spring of 2016 using a random 1% of each the four local WIC agencies caseload. The results of the pilot informed the survey design and ensured the viability of a multi-agency study design. Once the survey was finalized, the University of New Hampshire Institutional Review Board granted approval for data collection. The study was conducted in accordance with the Declaration of Helsinki and the protocol was approved by the University of New Hampshire Research Integrity Services Institutional Review Board as IRB#6491.

2.3. Survey Eligibility and Administration.

Study eligibility criteria required women be enrolled in the WIC program and the birth mother of their child or that their child was enrolled in the WIC Program. Each local WIC office's breastfeeding coordinator directed survey implementation at their respective agency. WIC participants were recruited by referrals from WIC staff, and flyers in the WIC offices. Surveys were offered to all women participating in the NH WIC program that visited local agency offices during August, September, and October of 2016. Surveys were administered in English and staff were available for respondent questions while completing the survey. Immediately prior to administration, respondents received instructions as to the purpose, audience, risks, benefits, and completion of the survey. Surveys were completed immediately onsite and took approximately 15 minutes to finish.

2.4. Sample Size

A total of 682 mothers responded to the survey. This degree of survey participation represents approximately 5.0% of the total WIC caseload in NH at the time of the study.

2.5. Data Collection

Paper surveys were completed during an office visit to WIC agencies while participants were at a WIC appointment receiving benefits or waiting to be called for their appointment. As the study proceeded, agency staff collected and periodically sent surveys to the research team. A student entered each respondent's data into an online version of the survey designed in Qualtrics Software to create an excel data file.

2.6. Variables

2.6.1. Demographics

Age was coded as 15 to 17, 18 to 34, and 35 and over. Race/ethnicity was coded as non-Hispanic White, and Other.

2.6.2. Breastfeeding

"Breastfeeding initiation" was based on three questions including: (1) declared breastfeeding status (currently breastfeeding, previously breastfed, planning to breastfeed, or never breastfed); (2) "One week after you gave birth, how were you feeding your baby?", with responses of breast milk only, formula only, both breast milk and formula; and (3) "How old was your baby when you stopped breastfeeding completely?", with responses of one through thirteen months or baby has not stopped breastfeeding. Ever having breastfed was defined as reporting currently breastfed, previously breastfed, feeding breast milk one week after birth (only or in combination with formula), having stopped breastfeeding, or having a baby that has not stopped breastfeeding. Never having breastfed was defined as reporting planning to breastfeed, never having breastfed, not feeding with breast milk the first week after birth, not having stopped breastfeeding, and not having a baby that continues to breastfeed.

"Duration of breastfeeding" was based on the declared breastfeeding status and the question: "How old was your baby when you stopped breastfeeding completely?" (see "Breastfeeding initiation" for all response categories). Breastfeeding for less than 4 months was defined conditionally on having reported previously breastfeeding and having stopped breastfeeding after one, two, or three months. Breastfeeding for greater than or equal to 4 months was defined conditionally on having reported previously breastfeeding and having stopped breastfeeding after four or months.

"Reason for stopping breastfeeding" was based on the question: "What were your reasons for stopping breastfeeding?" Responses were categorized as physiological (difficulty nursing or latching; not enough milk, milk dried up; too painful, too hard, nipples too sore; I got sick, my baby got sick, had to stop for medical reasons), other commitments (too much time, I went back to school, I went back to work), and met goal (I met my goal). More than one reason could be reported.

2.6.3. Employment and Industry

"Employment status" was based on the question: "What is your employment status?" Responses were categorized as full-time, part-time, and other. Other included individuals not in the labor force, unemployed, in school, disabled, seasonal workers, and/or stay at home mothers.

"Industry" was coded according to 2012 Census Industry Classification Codes. Industry responses were combined into broader categories to increase the number of responses in those categories for analysis purposes. "Accommodation, food, and hospitality" included responses from women working in restaurant, travel and hotel jobs. "Healthcare" included women working in healthcare or in a hospital setting as well as working in home healthcare, as a licensed nursing assistant, or in an assisted living or nursing home environment. "Retail" included women working in grocery, clothing, convenience, and department stores. "Other" included all other industries with sample sizes too small to consider separately. This included but was not limited to education, social assistance services, manufacturing, and other services. Study participants were asked to respond to the industry question only if they were currently employed or planning to return to work.

2.6.4. During Pregnancy

"Hoping to feed" was based on the question: "While you were pregnant, how had you hoped to feed your baby?", with responses of breastfeeding only, formula only, or a combination of breastfeeding and formula. "Received information" was based on the question: "Did you receive information about breastfeeding during pregnancy?", with responses of yes or no.

2.6.5. Total Worker Health Well-Being Domains

Policies and Culture

"Paid maternity leave" was based on the question: "Does your workplace offer paid maternity leave and is it separate from any other leave such as sick and or vacation leave?", with responses of yes, no, and "not sure." Conditional on having reported no to having paid maternity leave, "other maternity leave" was based on the question: "can employees take paid maternity leave using other leave such as sick time or vacation time?", with responses of yes, no, and "not sure." "Breastfeeding policy" was based on the question: "Does your workplace have a written policy on breastfeeding or pumping?", with responses of yes, no, and "not sure." "Seen policy" was conditional on having reported yes to having a breastfeeding policy at work and based on the question: "Have you seen or do you have a copy of the written policy on breastfeeding at your workplace?", with responses of yes, no, and "not sure." "Pumping break times" was based on the question: "Does your workplace provide break times to allow mothers to pump breastmilk?", with responses of yes, no, and "not sure." Conditional on having reported yes to having break times for pumping, "flexible breaks" was based on the question: "Is the break time flexible (e.g., you can take it when you need to)?", with responses of yes, no, and "not sure."

Physical environment and Safety Climate

"Private pumping space" was based on the question: "Does your workplace have a private space (NOT bathroom, or closet) for you to use a breast pump?", with responses of yes, no, and "not sure." "Onsite items" was based on the question: "Does your workplace offer the following items on-site for employees to use when expressing breastmilk?", with responses categorized as utilities (electrical outlet and/or nearby sink) and physical (chair and/or space with locked door). More than one item could be reported. "Supportive coworkers" was based on the question: "Are your co-workers supportive of mothers who need to use a breast pump during work?", with responses of yes, no, and "not sure." "Supportive supervisor" was based on the question: "Is your supervisor supportive of mothers who need to use a breast pump during work?", with responses of yes, no, and "not sure."

Health Behavior

"Pumped at work" was based on the question: "Have you had to use a breast pump at work?", with responses of yes, no, and "not sure."

Work Evaluation and Experience

"Reaction to pumping" was conditional on having reported yes to having pumped at work and based on the question: "What type of reaction, if any, have you received from those you work with?", with responses categorized as negative (negative reactions only or some positive and some negative reactions) and positive (no reactions given or positive reactions only). "Pumped longer if easier" was based on the question: "Would you have continued breastfeeding longer if it was easier to pump at work?", with responses of yes, no, and "not sure." Conditional on having reported yes to breastfeeding longer if it was easier at work, "factors" asked people to report what factors would have made it easier, with responses categorized as policy (a copy of the company policy, supportive coworkers, supportive supervisor, or flexible time/hours), and environment (a place to store breastmilk or a private space for pumping). More than one factor could be reported.

2.7. Statistical Analysis

All analyses were conducted using SAS Version 9.4 (SAS Institute Inc., Cary, NC, USA). Univariate and bivariate methods were used to estimate counts and percentages. Bivariate associations in contingency tables were tested either using Fisher's exact tests or Fisher's exact tests with Freeman and Halton's adaptations for non-standard RowxColumn tables [36]. Monte Carlo estimation with 10,000,000 samples was used to calculate Fisher–Freeman–Halton statistics for tables within industry. Statistical significance was determined based on an alpha of 0.05 with Bonferroni corrections dependent on the number of questions in a given worker well-being domain or survey topic. Estimates were considered marginally significant if they met the alpha criteria of 0.05 but were no longer significant after Bonferroni correction. Analyses and categorization of questions about demographics, employment status, and during pregnancy included not reported as a category to account for nonresponse. For Total Worker Health well-being questions, directed towards people who were employed, on maternity leave, or recently employed, nonresponse was not included.

3. Results

3.1. Breastfeeding Initiation

Table 1 presents the maternal demographic, employment, and pregnancy characteristics for the overall sample and stratified by never or ever having initiated breastfeeding. The majority of our sample was between the ages of 18 to 34, non-Hispanic White, and approximately 50% were employed full- or part-time. Greater percentages of women aged 35 and over had ever breastfed, compared to women who had never breastfed (13.5% vs. 8.4%, $p = 0.025$). There were no differences in race/ethnicity or employment status by breastfeeding initiation ($p = 0.123$ and $p = 0.723$, respectively). By industry, a greater percentage of women who had ever breastfed worked in healthcare (26.3% vs. 20.0%) and a smaller percentage worked in accommodation and retail (20.4% vs. 33.8% and 16.1% vs. 24.6%) than women who had never breastfed ($p = 0.011$). Among women who had breastfed, 64.2% had hoped to exclusively breastfeed during pregnancy, compared to 12.6% of women who had never breastfed ($p = 0.000$). Among women who had never breastfed, approximately 40.3% had hoped to breastfeed during pregnancy. There was no difference in the percentage of women who had received information about breastfeeding during pregnancy by breastfeeding initiation status ($p = 0.224$).

Table 1. Maternal Demographic, Employment, and Pregnancy Characteristics by Breastfeeding Initiation (Never versus Ever).

		Characteristic	Overall ($n = 669$)	Breastfed Never ($n = 119$)	Breastfed Ever ($n = 550$)	p-Value [1] Sig.[2]
Demographics	Age (years)	15 to 17	0.6% ($n = 4$)	2.5% ($n = 3$)	0.2% ($n = 1$)	0.025 *
		18 to 34	74.9% ($n = 501$)	78.2% ($n = 93$)	74.2% ($n = 408$)	
		35 and over	12.6% ($n = 84$)	8.4% ($n = 10$)	13.5% ($n = 74$)	
		Not Reported	12.0% ($n = 80$)	10.9% ($n = 13$)	12.2% ($n = 67$)	
	Race/Ethnicity	Other	14.9% ($n = 100$)	9.2% ($n = 11$)	16.2% ($n = 89$)	0.123
		Non-Hispanic White	84.9% ($n = 568$)	90.8% ($n = 108$)	83.6% ($n = 460$)	
		Not Reported	0.1% ($n = 1$)	0.0% ($n = 0$)	0.2% ($n = 1$)	
Employment	Status	Full time	26.9% ($n = 180$)	28.6% ($n = 34$)	26.5% ($n = 146$)	0.723
		Part time	25.6% ($n = 171$)	21.8% ($n = 26$)	26.4% ($n = 145$)	
		Other	47.2% ($n = 316$)	49.6% ($n = 59$)	46.7% ($n = 257$)	
		Not Reported	0.3% ($n = 2$)	0.0% ($n = 0$)	0.4% ($n = 2$)	
	Industry	Accommodation	22.8% ($n = 84$)	33.8% ($n = 22$)	20.4% ($n = 62$)	0.011 *
		Healthcare	25.2% ($n = 93$)	20.0% ($n = 13$)	26.3% ($n = 80$)	
		Retail	17.6% ($n = 65$)	24.6% ($n = 16$)	16.1% ($n = 49$)	
		Other	34.4% ($n = 127$)	21.5% ($n = 14$)	37.2% ($n = 113$)	
During Pregnancy	Hoping to Feed	Combination	29.0% ($n = 194$)	27.7% ($n = 33$)	29.3% ($n = 161$)	0.000 *
		Breastfeeding only	55.0% ($n = 368$)	12.6% ($n = 15$)	64.2% ($n = 353$)	
		Formula only	13.3% ($n = 89$)	56.3% ($n = 67$)	4.0% ($n = 22$)	
		Not Reported	2.7% ($n = 18$)	3.4% ($n = 4$)	2.5% ($n = 14$)	
	Received Information	Yes	95.1% ($n = 636$)	92.4% ($n = 110$)	95.6% ($n = 526$)	0.224
		No	4.0% ($n = 27$)	5.9% ($n = 7$)	3.6% ($n = 20$)	
		Not Reported	0.9% ($n = 6$)	1.7% ($n = 2$)	0.7% ($n = 4$)	

[1] p-Value based on Fisher's exact tests or Fisher's exact tests with Freeman and Halton's adaptations for RxC tables. [2] Statistical significance (*) was based on an alpha of 0.05 with Bonferroni correction based on the number of comparisons within each category or domain (with no correction for demographic variables). A Monte Carlo estimation with 10,000,000 samples was used to calculate Fisher–Freeman–Halton statistics for tables with industry. Estimates were considered marginally significant (^) if they met the alpha criteria of 0.05 but were no longer significant after Bonferroni correction.

Table 2 presents maternal workplace characteristics for the overall sample and stratified by never or ever having initiated breastfeeding. Within the policies and culture domain, a greater percentage of women who had ever breastfed had break times for pumping (49.7% vs. 25.9%, $p = 0.000$), compared to women who had never breastfed. There was no difference in having paid maternity leave, other maternity leave, a breastfeeding policy, having seen the workplace breastfeeding policy, or having flexible break times for pumping by breastfeeding initiation status (all $p > 0.400$). Within the physical environment and safety climate domain, by breastfeeding initiation status (ever vs. never), there were significant differences in having private spaces for pumping (40.8% vs. 19.0%, $p = 0.000$), supportive coworkers (51.6% vs. 36.6%, $p = 0.014$), and supportive supervisors (51.0% vs. 38.0%, $p = 0.011$).

Table 2. Maternal Workplace Characteristics by Breastfeeding Initiation (Never versus Ever).

TWH Domain [1]	Characteristic		Overall (n = 669)	Breastfed		p-Value [2] Sig.[3]
				Never (n = 119)	Ever (n = 550)	
Policies and Culture	Paid Maternity Leave	Yes	15.8% (n = 76)	13.8% (n = 12)	16.2% (n = 64)	0.764
		No	61.6% (n = 297)	60.9% (n = 53)	61.8% (n = 244)	
		Not Sure	22.6% (n = 109)	25.3% (n = 22)	22.0% (n = 87)	
	Other Maternity Leave	Yes	25.3% (n = 97)	23.0% (n = 17)	25.9% (n = 80)	0.821
		No	34.7% (n = 133)	33.8% (n = 25)	35.0% (n = 108)	
		Not Sure	39.9% (n = 153)	43.2% (n = 32)	39.2% (n = 121)	
	Breastfeeding Policy	Yes	10.9% (n = 49)	8.8% (n = 7)	11.3% (n = 42)	0.498
		No	37.7% (n = 170)	33.8% (n = 27)	38.5% (n = 143)	
		Not Sure	51.4% (n = 232)	57.5% (n = 46)	50.1% (n = 186)	
	Seen Policy	Yes	12.2% (n = 42)	8.5% (n = 5)	12.9% (n = 37)	0.480
		No	61.2% (n = 211)	59.3% (n = 35)	61.5% (n = 176)	
		Not Sure	26.7% (n = 92)	32.2% (n = 19)	25.5% (n = 73)	
Physical Environment and Safety Climate	Pumping Break Times	Yes	45.5% (n = 206)	25.9% (n = 21)	49.7% (n = 185)	0.000 *
		No	14.8% (n = 67)	17.3% (n = 14)	14.2% (n = 53)	
		Not Sure	39.7% (n = 180)	56.8% (n = 46)	36.0% (n = 134)	
	Flexible Breaks	Yes	81.1% (n = 163)	85.0% (n = 17)	80.7% (n = 146)	1.000
		No	12.4% (n = 25)	10.0% (n = 2)	12.7% (n = 23)	
		Not Sure	6.5% (n = 13)	5.0% (n = 1)	6.6% (n = 12)	
	Private Pumping Space	Yes	36.9% (n = 162)	19.0% (n = 15)	40.8% (n = 147)	0.000 *
		No	36.7% (n = 161)	39.2% (n = 31)	36.1% (n = 130)	
		Not Sure	26.4% (n = 116)	41.8% (n = 33)	23.1% (n = 83)	
	Supportive Coworkers	Yes	49.2% (n = 215)	36.6% (n = 26)	51.6% (n = 189)	0.014 *
		No	7.6% (n = 33)	4.2% (n = 3)	8.2% (n = 30)	
		Not Sure	43.2% (n = 189)	59.2% (n = 42)	40.2% (n = 147)	
	Supportive Supervisors	Yes	48.8% (n = 211)	38.0% (n = 27)	51.0% (n = 184)	0.011 *
		No	7.6% (n = 33)	2.8% (n = 2)	8.6% (n = 31)	
		Not Sure	43.5% (n = 188)	59.2% (n = 42)	40.4% (n = 146)	

[1] For the Total Worker Health well-being domain questions, survey participants were only instructed to reply for their current job, and if they were currently on maternity leave or recently left their job, they were asked to respond for their most recent job. [2] p-Value was based on Fisher's exact tests or Fisher's exact tests with Freeman and Halton's adaptations for RxC tables. [3] Statistical significance (*) based on an alpha of 0.05 with Bonferroni correction based on the number of comparisons within each category or domain (with no correction for demographic variables). A Monte Carlo estimation with 10,000,000 samples was used to calculate Fisher–Freeman–Halton statistics for tables with industry. Estimates were considered marginally significant (^) if they met the alpha criteria of 0.05 but were no longer significant after Bonferroni correction.

In addition, in Table 2, the percentage of women reporting "not sure" was notable for all workplace factors. Women who never breastfed consistently had greater percentages of "not sure" than women who had ever breastfed. Across significant associations for having break times for pumping, private pumping space, supportive coworkers, and supportive supervisors, the percentages of women reporting "not sure" was greater for women who had never breastfed (range: 41.8–59.2%) than women who had ever breastfed (range: 23.1–40.4%).

3.2. Duration of Breastfeeding

Table 3 presents the maternal demographic, employment, pregnancy, and breastfeeding characteristics stratified by duration of breastfeeding (less than 4 months or 4 months or longer). There was no difference in age, race/ethnicity, employment status, or industry by duration of breastfeeding (all $p > 0.099$). During pregnancy, 73.8% of women who breastfed for 4 months or longer hoped to only breastfeed, compared to 50.4% of women who breastfed less than 4 months ($p = 0.000$), and there was no difference in the percentage of women who receive information about breastfeeding during pregnancy by duration of breastfeeding ($p = 0.736$). Across reasons for stopping breastfeeding, compared to women who breastfed 4 months or longer, a greater percentage of women who breastfed for less than 4 months stopped breastfeeding for physiological reasons (86.6% vs. 64.7%, $p = 0.000$), a smaller percentage stopped breastfeeding when they met their breastfeeding goal (1.5% vs. 28.1%, $p = 0.000$), and there was no difference in the percentage of women who stopped breastfeeding due to other commitments ($p = 0.888$).

Table 3. Maternal Demographic, Employment, Pregnancy, and Breastfeeding Characteristics by Duration of Breastfeeding (<4 Months vs. ≥4 Months).

	Characteristic		Duration (Months, n = 307)		p-Value [1] Sig.[2]
			<4 (n = 139)	≥4 (n = 168)	
Demographics	Age (years)	15 to 17	0.7% (n = 1)	0.0% (n = 0)	0.270
		18 to 34	77.0% (n = 107)	72.6% (n = 122)	
		35 and over	11.5% (n = 16)	17.9% (n = 30)	
		Not Reported	10.8% (n = 15)	9.5% (n = 16)	
	Race/Ethnicity	Other	10.1% (n = 14)	16.7% (n = 28)	0.099
		Non-Hispanic White	89.9% (n = 125)	83.3% (n = 140)	
		Not Reported	0.0 % (n = 0)	0.0 % (n = 0)	
Employment	Status	Full time	25.2% (n = 35)	29.2% (n = 49)	0.773
		Part time	28.8% (n = 40)	28.0% (n = 47)	
		Other	46.0% (n = 64)	42.3% (n = 71)	
		Not Reported	0.0% (n = 0)	0.6% (n = 1)	
	Industry	Accommodation	23.8% (n = 19)	16.0% (n = 15)	0.650
		Healthcare	27.5% (n = 22)	29.8% (n = 28)	
		Retail	16.3% (n = 13)	18.1% (n = 17)	
		Other	32.5% (n = 26)	36.2% (n = 34)	
During Pregnancy	Hoping to Feed	Combination	42.4% (n = 59)	23.8% (n = 40)	0.000 *
		Breastfeeding only	50.4% (n = 70)	73.8% (n = 124)	
		Formula only	4.3% (n = 6)	0.6% (n = 1)	
		Not Reported	2.9% (n = 4)	1.8% (n = 3)	
	Received Information	Yes	96.4% (n = 134)	97.6% (n = 164)	0.736
		No	3.6% (n = 5)	2.4% (n = 4)	
		Not Reported	0.0 % (n = 0)	0.0 % (n = 0)	
Reason for Stopping Breastfeeding	Physiological	Yes	86.6% (n = 116)	64.7% (n = 99)	0.000 *
		No	13.4% (n = 18)	35.3% (n = 54)	
	Other Commitments	Yes	23.1% (n = 31)	22.2% (n = 34)	0.888
		No	76.9% (n = 103)	77.8% (n = 119)	
	Met Goal	Yes	1.5% (n = 2)	28.1% (n = 43)	0.000 *
		No	98.5% (n = 132)	71.9% (n = 110)	

[1] p-Value was based on Fisher's exact tests or Fisher's exact tests with Freeman and Halton's adaptations for RxC tables. [2] Statistical significance (*) was based on an alpha of 0.05 with Bonferroni correction based on the number of comparisons within each category or domain (with no correction for demographic variables). A Monte Carlo estimation with 10,000,000 samples was used to calculate Fisher–Freeman–Halton statistics for tables with industry. Estimates were considered marginally significant (^) if they met the alpha criteria of 0.05 but were no longer significant after Bonferroni correction.

Table 4 presents the maternal workplace characteristics stratified by duration of breastfeeding (less than 4 months or 4 months or longer). Within the policies and culture domain, there was one marginally significant difference by duration of breastfeeding. A greater percentage of women who breastfed 4 months or longer had break times for pumping, compared to women who breastfed less than 4 months (53.3% vs. 39.8%, $p = 0.032$, not significant after Bonferroni correction). Within the physical environment and safety climate domain, there were two marginally significant differences by duration of breastfeeding. Compared to women who breastfed less than 4 months, a greater percentage of women who breastfed 4 months or longer had private pumping spaces (46.2% vs. 33.0%, $p = 0.035$, not significant after Bonferroni correction) and utilities that supported breastfeeding (85.9% vs. 69.5%, $p = 0.022$, not significant after Bonferroni correction). Among women who breastfed 4 months or longer, 56.3% pumped at work, compared to 13.6% of women who breastfed less than 4 months ($p = 0.000$). Within the work evaluation and experience domain, there were no significant differences by duration of breastfeeding (all $p > 0.300$).

Table 4. Maternal Workplace Characteristics by Duration of Breastfeeding (<4 Months Versus ≥4 Months).

TWH Domain [1]	Characteristic		Duration (Months, n = 307) <4 (n = 139)	Duration (Months, n = 307) ≥4 (n = 168)	p-Value [2] Sig.[3]
Policies and Culture	Paid Maternity Leave	Yes No Not Sure	17.9% (n = 20) 55.4% (n = 62) 26.8% (n = 30)	16.2% (n = 21) 58.5% (n = 76) 25.4% (n = 33)	0.891
	Other Maternity Leave	Yes No Not Sure	31.9% (n = 29) 24.2% (n = 22) 44.0% (n = 40)	18.4% (n = 18) 36.7% (n = 36) 44.9% (n = 44)	0.055
	Breastfeeding Policy	Yes No Not Sure	8.3% (n = 9) 29.6% (n = 32) 62.0% (n = 67)	13.3% (n = 16) 35.0% (n = 42) 51.7% (n = 62)	0.240
	Seen Policy	Yes No Not Sure	13.0% (n = 10) 54.5% (n = 42) 32.5% (n = 25)	15.1% (n = 14) 62.4% (n = 58) 22.6% (n = 21)	0.361
	Pumping Break Times	Yes No Not Sure	39.8% (n = 43) 11.1% (n = 12) 49.1% (n = 53)	53.3% (n = 65) 14.8% (n = 18) 32.0% (n = 39)	0.032
	Flexible Breaks	Yes No Not Sure	76.2% (n = 32) 16.7% (n = 7) 7.1% (n = 3)	92.1% (n = 58) 6.3% (n = 4) 1.6% (n = 1)	0.077
Physical Environment and Safety Climate	Private Pumping Space	Yes No Not Sure	33.0% (n = 34) 33.0% (n = 34) 34.0% (n = 35)	46.2% (n = 54) 34.2% (n = 40) 19.7% (n = 23)	0.035
	Onsite Items	Utilities, Yes Utilities, No	69.5% (n = 41) 30.5% (n = 18)	85.9% (n = 73) 14.1% (n = 12)	0.022
		Physical, Yes Physical, No	96.6% (n = 57) 3.4% (n = 2)	89.4% (n = 76) 10.6% (n = 9)	0.200
	Supportive Coworkers	Yes No Not Sure	46.6% (n = 48) 6.8% (n = 7) 46.6% (n = 48)	56.2% (n = 68) 7.4% (n = 9) 36.4% (n = 44)	0.289
	Supportive Supervisors	Yes No Not Sure	46.1% (n = 47) 6.9% (n = 7) 47.1% (n = 48)	58.7% (n = 71) 6.6% (n = 8) 34.7% (n = 42)	0.155
Health Behavior	Pumped at Work	Yes No	13.6% (n = 14) 86.4% (n = 89)	56.3% (n = 67) 43.7% (n = 52)	0.000
	Reaction to Pumping	Any negative Positive/None	35.7% (n = 5) 64.3% (n = 9)	29.2% (n = 19) 70.8% (n = 46)	0.750
Work Evaluation and Experience	Pumped Longer if Easier	Yes No Not Sure	31.6% (n = 31) 29.6% (n = 29) 38.8% (n = 38)	36.5% (n = 42) 32.2% (n = 37) 31.3% (n = 36)	0.513
	Factors	Policy/Culture, Yes Policy/Culture, No	72.4% (n = 21) 27.6% (n = 8)	61.9% (n = 26) 38.1% (n = 16)	0.447
		Environment, Yes Environment, No	62.1% (n = 18) 37.9% (n = 11)	47.6% (n = 20) 52.4% (n = 22)	0.333

[1] For the Total Worker Health well-being domain questions, survey participants were only instructed to reply for their current job, and if they were currently on maternity leave or recently left their job, they were asked to respond for their most recent job. [2] p-Value was based on Fisher's exact tests or Fisher's exact tests with Freeman and Halton's adaptations for RxC tables. [3] Statistical significance (*) was based on an alpha of 0.05 with Bonferroni correction based on the number of comparisons within each category or domain (with no correction for demographic variables). A Monte Carlo estimation with 10,000,000 samples was used to calculate Fisher–Freeman–Halton statistics for tables with industry. Estimates were considered marginally significant (ˆ) if they met the alpha criteria of 0.05 but were no longer significant after Bonferroni correction.

Similar to Table 2, there was a consistent pattern of women with responses of "not sure" to workplace questions in Table 4. Except for other maternity leave, women who breastfed less than 4 months had greater percentages of "not sure" responses than women who breastfed 4 months or longer. Across marginally significant associations for having pumping break times, flexible times for pumping, private pumping spaces, and onsite utilities for pumping, the percentages of women "not sure" were greater for women who breastfed less than 4 months (range: 30.5–49.1%) than women who breastfed 4 months or longer (range: 14.1–32.0%).

3.3. Industry

Table 5 presents the maternal demographic, employment, pregnancy, and breastfeeding characteristics stratified by industry (accommodation, healthcare, retail, and other). By industry, the percentage of people aged 18 to 34 was largest and smallest for retail and other industries (84.6% and 73.2%, respectively) and the percentage of people aged 35 and over was largest and smallest for healthcare and accommodation (20.2% and 6.9%, respectively, $p = 0.023$). There was no association between industry and race/ethnicity ($p = 0.191$). Employment status varied significantly by industry with the largest and smallest percent of full-time workers in accommodation and retail (48.3% and 33.8%, respectively), and the largest and smallest percent of part-time workers in retail and healthcare (60.0% and 34.0%, respectively, $p = 0.017$).

Table 5. Maternal Demographic, Employment, Pregnancy, and Breastfeeding Characteristics by Industry.

Characteristic			Industry (n = 373)				p-Value [1] Sig.[2]
			Accommodation (n = 87)	Healthcare (n = 94)	Retail (n = 65)	Other (n = 127)	
Demographics	Age (years)	15 to 17	0.0% (n = 0)	0.0% (n = 0)	0.0% (n = 0)	0.0% (n = 0)	0.023 *
		18 to 34	77.0% (n = 67)	74.5% (n = 70)	84.6% (n = 55)	73.2% (n = 93)	
		35 and over	6.9% (n = 6)	20.2% (n = 19)	9.2% (n = 6)	17.3% (n = 22)	
		Not Reported	16.1% (n = 14)	5.3% (n = 5)	6.2% (n = 4)	9.4% (n = 12)	
	Race/Ethnicity	Other	17.2% (n = 15)	10.6% (n = 10)	6.2% (n = 4)	14.2% (n = 18)	0.191
		Non-Hispanic White	82.8% (n = 72)	88.3% (n = 83)	93.8% (n = 61)	85.8% (n = 109)	
		Not Reported	0.0% (n = 0)	1.1% (n = 1)	0.0% (n = 0)	0.0% (n = 0)	
Employment	Status	Full time	48.3% (n = 42)	46.8% (n = 44)	33.8% (n = 22)	39.4% (n = 50)	0.017 *
		Part time	41.4% (n = 36)	34.0% (n = 32)	60.0% (n = 39)	42.5% (n = 54)	
		Other	10.3% (n = 9)	19.1% (n = 18)	6.2% (n = 4)	18.1% (n = 23)	
		Not Reported	0.0% (n = 0)	0.0% (n = 0)	0.0% (n = 0)	0.0% (n = 0)	
During Pregnancy	Hoping to Feed	Combination	31.0% (n = 27)	34.0% (n = 32)	30.8% (n = 20)	26.8% (n = 34)	0.029 ^
		Breastfeeding only	42.5% (n = 37)	53.2% (n = 50)	49.2% (n = 32)	63.0% (n = 80)	
		Formula only	24.1% (n = 21)	9.6% (n = 9)	15.4% (n = 10)	7.1% (n = 9)	
		Not Reported	2.3% (n = 2)	3.2% (n = 3)	4.6% (n = 3)	3.1% (n = 4)	
	Received Information	Yes	90.8% (n = 79)	100.0% (n = 94)	96.9% (n = 63)	94.5% (n = 120)	0.017 *
		No	9.2% (n = 8)	0.0% (n = 0)	3.1% (n = 2)	4.7% (n = 6)	
		Not Reported	0.0% (n = 0)	0.0% (n = 0)	0.0% (n = 0)	0.8% (n = 1)	
Reason for Stopping Breastfeeding	Physiological	Yes	63.9% (n = 39)	73.9% (n = 51)	58.3% (n = 28)	60.7% (n = 54)	0.249
		No	36.1% (n = 22)	26.1% (n = 18)	41.7% (n = 20)	39.3% (n = 35)	
	Other Commitments	Yes	26.2% (n = 16)	14.5% (n = 10)	12.5% (n = 6)	28.1% (n = 25)	0.059
		No	73.8% (n = 45)	85.5% (n = 59)	87.5% (n = 42)	71.9% (n = 64)	
	Met Goal	Yes	6.6% (n = 4)	10.1% (n = 7)	14.6% (n = 7)	16.9% (n = 15)	0.256
		No	93.4% (n = 57)	89.9% (n = 62)	85.4% (n = 41)	83.1% (n = 74)	

[1] p-Value was based on Fisher's exact tests or Fisher's exact tests with Freeman and Halton's adaptations for RxC tables. [2] Statistical significance (*) was based on an alpha of 0.05 with Bonferroni correction based on the number of comparisons within each category or domain (with no correction for demographic variables). A Monte Carlo estimation with 10,000,000 samples was used to calculate Fisher–Freeman–Halton statistics for tables with industry. Estimates were considered marginally significant (^) if they met the alpha criteria of 0.05 but were no longer significant after Bonferroni correction.

Across industries, there were marginally significant differences in how women hoped to feed or if they received information about breastfeeding during pregnancy. The greatest and smallest percentage of women who hoped to only breastfeed were in other industries and accommodation (63.0% and 42.5%, respectively), and the greatest and smallest percentage of women who hoped to only feed with formula were in accommodation and other industries (24.1% and 15.4%, respectively, $p = 0.029$, not significant after Bonferroni correction). The greatest and smallest percentage of women who received information about breastfeeding were in healthcare and accommodation (100.0% and 90.8%, respectively, $p = 0.017$, not significant after Bonferroni correction). Reasons for stopping breastfeeding did not vary significantly by industry ($p = 0.256$).

Table 6 presents the maternal workplace characteristics stratified by industry (accommodation, healthcare, retail, and other). By industry, there were significant and marginally significant differences in policies and culture domain factors. Women working in healthcare and retail had the greatest and smallest percentages of other forms of maternity leave (44.4% and 15.1%, $p = 0.000$). Further, women working in healthcare and accommodation had the greatest and smallest percentages of other forms of maternity leave (20.0% and 3.9%, $p = 0.003$). In addition, there were marginally significant differences in paid maternity leave by industry. The greatest percentages of paid maternity were found among women working in healthcare and other industries and the smallest percentages were found among women working in accommodation and retail (22.1% and 23.3% vs. 7.3% and 15.9%, respectively, $p = 0.021$, not significant after Bonferroni correction).

Table 6. Maternal Workplace Characteristics by Industry.

TWH Domain [1]	Characteristic		Industry ($n = 373$)				p-Value [2] Sig. [3]
			Accommodation ($n = 87$)	Health care ($n = 94$)	Retail ($n = 65$)	Other ($n = 127$)	
Policies and Culture	Paid Maternity Leave	Yes No Not Sure	7.3% ($n = 6$) 79.3% ($n = 65$) 13.4% ($n = 11$)	22.1% ($n = 19$) 58.1% ($n = 50$) 19.8% ($n = 17$)	15.9% ($n = 10$) 61.9% ($n = 39$) 22.2% ($n = 14$)	23.3% ($n = 27$) 62.9% ($n = 73$) 13.8% ($n = 16$)	0.021 ˆ
	Other Maternity Leave	Yes No Not Sure	16.4% ($n = 12$) 53.4% ($n = 39$) 30.1% ($n = 22$)	44.4% ($n = 28$) 17.5% ($n = 11$) 38.1% ($n = 24$)	15.1% ($n = 8$) 35.8% ($n = 19$) 49.1% ($n = 26$)	25.9% ($n = 22$) 47.1% ($n = 40$) 27.1% ($n = 23$)	0.000 *
	Breastfeeding Policy	Yes No Not Sure	3.9% ($n = 3$) 49.4% ($n = 38$) 46.8% ($n = 36$)	20.0% ($n = 17$) 36.5% ($n = 31$) 43.5% ($n = 37$)	8.5% ($n = 5$) 28.8% ($n = 17$) 62.7% ($n = 37$)	17.0% ($n = 19$) 43.8% ($n = 49$) 39.3% ($n = 44$)	0.003 *
	Seen Policy	Yes No Not Sure	3.3% ($n = 2$) 73.8% ($n = 45$) 23.0% ($n = 14$)	18.2% ($n = 12$) 65.2% ($n = 43$) 16.7% ($n = 11$)	11.4% ($n = 5$) 68.2% ($n = 30$) 20.5% ($n = 9$)	19.8% ($n = 16$) 61.7% ($n = 50$) 18.5% ($n = 15$)	0.096
	Pumping Break Times	Yes No Not Sure	35.8% ($n = 29$) 18.5% ($n = 15$) 45.7% ($n = 37$)	59.0% ($n = 49$) 8.4% ($n = 7$) 32.5% ($n = 27$)	44.4% ($n = 28$) 14.3% ($n = 9$) 41.3% ($n = 26$)	54.0% ($n = 61$) 13.3% ($n = 15$) 32.7% ($n = 37$)	0.071
	Flexible Breaks	Yes No Not Sure	72.4% ($n = 21$) 17.2% ($n = 5$) 10.3% ($n = 3$)	83.3% ($n = 40$) 12.5% ($n = 6$) 4.2% ($n = 2$)	85.2% ($n = 23$) 11.1% ($n = 3$) 3.7% ($n = 1$)	84.7% ($n = 50$) 8.5% ($n = 5$) 6.8% ($n = 4$)	0.788
Physical Environment and Safety Climate	Private Pumping Space	Yes No Not Sure	26.0% ($n = 20$) 54.5% ($n = 42$) 19.5% ($n = 15$)	55.0% ($n = 44$) 21.3% ($n = 17$) 23.8% ($n = 19$)	24.2% ($n = 15$) 50.0% ($n = 31$) 25.8% ($n = 16$)	46.3% ($n = 50$) 34.3% ($n = 37$) 19.4% ($n = 21$)	0.000 *
	Onsite Items	Utilities, Yes Utilities, No	76.1% ($n = 35$) 23.9% ($n = 11$)	79.4% ($n = 50$) 20.6% ($n = 13$)	79.3% ($n = 23$) 20.7% ($n = 6$)	83.3% ($n = 60$) 16.7% ($n = 12$)	0.797
		Physical, Yes Physical, No	91.3% ($n = 42$) 8.7% ($n = 4$)	93.7% ($n = 59$) 6.3% ($n = 4$)	86.2% ($n = 25$) 13.8% ($n = 4$)	93.1% ($n = 67$) 6.9% ($n = 5$)	0.602
	Supportive Coworkers	Yes No Not Sure	42.5% ($n = 34$) 8.8% ($n = 7$) 48.8% ($n = 39$)	63.9% ($n = 53$) 4.8% ($n = 4$) 31.3% ($n = 26$)	42.6% ($n = 26$) 6.6% ($n = 4$) 50.8% ($n = 31$)	61.1% ($n = 66$) 6.5% ($n = 7$) 32.4% ($n = 35$)	0.034 ˆ
	Supportive Supervisors	Yes No Not Sure	41.6% ($n = 32$) 14.3% ($n = 11$) 44.2% ($n = 34$)	58.5% ($n = 48$) 3.7% ($n = 3$) 37.8% ($n = 31$)	47.5% ($n = 29$) 8.2% ($n = 5$) 44.3% ($n = 27$)	62.0% ($n = 67$) 5.6% ($n = 6$) 32.4% ($n = 35$)	0.044 ˆ
Health Behavior	Pumped at Work	Yes No	23.7% ($n = 18$) 76.3% ($n = 58$)	42.2% ($n = 35$) 57.8% ($n = 48$)	23.7% ($n = 14$) 76.3% ($n = 45$)	41.3% ($n = 45$) 58.7% ($n = 64$)	0.010 *
Work Evaluation and Experience	Reaction to Pumping	Any negative Positive / None	55.6% ($n = 10$) 44.4% ($n = 8$)	34.3% ($n = 12$) 65.7% ($n = 23$)	53.8% ($n = 7$) 46.2% ($n = 6$)	26.7% ($n = 12$) 73.3% ($n = 33$)	0.095
	Pumped Longer if Easier	Yes No Not Sure	35.8% ($n = 24$) 28.4% ($n = 19$) 35.8% ($n = 24$)	38.6% ($n = 27$) 30.0% ($n = 21$) 31.4% ($n = 22$)	20.4% ($n = 10$) 30.6% ($n = 15$) 49.0% ($n = 24$)	36.6% ($n = 34$) 34.4% ($n = 32$) 29.0% ($n = 27$)	0.250
	Factors	Policy/Culture, Yes Policy/Culture, No	69.6% ($n = 16$) 30.4% ($n = 7$)	53.8% ($n = 14$) 46.2% ($n = 12$)	60.0% ($n = 6$) 40.0% ($n = 4$)	69.7% ($n = 23$) 30.3% ($n = 10$)	0.554
		Environment, Yes Environment, No	60.9% ($n = 14$) 39.1% ($n = 9$)	34.6% ($n = 9$) 65.4% ($n = 17$)	50.0% ($n = 5$) 50.0% ($n = 5$)	48.5% ($n = 16$) 51.5% ($n = 17$)	0.335

[1] For the Total Worker Health well-being domain questions, survey participants were only instructed to reply for their current job, and if they were currently on maternity leave or recently left their job, they were asked to respond for their most recent job. [2] p-Value was based on Fisher's exact tests or Fisher's exact tests with Freeman and Halton's adaptations for RxC tables. [3] Statistical significance (*) was based on an alpha of 0.05 with Bonferroni correction based on the number of comparisons within each category or domain (with no correction for demographic variables). A Monte Carlo estimation with 10,000,000 samples was used to calculate Fisher–Freeman–Halton statistics for tables with industry. Estimates were considered marginally significant (ˆ) if they met the alpha criteria of 0.05 but were no longer significant after Bonferroni correction.

Within the physical environment and safety climate domain, there were significant and marginally significant differences by industry. Women in healthcare and other industries had the greatest percentages of private pumping spaces in the workplace, compared to accommodation and retail

(55.0% and 46.3% vs. 26.0% and 24.2%, respectively, $p = 0.000$). Further, women in healthcare and "other" industries had the greatest percentages of supportive coworkers in the workplace, compared to accommodation and retail (63.9% and 61.1% vs. 42.5% and 42.6%, respectively, $p = 0.034$, not significant after Bonferroni correction), and women in healthcare and "other" industries had the greatest percentages of supportive supervisors in the workplace, compared to accommodation and retail (58.5% and 62.0% vs. 41.6% and 47.5%, respectively, $p = 0.044$, not significant after Bonferroni correction). Within the health behavior domain, greater percentages of women in healthcare and other industries pumped at work, compared to women in accommodation and retail (42.2% and 41.3% vs. 23.7% and 23.7%, respectively, $p = 0.010$). There were no significant differences within the work evaluation and experience domain factors by industry (all $p > 0.095$)

Similar to Tables 2 and 4, patterns emerged when examining responses of "not sure" in Table 6. Across significant effects, women working in retail had the greatest percentages of "not sure" and women working in other industries had the smallest percentages of "not sure."

4. Discussion

4.1. Findings

Based on previous research and the TWH model, this study explored, among WIC participants and by industry, factors that encourage and/or discourage the initiation and continuation of breastfeeding; pumping at work; and the workplace behaviors, policies, culture, environment, and safety climate associated with breastfeeding and pumping. Our study confirmed the results of a previous study of WIC participants and found that breastfeeding initiation was associated with age, race/ethnicity, and hoping or planning to breastfeed [13]. Further, also similar to this previous study, we found that breastfeeding initiation was not associated with employment status.

Our study did find, however, significant associations between industry and breastfeeding initiation, pumping at work, and the policies and physical environment related to breastfeeding and pumping. Confirming previous findings, we found that women in specific service-oriented industries (i.e., accommodation and retail) reported the lowest rates of breastfeeding initiation and workplace supports for breastfeeding and pumping [12]. Compared to healthcare and all other industries, women who worked in accommodation or retail had the smallest percentages of ever having breastfed, planning to only breastfeed, receiving information on breastfeeding while pregnant, paid maternity leave, a breastfeeding policy, private pumping spaces, and having pumped at work.

Notably, workplace policy factors supporting breastfeeding (i.e., having paid maternity leave, other maternity leave, and a breastfeeding policy) varied by industry but were not associated with breastfeeding initiation or duration. Further, how a woman hoped to feed and having a private pumping space at work were significantly associated with industry, breastfeeding initiation, and breastfeeding duration.

Our study confirms previous findings by Snyder et al. (2018) that having a breastfeeding policy, a space to pump, and coworker and supervisor support towards pumping at work vary by industry with the highest rates found among women in a professional industry (i.e., healthcare) [12]. Further, we also found women in service-oriented industries reported the lowest rates of having breastfed for four or more months. In contrast to Snyder et al. (2018), the majority of women in our study did not have or were "not sure" about each of these factors. Further, also unlike Synder et al. (2018), the majority of women in our study had not met their goal when they stopped breastfeeding.

4.2. Limitations

This study was cross-sectional and we were unable to assess the temporality of associations such as having received information on breastfeeding, how a woman hoped to feed her child, and subsequent breastfeeding behavior. We were also unable to assess supervisor or coworker support of pumping in the workplace pre-partum and its impact on pumping behavior. Survey responses were based on self-report and subject to several biases including but not limited to response bias, nonresponse bias, recall bias, and observation bias. Women who were employed, initiated breastfeeding, or had difficulty breastfeeding may have been more likely to take the survey, respond to all survey questions, and more accurately remember their breastfeeding experiences.

The survey also directed women who were currently on maternity leave or who had recently left their job to also respond to workplace questions. This may have resulted in increased rates of employment, having breastfed, and difficulties breastfeeding than in the entire WIC population. Due to this design effect, we were also unable to reliably identify and analyze the rates of women who were pregnant or gave birth and decided to no longer work (and their workplace environment).

Income, a key factor in the initiation and duration of breastfeeding, was not collected in this study. However, we assumed study participants were of a similar, lower socioeconomic status given they had qualified for the WIC program. All WIC families are at or below 185% of the family poverty level unless they adjunctively qualified through participation in the Supplemental Nutrition Assistance Program, Temporary Assistance for Needy Families Program, and/or Medicaid. The types of jobs and industries reported in our study reflect the low to moderate income of WIC participants. Our study also did not collect the age of the child and we were unable to determine who was still on paid maternity leave at the time of survey administration. Categories for industry were especially broad due to small sample sizes and we were not able to calculate numerous factors related to industry and occupation, employment, and the workplace including occupation alone, additional industries, size of the workplace (greater than or less than 50 people), and exempt versus non-exempt jobs.

Many breastfeeding studies focusing on workplace support by employment type are limited to their sample population [12,21]. This study is limited to women participating in the WIC program and/or mothers with children participating in the WIC program and our findings may not be generalizable outside of this population.

5. Conclusions

5.1. Implications

Our study illustrates how breastfeeding worksite supports are critical to TWH and well-being and suggests that women with a supportive environment are more likely to initiate breastfeeding and breastfeed longer compared to those without a supportive environment. When women begin the WIC program, they are often overwhelmed with the demands of working and caring for their family on a limited income. Although women are encouraged to explore their specific workplace policies and environment during breastfeeding education sessions and counseling appointments, these factors may contribute to the high rates of "not sure" reported in this study. Recently, there has been increased attention to breastfeeding support within the workplace to ensure compliance with the Patient Protection and Affordable Care Act (2010), which amended Section 7 of the Fair Labor Standards Act to require employers to provide: (1) "reasonable break time for an employee to express breast milk for her nursing child for 1 year after the child's birth each time such employee has need to express the milk," and (2) "a place, other than a bathroom, that is shielded from view and free from intrusion from coworkers and the public, which may be used by an employee to express breast milk." [37,38]. This study was conducted six years after the law was enacted and women still reported not having space or flexible time at work to express breast milk.

5.2. Recommendations

Currently, there are numerous ambiguities across breastfeeding research, policies, and practice at the state and federal level. There is a need to make clear connections between federal statutes, public health research, official company-specific policies, and actual practices in the workplace, especially the transparent designation of a workplace contact for breastfeeding policies and practice. Human resource or occupational health personnel in the workforce who write policies or design lactation space should be educated on core components that make up comprehensive lactation programs. Managers and supervisors need to be aware of the unique, acute, and transient needs of breastfeeding mothers returning to work specific to their job class, duties, schedules, and locations. Providing education and training directed toward leadership, supervisors, and human resource personnel regarding the benefits of breastfeeding for both employees and employers and the supports needed when returning to work should be included in any TWH framework. In addition, our study found that many women were unaware of their employer's benefits for lactation support after returning to work, demonstrating the need for improved communication and awareness about the benefits of health-related employer policies in the context of the TWH framework.

5.3. Future Research

Additional studies with larger sample sizes of women participating in WIC, characterizing the barriers to breastfeeding associated with specific industries and subpopulations, would inform future interventions, policy development, and education for employers of this population. Currently, lack of support for breastfeeding across industries is only discussed anecdotally, especially within the WIC program. Given our sample population, we suggest that an equality lens be considered in providing and communicating lactation support; studies should examine whether or not women are afraid to ask about the breastfeeding policies in their workplace, how employers disseminate health benefit information, and the availability and visibility of spaces for breastfeeding in the workplace. More broadly, learning about workplace policies and attitudes towards breastfeeding often involves speaking with coworkers and supervisors suggesting worksite power imbalances between employee and employer be examined. Future studies should also consider the high rates of "not sure" reported in this study in response to questions about workplace support and policies for breastfeeding. In order to better educate WIC participants, methods to improve the provision or dissemination of informational materials should be explored.

5.4. Final Remarks

In breastfeeding research, policy, and practice a variety of social justices are being addressed by agencies, leaders, and grass roots groups that believe breastfeeding is a human right that should not be denied or sacrificed when returning to work after having a baby. The priorities for these organizations include equal access to prenatal and postpartum lactation care and support, as well as targeted, evidence-based approaches to address the large disparities in workplace accommodations found in this study.

Author Contributions: E.A.L. cleaned and curated the data, conducted the formal data analyses using statistical software, and wrote and edited the original article draft (sections including the introduction, methodology, results, discussion, and conclusion). K.A., M.H., and L.S. conceptualized the overarching research goals and aims; led the investigation, project administration, and collection of survey data; and participated in the survey development. K.A., M.H., and L.S. also assisted with writing and reviewing the introduction, methods, discussion, and conclusions of the article.

Funding: This research was funded by the National Institute for Occupational Safety and Health Cooperative Agreement #U60 OH010910, NH Occupational Health Surveillance Program: Fundamental.

Acknowledgments: We would like to thank the efforts of University of New Hampshire Master of Public Health Program Field Study students Ashley Valdes and Kyle Dopfel and the New Hampshire Breastfeeding Task Force Board of Directors.

Conflicts of Interest: The authors have no conflicts of interest to disclose. The funder had no role in the design of the study; the collection, analyses, and interpretation of data; the writing of the manuscript; or the decision to publish the results.

References

1. Fein, S.B.; Roe, B. The effect of work status on initiation and duration of breast-feeding. *Am. J. Public Health* **1998**, *88*, 1042–1046. [CrossRef] [PubMed]

2. Gielen, A.C.; Faden, R.R.; O'Campo, P.; Brown, C.H.; Paige, D.M. Maternal employment during the early postpartum period: Effects on initiation and continuation of breast-feeding. *Pediatrics* **1991**, *87*, 298–305. [PubMed]
3. Hawkins, S.S.; Griffiths, L.J.; Dezateux, C.; Law, C.; Millennium Cohort Study Child Health Group. Maternal employment and breast-feeding initiation: Findings from the Millennium Cohort Study. *Paediatr. Perinat. Epidemiol.* **2007**, *21*, 242–247. [CrossRef] [PubMed]
4. Kimbro, R.T. On-the-job moms: Work and breastfeeding initiation and duration for a sample of low-income women. *Matern. Child Health J.* **2006**, *10*, 19–26. [CrossRef] [PubMed]
5. Horta, B.L.; Victora, C.G. Long-Term Effects of Breastfeeding: A Systematic Review. Available online: http://apps.who.int/iris/bitstream/handle/10665/79198/9789241505307_eng.pdf?sequence=1 (accessed on 17 December 2018).
6. National Center for Chronic Disease Prevention and Health Promotion. Breastfeeding Report Card. Available online: https://www.cdc.gov/breastfeeding/pdf/2014breastfeedingreportcard.pdf (accessed on 6 November 2018).
7. Mirkovic, K.R.; Perrine, C.G.; Scanlon, K.S.; Grummer-Strawn, L.M. In the United States, a Mother's Plans for Infant Feeding Are Associated with Her Plans for Employment. *J. Hum. Lact.* **2014**, *30*, 292–297. [CrossRef]
8. Lindberg, L. Trends in the relationship between breastfeeding and postpartum employment in the United States. *Soc. Biol.* **1996**, *43*, 191–202. [CrossRef] [PubMed]
9. Ryan, A.S.; Zhou, W.; Arensberg, M.B. The effect of employment status on breastfeeding in the United States. *Women's Health Issues* **2006**, *16*, 243–251. [CrossRef] [PubMed]
10. Roe, B.; Whittington, L.A.; Fein, S.B.; Teisl, M.F. The conflict between breast-feeding and maternal employment: Expectations and realities. Presented at the Annual Meeting of the Population Association of America, New Orleans, LA, USA, 9–11 May 1996; pp. 2, 27.
11. Mirkovic, K.R.; Perrine, C.G.; Scanlon, K.S.; Grummer-Strawn, L.M. Maternity leave duration and full-time/part-time work status are associated with US mothers' ability to meet breastfeeding intentions. *J. Hum. Lact.* **2014**, *30*, 416–419. [CrossRef]
12. Snyder, K.; Hansen, K.; Brown, S.; Portratz, A.; White, K.; Dinkel, D. Workplace Breastfeeding Support Varies by Employment Type: The Service Workplace Disadvantage. *Breastfeed. Med.* **2018**, *13*, 23–27. [CrossRef]
13. Murtagh, L.; Moulton, A.D. Working mothers, breastfeeding, and the law. *Am. J. Public Health* **2011**, *101*, 217–223. [CrossRef]
14. Haviland, B.; James, K.; Killman, M.; Trbovich, K. Policy Brief: Supporting Breastfeeding in the Workplace. Available online: http://www.asphn.org/resource_files/657/657_resource_file2.pdf (accessed on 11 November 2018).
15. Dagher, R.K.; McGovern, P.M.; Schold, J.D.; Randall, X.J. Determinants of breastfeeding initiation and cessation among employed mothers: A prospective cohort study. *BMC Preg. Childbirth* **2016**, *16*, 194. [CrossRef] [PubMed]
16. United States Public Health Service, Office of the Surgeon General; Centers for Disease Control and Prevention (U.S.); United States Department of Health and Human Services, Office on Women's Health. *The Surgeon General's Call to Action to Support Breastfeeding 2011*; U.S. Department of Health and Human Services, U.S. Public Health Service, Office of the Surgeon General: Rockville, MD, USA, 2011; (pp. 1 online resource (1 PDF file (vi, 88 p). Available online: http://www.ncbi.nlm.nih.gov/books/NBK52682 (accessed on 12 February 2019).
17. Centers for Disease Control and Prevention. Breastfeeding Among U.S. Children Born 2009–2015, CDC National Immunization Survey: Rates of Any and Exclusive Breastfeeding by Socio-Demographics among Children Born in 2015 (Percentage +/- Half 95% Confidence Interval). Available online: https://www.cdc.gov/breastfeeding/data/nis_data/rates-any-exclusive-bf-socio-dem-2015.htm (accessed on 17 December 2018).
18. Briefel, R.R.; Deming, D.M.; Reidy, K.C. Parents' Perceptions and Adherence to Children's Diet and Activity Recommendations: The 2008 Feeding Infants and Toddlers Study. *Prev. Chron. Dis.* **2015**, *12*, E159. [CrossRef] [PubMed]
19. Houghtaling, B.; Byker Shanks, C.; Jenkins, M. Likelihood of Breastfeeding Within the USDA's Food and Nutrition Service Special Supplemental Nutrition Program for Women, Infants, and Children Population. *J. Hum. Lact.* **2017**, *33*, 83–97. [CrossRef] [PubMed]

20. Jenkins, A.L.; Tavengwa, N.V.; Chasekwa, B.; Chatora, K.; Taruberekera, N.; Mushayi, W.; Madzima, R.C.; Mbuya, M.N. Addressing social barriers and closing the gender knowledge gap: Exposure to road shows is associated with more knowledge and more positive beliefs, attitudes and social norms regarding exclusive breastfeeding in rural Zimbabwe. *Matern. Child Nutr.* **2012**, *8*, 459–470. [CrossRef] [PubMed]
21. Dunn, R.L.; Kalich, K.A.; Fedrizzi, R.; Phillips, S. Barriers and Contributors to Breastfeeding in WIC Mothers: A Social Ecological Perspective. *Breastfeed. Med.* **2015**, *10*, 493–501. [CrossRef] [PubMed]
22. Darfour-Oduro, S.A.; Kim, J. WIC mothers' social environment and postpartum health on breastfeeding initiation and duration. *Breastfeed. Med.* **2014**, *9*, 524–529. [CrossRef] [PubMed]
23. Hedberg, I.C. Barriers to breastfeeding in the WIC population. *MCN Am. J. Matern. Child Nurs.* **2013**, *38*, 244–249. [CrossRef]
24. Holmes, A.V.; Chin, N.P.; Kaczorowski, J.; Howard, C.R. A barrier to exclusive breastfeeding for WIC enrollees: Limited use of exclusive breastfeeding food package for mothers. *Breastfeed. Med.* **2009**, *4*, 25–30. [CrossRef]
25. Chaudry, A.; Pedroza, J.; Sandstrom, H. How Employment Constraints Affect Low-Income Working Parents' Child Care Decisions. Available online: https://www.urban.org/sites/default/files/publication/32731/412513-How-Employment-Constraints-Affect-Low-Income-Working-Parents-Child-Care-Decisions.PDF (accessed on 18 December 2018).
26. New Hampshire Health Wisdom. New Hampshire WIC Pediatric Nutrition Surveillance (PedNSS): Breastfeeding. Available online: https://wisdom.dhhs.nh.gov/c10/epht/pediatricnutrition/wic1.html#breastfeeding (accessed on 1 January 2018).
27. Centers for Disease Control and Prevention. Breastfeeding Report Card. Available online: https://www.cdc.gov/breastfeeding/data/reportcard.htm (accessed on 1 January 2018).
28. Dunn, R.L.; Kalich, K.A.; Henning, M.J.; Fedrizzi, R. Engaging field-based professionals in a qualitative assessment of barriers and positive contributors to breastfeeding using the social ecological model. *Matern. Child Health J.* **2015**, *19*, 6–16. [CrossRef]
29. National Institute for Occupational Safety and Health. Total Worker Health. Available online: https://www.cdc.gov/niosh/twh/default.html (accessed on 18 December 2018).
30. Chari, R.; Chang, C.C.; Sauter, S.L.; Petrun Sayers, E.L.; Cerully, J.L.; Schulte, P.; Schill, A.L.; Uscher-Pines, L. Expanding the Paradigm of Occupational Safety and Health: A New Framework for Worker Well-Being. *J. Occup. Environ. Med.* **2018**, *60*, 589–593. [CrossRef]
31. Stuebe, A.M. Enabling women to achieve their breastfeeding goals. *Obstet. Gynecol.* **2014**, *123*, 643–652. [CrossRef] [PubMed]
32. Carothers, C.; Hare, I. The business case for breastfeeding. *Breastfeed. Med.* **2010**, *5*, 229–231. [CrossRef] [PubMed]
33. Tsai, S.Y. Employee perception of breastfeeding-friendly support and benefits of breastfeeding as a predictor of intention to use breast-pumping breaks after returning to work among employed mothers. *Breastfeed. Med.* **2014**, *9*, 16–23. [CrossRef] [PubMed]
34. Ball, T.M.; Wright, A.L. Health care costs of formula-feeding in the first year of life. *Pediatrics* **1999**, *103*, 870–876.
35. Centers for Disease Control and Prevention. The CDC Worksite Health ScoreCard: An Assessment Tool for Employers to Prevent Heart Disease, Stroke, and Related Health Conditions. Available online: https://www.cdc.gov/workplacehealthpromotion/pdf/hsc-manual.pdf (accessed on 15 September 2018).
36. Freeman, G.H.; Halton, J.H. Note on an exact treatment of contingency, goodness of fit and other problems of significance. *Biometrika* **1951**, *38*, 141–149. [CrossRef]
37. 111th Congress. Patient Protection and Affordable Care Act. Public Law 111-148 2010. Available online: http://www.gpo.gov/fdsys/pkg/PLAW-111publ148/pdf/PLAW111publ148.pdf (accessed on 24 September 2018).
38. U.S. Department of Labor Wage and Hour Division. Frequently Asked Questions—Break Time for Nursing Mothers. Available online: https://www.dol.gov/whd/nursingmothers/faqBTNM.htm (accessed on 17 December 2018).

© 2019 by the authors. Licensee MDPI, Basel, Switzerland. This article is an open access article distributed under the terms and conditions of the Creative Commons Attribution (CC BY) license (http://creativecommons.org/licenses/by/4.0/).

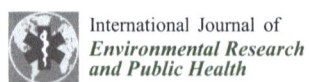

Article

A Cluster Randomized Controlled Trial of a Total Worker Health® Intervention on Commercial Construction Sites

Susan E. Peters [1], **Michael P. Grant [1]**, **Justin Rodgers [2]**, **Justin Manjourides [2]**, **Cassandra A. Okechukwu [1]** and **Jack T. Dennerlein [1,3,*]**

1. Harvard Center for Work, Health and Wellbeing, Harvard T.H. Chan School of Public Health, Boston, MA 02115, USA; sepeters@hsph.harvard.edu (S.E.P.); mgrant@hsph.harvard.edu (M.P.G.); cassandrao@post.harvard.edu (C.A.O.)
2. Department of Health Sciences, Bouvé College of Health Sciences, Northeastern University, Boston, MA 02115, USA; j.rodgers@northeastern.edu (J.R.); j.manjourides@northeastern.edu (J.M.)
3. Department of Physical Therapy, Movement and Rehabilitation Science, Bouvé College of Health Sciences, Northeastern University, Boston, MA 02115, USA
* Correspondence: j.dennerlein@northeastern.edu

Received: 7 October 2018; Accepted: 23 October 2018; Published: 25 October 2018

Abstract: This study evaluated the efficacy of an integrated Total Worker Health® program, "All the Right Moves", designed to target the conditions of work and workers' health behaviors through an ergonomics program combined with a worksite-based health promotion Health Week intervention. A matched-pair cluster randomized controlled trial was conducted on ten worksites (five intervention (n = 324); five control sites (n = 283)). Worker surveys were collected at all sites pre- and post-exposure at one- and six-months. Linear and logistic regression models evaluated the effect of the intervention on pain and injury, dietary and physical activity behaviors, smoking, ergonomic practices, and work limitations. Worker focus groups and manager interviews supplemented the evaluation. After controlling for matched intervention and control pairs as well as covariates, at one-month following the ergonomics program we observed a significant improvement in ergonomic practices (B = 0.20, p = 0.002), and a reduction in incidences of pain and injury (OR = 0.58, p = 0.012) in the intervention group. At six months, we observed differences in favor of the intervention group for a reduction in physically demanding work (B = −0.25, p = 0.008), increased recreational physical activity (B = 35.2, p = 0.026) and higher consumption of fruits and vegetables (B = 0.87, p = 0.008). Process evaluation revealed barriers to intervention implementation fidelity and uptake, including a fissured multiemployer worksite, the itinerant nature of workers, competing production pressures, management support, and inclement weather. The All the Right Moves program had a positive impact at the individual level on the worksites with the program. For the longer term, the multi-organizational structure in the construction work environment needs to be considered to facilitate more upstream, long-term changes.

Keywords: organizational intervention; health promotion; injury prevention; musculoskeletal; ergonomics; mixed-methods study; construction industry; safety management; health risk behaviors; occupational health

1. Introduction

Internationally, construction workers have higher rates of musculoskeletal disorders, and chronic diseases related to obesity, lack of physical activity and smoking than workers in other industries [1–4]. In construction workers, musculoskeletal disorders have a one-year pain prevalence rate (at least one episode of pain in the last year) of 51% for the back, 37% for the lower extremities, 32% for the upper extremities, and 24% for the neck in construction workers [5]. The high prevalence of musculoskeletal and cardiovascular disorders causes a sizable burden to employers, insurers, and society as a whole, attributing to work absenteeism, healthcare costs, work schedule delays, and high turnover [6–8]. In 2014, approximately 33% of absenteeism was attributed to musculoskeletal symptoms [9].

Construction workers also have high rates of chronic health issues. Over 70% of construction workers are overweight [10]. Obese construction workers are at increased risk of receiving disability benefits for cardiovascular disease and musculoskeletal disorders [11,12]. This risk is even higher for obese workers with high physical job demands, especially for those with musculoskeletal disorders [11]. Specifically, construction workers also have the highest prevalence of smoking (39%) of all occupational groups [1]. The risk of chronic lung disease and cancers is also amplified by the combined effects of smoking with other respiratory exposures, such as dust, silica, and asbestos [13–15].

Extensive research has linked these injury and poor health outcomes to individual factors, as well as the conditions of work, including job demands, physical work environment and psychosocial work factors (e.g., supervisor support and worker collegiality) [7]. Construction workers' injuries and poor health have been associated with the high physical demands, prolonged exposure to awkward postures, whole body vibration, long working hours, and psychosocial hazards in the work environment [2,16].

While these factors are prevalent in the construction industry, the complex work organization of construction work provides additional challenges for implementing traditional workplace prevention programs. The hierarchical structure between the site owners, general contractors, and subcontracting companies results in a fissured workplace [17]. The dynamic nature of these worksites results in workers moving on and off the site day-to-day. In addition, construction has high workforce turnover within the company, further complicating the number of workers transitioning in and out of the workforce, which has been linked to higher injury rates [18,19].

Integrated approaches that address the work environment to improve both occupational safety and health outcomes, and worker wellbeing outcomes, are acknowledged as being the most successful [20,21]. However, these integrated and comprehensive interventions for construction worksites need further investigation [20–25]. To date, most integrated approaches for construction workers have been individual-based, or those provided through labor unions [24,26]. Many worksite-based safety interventions for construction worksites have focused on using simple campaigns (such as poster and leaflet educational material) [27,28], training programs [29,30], behavioral management programs [10,31,32], or new, task-specific ergonomic tools and methods [33,34]. The intervention, "All the Right Moves" (ARM) described in this study, tested a different approach based on integrated approaches promoted by The National Institute for Occupational Safety and Health (NIOSH) Total Worker Health® program. Such approaches target the conditions of work that affect workers injuries and health outcomes [7,35]. The ARM intervention targeted the conditions of work through a worksite-based ergonomics program integrated into current work practices and on-site opportunities for workers to improve their health behaviors. The project's goal was to develop and determine the feasibility of an integrated health promotion and health protection worksite-based program designed specifically for the dynamic nature of a commercial construction work site.

The purpose of this study was to examine the intervention—ARM, on commercial construction sites, using a mixed methods approach. The specific aims of this project were to examine the efficacy of an integrated program including: (1) a soft tissue injury prevention program on workers' perception of worksite ergonomic practices, new pain and injury incidences, and work limitations; and (2) a health promotion/health coaching (Health Week) program for diet, leisure time physical activity, and reduced smoking behaviors.

2. Materials and Methods

2.1. Study Design and Randomization

We conducted a cluster randomized control trial on ten (five matched pairs) commercial construction sites (five intervention; five control) across the Boston metropolitan area, Massachusetts, United States between 2014 and 2015. Construction sites were matched within each general contracting company that agreed to participate in the study. Each pair of worksites was matched based on approximate size, scope, and phase of construction. This ensured that each matched pair consisted of similar organizational and worksite factors, such as similar existing company health and safety management systems [36]. Within each matched pair, one site was randomly assigned to either an intervention or a control group. A blocked randomization sequence was generated using a web-based random number generator by a member of the research team, who then allocated the pairs to either intervention or control. All workers within a specific worksite received the same intervention (or control) as allocated. Randomization and allocation of randomization sequence occurred as soon as two construction sites within a general contractor agreed to participate regardless of their assignment to control or intervention. The intervention groups received the intervention, ARM, whilst the control group received no intervention. Due to the pragmatic nature of the intervention, neither interventionists nor participants were blinded.

2.2. Recruitment and Eligibility

Construction sites were recruited through construction site owners and general contractors. To be eligible to participate in the study, worksites had to be in operation for 4 months or longer, and have 30 or more workers. Before the intervention commenced, a recruitment meeting was conducted with each site owner or general contractor to provide an overview of the study, programmatic activities, and to obtain leadership commitment. These recruitment meetings were conducted by the intervention primary investigator (J.T.D). Once a general contractor agreed, additional meetings with the leadership of each of the selected sites provided further leadership commitment and agreement for the study to take place on their sites.

Workers were introduced to the study by the research team and the general contractor safety manager, at a "safety stand-down" or toolbox talk. During the study, all new workers on a site were oriented to the study at their new-worker onsite safety orientation. Individual construction workers were surveyed within each site after a study launch meeting and at new-hire safety orientations for those workers who started after study commencement. Surveyed workers at each site were eligible if they were aged 18–65, and were English literate. All surveyed workers self-nominated and provided verbal consent during the survey process

All subjects gave their informed consent for inclusion before they participated in any data collection activities. The study was conducted in accordance with the Declaration of Helsinki, and the protocol was approved by the Ethics Committee of Harvard T.H. Chan School of Public Health Institutional Review Board (IRB-13-1948).

2.3. The "All the Right Moves" (ARM) Intervention

The ARM intervention was designed to integrate intervention components into the companies' existing safety and health practices on the sites. The intervention components were first developed and vetted with researchers and construction safety professionals, based on evidence-based organizational interventions and our own studies in the construction industry [4,18,37]. Following this process, the components of the interventions were piloted on commercial construction sites not involved in this trial. Managers and workers from the pilot sites provided qualitative feedback on program components, and the feedback was used to modify the intervention components. The changes were again vetted with these workers to refine the intervention components. This feedback was crucial to ensure intervention-organization fit, worker buy-in, and feasibility of implementing the components.

The ARM intervention contained two main intervention components: (1) the Soft Tissue Injury Prevention Program (StIPP) which focused on improving ergonomics practices at the site and worker level to improve musculoskeletal health; and (2) Health Week, that integrated key messages and provided integrated health coaching opportunities for individual workers to improve ergonomic practices and improved health behaviors (diet, physical activity, and smoking) associated with cardiovascular health. Both of these activities were based on industry safety practices with the ergonomics program using a structure similar to current safety management systems [38], and the health week based on the industry's practice of Safety Week campaigns and training. Refer to Figure 1 for the intervention's logic model.

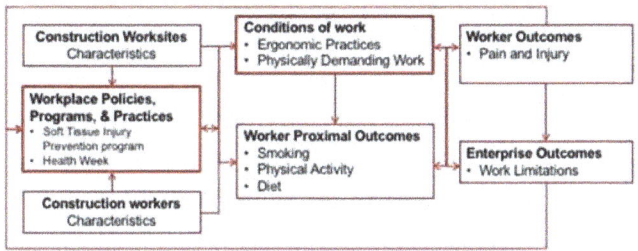

Figure 1. Logic model for the All the Right Moves (ARM) intervention.

The StIPP intervention component: This consisted of worksite inspections and feedback, task pre-planning, supervisor training, and worker training implemented for six weeks prior to the health week. The ergonomics-focused program targeted organizational practices and physical job demands by creating a systematic process to control worksite hazards.

Worksite Inspections and Feedback: The inspection process utilized a standardized worksite walkthrough inspection process augmented from an existing safety inspection process adapted from the successful Building Safety for Everyone program [18,36]. Photographs were taken of the injury hazards and ergonomic solutions which could be uploaded through an internet-based platform. The internet-based platform allowed data from all observations in a given date range to be aggregated and a report generated. A pre-intervention worksite inspection was conducted for each site one-week before the intervention activities were launched in order to customize foreman training as well as provide one-on-one training for the safety manager to identify soft tissue injury hazards and ergonomic practices. The walkthrough was conducted by an experienced ergonomist (J.T.D or M.P.G.), who was accompanied by a research assistant and the site safety manager from the general contractor. During the following six-week intervention periods, the safety manager conducted safety inspections on their own documenting their inspections using a custom-made web-based inspection tool. The tool allowed the safety manager to upload observations, including date, location, photo, hazard identified, solutions.

Each week the research team working with the safety manager compiled an inspection report and materials to provide critical feedback to the foreman and to the work crews. Based on our learnings from the Building Safety for Everyone program [18], detailed reports were communicated to foreman at weekly meetings and posters highlighting examples of hazards and solutions from these reports were placed in highly-visible areas around the worksite.

Task pre-planning: In addition to the inspection and feedback, we adapted existing pre-task planning checklists to incorporate soft-tissue injury hazards and the application of ergonomics solutions. These checklists identified task that involved manual materials handling, overhead work, and ground work. Ergonomic solutions included the NIOSH Simple Ergonomics Solutions for Construction Workers [39], as well as various trade specific solutions publicly available, which we compiled in a manual for the safety managers.

Supervisor training: This took place at the start of the intervention to report information from the pre-intervention walkthrough to the site foreman for the subcontractor companies currently on the site.

The training curriculum included information about the intervention, programmatic activities, injury hazards and ergonomic solutions identified from the first worksite inspection, and a few basic solutions from the NIOSH Simple Solutions [39], as well as expectations for the duration of the intervention implementation. The training was conducted during a mandatory weekly foreman meeting. Safety managers for each site also received this training, as well as trainings on how to use the web-based worksite inspection tool.

Worker training consisted of an "Ergonomics Toolbox Talk" (i.e., full company break in normal work to discuss an observed safety concern) that consisted of providing a few of the key messages from the supervisor training. The toolbox talk took place at the start of the intervention for workers already on the worksite and during new worker safety orientations, for workers coming onto the site after the initial launch meetings.

Health Week: This health promotion intervention was modeled after the existing safety week in construction (one week each year that is dedicated to raising awareness of workplace safety). The key goal of Health Week was to provide health education through toolbox talks and engage workers in programs to facilitate health behaviors through an opt-in health coaching program. Health Week targeted psychosocial factors and individual health-related behaviors by engaging workers in one-on-one discussions about their health and connecting them with relevant resources to improve their health behaviors. Toolbox talks were held during workers' break times each day of Health Week. Scripts and one-page toolbox cards were developed by the research team and a health promotion consultant, and then vetted with construction companies before being used. Topics included benefits of health coaching, soft tissue injury prevention, smoking cessation, energy balance (diet and physical activity) and a wrap-up session. Free web-based and phone resources were provided for each relevant topic. In addition, resources included free telephone-based health coaching provided by a large health-care organization. For active smokers, nicotine replacement therapy (NRT) (two-week supply) was provided free of charge.

Because of the success of individualized health coaching in construction workers, and prior results demonstrating dynamic workers movement between sites, Health Week encouraged workers to sign up and participate in health coaching program [40,41]. The health coaching program consisted of up to four telephone sessions by a trained health coach at no cost to the worker. The focus of these sessions was soft tissue injury prevention, dietary behaviors, physical activity and smoking cessation. Workers were able to select which of these topics they would receive coaching for. Each day workers were reminded to sign up for health coaching and those who did sign up were put into a lottery to win a USD$50 gift card to a large hardware-chain store.

2.4. Control Site Activities

For the control sites, all workers completed surveys at the same time intervals as the intervention sites. Workers were introduced to the study at an initial toolbox talk or at new worker orientation. They were also asked to complete surveys, at the same time intervals as the intervention sites. For the data collection periods, a banner with the program's logo was posted on the control group sites, similar to the intervention sites. No other information was provided, and no other activities were completed on control sites.

2.5. Worker Survey Data Collection

Workers completed surveys on-site at baseline—either at the initial work-site toolbox talk or at new worker orientations for workers joining the site after the launch of the project. Workers also completed surveys at two follow-up intervals, after completion of the StIPP program and one week prior to health week (FU1), and six months after health week (FU2). Due to the flow of workers on site, follow-up 1 occurred from 1 to 5 weeks post baseline survey. Baseline and FU1 surveys were collected on site and FU2 was collected via mail delivery. Workers were incentivized with a USD$5 gift card for completion of FU1 surveys, and USD$20 for FU2 surveys. The surveys contained questions on perceived work environment, ergonomic practices, health behaviors and worker health outcomes. The baseline survey also contained additional sociodemographic questions. The primary outcomes were health outcomes (pain and work limitations). Secondary worker proximal outcomes included health behaviors and safety practices. Workers who consented to participate were tracked via phone call or text to complete follow-up surveys at one (FU1) and six months (FU2) if they were no longer at the original study site.

2.6. Primary and Secondary Outcome Measures

Musculoskeletal pain and injury was measured with items adapted from the Nordic MSK Pain instrument [42]. We examined the probability of a worker having a new incidence of pain and/or injury at the follow-up time points using the question: "Have you needed to reduce or alter your work because of injury or musculoskeletal pain?" The questionnaire timeframe was adapted for the three different surveys to allow us to capture a change in pain and/or injury incidence following intervention roll-out. For baseline, the respondents were asked to answer the question with respect to last 12 months. For FU1, this was since they started work on the control/intervention site, and for FU2, it was for the preceding 6 months. Pain (without injury) was measured by asking: "During the past 3 months, have you had pain or aching in any of the areas shown on the diagram?"

Dietary behaviors were measured with three variables: "healthy diet", "unhealthy diet", and "dietary balance" at FU2 only [43,44]. Healthy diet was measured using six questions about the weekly frequency with which participants consumed the following types of foods and beverages: fruits, 100% orange or grapefruit juice, other 100% fruit juices, vegetables, baked potatoes, and salad. Unhealthy diet was measured with questions on the weekly consumption of fried foods, sugared snacks, fast foods, and sugar-sweetened beverages. Dietary balance was calculated as the sum of healthy diet and unhealthy diet multiplied by negative one, so that positive dietary balance indicated a healthier diet and negative dietary balance indicated a less healthy diet.

Physical activity was measured using a modified version of the Centers for Disease Control and Prevention Behavioral Risk Factor and Surveillance System Physical Activity Measure at FU2 only [45]. It included items on time spent walking and participating in both vigorous and moderate physical activities both at home and work during the last seven days.

Smoking status was categorized as a current smoker, former smoker, or never smoker [46]. Current smokers were those who currently smoke and have smoked at least 100 cigarettes in their lifetime. Former smokers were those who had smoked at least 100 cigarettes in their lifetime but do not currently smoke. Never smokers were those who had smoked less than 100 cigarettes and do not currently smoke. Current smokers were further differentiated according to the magnitude of their smoking behavior, measured by smoking frequency, smoking quantity, and contemplation.

2.7. Other Variables Measured

Ergonomic Practices were measured using three items from Amick et al. [47]: "Ergonomic strategies are used to improve the design of work", "Ergonomic factors are considered in task pre-planning and in purchasing new tools or equipment", and "Ergonomic factors are considered in safety and health inspections". These were rated on a 5-point scale ranging from 1 = strongly agree to 5 = strongly disagree. Ergonomic practice items were coded for the analysis so that higher scores of ergonomic practices represented better ergonomic practices.

Work limitations were measured using the eight question short-form Work Limitations Questionnaire, which contained domains on time, physical, mental and interpersonal demands [48]. Responses on a 5-point Likert scale were coded for the analysis so that higher values on the work limitations scale represented more or higher work limitations.

Physically demanding job demands were measured by two ordinal variables stemming from the following questions: "Please indicate how physically demanding your job is over the last 7 days", on a scale ranging from 1 = "not at all physically demanding" to 5 = "extremely physically demanding".

Sociodemographic variables included age (years), sex (male/female), race (white, black/African American, Latino/Hispanic, other), education level, job title (apprentice, journeyman, foreman and supervisor), and construction trade (carpenters, electricians, drywallers, ironworkers, laborers, painters, pipefitters, and plumbers). Race and ethnicity were later combined into the following two categories: "white" and "not white" for the analysis. Job title was later categorized into two categories for the analysis: "apprentice/journeyman", and "foreman/supervisor". Trade was categorized into the following four categories based on workers' job demands: (1) mechanical; (2) finishing; (3) ironwork; and, (4) labor. These categorizations have been used previously [36].

2.8. Process Evaluation

Process evaluation data collection focused on collecting information on uptake and exposure to the intervention components, as well as barriers and facilitators to implementation. Qualitative data was collected at the completion of the intervention through focus groups with workers and interviews with managers. All interviews and focus groups were recorded and transcribed. To maintain confidentiality, participants were instructed to avoid identifying themselves, their coworkers or the company they worked for, during the interviews and focus groups. In addition, data were collected on uptake and exposure to the intervention components through checklists completed for each intervention activity by members of the research team.

Post-intervention worker focus groups were conducted at four of the five intervention sites. One site did not participate due to a scheduling conflict. The aims of the focus groups were to: (1) explore workers perceptions of health and safety at their sites; (2) explore workers' perceptions of intervention activities including facilitators and barriers to uptake of the intervention, feasibility, and success of the intervention; and (3) identify how health and safety was handled onsite considering the fissured nature of the worksites and workforce.

Post-intervention interviews with safety managers from the general contractors were conducted at the same seven worksites in which worker focus groups were conducted. The aim was to: (1) explore their perceptions of intervention activities including facilitators and barriers to uptake of the intervention and intervention delivery, feasibility, and success of the intervention; (2) investigate mechanisms that enable foremen and site management to support worker participation in health and safety interventions; and, (3) identify areas for improvement for future interventions.

2.9. Hypotheses

We tested the following hypotheses for the primary outcomes: (1a) At FU1 and FU2, workers on intervention sites will report lower incidences of pain or injury compared to workers on the control sites; (1b) At FU2, workers on intervention sites will report improved diet and leisure time physical activity behaviors compared to workers on the control sites; and (1c) At FU2, workers on intervention sites will smoke on fewer days and with fewer cigarettes per month.

We also tested hypotheses for secondary outcomes: (2a) Workers on intervention sites will report improved ergonomic and safety practices at FU1, and lower physical job demands at FU1 and FU2, compared to workers on control sites at follow up; and (2b) At FU1 and FU2, workers on intervention sites will report improved work limitations at follow up than workers on the control sites.

2.10. Data Analysis

All data analyses were completed in SAS Version 9.3 (SAS Institute Inc., Cary, NC, USA). First, we compared worker demographics between control and intervention sites using chi-squared tests of homogeneity for categorical variables and *t*-tests for continuous variables. A priori power calculations were conducted for the primary outcome, pain and injury, adjusting for potential intra-class correlation, ICC = 0.05 due to the cluster-based design, and using a two-sided test at $\alpha = 0.05$. We have sufficient power (>0.8) to detect at effect size greater than 0.6 with an estimated sample size of 176.

As pain and injury outcomes were binary measures, we first performed logistic regression models accounting only for the baseline level of the outcome variables. Each model also utilized cluster robust standard errors to account for individual correlation within worksites. Second, we included fixed effects for the matched pairs within each company, and adjusted the models for age, race, and job title.

All other variables were continuous. We conducted linear regression models on the change scores between baseline and FU1 and, baseline and FU2 as the dependent variables and treatment status (intervention; control) as the independent variable. We used cluster robust standard errors to account for individual clustering within worksites. We then adjusted for matched pairs within the companies through the addition of a fixed effect and also accounted for the possibility of post-randomization, and residual confounding by adjusting for age, sex, race, job title, and trade. No analyses were conducted for smoking as there were too few smokers who changed their smoking status over the course of the intervention on the sites.

We conducted sensitivity analyses to observe initially whether the removal of the one matched pair for the site that did not perform the intervention activities for the soft tissue ergonomics program, resulted in any differences in effect of the intervention on the primary and secondary outcomes. We then sequentially removed each pair per analysis to evaluate whether removal of any pair resulted in differences in the effectiveness evaluation.

3. Results

3.1. Study Characteristics and Response Rates

Six construction companies operating in the Boston metropolitan area, Massachusetts, were invited to participate, and five agreed. Within each of these companies two worksites per company were randomly assigned to the intervention or the control, resulting in a total of 10 worksites. The participation rates for the follow-up surveys (of those who completed the baseline surveys) were 69% ($n = 228/332$) for FU1 and 78% ($n = 118/151$) for FU2, and were included in the analyses (Figure 2). At baseline, it was difficult to determine the total number of eligible workers on site and hence response rates of those eligible. We were able to record the number of workers at the site orientations and were able to capture almost all of the new workers that came on to the site after the orientation.

There were no significant differences between the intervention and control sites at baseline (Table 1), FU1 or FU2 for age, sex, race/ethnicity or education at any data collection interval. There were no significant differences ($p \geq 0.05$) for those who completed surveys at baseline and those who did not at FU1 or FU2, with respect to age, sex, ethnicity/race, education level or job title.

Table 1. Distribution of demographic characteristics at baseline ($N = 607$).

	Total ($N = 607$)		Control ($n = 283$)		Intervention ($n = 324$)		Test of Equivalence, p-Value
	N	Mean (SD)	N	Mean (SD)	N	Mean (SD)	
Age	586	40.42 (10.78)		40.28 (11.05)		40.55 (10.55)	0.7643
	N	n (%)	N	n (%)	N	n (%)	
Gender							
Male	592	573 (97%)	275	270 (98%)	317	303 (96%)	0.0736
Female		19 (3%)		5 (2%)		14 (4%)	
Race/Ethnicity							
White		457 (77%)		214 (77%)		243 (77%)	
Black/AA	595	57 (10%)	244	24 (9%)	351	33 (11%)	0.7883
Latino/Hispanic		35 (6%)		16 (6%)		19 (6%)	
Other		46 (8%)		24 (9%)		22 (7%)	

Table 1. *Cont.*

	Total (N = 607)		Control (n = 283)		Intervention (n = 324)		Test of Equivalence, *p*-Value
	N	Mean (SD)	N	Mean (SD)	N	Mean (SD)	
Education							
<H.S.		33 (6%)		17 (6%)		16 (5%)	
H.S./G.E.D.	587	317 (54%)	274	151 (55%)	313	166 (53%)	0.5762
Some college		194 (33%)		90 (33%)		104 (33%)	
College graduate		43 (7%)		16 (6%)		27 (9%)	
Title							
Apprentice		104 (19%)		40 (16%)		64 (22%)	
Journeyman	554	330 (59%)	256	156 (61%)	298	174 (58%)	0.3400
Foreman		100 (18%)		50 (19%)		50 (17%)	
Supervisor		20 (4%)		10 (4%)		10 (3%)	
Trade							
Finishing		59 (12%)		25 (11%)		34 (12%)	
Mechanical	499	366 (73%)	226	168 (74%)	273	198 (73%)	0.1643
Laborers		30 (6%)		18 (8%)		12 (4%)	
Ironworkers		44 (9%)		15 (7%)		29 (11%)	

AA = African American, H.S. = High School, G.E.D. = General Equivalency Diploma; SD = Standard Deviation.

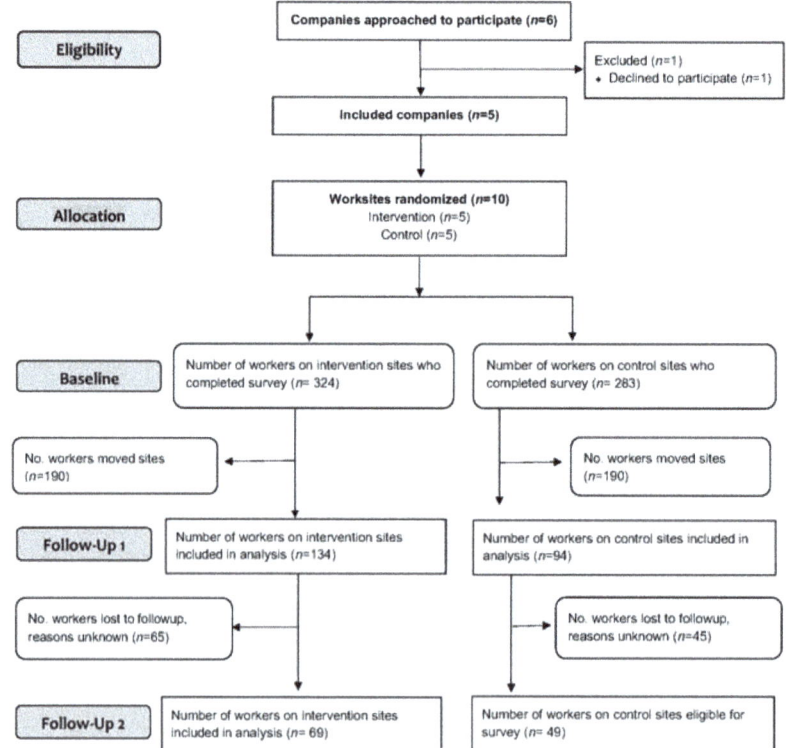

Figure 2. Participant flow through the trial.

3.2. Outcomes

Similar to demographic characteristics, all the outcome variables were not statistically different between the workers in the intervention and control groups at baseline, except for physical demanding work ($p < 0.001$) (Table 2). However, as described in Section 2.10, models testing the hypotheses examined changes from baseline in the cohort accounting for baseline measurements.

Table 2. Descriptive statistics for primary and secondary outcome variables.

Outcome Variable	Control			Treatment		
	Baseline (N = 283)	FU1 (N = 94)	FU2 (N = 49)	Baseline (N = 324)	FU1 (N = 134)	FU2 (N = 69)
Worker Outcomes						
	n (%)[N]	n (%)[N]	n (%)[N]	n (%)[N]	n (%)[N]	n (%)[N]
New pain or injury [2]	83 (30.0%)[277]	20 (21.5%)[93]	15 (31.3%)[48]	115 (36.4%)[316]	27 (20.6%)[131]	15 (21.7%)[69]
Pain interfering with work	197 (69.9%)[282]	54 (57.5%)[94]	37 (75.5%)[49]	234 (72.4%)[323]	78 (58.2%)[134]	48 (69.6%)[69]
Current Smoker	82 (30.4%)[269]		12 (24.5%)[49]	99 (33.9%)[292]		18 (26.1%)[69]
	Mean (SD)[N]	Mean (SD)[N]	Mean (SD)[N]	Mean (SD)[N]	Mean (SD)[N]	Mean (SD)[N]
Physical activity	76.57 (76.70)[229]		67.69 (95.55)[45]	67.76 (61.95)[270]		69.04 (93.66)[66]
Healthy diet	5.60 (2.32)[276]		5.42 (1.67)[48]	5.62 (2.24)[318]		5.48 (2.01)[69]
Unhealthy diet	2.05 (1.21)[274]		2.12 (1.37)[47]	2.25 (1.31)[317]		1.76 (1.15)[69]
Diet balance	3.57 (2.48)[274]		3.24 (1.92)[47]	3.36 (2.46)[317]		3.72 (2.25)[69]
Enterprise Outcomes						
Work limitations	1.51 (0.64)[277]	1.39 (0.57)[91]	1.27 (0.41)[49]	1.53 (0.67)[321]	1.46 (0.62)[128]	1.27 (0.54)[68]
Conditions of Work						
	n (%)[N]	n (%)[N]	n (%)[N]	n (%)[N]	n (%)[N]	n (%)[N]
Demanding Work [1,3]	213 (79.3%)[269]	43 (47.3%)[91]	30 (61.2%)[49]	206 (66.9%)[308]	60 (46.2%)[130]	31 (45.6%)[68]
	Mean (SD)[N]	Mean (SD)[N]	Mean (SD)[N]	Mean (SD)[N]	Mean (SD)[N]	Mean (SD)[N]
Ergonomic practices	3.89 (0.67)[276]	3.69 (0.78)[93]		3.8 (0.62)[313]	3.68 (0.80)[132]	

FU1 = Follow-up 1; FU2 = Follow-up 2; SD = Standard Deviation. [1] Differences between treatment and control groups at baseline, $p < 0.05$; [2] At baseline, this was measured as the number of workers who had pain or injury, at follow-up intervals this was measured as new pain or injury since baseline; [3] Physical demanding work was categorized as those nominating a 4 or 5 on the physically demanding scale.

3.2.1. Pain and Injury

Hypothesis 1a tested differences in pain incidence between intervention and control group workers. Model results revealed no significant differences at FU1 in the unadjusted model. However, after adjusting for covariates, in addition to the matched pairs, there was approximately 42% reduction in risk of having new pain or injury compared to the control sites (p = 0.012) (Table 3). While the magnitude of this risk reduction was maintained at FU2 there were fewer participants and an increase in variability that made this reduction not statistically significant. Thus, hypothesis 1a was partially supported at FU1.

Table 3. Effects of ARM intervention on Pain and Injury at 1-month and 6-months post-intervention while adjusting for baseline level of outcome variable.

Outcome Variable	Unadjusted			Adjusted [1]		
	N	OR (95% CI)	p-Value	N	OR (95% CI)	p-Value
FU1 (1 month)						
New pain or injury [2]	216	1.01 (0.49, 2.07)	0.982	208	0.58 (0.39, 0.86)	0.012 **
Pain in last 3 months	228	1.03 (0.65, 1.63)	0.884	219	0.85 (0.63, 1.15)	0.252
FU2 (6 months)						
New pain or injury [2]	115	0.48 (0.13, 1.73)	0.227	112	0.60 (0.24, 1.49)	0.236
Pain in last 3 months	116	0.74 (0.32, 1.69)	0.429	116	0.85 (0.37, 1.99)	0.683

CI = confidence intervals; OR = odds ratio. Results from logistic regression models with cluster robust standard errors to account for individual clustering within worksites (** p < 0.05); [1] Adjusted model with fixed effects for matched pairs and for age, race, and job title. [2] New injury or pain reported by the worker on FU1 /FU2 survey since baseline survey.

3.2.2. Physical Activity and Dietary Behaviors

The number of minutes that participants spent performing recreational physical activity decreased on average in the control groups, but increased in the intervention groups. This difference was non-significant in the unadjusted model, but became significant in the adjusted model (B = 31.03, p = 0.03) (Table 4).

There were no observable differences at FU2 between the intervention and control sites for unhealthy diet (i.e., eating fatty or sugary foods) for the unadjusted or adjusted models respectively (Table 4). For healthy diet, we observed no differences between the intervention and control groups in the unadjusted model. However, when accounting for the matched intervention and control pairs within each company, and adjusting for covariates, we found a significant small positive influence on healthier diet behaviors in the intervention compared to the control groups (B = 0.87; p = 0.008). Overall, we saw a small improvement in having a more balanced diet nearing significance due to the improvement in healthy eating behaviors (B = 1.05, p = 0.054). Thus, hypothesis 1b was partially supported.

Table 4. Effects of the ARM intervention on physical activity and dietary behaviors from baseline to FU2 (6 months).

Outcome Variable	Unadjusted			Adjusted [1]		
	N	B (95% CI)	p-Value	N	B (95% CI)	p-Value
Recreational physical activity	97	12.54 (−24.42, 49.51)	0.462	84	35.20 (5.35, 65.04)	0.026 **
Dietary balance	116	0.83 (−0.62, 2.28)	0.229	100	1.05 (−0.02, 2.13)	0.054 *
Healthy diet	118	0.63 (0.33, 1.59)	0.173	101	0.63 (−0.17, 1.43)	0.008 **
Unhealthy diet	116	−0.07 (−1.11, 0.99)	0.89	100	−0.12 (−0.81, 0.56)	0.691

B = regression coefficient; CI = confidence intervals. Results from linear regression models with cluster robust standard errors to account for individual clustering within worksites (* p <0.1, ** p <0.05). [1] Adjusted with fixed effects for matched pairs and age, sex, race, title, and trade.

3.2.3. Tobacco Use

Changes in smoking and tobacco used were small in both groups. Two people in the intervention group quit smoking, while in the control group, one person quit and one started smoking.

3.2.4. Ergonomic Practices and Work Limitations

After the StIPP intervention activities, we observed a small but significant improvement in the intervention, compared to the control sites, for ergonomic practices, after adjusting for matched pairs, and age, gender, race, job title and trade (B = 0.20, p = 0.002) (Table 5). We also saw a significant small reduction in physical job demands at FU2 (B= −0.25, p = 0.008). Hypothesis 2a was therefore partially supported. There were no observable differences between the intervention and control sites in the worker's perceptions of their work limitations at FU1 or FU2 for the unadjusted or adjusted models (Table 5). Thus, hypothesis 2b was not supported.

Table 5. Effects of the ARM intervention on Working Conditions and Enterprise Outcomes from baseline to FU1 (1 month) and FU2 (6 months).

Outcome Variable		Unadjusted			Adjusted [1]	
	N	B (95% CI)	p-Value	N	B (95% CI)	p-Value
		FU1 (1 month)				
Ergonomic practices	182	0.00 (−0.21, 0.20)	0.953	182	0.20 (0.09, 0.31)	0.002 **
Physically demanding work	208	0.17 (−0.05, 0.37)	0.121	174	0.17 (−0.06, 0.40)	0.129
Work limitations (8-item)	216	0.11 (−0.08, 0.30)	0.225	179	0.09 (−0.06, 0.24)	0.212
		FU2 (6 months)				
Physically demanding work	114	−0.14 (−0.51, 0.23)	0.407	100	−0.25 (−0.41, −0.08)	0.008 **
Work limitations (8-item)	119	0.02 (−0.08, 0.13)	0.641	102	0.04 (−0.07, 0.15)	0.432

B = regression coefficient; CI = confidence intervals. Results from linear regression models with cluster robust standard errors to account for individual clustering within worksites (** p < 0.05). [1] Adjusted with fixed effects for matched pairs and age, gender, race, title, and trade.

3.2.5. Sensitivity Analysis

We conducted analyses by removing each matched pair across intervention and control sites. We observed that when we removed the matched pair which included the intervention site that had limited participation in the ergonomic intervention activities, the strength of the significant findings increased.

3.3. *Process Evaluation*

3.3.1. Intervention Fidelity and Uptake

Soft Tissue Injury Prevention Program: Foreman training ranged from 25–45 min per site, and was delivered as per the protocol on the five intervention sites. The number of foreman who attended per site varied (median: 6; range: 5–25). Baseline participation rates for the project launch (range: 25–93%) and orientation (range: 75–90%) also varied significantly across sites. The number of ergonomic inspections and feedback reports differed greatly across the five intervention sites (median: 15; range: 0–19). At best, sites had three ergonomic observations per week during the six weeks of the program. At worst, one site completed no inspections and feedback reports to the foreman, due to severe weather conditions causing the site to shut down during the intervention period. Many of the improvements recorded concentrated on how workers were setting up their own work areas rather than systems level changes, e.g., getting equipment off the ground and performing tasks at heights around waist level, rather than below the knee.

Health Week and Coaching: 45 workers (14%) signed up for health coaching. Most workers had favorable responses to engaging in the toolbox talks during health week. However, only 7 out of the

45 workers who signed up for health coaching participated in the first phone call, and only three completed four weeks of health coaching.

Workers signed up for health coaching for dietary behaviors, physical activity and smoking cessation. No workers signed up for coaching on soft tissue injury prevention. Qualitatively, workers reported getting benefit from the smoking cessation toolbox talks. Providing NRT kits was popular; however, due to privacy issues and poor follow-up rates, we were unable to link the NRT distribution to the surveys and effects on smoking quit rates. One worker reported: "I think tobacco was good for me and my guys. Most of them smoke, so I think it was good for them. The NRT inspired some of the workers to give quitting a try." Other topics of interest raised in the focus groups included stress management, alcohol consumption and appropriate pain management.

There were no adverse events reported by the participants for participating in either StIPP or Health Week.

3.3.2. Barriers to Intervention Implementation

Based on key informant interviews on the intervention sites, while indicating it was good to have the ergonomics inspections and topics at the forefront of the workers' and subcontractors' activities, workers mentioned a number of barriers to fully implementing the intervention.

Fissured workplace issues: A key barrier was the capability of subcontractor companies to make changes in working conditions. While the program trained the foreman of the subcontractors with a focus on pre-task planning, the subcontractors did not have the systems in place or the available tools to assist in changing the working conditions.

Production pressures and unpredictable schedules: The site that conducted no ergonomics inspections had large production pressures as the construction schedule was delayed significantly due to unusual winter weather. For example, one safety manager observed that production pressures could be a driving factor: "I think it's the schedules . . . Because they rush around, it's hard for them to take a step back and really evaluate how they're doing things. They're just trying to do it as quickly as possible."

Management support and worker buy-in: Focus group participants and key informants reported that programs needed buy-in and support from upper management for interventions to be successful. This is especially true with respect to training and data collection which, by necessity, must be conducted on the worksite during working hours. For instance, general contractors could allow for extra training related to the ARM program and build it into the contracts of the subcontractors. That way, the time needed for training purposes and intervention delivery would be agreed to ahead of time and budgeted into the contracts signed by both parties. To illustrate this point, one safety manager noted: "A health and safety program would have a lot more buy-in and success on a site if it was written into the contract... An owner or GC [general contractor] would have to financially support the program running on their site."

4. Discussion

The goal of this study was to evaluate the efficacy of a construction worksite-based integrated intervention targeting both the conditions of work, and workers' health behaviors, simultaneously. We observed short-term improvements in ergonomic practices and in incidences of pain and injury after an injury prevention program. We also observed an improvement in physical activity and healthier dietary behaviors, such as increased consumption of fruits and vegetables, after a health promotion Health Week program.

At the individual level, we found a significant improvement in ergonomic practices, and a reduction in incidences of pain and injury, which supported the hypothesized pathways for the program. As promoted by NIOSH, ergonomic practices focus on workers modifying or establishing work procedures to reduce the risk of injuries [39,49]. While we did not quantify exposure to specific ergonomic hazards, the StIPP focused on workers' setting up their work more ergonomically.

For example, working at knuckle level instead of on the ground, and using appropriate tools to reduce extreme postures associated with overhead work and manual materials handling. The program targeted the conditions of work directly controlled by the workers themselves (Figure 2) [7]. Giving such control to workers is important in reducing disability, as it gives workers opportunities to adapt their work in order to better manage their own musculoskeletal symptoms and health [50,51].

While we were encouraged that an improvement in ergonomics practices occurred, results also indicated that the program was not successful at addressing system level components. For example, while we saw ergonomics practices improve, we saw no significant change in the physical demands on the workers. Hence, we suspect that the intervention changed the way people completed their work but had limited effect on the physical demands of the job. In addition, the process evaluation revealed several important barriers and facilitators to our program at the organizational level. First, management and worker buy-in were identified to be integral to the success of the soft tissue injury prevention program. This was perceived to be key in a work environment that is fast-paced, unpredictable, and with tight production schedules tied to the requirements of the general contractor. For example, there was little time to complete task preplanning or for the safety manager to complete inspection protocols for injury hazards and ergonomic solutions. When management support for health and safety programs is not observed by the workers, other competing factors are often prioritized over health and safety, especially ergonomic practices [52]. This was quite evident on one site which had major delays due to the winter storms of 2015 in the Boston metropolitan area. Due to the loss of almost a month of production, competing safety and schedule priorities would supersede program delivery. Similar challenges to program delivery have been reported by others in the construction industry [53].

While we have had past success with a worksite safety program integrated within the complex structure associated with multiple employers, a large barrier to a systems approach ergonomics program was the challenge faced by subcontractors to make changes, even those changes that could improve site safety on their own worksite. Unlike our previous program that was designed to re-enforce existing safety practices [36], the ARM program required subcontractors to implement new, or modify existing practices and tools, that may be specific to their trade. Our program focused on simple ergonomics solutions that individual workers could implement to their own work [39]. However, more complex or system-level changes would require the involvement of multiple groups or stakeholders [54]. Ergonomics solutions in a fissured workplace require all site employers to take on elements of the program to effectively and systematically influence the overall conditions of work [17].

Moreover, system-level changes require better upfront planning before construction begins, such as during the bidding process for a job by setting out requirements from the multiple employers, and in the contracts for the jobs. The key informant interviews supported this concept. Expectations regarding safety programs in the contract is standard procedure in larger projects, especially owner-insured programs. An example is with respect to safety training, in which owners, especially public entities, require that construction workers have a minimum of OSHA-10 training to be onsite [55]. Whilst others require their contracting companies complete safety prequalification safety surveys, or have written safety management programs. Thus, including ergonomics in the contractual language may set up better expectations for a program.

Other researchers in the construction industry have also found mixed findings with respect to improvements in pain and injury and perceived physical effort after implementing ergonomic interventions, including participatory ergonomics programs [33,56–58]. In these studies, reasons for intervention failure were generally associated with the intervention not being delivered as intended or implemented at all of the sites [28,57]. In our study, intervention delivery occurred as per the protocol in four of the five sites during the intervention period. However, since the ergonomics program stopped after six weeks and workers often moved from sites before the follow-up data collection was completed, we also attributed this to our loss of significance at the six-month follow-up. Although we observed that on average the reduction in pain and injury incidences, and improvements in ergonomic practices were maintained, there was reduction in power due to loss to follow up.

In contrast, the Health Week had many successes in overcoming some of these barriers associated with the multiemployer structure. For one, it simply required the participation of the workers and little, if any, infrastructure. In theory, the Health Week might have addressed some conditions of work regarding psychosocial factors around health, like supervisor or co-worker support. Anecdotally, we observed foremen and co-workers being supportive of ensuring their co-workers signed up for health coaching or NRT. Some foremen would cover for their workers to allow them to participate in the week's activities. We also observed workers talking about eating healthier food with their coworkers during the week.

Another major strength of the Health Week was how it aligned with companies' current practices on the worksite and also with the interests and goals of the workers. This was also found in previous formative work we completed that found that policies, programs and practices are supported by management and workers alike if they can be easily integrated into company's business structures and align with workers' goals and needs [59,60]. Health Week was in a familiar format for the workers and companies alike. We modelled Health Week after the industry's standard practice of safety week where contractors have a specific theme and perform a series of outreach activities for workers to provide information on resources and best practices. Thus, due to the familiar format, workers may have been more receptive to the daily topics. Although the uptake on NRT and individualized health coaching was low, we did see improvements in workers' health behaviors, including higher intake of fruits and vegetables, and increased amount of time per week engaged in recreational physical activity. This finding is similar to the results of a health promotion intervention conducted in the Netherlands, which found that onsite group coaching sessions resulted in changes in physical activity, and dietary behaviors, but did not improve musculoskeletal symptoms [61].

Methodological Considerations

Research in construction has challenges with loss to follow up due to the dynamic nature of construction with workers coming and going on worksites as the construction job requires specific trades during the timeline of the study [18,36]. The issue of poor follow-up rates can lead to bias; however, usually towards the null [62]. This is predominately due to the itinerant nature of construction workers [18]. This resulted in our analyses at FU2 being underpowered for some of our outcomes (such as pain and injury) where the effect size was similar to FU1. Similar findings have been found in related interventions [63].

Another challenge was the success of integrating the injury prevention and health promotion activities in this environment. Integration was achieved by linking the two programs by name and key messaging in the planning and implementation phases. In addition, messaging around Health Week included training on both injury prevention and health promotion giving workers the tools to improve their working conditions, as well as giving them control for their health. The ergonomics program prior to Health Week did have health messaging but without any specific health promotion activities.

One limitation was that our intervention depended on the participation of the general contractor safety managers, whose involvement and dedication to the study varied across sites and between general contractors. This aspect of the intervention was by design, as we considered it important for integration and sustainability into current company processes, that the ergonomics inspections were performed by the safety managers. Giving the safety managers latitude to decide how invested they were in the program allowed us to assess the feasibility of the intervention being adopted without the aid of study staff. This would ensure that our observations were realistic and representative of barriers and facilitators to the intervention's delivery by non-study staff.

Further, this study involved worksites in commercial construction only. Thus, the results may not be generalizable to other types of construction (i.e., residential or industrial). However, commercial construction accounts for a large portion of U.S. construction activities, and represents an important area for injury prevention research. Similarly, the construction workforce in the Boston metropolitan area may not be representative of commercial construction workers in other parts of the country or world, where work practices, demographics, and union membership differ.

Despite these limitations, our study had several strengths, most notably the study design and the wide variety of general contractors and sites recruited into the study. The cluster randomized control trial design is a novel approach in commercial construction. Typically, approaches to improve the health and safety of construction workers have often focused on the individual worker, targeting workers when they are enrolled in apprentice programs [64,65], targeting workers through social media campaigns via posters at worksites and/or brochures sent to union members [66,67], and engineering controls for specific tasks [68]. However, best practice involves system-level approaches that comprehensively address workplace systems relevant to the control of hazards and worker safety, health, and well-being [20]. This study was fortunate to be able to recruit five major general contractors operating in the Boston metropolitan area and gain access to ten different construction sites for the purpose of evaluating the ARM intervention. Furthermore, delivering the intervention through mid-level managers (through a combination of the general contractor safety managers and subcontractor foremen) was a strength of the study. This focused intervention efforts on those who were in the best positions to make changes to the conditions of work.

The ergonomics inspection and communication protocol provided a method to identify broad areas for improving ergonomics in the dynamic construction work environment. It is important to understand the challenges and successes of intervention delivery in order to inform and improve future worksite-based interventions. It appears that the largest barriers to the success of the intervention were the inability of subcontractors to make changes to their worksite and the variability in the involvement and dedication to the study across different worksites and general contractors. These are real-world, as well as research study challenges. Subcontractors did not have the systems in place, or the available tools, to assist in changing their working conditions. Competing safety and production priorities also influenced the level of management commitment to the study. Additionally, construction safety research may have broader implications for an increasing number of industries that are becoming as dynamic and variable as construction, as more services once housed in a single facility are outsourced to multiple employers [17].

5. Conclusions

The ARM program had a positive impact at the individual level on the worksites that implemented the program. The trial saw improved ergonomics practices, as well as, reduction in new pain and injury, and improved diet and physical activity, as reported by the workers. A number of obstacles were encountered which made integrating a health promotion and injury prevention intervention into the multi-employer, outcome-driven, dynamic work environment challenging. Process tracking suggested that our intervention had less impact at the systems/organizational level in terms of changing organizational programs and practices, due to the complex organizational structures on site. For the longer term, more organizations in the multiple employer environment should be involved in the implementation to facilitate more upstream changes.

Author Contributions: Conceptualization, J.T.D., C.A.O. and M.P.G.; Methodology, J.T.D., C.A.O. and M.P.G.; Formal Analysis, S.E.P., J.M., J.R.; Investigation, J.T.D., M.P.G. and C.A.O.; Resources, J.T.D.; Data Curation, M.P.G.; Writing—Original Draft Preparation, S.E.P.; Writing—Review & Editing, S.E.P., J.T.D., M.P.G., J.R., J.M. and C.A.O.; Visualization, S.E.P. and J.T.D.; Project Administration, J.T.D.; Funding Acquisition, J.T.D., C.A.O. and J.M.

Funding: This research was funded by a grant from the National Institute for Occupational Safety and Health (NIOSH) for the Center for Work, Health and Well-being at the Harvard T.H. Chan School of Public Health, grant number U19 OH008861. Additional funding was provided by the NIOSH Education and Research Center at the Harvard Chan School, grant number T42OH008416.

Acknowledgments: The authors thank Glorian Sorensen, Greg Wagner, Jeffrey Katz, Emily Sparer, Kristin Ironside, Andrea Sheldon, Kincaid Lowe, and Mia Goldwasser from the Harvard T.H. Chan School of Public

Health Center for Work, Health, and Wellbeing. The authors also provide a special and extra thank you to all of our construction company partners in the Boston metropolitan area.

Conflicts of Interest: The authors declare no conflict of interest. The funders had no role in the design of the study; in the collection, analyses, or interpretation of data; in the writing of the manuscript, or in the decision to publish the results.

References

1. Bush, D.M.; Lipari, R.N. *The CBHSQ Report: Short Report—Substance Use and Substance Use Disorder by Industry*; Substance Abuse and Mental Health Services Administration: Rockville, MD, USA, 2015.
2. The Center for Construction Research and Training. *The Construction Chart Book. The U.S. Construction Industry and Its Workers*, 6th ed.; The Center for Construction Research and Training: Silver Spring, MD, USA, 2018.
3. Punnett, L.; Warren, N.; Henning, R.; Nobrega, S.; Cherniack, M. CPH-NEW Research Team. Participatory ergonomics as a model for integrated programs to prevent chronic disease. *J. Occup. Environ. Med.* **2013**, *55*, S19–S24. [CrossRef] [PubMed]
4. Caban-Martinez, A.J.; Lowe, K.A.; Herrick, R.; Kenwood, C.; Gagne, J.J.; Becker, J.F.; Schneider, S.P.; Dennerlein, J.T.; Sorensen, G. Construction workers working in musculoskeletal pain and engaging in leisure-time physical activity: Findings from a mixed-methods pilot study. *Am. J. Ind. Med.* **2014**, *57*, 819–825. [CrossRef] [PubMed]
5. Umer, W.; Antwi-Afari, M.F.; Li, H.; Szeto, G.P.Y.; Wong, A.Y.L. The prevalence of musculoskeletal symptoms in the construction industry: A systematic review and meta-analysis. *Int. Arch. Occup. Environ. Health* **2018**, *91*, 125–144. [CrossRef] [PubMed]
6. Pronk, N.P.; McLellan, D.L.; McGrail, M.P.; Olson, S.M.; McKinney, Z.J.; Katz, J.N.; Wagner, G.R.; Sorensen, G. Measurement tools for integrated worker health protection and promotion: Lessons learned from the Safewell Project. *J. Occup. Environ. Med.* **2016**, *58*, 651–658. [CrossRef] [PubMed]
7. Sorensen, G.; McLellan, D.L.; Sabbath, E.L.; Dennerlein, J.T.; Nagler, E.M.; Hurtado, D.A.; Pronk, N.P.; Wagner, G.R. Integrating worksite health protection and health promotion: A conceptual model for intervention and research. *Prev. Med.* **2016**, *91*, 188–196. [CrossRef] [PubMed]
8. McLellan, D.; Moore, W.; Nagler, E.; Sorensen, G. *Implementing an Integrated Approach Weaving Worker Health, Safety, and Well-being into the Fabric of Your Organization*; Harvard Center for Work, Health and Wellbeing: Boston, MA, USA, 2017; pp. 1–141.
9. Bureau of Labor Statistics. Nonfatal Occupational Injuries and Illnesses Requiring Days Away from Work. Available online: https://www.bls.gov/news.release/osh2.toc.htm (accessed on 1 June 2018).
10. Viester, L.; Verhagen, E.; Bongers, P.M.; van der Beek, A.J. Effectiveness of a Worksite Intervention for Male Construction Workers on Dietary and Physical Activity Behaviors, Body Mass Index, and Health Outcomes: Results of a Randomized Controlled Trial. *Am. J. Health Promot.* **2018**, *32*, 795–805. [CrossRef] [PubMed]
11. Robroek, S.J.W.; Jarvholm, B.; van der Beek, A.J.; Proper, K.I.; Wahlstrom, J.; Burdorf, A. Influence of obesity and physical workload on disability benefits among construction workers followed up for 37 years. *Occup. Environ. Med.* **2017**, *74*, 621–627. [CrossRef] [PubMed]
12. Viester, L.; Verhagen, E.A.; Oude Hengel, K.M.; Koppes, L.L.; van der Beek, A.J.; Bongers, P.M. The relation between body mass index and musculoskeletal symptoms in the working population. *BMC Musculoskelet. Disord.* **2013**, *14*, 238. [CrossRef] [PubMed]
13. Dietz, A.; Ramroth, H.; Urban, T.; Ahrens, W.; Becher, H. Exposure to cement dust, related occupational groups and laryngeal cancer risk: Results of a population based case-control study. *Int. J. Cancer* **2004**, *108*, 907–911. [CrossRef] [PubMed]
14. Kurihara, N.; Wada, O. Silicosis and smoking strongly increase lung cancer risk in silica-exposed workers. *Ind. Health* **2004**, *42*, 303–314. [CrossRef] [PubMed]
15. Lee, P.N. Relation between exposure to asbestos and smoking jointly and the risk of lung cancer. *Occup. Environ. Med.* **2001**, *58*, 145–153. [CrossRef] [PubMed]
16. Institute of Medicine and National Research Council. *Musculoskeletal Disorders and the Workplaces: Low Back and Upper Extremities*; The National Academies Press: Washington, DC, USA, 2001; pp. 1–512. ISBN 978-0-309-13200-2.

17. Weil, D. *The Fissured Workplace: Why Work Became So Bad for So Many and What Can Be Done to Improve it*; Harvard University Press: Cambridge, MA, USA, 2014; pp. 1–424. ISBN 9780674975446.
18. Sparer, E.H.; Herrick, R.F.; Dennerlein, J.T. Development of a safety communication and recognition program for construction. *New Solut.* **2015**, *25*, 42–58. [CrossRef] [PubMed]
19. Breslin, F.C.; Smith, P. Trial by fire: A multivariate examination of the relation between job tenure and work injuries. *Occup. Environ. Med.* **2006**, *63*, 27–32. [CrossRef] [PubMed]
20. Sorensen, G.; Barbeau, E.M. Integrating occupational health, safety and worksite health promotion: Opportunities for research and practice. *Med. Lav.* **2006**, *97*, 240–257. [PubMed]
21. Magnavita, N. Obstacles and future prospects: Considerations on health promotion activities for older workers in Europe. *Int. J. Environ. Res. Public Health* **2018**, *15*, 662. [CrossRef] [PubMed]
22. Bradley, C.J.; Grossman, D.C.; Hubbard, R.A.; Ortega, A.N.; Curry, S.J. integrated interventions for improving total worker health: A panel report from the national institutes of health pathways to prevention workshop: Total Worker Health-What's work got to do with it? *Ann. Intern. Med.* **2016**, *165*, 279–283. [CrossRef] [PubMed]
23. De Boer, A.G.; Burdorf, A.; van Duivenbooden, C.; Frings-Dresen, M.H. The effect of individual counselling and education on work ability and disability pension: A prospective intervention study in the construction industry. *Occup. Environ. Med.* **2007**, *64*, 792–797. [CrossRef]
24. Okechukwu, C.A.; Krieger, N.; Chen, J.; Sorensen, G.; Li, Y.; Barbeau, E.M. The association of workplace hazards and smoking in a U.S. multiethnic working-class population. *Public Health Rep.* **2010**, *125*, 225–233. [CrossRef] [PubMed]
25. Oude Hengel, K.M.; Blatter, B.M.; Joling, C.I.; van der Beek, A.J.; Bongers, P.M. Effectiveness of an intervention at construction worksites on work engagement, social support, physical workload, and need for recovery: Results from a cluster randomized controlled trial. *BMC Public Health* **2012**, *12*, 1008. [CrossRef] [PubMed]
26. Okechukwu, C.A.; Krieger, N.; Sorensen, G.; Li, Y.; Barbeau, E.M. MassBuilt: Effectiveness of an apprenticeship site-based smoking cessation intervention for unionized building trades workers. *Cancer Cause. Control* **2009**, *20*, 887–894. [CrossRef] [PubMed]
27. Saarela, K.L. A poster campaign for improving safety on shipyard scaffolds. *J. Saf. Res.* **1989**, *20*, 177–185. [CrossRef]
28. Van der Molen, H.F.; Basnet, P.; Hoonakker, P.L.; Lehtola, M.M.; Lappalainen, J.; Frings-Dresen, M.H.; Haslam, R.; Verbeek, J.H. Interventions to prevent injuries in construction workers. *Cochrane Database Syst. Rev.* **2018**, *2*, CD006251. [CrossRef] [PubMed]
29. Bena, A.; Berchialla, P.; Coffano, M.E.; Debernardi, M.L.; Icardi, L.G. Effectiveness of the training program for workers at construction sites of the high-speed railway line between Torino and Novara: Impact on injury rates. *Am. J. Ind. Med.* **2009**, *52*, 965–972. [CrossRef] [PubMed]
30. Caban-Martinez, A.J.; Moore, K.J.; Clarke, T.C.; Davila, E.P.; Clark, J.D.; Lee, D.J.; Fleming, L.E. Health Promotion at the Construction Work Site: The Lunch Truck Pilot Study. *Workplace Health Saf.* **2018**. [CrossRef] [PubMed]
31. Lingard, H.; Rowlinson, S. Behavior-based safety management in Hong Kong's construction industry. *J. Saf. Res.* **1997**, *28*, 243–256. [CrossRef]
32. Wickizer, T.M.; Kopjar, B.; Franklin, G.; Joesch, J. Do drug-free workplace programs prevent occupational injuries? Evidence from Washington State. *Health Serv. Res.* **2004**, *39*, 91–110. [CrossRef] [PubMed]
33. Van der Molen, H.F.; Sluiter, J.K.; Hulshof, C.T.; Vink, P.; van Duivenbooden, C.; Holman, R.; Frings-Dresen, M.H. Implementation of participatory ergonomics intervention in construction companies. *Scand. J. Work Environ. Health* **2005**, *31*, 191–204. [CrossRef] [PubMed]
34. Hess, J.A.; Hecker, S.; Weinstein, M.; Lunger, M. A participatory ergonomics intervention to reduce risk factors for low-back disorders in concrete laborers. *Appl. Ergon.* **2004**, *35*, 427–441. [CrossRef] [PubMed]
35. Sorensen, G.; McLellan, D.; Dennerlein, J.T.; Pronk, N.P.; Allen, J.D.; Boden, L.I.; Okechukwu, C.A.; Hashimoto, D.; Stoddard, A.; Wagner, G.R. Integration of health protection and health promotion: Rationale, indicators, and metrics. *J. Occup. Environ. Med.* **2013**, *55*, S12–S18. [CrossRef] [PubMed]
36. Sparer, E.H.; Catalano, P.J.; Herrick, R.F.; Dennerlein, J.T. Improving safety climate through a communication and recognition program for construction: A mixed methods study. *Scand. J. Work Environ. Health* **2016**, *42*, 329–337. [CrossRef] [PubMed]

37. Sparer, E.H.; Okechukwu, C.A.; Manjourides, J.; Herrick, R.F.; Katz, J.N.; Dennerlein, J.T. Length of time spent working on a commercial construction site and the associations with worker characteristics. *Am. J. Ind. Med.* **2015**, *58*, 964–973. [CrossRef] [PubMed]
38. American National Standards Institute. *ANSI Essential Requirements: Due Process Requirements for American National Standards*; American National Standards Institute: New York, NY, USA, 2012; pp. 1–27.
39. The National Institute for Occupational Safety and Health. Simple Solutions: Ergonomics for Construction Workers. DHHS (NIOSH) Publication No. 2007-122. Available online: https://www.cdc.gov/niosh/docs/2007-122/default.html (accessed on 1 June 2018).
40. Oude Hengel, K.M.; Joling, C.I.; Proper, K.I.; Blatter, B.M.; Bongers, P.M. A worksite prevention program for construction workers: Design of a randomized controlled trial. *BMC Public Health* **2010**, *10*, 336. [CrossRef] [PubMed]
41. Viester, L.; Verhagen, E.A.; Proper, K.I.; van Dongen, J.M.; Bongers, P.M.; van der Beek, A.J. VIP in construction: Systematic development and evaluation of a multifaceted health programme aiming to improve physical activity levels and dietary patterns among construction workers. *BMC Public Health* **2012**, *12*, 89. [CrossRef] [PubMed]
42. Kuorinka, I.; Jonsson, B.; Kilbom, A.; Vinterberg, H.; Biering-Sorensen, F.; Andersson, G.; Jorgensen, K. Standardized Nordic Questionnaires for the analysis of musculoskeletal symptoms. *Appl. Ergon.* **1987**, *18*, 233–237. [CrossRef]
43. Harley, A.E.; Yang, M.; Stoddard, A.M.; Adamkiewicz, G.; Walker, R.; Tucker-Seeley, R.D.; Allen, J.D.; Sorensen, G. Patterns and Predictors of Health Behaviors Among Racially/Ethnically Diverse Residents of Low-Income Housing Developments. *Am. J. Health Promot.* **2014**, *29*, 59–67. [CrossRef] [PubMed]
44. Prochaska, J.J.; Velicer, W.F.; Nigg, C.R.; Prochaska, J.O. Methods of quantifying change in multiple risk factor interventions. *Prev. Med.* **2008**, *46*, 260–265. [CrossRef] [PubMed]
45. Pierannunzi, C.; Hu, S.S.; Balluz, L. A systematic review of publications assessing reliability and validity of the Behavioral Risk Factor Surveillance System (BRFSS), 2004–2011. *BMC Med. Res. Methodol.* **2013**, *13*, 49. [CrossRef] [PubMed]
46. Cigarette Smoking among Adults—United States, 1992, and Changes in the Definition of Current Cigarette Smoking. *MMWR. Morb. Mortal. Wkly. Rep.* **1994**, *43*, 342. Available online: https://www.cdc.gov/mmwr/preview/mmwrhtml/00033250.htm (accessed on 1 June 2018).
47. Amick, B.C.; Habeck, R.V.; Hunt, A.; Fossel, A.H.; Chapin, A.; Keller, R.B.; Katz, J.N. Measuring the impact of organizational behaviors on work disability prevention and management. *J. Occup. Rehabil.* **2000**, *10*, 21–38. [CrossRef]
48. Lerner, D.; Amick, B.C.; Rogers, W.H.; Malspeis, S.; Bungay, K.; Cynn, D. The Work Limitations Questionnaire. *Med. Care* **2001**, *39*, 72–85. [CrossRef] [PubMed]
49. Marras, W.S.; Lavender, S.A.; Leurgans, S.E.; Fathallah, F.A.; Ferguson, S.A.; Allread, W.G.; Rajulu, S.L. Biomechanical risk factors for occupationally related low back disorders. *Ergonomics* **1995**, *38*, 377–410. [CrossRef] [PubMed]
50. Tveito, T.H.; Shaw, W.S.; Huang, Y.H.; Nicholas, M.; Wagner, G. Managing pain in the workplace: A focus group study of challenges, strategies and what matters most to workers with low back pain. *Disabil. Rehabil.* **2010**, *32*, 2035–2045. [CrossRef] [PubMed]
51. Dennerlein, J.T. Chronic low back pain: A successful intervention for desk-bound workers. *Occup. Environ. Med.* **2018**, *75*, 319–320. [CrossRef] [PubMed]
52. Harvard Business Review. 7 Ways to Improve Operations without Sacrificing Worker Safety by David Michaels. Available online: https://hbr.org/2018/03/7-ways-to-improve-operations-without-sacrificing-worker-safety (accessed on 21 March 2018).
53. Dasgupta, P.; Sample, M.; Buchholz, B.; Brunette, M. Is worker involvement an ergonomic solution for construction intervention challenges: A systematic review. *Theory Issues Ergon. Sci.* **2017**, *18*, 433–441. [CrossRef]
54. Dale, A.M.; Jaegers, L.; Welch, L.; Barnidge, E.; Weaver, N.; Evanoff, B.A. Facilitators and barriers to the adoption of ergonomic solutions in construction. *Am. J. Ind. Med.* **2017**, *60*, 295–305. [CrossRef] [PubMed]
55. Occupational Safety and Health Administration. Training Requirements in OSHA Standards. OSHA 2254-09R 2015. Available online: https://www.osha.gov/Publications/osha2254.pdf (accessed on 1 June 2018).

56. Boschman, J.S.; Frings-Dresen, M.H.W.; van der Molen, H.F. Use of Ergonomic Measures Related to Musculoskeletal Complaints among Construction Workers: A 2-year Follow-up Study. *Saf. Health Work* **2015**, *6*, 90–96. [CrossRef] [PubMed]
57. Visser, S.; van der Molen, H.F.; Sluiter, J.K.; Frings-Dresen, M.H.W. The process evaluation of two alternative participatory ergonomics intervention strategies for construction companies. *Ergonomics* **2018**, *61*, 1156–1172. [CrossRef] [PubMed]
58. Dale, A.M.; Jaegers, L.; Welch, L.; Gardner, B.T.; Buchholz, B.; Weaver, N.; Evanoff, B.A. Evaluation of a participatory ergonomics intervention in small commercial construction firms. *Am. J. Ind. Med.* **2016**, *59*, 465–475. [CrossRef] [PubMed]
59. Dennerlein, J.T.; O'Day, E.T.; Mulloy, D.F.; Somerville, J.; Stoddard, A.M.; Kenwood, C.; Teeple, E.; Boden, L.I.; Sorensen, G.; Hashimoto, D. Lifting and exertion injuries decrease after implementation of an integrated hospital-wide safe patient handling and mobilisation programme. *Occup. Environ. Med.* **2017**, *74*, 336–343. [CrossRef] [PubMed]
60. Sorensen, G.; Sparer, E.; Williams, J.A.R.; Gundersen, D.; Boden, L.I.; Dennerlein, J.T.; Hashimoto, D.; Katz, J.N.; McLellan, D.L.; Okechukwu, C.A.; et al. Measuring best practices for workplace safety, health and wellbeing: The Workplace Integrated Safety and Health assessment. *J. Occup. Environ. Med.* **2018**, *60*, 430–439. [CrossRef] [PubMed]
61. Viester, L.; Verhagen, E.A.; Bongers, P.M.; van der Beek, A.J. The effect of a health promotion intervention for construction workers on work-related outcomes: Results from a randomized controlled trial. *Int. Arch. Occup. Environ. Health* **2015**, *88*, 789–798. [CrossRef] [PubMed]
62. Manjourides, J.; Sparer, E.H.; Okechukwu, C.A.; Dennerlein, J.T. The Effect of Workforce Mobility on Intervention Effectiveness Estimates. *Ann. Work Expo. Health* **2018**, *62*, 259–268. [CrossRef] [PubMed]
63. Magnavita, N. Medical surveillance, continuous health promotion and a participatory intervention in a small company. *Int. J. Environ. Res. Public Health* **2018**, *15*, 662. [CrossRef] [PubMed]
64. Sokas, R.K.; Jorgensen, E.; Nickels, L.; Gao, W.; Gittleman, J.L. An intervention effectiveness study of hazard awareness training in the construction building trades. *Public Health Rep.* **2009**, *124*, 160–168. [CrossRef] [PubMed]
65. The Center for Construction Research and Training. Diffusing Ergonomic Innovations in Construction (Completed—2004–2009). Available online: http://orcehs.org/wiki/display/orcehs/Construction+Ergonomics (accessed on 31 October 2010).
66. Strickland, J.R.; Smock, N.; Casey, C.; Poor, T.; Kreuter, M.W.; Evanoff, B.A. Development of targeted messages to promote smoking cessation among construction trade workers. *Health Educ. Res.* **2015**, *30*, 107–120. [CrossRef] [PubMed]
67. Dale, A.M.; Strand, J.; Schneider, S.; Cain, C.; Rempel, D. Piloting of a social marketing campaign to reduce musculoskeletal risks related to manual materials handling on construction projects. *Occup. Environ. Med.* **2018**, *75*. [CrossRef]
68. Rempel, D.; Star, D.; Barr, A.; Janowitz, I. Overhead drilling: Comparing three bases for aligning a drilling jig to vertical. *J. Saf. Res.* **2010**, *41*, 247–251. [CrossRef] [PubMed]

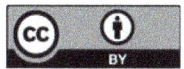

© 2018 by the authors. Licensee MDPI, Basel, Switzerland. This article is an open access article distributed under the terms and conditions of the Creative Commons Attribution (CC BY) license (http://creativecommons.org/licenses/by/4.0/).

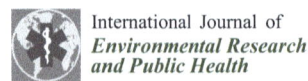

Article

From Research-to-Practice: An Adaptation and Dissemination of the COMPASS Program for Home Care Workers

Ryan Olson [1,2,3,*], Jennifer A. Hess [4], Kelsey N. Parker [1], Sharon V. Thompson [1,5], Anjali Rameshbabu [1], Kristy Luther Rhoten [1] and Miguel Marino [6]

1. Oregon Institute of Occupational Health Sciences, Oregon Health & Science University (OHSU), Portland, OR 97239, USA; kelsnparker@gmail.com (K.N.P.); svthomp2@illinois.edu (S.V.T.); rameshba@ohsu.edu (A.R.); luther.kristy@gmail.com (K.L.R.)
2. Oregon Health & Science University (OHSU)-Portland State University School of Public Health, Portland, OR 97239, USA
3. Department of Psychology, Portland State University, Portland, OR 97201, USA
4. Labor Education and Research Center, University of Oregon, Eugene, OR 97403, USA; jhessdc@gmail.com
5. Division of Nutritional Sciences, University of Illinois at Urbana-Champaign, Urbana, IL 61801, USA
6. Department of Family Medicine, Oregon Health & Science University, Portland, OR 97239, USA; marinom@ohsu.edu
* Correspondence: olsonry@ohsu.edu; Tel.: +1-503-494-2501

Received: 18 October 2018; Accepted: 24 November 2018; Published: 7 December 2018

Abstract: The COMmunity of Practice And Safety Support (COMPASS) program was developed to prevent injuries and advance the health and well-being of home care workers. The program integrates elements of peer-led social support groups with scripted team-based programs to help workers learn together, solve problems, set goals, make changes, and enrich their supportive professional network. After a successful pilot study and randomized controlled trial, COMPASS was adapted for the Oregon Home Care Commission's training system for statewide dissemination. The adapted program included fewer total meetings (7 versus 13), an accelerated meeting schedule (every two weeks versus monthly), and a range of other adjustments. The revised approach was piloted with five groups of workers (total n = 42) and evaluated with pre- and post-program outcome measures. After further adjustments and planning, the statewide rollout is now in progress. In the adaptation pilot several psychosocial, safety, and health outcomes changed by a similar magnitude relative to the prior randomized controlled trial. Preliminary training evaluation data (n = 265) show high mean ratings indicating that workers like the program, find the content useful, and intend to make changes after meetings. Facilitating factors and lessons learned from the project may inform future similar efforts to translate research into practice.

Keywords: home care workers; workplace; occupational; safety; health; well-being; dissemination

1. Introduction

For many Americans, especially older adults, home care workers (HCWs) are a vital source of daily personal support that facilitates their ability to "age in place." With a growing proportion of aging adults in the US population in coming years, the currently estimated 2.9 million home care and personal care aides is projected to increase by 41% between 2016 and 2026. This growth rate is considerably higher than the 7% average growth for all US occupations [1].

HCWs face job demands that are unique and multi-faceted, and they often lack resources or supports to help them meet such demands [2]. Despite the important service they provide in communities, HCWs remain poorly compensated with a median income of $23,130 that is considerably lower than the median for all US workers [1]. Nearly half the nation's HCWs rely on low-income tax credits and federal assistance programs to make ends meet [3]. HCWs face a number of physical demands and exposures as they assist older adults with activities of daily living, such as walking and other movements, personal hygiene, dressing, bathing, cooking, and housekeeping. Thus, HCWs often suffer from musculoskeletal strain, are exposed to infectious agents and hazardous chemicals, and are at-risk for puncture injuries from sharps when clients do not discard them properly [4]. Further, because they work alone within the homes of their clients, HCWs lack many occupational safety and health protections that are commonly available for employees in more traditional workplaces (e.g., supervision, environmental safety audits, employer assessment and correction of hazards, co-worker support, safety committees, and safety training) [2]. The degree of worker vulnerability differs for independent contractors compared to those who work for home care agencies, but most all HCWs experience deficits in protections to some degree.

Although HCWs report high satisfaction from the close relationships they develop with clients [4], some home care clients may engage in very challenging behaviors, including verbal and physical aggression. HCWs report incidents of verbal and sexual harassment, which are associated with stress, depression, sleep problems, and burnout [5]. The unique profile of challenges for HCWs points to the critical need for interventions geared toward protecting their safety, health, and well-being.

Research with this socially important workgroup has led to the development of effective interventions to reduce blood and body fluid exposures [6], reduce musculoskeletal pain [7], and improve physical fitness and work ability [8]. Socially supportive group interventions have produced long-term improvements in well-being for family caregivers [9] and improved a range of safety, health, and well-being factors among independent HCWs serving consumer-employers in publicly funded programs in Oregon [10]. In addition to experimentally evaluated programs, there are valuable resources for HCWs developed through participatory methods. For example, the Safe Home Care Project provides resources on safe cleaning and disinfection and on safe practices to reduce risk of injuries from sharps and blood-borne exposures (University of Massachusetts, Lowell, Safe Home Care, n.d. [11]). The Caring for Yourself While Caring for Others handbook (National Institute for Occupational Safety and Health [NIOSH] n.d. [12]) provides a checklist of potentially hazardous work tasks, along with tips and tools for preventing exposures and injuries for each family of tasks. The handbook also addresses communication strategies and workplace stress. Helpful illustrations show workers examples and non-examples of safe practices and tool use, and overall, the book is designed to help facilitate conversations between workers and their clients (or with their family members or workplace supervisors) about improving workplace safety.

1.1. Translating Evidence-Based Interventions into Practice

In the healthcare domain, Balas and Boren [13] stated that " ... it takes an average of 17 years for research evidence to reach clinical practice" (p. 66). For nine clinical procedures established effective in landmark trials, the authors reported current rates of procedure use between 17.0% to 70.4%. Even in medicine, there are very long time lines to realize variable degrees of adoption.

Typically, an intervention's reach beyond the research setting is limited by constraints such as a lack of funding to facilitate its usability and scalability or the absence of structures or partners to market it to potential adopters. In some cases, an intervention's features may not encourage its transfer to practice (e.g., too complex, costly, or effortful to implement). Moreover, intervention researchers are typically evaluated and rewarded for obtaining competitive grants, conducting innovative and high quality research, and publishing research findings. Occupational incentives are not typically aligned for investigators to adapt, commercialize, market, and disseminate the evidence-based programs they create or study. These types of barriers include the overarching culture of peer review, which tends to emphasize factors related to the internal validity of intervention studies over issues related to external validity (e.g., factors that influence participation, adoption, and implementation). To illustrate, in a review of health promotion intervention research using the widely recognized RE-AIM framework,

Bull and colleagues [14] reported that just 25% of studies reported information on adoption, and only 12.5% reported implementation data.

In order to overcome some of these barriers, Harris and colleagues [15] proposed a dissemination framework that addresses the gap between scientists and end users of evidence-based health promotion interventions. Their approach relies on a motivated "disseminator" or intermediary organization to help researchers adapt, market, and disseminate interventions. In their model, researchers and intermediary disseminating organizations form a reciprocal relationship that generates "Dissemination Resources" that are then marketed to end users—primarily by the disseminating organization. The authors provided two examples of interventions that were successfully disseminated through this approach that had reached nearly 2000 employers and community based adopters at the time of the publication.

Systematic reviews of research on the translation of community-based interventions into practice suggest additional facilitators for success. Matthews and colleagues [16] shared that translating physical activity interventions into practice was facilitated by tailoring an intervention to suit the intended adopter, partnering strategically with receptive organizations, and adequately training implementers. In another review, Estabrooks and Glasgow [17] shared that interventions are more translation-friendly if they are perceived by the intended users as being more advantageous than existing practices, compatible with their current needs and values, feasible to deliver and implement, able to be tested for potential adoption, and have demonstrated effectiveness among stakeholders [18].

Other dissemination research highlights the importance of commitment from organizational leaders (including financial support) and the presence of workplace champions. The successful large-scale adoption of the evidence-based Stand Up Australia intervention (disseminated as the BeUpstanding Program^{TM}) was attributed by researchers in part to a strong partnership with and timely funding support from the adopter (government, in this case). The authors also reported the importance of packaging the intervention into an online toolkit, and then transferring the toolkit to a workplace champion. The toolkit helped champions by providing practical strategies for making a business case for the intervention, obtaining buy-in from organizational leaders, and how to deliver and evaluate the program [19]. Qualitative research with adopters and non-adopters of the evidence-based PHLAME wellness program for firefighters highlighted the importance of a committed chief and the presence of a workplace wellness champion at adopting fire stations (i.e., the "champ-and-chief" model of adoption) [20].

1.2. Translating Home Care Worker Interventions for Practice

Although evidence-based and useful interventions for HCWs and other caregivers are available, we were unable to find any peer-reviewed publications regarding their dissemination. Therefore, we reached out for phone interviews with contacts for caregiver programs or resources we were familiar with. The principal investigator for the Safe Home Care Project (M. Quinn, personal communication, 5 October 2018) indicated that its dissemination occurs via fact sheets containing safety and health education, publications in scientific journals, and articles within HCW trade association magazines. The Health Education Program, a supportive group program for family caregivers, is distributed by the principal investigator when requested by caregiver agencies (R. Toseland, 26 September 2018). The Caring For Yourself While Caring For Others handbook, developed by the Labor Occupational Health Program in partnership with NIOSH for Alameda County workers in California, was later adopted within the Alameda County Health Consortium. However, its current dissemination channels outside of being downloadable through its website are unknown (L. Stock, 26 September 2018). In these selected cases, translation, dissemination, and adoption efforts have not been systematically described, and appear to have been supported by dedicated principal investigators or partners without funding or formal systemic support following initial development and evaluation research.

In our view, an important way to address this gap and inform future translation and dissemination efforts, is to publish qualitative and quantitative descriptions of barriers, facilitators, and successes in dissemination after interventions are established to be effective. On this theme, the current paper reports the process and results of a successful intervention adaptation and dissemination effort in progress. The COMmunity of Practice And Safety Support (COMPASS) program was designed to advance the safety, health, and well-being of HCWs. The intervention's peer-led and supportive group tactics are aimed at creating a protective occupational social support structure for typically isolated HCWs. Developed using a *Total Worker Health*® approach, COMPASS simultaneously focused on reducing hazards for injuries and illnesses, while also promoting factors to advance workers' health and well-being. The intervention was developed with labor and governmental partners, and was demonstrated effective through a cluster randomized controlled trial (RCT). A range of factors showed significant improvements, including workers' experienced community of practice, safety behaviors (including ergonomic tool use), and health factors (such as fruit and vegetable consumption [10]). Following the RCT, COMPASS was adapted for dissemination with the Oregon Home Care Commission (OHCC), pilot tested in its adapted form, and is now being rolled out statewide by the OHCC as a paid training opportunity available to roughly 60% of Oregon's home care workforce. The current project describes original and adapted programs, results from the pilot test of the adapted program, and preliminary training evaluation data from the COMPASS rollout by the OHCC.

2. Materials and Methods

The COMPASS research program began formally in 2011 as a research project within the Oregon Healthy Workforce Center, a Center of Excellence in *Total Worker Health*® (NIOSH U19OH010154). Over the life of the program, all COMPASS research procedures have been reviewed and approved by the Oregon Health & Science University Human Subjects Institutional Review Board. Research partners include the Service Employees International Union Local 503 and the OHCC. After supporting initial development and evaluation research, both the union and the OHCC continued support for the intervention's translation into practice, with the OHCC as the ultimate adopting organization. The OHCC is housed within Oregon's Department of Human Services as a component of state-supported Services for Seniors and People with Disabilities. The OHCC is charged with defining qualifications for HCWs and other caregivers who provide services for consumers who qualify for publicly funded care. These HCWs work as independent contractors without a supporting home care agency, supervisor, or co-workers, and are employed directly by their clients who are referred to as "consumer-employers." The OHCC operates a training system offering over 20 course topics for HCWs and personal support workers throughout the state, manages a registry to match workers with consumer-employers (or consumer-employers with workers), and serves as the employer of record for collective bargaining with the union.

The original three-year long COMPASS research project [21] included intervention development followed by a pilot study [22] and cluster RCT [10]. The original trial design involved baseline, 6 month, and 12 month measurements. Participants were recruited from among the population of HCWs caring for consumer-employers who qualified for publicly funded home care services through the OHCC managed system. As the RCT was underway, the Oregon Healthy Workforce Center applied for and was awarded an additional two years of funding. In that extended two-year agenda an additional follow-up measurement was added (≈24 months post-baseline), as well as qualitative research focused on caregivers' experiences at work and in the COMPASS program [2]. Further research was planned to conduct interviews with leaders and workers at private home care agencies to inform future dissemination in that industry segment. However, when the opportunity arose to adapt and potentially disseminate COMPASS within the OHCC training system, dissemination aims with private agencies were postponed and the intervention was adapted and piloted for dissemination in the Commission's training program. Translation and dissemination efforts continued after research grant funding for COMPASS ended in 2016. Further adaptation of the intervention materials and process was completed with financial support from the Commission and the Oregon Institute of Occupational

Health Sciences at Oregon Health & Science University. In the Fall of 2017 COMPASS was added to the OHCC's training system as a paid course offering for workers. Below we describe the methods for each phase of the COMPASS research with an emphasis on how intervention materials and processes were adapted, piloted, and translated into practice.

2.1. COMPASS Pilot and Randomized Controlled Trial

The original COMPASS intervention development and evaluation has been described in previous publications in detail. However, a high-level summary is needed to understand how materials and processes were modified for translation into practice. COMPASS is a supportive group program that is peer-led and scripted. Intervention tactics employed were modeled on effective social support groups [9,23,24] and scripted team-based health promotion programs [25–28]. Original intervention resources developed included two types of guidebooks: a group leader guidebook with additional instructions and activity answers, and a group member guidebook without those group-leader specific instructions and activity answers. In both the pilot and RCT, groups met monthly to complete a scripted meeting that followed a ritualized structure. Each meeting involved a WorkLife check-in, educational lesson, goal setting and follow-up, a healthy meal break, and a WorkLife support activity.

The curriculum was developed in two phases so the RCT could begin while investigators continued to develop and pilot test additional scripted meetings. In the first phase, leader and member versions of guidebook one were developed with seven scripted meetings that were evaluated by workers ($n = 16$) in the published pilot study, and then revised and evaluated in the first half of the RCT intervention phase (16 clusters of workers, $n = 149$). In addition to the scripted meetings, guidebook one included an "Extras" section with additional resources for workers, including the Gershon Home Hazard Checklist, the NIOSH Caring for Yourself While Caring for Others handbook, and perforated cards printed with templates for behavioral self-monitoring activities. Pages for tracking attendance and goals were also included. In an unpublished phase of the pilot study, guidebook two (six additional meetings) was developed and then evaluated with a subgroup of pilot participants ($n \approx 6$) as the RCT began using guidebook one. Guidebook two was also modified based on pilot results, and then used in the second half of the RCT intervention phase. The second guidebook included a slightly different structure. In the educational lesson component, groups chose from a menu of homework reading topic options to read before the next meeting; these topics were then discussed at the next meeting using a structured discussion guide. Like the first guidebook, the second guidebook included forms for tracking attendance and goal completion and perforated cards printed with templates for behavioral self-monitoring activities.

Seven of the eight original RCT intervention groups were led by a permanent peer-leader who was involved in the published pilot study. The eighth group lacked a peer-leader from the pilot, and was therefore led by two peer co-leaders who volunteered for this role at their group's first meeting. Guidebook materials were supported with a peer leader toolkit of ergonomic tools and objects for activities (slide boards, transfer belts, anti-friction disks, Gimme-A-Lift, and tennis balls), as well as resource giveaways used for completing "take home goals" (knee pads, step counters, and wrist bead counters for behavioral self-monitoring). Workers also received pay and incentives for attending meetings and research data collection waves, and were recognized with participation-based incentives for earning individual and/or group certification. During the first six months, participants obtained individual certification if they attended five team meetings and completed five individual goals; teams were certified if the entire team completed five team goals. During the second six months individual certification was earned if the participant attended at least four meetings and completed eight individual goals (one repeat goal and one new goal were selected each meeting); team certification was awarded if all team members completed four or more team goals. Those who earned individual certification obtained a $60 gift certificate and certified teams received COMPASS jackets (first six months) and COMPASS umbrellas or a team patch (second six months). Participants were paid $11 an hour through the grant for study-related activities prior to October 2013, and $15 an hour thereafter following a state-wide wage increase. Supplemental incentives included a $30 retention bonus at follow-up research data collection periods, lottery drawings for supplemental compensation awards totaling $1000 (many small awards were drawn), and additional gifts at baseline (COMPASS tote bag), 6 months (COMPASS t-shirt), and 12 months (COMPASS lunch bag).

2.2. COMPASS Adaptation and Pilot for the OHCC

During the development and research phases for COMPASS investigators solicited union and OHCC input, provided regular updates to the OHCC training committee and the union to inform them of progress and findings, and periodically discussed the future of the program. Following the successful RCT, and in response to ongoing dialogue about the program, the OHCC requested that investigators adapt COMPASS to be offered as a paid training course in their system. One motivation for this decision expressed by OHCC leaders was an interest in cultivating leadership skills among HCWs. A plan for adapting COMPASS guidebook one was worked out collaboratively, implemented by researchers, and then pilot tested. Adjustments to the approach were guided by OHCC practical needs, but with a commitment to retaining core evidence-based tactics. Adjustments included: a faster cycle time, where groups met every other week instead of once a month; reduction of total meetings to seven (e.g., only topics from guidebook one); the use of professional OHCC-contracted trainers to serve as group facilitators who would lead the first meeting and then support each group as a "guide on the side" thereafter; using rotating volunteer peer-leaders at meetings two through seven; removing the meal served during breaks; replacing some original group and individual goals to attend related OHCC trainings with new goals focused on workers making targeted work-environment and behavior changes; and incentive adjustments. The long-term strategic plan also included proposed adjustments to training evaluation questions for all OHCC training courses in order to accommodate a peer-led course series like COMPASS. Table 1 summarizes COMPASS guidebook one original topics and goals, as well as adaptations (most adaptations were made prior to the adaptation pilot, but some were made afterward).

The adaptation pilot involved five COMPASS groups led by four OHCC facilitators in three Oregon cities. This sampling approach was selected to provide a check that the adjusted process was functional across multiple facilitators and groups, and that the intervention was changing targeted outcomes by a similar magnitude (effect size) relative to the effective version evaluated in the RCT. Workers received hourly wages for attending COMPASS adaptation pilot meetings, just as they would for attending other courses offered by the OHCC (workers receive wages for any non-duplicated course annually). Pilot participants received an additional $15 for completing surveys and/or taking part in an interview with study staff. Plans were also made for COMPASS to satisfy safety training requirements (completion of two safety courses every two years) for workers to be listed on the OHCC registry for finding (or being found by) potential new Medicaid/Medicare-funded consumer-employers. The adapted program was supported with the same ergonomic toolkit and resource giveaways as the intervention as implemented in the RCT. However, no incentives were provided for individual or group certification. Instead, printed paper certificates were awarded based on attendance. As noted above, professional trainers under contract with the OHCC were identified to serve as COMPASS facilitators. The research team created a half-day orientation and facilitator training workshop to prepare facilitators for their role. This training included a history of the program and research findings, description and handouts on the role of facilitators, and practice with scripted guidebook activities with coaching from researchers. Guidebooks and other materials for implementation were provided to facilitators before their first group meeting.

Table 1. COMmunity of Practice And Safety Support (COMPASS) guidebook one: Topics with original and adapted goal options (adaptations are in **bold italics**).

	Meeting and Topic	Content and/or Sample Activities	Original Goals	Adjusted Goals (as of Fall 2018)
1.	Team Building Workshop	• Team building activities • How safety and health are related • How COMPASS teams work	Group Goal • Odds and Evens Step Challenge Individual Goal Options • Watch a "23 and ½ h" video • Daily activity tracking with app • Take an OHCC class on any topic	Group Goal • Odds and Evens *Walking Minutes* Challenge Individual Goal Options ***Aim for 30 min daily walking via:*** • *Workday walks* • *Errand/commute walks* • *Free time walks*
2.	Fruits & Vegetables *More Plants on the Plate*	• Fruit and vegetable serving sizes and recommendations • Nutrition information and game(s) • *Harvard Healthy Eating Plate and whole foods*	Group Goal • Bring healthy recipe to share with group Individual Goal Options • Track fruit and veggie servings and strive for 5 daily • Try four new fruits or veggies or prepare them in a new way • Swap out sugary drinks and replace with water or zero calorie drinks	Group Goal • *Fruit and veggie challenge to track and eat 5 servings daily for two weeks* Individual Goal Options • *Fill half of plate at meals with fruits and vegetables* • *Swap out high-calorie snacks and replace with fruit or veggie snacks* • *Swap out sugary drinks and replace with water or zero calorie drinks*
3.	Back to Healthy Postures	• Practice finding neutral spine • Tips for maintaining neutral spine during common activities	Group Goal • Track neutral spine postures by task or alarm Individual Goal Options • Track neutral spine by alarm • Track neutral spine by task • Attend OHCC class titled "Protecting Against Sprains and Strains"	Group Goal • *Identify a housekeeping task and do in a new way that protects neutral spine posture* Individual Goal Options • Track neutral spine by task • Track neutral spine by alarm • *Deleted OHCC course goal*

Table 1. Cont.

	Meeting and Topic	Content and/or Sample Activities	Original Goals	Adjusted Goals (as of Fall 2018)
4.	Functional Fitness	<ul><li>Core strength and practical/functional fitness</li><li>Anywhere core exercises</li><li>Healthy Hobbies</li></ul>	Group Goal<ul><li>Repeat Odds and Evens Step Challenge</li></ul>Individual Goal Options<ul><li>Core exercise scavenger hunt</li><li>Pair with group member and do a healthy hobby activity</li><li>Find and take part in an exercise class/resource in the community</li></ul>	Group Goal<ul><li>Repeat Odds and Evens *Walking Minutes* Challenge</li></ul>Individual Goal Options<ul><li>Core exercise scavenger hunt</li><li>*Strength training twice a week*</li><li>Find and take part in an exercise class/resource in the community</li></ul>
5.	Take a Load Off With Tools	<ul><li>Safety traps that lead to injuries</li><li>Common injuries</li><li>Low tech tool introduction and practice</li></ul>	Group Goal<ul><li>Complete the "Gershon Home Hazard Checklist" in consumer-employers' homes</li></ul>Individual Goal Options<ul><li>Attend relevant OHCC class like "Durable Medical Equipment" or "Protect Against Sprains and Strains"</li><li>Research tools online or at a medical supply store</li><li>Watch video on Gimme-a-Lift or Slide Boards with Transfer Belts</li></ul>	Group Goal<ul><li>*Complete the NIOSH "Caring for Yourself While Caring for Others" hazard checklist*</li></ul>Individual Goal Options<ul><li>*Increase use of tools already on hand*</li><li>*Use the "Caring for Yourself While Caring for Others" booklet to identify tools needed*</li><li>*Talk to a case manager about needed tools or training*</li></ul>

Table 1. Cont.

Meeting and Topic	Content and/or Sample Activities	Original Goals	Adjusted Goals (as of Fall 2018)
6. Communicating for Hazard Correction	<ul><li>Learn effective and less effective ways to communicate about hazards</li><li>Learn PRAISE mnemonic communication strategy</li><li>Role play communication with consumer-employer</li></ul>	Group Goal<ul><li>Use the NIOSH "Caring for Yourself While Caring for Others" booklet and discuss relevant hazards with your consumer-employer</li></ul>Individual Goal Options<ul><li>Good day/bad day interview with consumer-employer</li><li>Attend OHCC class on communication such as "Challenging Behaviors", Keeping it Professional", or "Working Together"</li><li>Use PRAISE strategy with others</li></ul>	Group Goal<ul><li>Discuss relevant hazards with your consumer-employer *that you identified previously using the NIOSH "Caring for Yourself While Caring for Others" booklet*</li></ul>Individual Goal Options<ul><li>Good day/bad day interview with consumer-employer</li><li>Use PRAISE *skills with a friend or co-worker*</li><li>*Find and correct a hazard in your own home*</li></ul>
7. Mental Health	<ul><li>Practice guided relaxation</li><li>Three good things activity</li><li>*Positive/negative talk activity and healthy stress coping*</li></ul>	Group Goal<ul><li>Set a personal safety or health goal from any area COMPASS covered</li></ul>Individual Goal Options<ul><li>Gratitude journal</li><li>Progressive muscle relaxation daily for one week</li><li>Attend OHCC class "Stress Management and Relaxation Techniques"</li></ul>	Group Goal<ul><li>*COMPASS mental health book club*</li></ul>Individual Goal Options<ul><li>Gratitude journal</li><li>Progressive muscle relaxation daily for one week</li><li>*Track stressful events and practice healthy stress coping strategies learned in COMPASS*</li></ul>

Note: Guidebook adjustments are noted with **bold italics**. NIOSH: National Institute for Occupational Safety and Health; OHCC: Oregon Home Care Commission. All goals had "short hand" names for workers to remember and name their choice easily, but in the table, are written out in descriptive form. In the randomized trial version of COMPASS, groups used a poster with the image of a house with doors and windows to track group and individual goal completion. In the adapted version of COMPASS the poster was not used due to removal of the certification incentives (a simple attendance requirement for getting COMPASS safety class credits was instituted instead). The PRAISE mnemonic was created by Dr. Robert Wright, and stood for: Plan, Respect, Ask open ended questions, use "I" statements, and Express empathy.

At baseline researchers collected direct measures of height (SECA 213 stadiometer; SECA, Chino, CA, USA) and weight (Tanita TBF-310GS; Tanita Corp, Arlington Heights, IL, USA), and survey measures of demographics, work history, and current work characteristics. Pre- and post-program evaluation measures emphasized outcomes from the prior RCT [10]. Survey scales/items included experienced community of practice [29]; frequency counts for five types of safety behaviors [10]; fruit and vegetable consumption (single item 1–10+ servings daily, created for adaptation pilot); consumption of sugary drinks, snacks, and fast food meals [30]; frequency of meals brought from home [30]; weekly healthy physical activity levels [26]; and physical and psychological well-being [31].

2.3. Statewide Rollout of COMPASS in the OHCC Training System

In parallel with and following the adaptation pilot test, several efforts were initiated to support eventual adoption and statewide rollout of COMPASS within the OHCC's training system. These efforts included initiating negotiations for an interagency agreement between Oregon Health & Science University (OHSU) and the Oregon Department of Human Services to govern the terms of use of guidebooks; investigators requesting adjustments to the standard OHCC training evaluation questions to accommodate a course series like COMPASS; and revisions to the OHCC version of the COMPASS guidebook in response to observing the pilot and in response to guidance from OHSU Technology Transfer and Business Development. We also explored whether other stakeholders, such as the relevant workers' compensation insurer or an SEIU Health Trust, would support or fund parts of the dissemination effort. These conversations did not result in direct financial support for dissemination efforts, but helped guide sustainability decisions and resulted in in the addition of information about an Employee Assistance Program available to HCWs to the Extras section of COMPASS guidebooks.

Negotiations for terms of use of the program took quite a long time, in part due to the timing of the retirement of the OHCC's Training Director and other staff turnover. Other hurdles involved navigating unclear review and approval steps within the state government, and some long inter-agency response times for document review requests. At the conclusion of over a year of episodic back-and-forth work and hand-offs on the inter-agency research agreement, the ultimate terms granted the OHCC non-exclusive rights to print and use COMPASS guidebooks in exchange for sharing long-term evaluation data with OHSU (5+ years). Evaluation data would include class attendance for COMPASS and non-COMPASS courses, class evaluations, and assisting OHSU in coordinating with the workers' compensation insurer to obtain injury claims data for workers who took COMPASS over the years and cross-sectional comparison groups of workers who either had not taken any training, and those who had taken some training classes (but not COMPASS).

Within the OHCC training system, at the end of each class HCWs are asked to complete a training evaluation (no names recorded) and leave it for their trainer to collect. Some of these original evaluation items did not clearly apply to a peer-led and scripted program. For example, one item asked workers to rate the degree to which "Information was presented in a variety of ways to facilitate learning." In COMPASS, all of the material is presented using a single scripted and peer-led method, and past research showed that this method produced large knowledge gains [22]. Two additional items asked students to rate the trainer's performance (preparedness and communication effectiveness), but in COMPASS, there is a supporting facilitator rather than a traditional trainer. In addition to recommending adjustments to questions like those above, researchers also requested additional questions that asked workers to rate their intentions to make changes as a result of the training.

To further strengthen the program and streamline dissemination, COMPASS guidebooks were further adjusted in ways to support their use in the OHCC training system. Giveaways for students that had no funding stream within the state (or potential funding stream) to support their use in the OHCC version of COMPASS, and homework assignments facilitated with such giveaways (e.g., small knee pads), were removed from the program. Investigators also replaced some activities with new ones, and made adjustments to other activities to make them run more smoothly. With guidance from

OHSU Technology Transfer and Business Development, investigators also worked with an OHSU graphic design specialist to create a professional design and layout for the guidebooks.

After the agreement was settled and signed, and the revised OHCC guidebooks with the new design were ready, the OHCC and investigators planned a "soft launch" of COMPASS by two facilitators in two cities. One facilitator had participated in the original adaptation pilot, and the other was new to the COMPASS program. The new facilitator and other OHCC staff received in-person training from investigators regarding COMPASS group facilitation, and the facilitator with previous experience had a meeting with investigators to be refreshed on the program and be informed of changes and adjustments made. Following the soft launch further technical corrections were made to the guidebooks (fixing typos, clarifying arrangements) and we removed all remaining giveaways for students and replaced them with alternatives (e.g., step counter giveaways used for walking challenges were removed, and activities/goals were altered to focus on "walking minutes per day/week"). As of October 2018, 2 additional facilitators were trained by OHCC training department staff and 12 groups have been completed or initiated in 7 different cities.

3. Results

3.1. Adaptation Pilot Results

Four facilitators (n = 3 female) were recommended by the OHCC Training Director and trained by investigators for the adaption pilot. Forty-two home care workers registered for five COMPASS groups (one facilitator ran two groups) offered in the following cities: Albany (k = 2), Salem (k = 2), and Corvallis (k = 1). The groups were offered at varied times to maximize opportunities for workers, with one in the late morning, three in the early afternoon, and one in the evening.

Participants were predominantly older (mean age = 49.23 years), female (80.56%), and Caucasian (77.78%). Workers reported an average tenure in home care of 7.12 years and an average of 22.37 weekly work hours. The reported lifetime prevalence of a diagnosis of depression or anxiety was 41.67% and 44.44%, respectively. For additional demographic details please see Table 2.

Table 2. Home care worker participants in the pilot study of the COMPASS adaptation for the Oregon Home Care Commission: Characteristics at baseline.

Measure	n	OHCC-Pilot Sample n = 36 [a]
Age, Mean (SD)	35	49.23 (12.16)
Female, n (%)	36	29 (80.56)
BMI Mean (SD)	35	31.38 (7.41)
Race, n (%)	36	
Caucasian		28 (77.78)
American Indian/Alaskan Native		1 (2.78)
Asian		1 (2.78)
Native Hawaiian/Pacific Islander		1 (2.78)
Black/African American		0 (0.00)
More than one race		3 (8.33)
Other		2 (5.56)
Relationship status, n (%) [b]	35	
Married		19 (54.29)
Divorced/Separated		8 (22.86)
Living with Sig. Other		4 (11.45)
Never Married		4 (11.45)

Table 2. Cont.

Measure	n	OHCC-Pilot Sample n = 36 [a]
Highest degree completed, n (%)	35	
No certificate or degree		2 (5.71)
High School Diploma		8 (22.86)
Vocational/Tech. Certificate		5 (14.29)
Associates Degree		6 (17.14)
College Degree		11 (31.43)
Graduate School Degree		3 (8.57)
Tenure as home care worker	36	
Mean (SD)		7.12 (7.92)
Range		0.25–38.00
Daily work hours	19	
Mean (SD)		8.74 (7.24)
Range		2.00–24.00
Weekly work hours	29	
Mean (SD)		22.37 (17.25)
Range		2.00–64.00
Number of public consumer-employers [c]	29	
Mean (SD)		1.72 (1.03)
Range		0.00–4.00
Number of private consumer-employers	13	
Mean (SD)		0.77 (0.60)
Range		0.00–2.00
Number of dependent children	36	
Mean (SD)		0.36 (0.83)
Range		0.00–4.00
Ever diagnosed w/ depression, n (%)	36	15 (41.67)
If yes, taking meds, n (%)		7 (46.67)
Ever diagnosed w/ anxiety, n (%)	36	16 (44.44)
If yes, taking meds, n (%) [d]		7 (43.75)
Ever diagnosed w/ chronic pain, n (%)	36	8 (22.22)
If yes, taking meds, n (%) [e]		4 (50.00)
Ever diagnosed w/ diabetes, n (%)		9 (25.00)
If yes, taking meds, n (%)		7 (77.78)
Ever diagnosed w/ hypertension, n (%)	36	11 (30.56)
If yes, taking meds, n (%) [f]		9 (81.82)

Note: OHCC = Oregon Home Care Commission. [a] This sample size represents workers who enrolled at baseline and returned for post-intervention measurements. When percentages are reported they reflect the percent of those reporting for that variable. [b] The survey failed to provide an option for participants to select "single", or to set a time frame for the recency of divorce or separation status. [c] An outlier data point of 78 reported current public consumer-employers was removed for analysis of this variable due to the improbability that such a number could be correct. [d] 3 did not report yes or no for medication. [e] 1 did not report yes or no for medication. [f] 1 did not report yes or no for medication.

Changes in primary outcomes were evaluated with descriptive effect sizes (Cohen's d) and two-tailed t tests. Given that the pilot was designed to evaluate feasibility and check effect sizes, and not to be a fully statistically powered effectiveness study, inferential t-test results should be viewed as supplementary and interpreted with the understanding that type II errors were probable. Pre- and post-program means, mean changes, effect sizes, and p values are reported in Table 3. Moderate-to-large effect sizes and statistically significant changes were observed for experienced community of practice, using new tools/techniques for housecleaning, fruit and vegetable consumption, meals brought from home, and healthy physical activity. All other outcomes changed in expected directions with the exception of two safety outcomes that had very small negative effect sizes (<0.10).

Table 3. COMPASS adaptation pilot intervention effects on primary outcomes.

Primary Outcomes (Time Anchor)	N	Pre Mean (SD)	Post Mean (SD)	Mean Effect	Effect Size (d)	p-Value
Experienced community of practice [a] (3 mo)	35	35.56 (5.03)	39.67 (4.48)	+4.11	+0.86	<0.000
Safety Behaviors [b] (3 mo)						
Talked with CE about improving unsafe conditions	34	2.15 (1.71)	2.08 (1.73)	−0.07	−0.04	0.865
Corrected slip/trip/fall hazards	34	1.62 (1.44)	1.50 (1.38)	−0.12	−0.09	0.714
Corrected other hazards	34	0.91 (1.00)	0.71 (1.00)	−0.20	−0.20	0.292
Used new tool/techniques for moving objects or CEs	35	1.31 (1.47)	1.43 (0.96)	+0.12	+0.10	0.701
Used new tools/techniques for housecleaning	35	1.11 (0.96)	1.69 (0.99)	+0.58	+0.59	0.009
Daily Diet/Exercise Behaviors (1 mo)						
Fruit & vegetable servings	35	4.05 (1.71)	4.87 (1.60)	+0.82	+0.49	0.026
Sugary snacks [c]	35	3.91 (1.87)	3.20 (1.55)	−0.71	−0.42	0.865
Sugary drinks [c]	35	3.14 (2.33)	2.51 (1.60)	−0.63	−0.32	0.714
Fast food [c]	35	2.14 (1.09)	1.97 (1.01)	−0.17	−0.16	0.292
Meals brought from home [c]	35	5.18 (2.39)	6.14 (2.70)	+0.96	+0.38	0.009
Healthy physical activity [d]	34	2.44 (1.52)	3.65 (1.58)	+1.21	+0.78	<0.000
Well-Being (1 mo)						
SF-12 physical composite score	31	48.05 (11.51)	48.38 (8.23)	+0.33	+0.03	0.834
SF-12 mental composite score	31	50.37 (10.17)	51.18 (6.75)	+0.81	+0.10	0.699

Note: Sample size varied due to missing responses for certain questions. Cohen's d effect sizes were computed using the pooled standard deviation for pre and post-test time points. p-values are for two tailed t-tests. CE = Consumer-employer. SF-12 = 12-item short form health survey. [a] Sum of nine items rated on a five-point scale, responses range from 1 (strongly disagree) to 5 (strongly agree). [b] Six-point frequency scales, responses ranged from 0 (never) to 5 (5+ times). [c] Items related to sugary snacks, drinks, fast food, and meals from home were reported on 10 frequency intervals: 1, never | 2, 1–3 times per month | 3, 1–2 times per week | 4, 3–4 times per week | 5, 5–6 times per week | 6, Once per day | 7, 2 times per day | 8, 3 times per day | 10, 5 or more times per day. Thus, a mean score of 3 would equal the behavior occurring 1–2 times per week. [d] Mean of four items asking about days per week with 30 min of different moderate-to-vigorous physical activities. Eight-point response scale ranged from 0 (none) to 7 (daily).

3.2. Statewide Rollout: Additional Adaptations in Progress and Preliminary Training Evaluation Results

As the statewide rollout of COMPASS was being planned and initiated, the OHCC expressed interest in further adaptations being made to COMPASS so that it would be inclusive of personal support workers. Within Oregon's publicly funded programs, personal support workers provide care for individuals with cognitive and developmental disabilities who qualify for publicly funded support services. Service recipients' ages range across the lifespan. This type of work was viewed to share many similarities with home care work, but also pose some different safety, health, well-being demands that might suggest new or revised guidebook activities and content. Investigators contracted with the OHCC to conduct formative research with personal support workers (e.g., survey, qualitative interviews) and make tailored curriculum adjustments based on findings. Bundled in this new phase of dissemination work included the development of interactive online orientation training for new COMPASS facilitators and creating promotional videos for the program. It is anticipated that after COMPASS is revised to accommodate personal support workers, the OHCC will then translate the guidebooks into several non-English languages to encourage non-native English speakers to participate in higher numbers.

As noted in the methods section, 12 COMPASS groups have been completed or are in progress in the statewide rollout. For the current analysis, the OHCC provided training evaluations ($n = 265$) from workers who participated in COMPASS group meetings from summer 2017 to summer 2018. Two different training evaluation question sets were completed by workers in the data set. An older version (but more recent than the original OHCC training evaluation questions prior to the adaptation pilot) was completed by 229 workers. A newer version, adjusted to better accommodate evaluations of the COMPASS dissemination, was completed by 36 workers. Table 4 provides mean ratings and standard deviations for the older evaluation questions for each COMPASS meeting, as well as an overall average rating for each question across meetings. All mean ratings were above 4 (max = 5) on a scale where 1 = poor, 2 = fair, 3 = average, 4 = good, and 5 = excellent. Table 5 reviews mean ratings and standard deviations for each question in the new format, but not for each meeting due to insufficient data. For those questions mean ratings all averaged above 3 (max = 4) on a scale where 1 = strongly disagree, 2 = disagree, 3 = agree, and 4 = strongly agree. Attendance data and evaluation data for other comparable OHCC classes are not yet available for analysis.

Table 4. Worker evaluations for COMPASS groups in the Oregon Home Care Commission training system: Mean (*SD*) ratings for quantitative questions in the original evaluation format.

Question	Meeting Number (Sample Size)								
	Unknown (n = 33)	1 (n = 26)	2 (n = 41–42)	3 (n = 30)	4 (n = 14)	5 (n = 15–16)	6 (n = 27–28)	7 (n = 39–40)	Overall (n = 229)
The training met my expectations and needs	4.69 (0.66)	4.36 (0.63)	4.41 (0.59)	4.60 (0.56)	4.64 (0.63)	4.75 (0.44)	4.75 (0.44)	4.80 (0.46)	4.67 (0.55)
The information will be useful in my work	4.67 (0.65)	4.36 (0.74)	4.69 (0.56)	4.67 (0.61)	4.79 (0.43)	4.80 (0.41)	4.79 (0.42)	4.90 (0.38)	4.74 (0.53)
Info. was presented in ways that facilitated learning	4.64 (0.65)	4.43 (0.85)	4.67 (0.57)	4.67 (0.48)	4.64 (0.63)	4.88 (0.34)	4.75 (0.44)	4.76 (0.48)	4.70 (0.55)
The trainer/facilitator was well prepared and organized	4.45 (0.79)	4.36 (0.74)	4.57 (0.59)	4.73 (0.45)	4.79 (0.43)	4.81 (0.40)	4.75 (0.44)	4.83 (0.45)	4.68 (0.56)
The trainer/facilitator communicated effectively	4.48 (0.76)	4.50 (0.65)	4.62 (0.58)	4.77 (0.43)	4.86 (0.36)	4.81 (0.40)	4.75 (0.44)	4.85 (0.43)	4.72 (0.53)
The handouts (or written materials) are helpful	4.57 (0.68)	4.54 (0.88)	4.67 (0.48)	4.66 (0.55)	4.57 (0.65)	4.88 (0.34)	4.74 (0.44)	4.86 (0.41)	4.71 (0.53)
I would recommend this training to others	4.70 (0.64)	4.46 (0.88)	4.69 (0.56)	4.71 (0.53)	4.71 (0.47)	4.88 (0.34)	4.75 (0.44)	4.90 (0.38)	4.75 (0.53)

Note: "Info." = information. Rating scale was 1 = poor, 2 = fair, 3 = average, 4 = good, and 5 = excellent.

Table 5. Worker evaluations for COMPASS groups in the Oregon Home Care Commission training system: Mean (SD) ratings for quantitative questions in the revised/new format.

Question	Overall (n = 36)
The training met my expectations and needs	3.58 (0.50)
The information will be useful in my work	3.56 (0.50)
Information was presented in ways that facilitated learning	3.61 (0.50)
The trainer/facilitator was well prepared and organized	3.63 (0.48)
The trainer/facilitator communicated effectively	3.58 (0.50)
The handouts (or written materials) are helpful	3.55 (0.51)
I would recommend this training to others	3.62 (0.65)
I enjoyed this training	3.58 (0.66)
I will do something new, different, or better in order to be safer at work because of this training	3.53 (0.51)
I will do something new, different, or better in order to improve my health and well-being because of this training	3.66 (0.48)
I will do something new, different, or better in order to improve my consumer-employers' health and well-being because of this training	3.60 (0.50)

Note: rating scale was 1 = strongly disagree, 2 = disagree, 3 = agree, 4 = strongly agree, and also a "does not apply" option. If participants marked "does not apply" this was coded as missing data and was not included in calculations.

4. Discussion

The current project represents a rare, and thus far successful, effort to translate an evidence-based intervention into practice for HCWs. A pilot test of the adapted program confirmed that adjusted intervention processes were functional, and that outcomes were changing with effect sizes resembling those from the prior randomized controlled trial. Preliminary evaluation data suggest the program is well liked, rated as useful, and that workers report intentions to make safety and health changes as a result of participating. An additional strength of the dissemination effort includes an inter-agency research agreement that will generate long-term evaluation data for COMPASS participants (attendance, course evaluations, workers' compensation injury claims) with potential for some cross-sectional analyses of HCWs within the state. Several factors facilitated this successful dissemination effort and its probable long-term sustainability, but key factors included engagement and collaboration with the adopting partner (the OHCC) in initial intervention development, continued dialogue and discussion during research phases, flexibility from both investigators and the OHCC while adjusting the program to meet training system needs, and sustained top level commitment at the OHCC. Other researchers may consider following a similar model of sustained partnership across research phases in order to enhance a sense of ownership from the adopting partner and promote dissemination sustainability. Considering the factors Rogers [18] pointed out as being important for successful dissemination, we believe the OHCC perceived COMPASS as compatible with their current needs and values, feasible to deliver and implement, able to be tested for potential adoption (e.g., our adaptation pilot), and to have demonstrated effectiveness among stakeholders (this included early and consistent collaboration with and commitment from the union). Consistent with dissemination research findings of Kuehl et al. [20], leadership support included both committed chiefs (the Executive Director of the OHCC, Senior Director of Technology Transfer at OHSU) and champions (OHCC Training Directors and key members of the OHCC Training Committee).

While many facilitating factors were present, the dissemination effort faced some barriers to success. Some of these barriers included turnover of key staff at various time points, gaps in funding, and complexities in navigating government and university processes. Into the future, the long-term success of the adoption of COMPASS in the OHCC will depend on some level of continued support from OHSU, the Oregon Institute of Occupational Health Sciences, and the Oregon Healthy Workforce Center (e.g., to update and adapt the curriculum) as well as continued financial commitment from the

OHCC/state of Oregon to fund guidebook printing and wages for facilitators and workers. Stable state funding for both the OHCC and the Oregon Institute of Occupational Health Sciences will be key, as well as continued NIOSH funding for the Oregon Healthy Workforce Center. Thus, investigators and partners at the OHCC will need to plan ahead, anticipating courses of action if any one of these sources of support is disrupted. This includes evolving structures at the Oregon Institute of Occupational Health Sciences to support translation and dissemination of evidence-based programs created by its investigators and their collaborators.

Looking outside of the state of Oregon in the US, we recommend that researchers who aim to develop, evaluate, and disseminate interventions for similar populations investigate institutional structures and potential partners within their target region. For publicly funded HCWs in Oregon, both union and governmental partners were equally engaged through intervention development and evaluation phases, but governmental partners played the most central role in the dissemination phase because of their ownership of the training system for publicly funded HCWs. In contrast, in our neighboring state of Washington, an SEIU 775 Benefits Group "owns" and operates training programs for publicly funded HCWs. Therefore, development and evaluation phases of an intervention for HCWs in Washington would similarly need to involve both government and labor partners, but during a dissemination phase, the union benefits group would play the most central collaborative role.

Given that the literature on translation of *Total Worker Health*® interventions into practice is in its infancy, future dissemination and implementation science with effective programs is strongly encouraged. For example, if interest in COMPASS expanded and resources are available to study a new dissemination effort, research could systematically evaluate organizational readiness factors and measure adoption and implementation of the program across multiple new organizations. Such future dissemination science with any particular *Total Worker Health*®-informed intervention may be fruitfully guided by recommendations and tools from Dugan and Punnett [32]. Based on their experience developing the Healthy Workplace Participatory Program, the authors provide examples of potential dissemination and implementation studies and tools, such as the Five and Ten D&I Evaluation Tool to assess specific implementation outcomes.

5. Conclusions

HCWs are a priority population for protective interventions that advance their safety, health, and well-being. Rapidly growing in number, HCWs help some of our most vulnerable citizens remain in their homes and enjoy a higher quality of life. In-home care may also create critical cost-savings in the healthcare system by preventing older adults from transitioning prematurely to long-term care facilities. While some interventions have research evidence for their effectiveness, and other valuable tools and resources are available, we could not find a descriptive or empirical paper about a successful research-to-practice intervention dissemination effort with HCWs. In this regard, the current description of the adaptation and dissemination of COMPASS with the OHCC may help guide future similar efforts with other partners or in other states. Consistent with previous findings in the dissemination science literature, the success of the current effort was facilitated by several favorable factors that can be cultivated in future projects by other intervention scientists. These include early engagement and collaboration with industry and labor in the development of interventions, designing for feasibility and repeatability of intervention tactics, and sustained engagement over time to foster strong relationships and top-level leadership commitment over the long term. We also believe flexibility and persistence from all parties was essential for overcoming barriers as they arose. This persistence included a commitment to the effort during times when resources for dissemination efforts were scarce or uncertain. We are optimistic with continued contingency and structural planning that the rollout of COMPASS will be sustained within the OHCC, with the ultimate potential to improve the safety, health, and well-being of approximately 60% of the Oregon home care work force.

Author Contributions: All authors contributed substantially to the work reported. Conceptualization, R.O., J.A.H., S.V.T., K.L.R., and M.M.; Methodology, R.O., J.A.H., S.V.T., K.L.R, K.N.P., and M.M.; Formal Analysis, K.N.P. and R.O.; Investigation, S.V.T., K.L.R., K.N.P. and R.O.; Data Curation, S.V.T., K.L.R., K.N.P. and R.O.; Writing-Original Draft Preparation, R.O. and A.R.; Writing-Review & Editing, R.O., J.A.H., S.V.T., A.R., K.N.P., and K.L.R.; Visualization, R.O. and A.R.; Supervision, R.O.; Project Administration, S.V.T. and K.N.P.; Funding Acquisition, R.O., J.A.H., S.V.T., K.N.P, and M.M.

Funding: This research was funded by the National Institute for Occupational Safety & Health grant number (U19 OH010154), a contract from the Oregon Home Care Commission, and the Oregon Institute of Occupational Health Sciences.

Acknowledgments: We thank the leadership and staff at the Oregon Home Care Commission for their long-term collaboration and commitment to the project (Cheryl Miller, Roberta Lilly, Kristen Eisenman, Leslie Houston, Kelly Rosenau, and many others). The Service Employees International Union Local 503 provided critical support during the development and evaluation of COMPASS, including feedback, guidance, and use of meeting spaces for groups. We are grateful for Diane Elliot's collaboration and contributions as a Co-Investigator during the pilot and RCT phases of the project. The "Fruits & Vegetables" and "Jeopardy" activities in the second meeting of COMPASS guidebook one (pre-dissemination editions) were developed by Diane Elliot, MD, FACSM, Kerry Kuehl, MD, DrPH, and Linn Goldberg, MD, FACSM, Division of Health Promotion and Sports Medicine, OHSU. Brad Wipfli and Robert Wright made important contributions to scripted content in Communication for Hazard Correction and Mental Health meetings in COMPASS guidebook one, and we thank Brian Luke Seaward for his permission to adapt a stress coping activity for the disseminated version of the guidebooks. We thank Kristen Eisenman, Paul Weaver, Sydney Running, Vinesa Faaogea, and Lisa Olson for training evaluation data entry and processing. We also thank student interns and volunteers involved with the adaptation and dissemination phases of the project, including Teala Alvord and Claire Boenisch.

Conflicts of Interest: The authors declare no conflict of interest. The funders had no role in the design of the study; in the analyses or interpretation of data; in the writing of the manuscript, and in the decision to publish the results. The Oregon Home Care Commission played a collaborative role in planning COMPASS adaptations and dissemination strategies, and also collected and shared training evaluation data for the dissemination phase of the project.

References

1. Bureau of Labor Statistics. Occupational Outlook Handbook. Home Health Aides and Personal Care Aides. Available online: https://www.bls.gov/ooh/healthcare/home-health-aides-and-personal-care-aides.htm (accessed on 19 September 2018).
2. Mabry, L.; Parker, K.N.; Thompson, S.V.; Bettencourt, K.M.; Haque, A.; Luther Rhoten, K.; Wright, R.R.; Hess, J.A.; Olson, R. Protecting workers in the home care industry: Workers' experienced job demands, resource gaps, and benefits following a socially supportive intervention. *Home Health Care Serv. Q.* **2018**, 1–18. [CrossRef] [PubMed]
3. Jacobs, K.; Perry, I.; MacGillvary, J. *The High Public Cost of Low Wages*; UC Berkeley: Berkeley, CA, USA, 2015.
4. Quinn, M.M.; Markkanen, P.K.; Galligan, C.J.; Sama, S.R.; Kriebel, D.; Gore, R.J.; Brouillette, N.M.; Okyere, D.; Sun, C.; Punnett, L.; et al. Occupational health of home care aides: Results of the safe home care survey. *Occup. Environ. Med.* **2016**, *73*, 237–245. [CrossRef] [PubMed]
5. Hanson, G.C.; Perrin, N.A.; Moss, H.; Laharnar, N.; Glass, N. Workplace violence against homecare workers and its relationship with workers health outcomes: A cross-sectional study. *BMC Public Health* **2015**, *15*, 11. [CrossRef] [PubMed]
6. Amuwo, S.; Lipscomb, J.; McPhaul, K.; Sokas, R.K. Reducing occupational risk for blood and body fluid exposure among home care aides: An intervention effectiveness study. *Home Health Care Serv. Q.* **2013**, *32*, 234–248. [CrossRef] [PubMed]
7. Horneij, E.; Hemborg, B.; Jensen, I.; Ekdahl, C. No significant differences between intervention programmes on neck, shoulder and low back pain: A prospective randomized study among home-care personnel. *J. Rehabil. Med.* **2001**, *33*, 170–176. [CrossRef] [PubMed]
8. Pohjonen, T.; Ranta, R. Effects of worksite physical exercise intervention on physical fitness, perceived health status, and work ability among home care workers: Five-year follow-up. *Prev. Med.* **2001**, *32*, 465–475. [CrossRef] [PubMed]
9. Toseland, R.W. Long-term effectiveness of peer-led and professionally led support groups for caregivers. *Soc. Serv. Rev.* **1990**, *64*, 308–327. [CrossRef]

10. Olson, R.; Thompson, S.V.; Elliot, D.L.; Hess, J.A.; Rhoten, K.L.; Parker, K.N.; Wright, R.R.; Wipfli, B.; Bettencourt, K.M.; Buckmaster, A.; et al. Safety and health support for home care workers: The COMPASS randomized controlled trial. *Am. J. Public Health* **2016**, *106*, 1823–1832. [CrossRef]
11. UMassLowell Safe Home Care and Sustainable Hospitals Program. Safe Care Resources. Available online: https://www.uml.edu/Research/SHCH/Safe-Home-Care/Research-Areas/ (accessed on 7 October 2018).
12. National Institute for Occupational Safety and Health. Caring for Yourself While Caring for Others. Available online: https://www.cdc.gov/niosh/docs/2015-102/default.html (accessed on 7 October 2018).
13. Balas, E.A.; Boren, S.A. Managing Clinical Knowledge for Health Care Improvement. In *Yearbook of Medical Informatics*; Schattauer Verlagsgesellschaft mbH: Stuttgart, Germany, 2000; pp. 65–70.
14. Bull, S.S.; Gillette, C.; Glasgow, R.E.; Estabrooks, P. Work site health promotion research: To what extent can we generalize the results and what is needed to translate research to practice? *Health Educ. Behav.* **2003**, *30*, 537–549. [CrossRef]
15. Harris, J.R.; Cheadle, A.; Hannon, P.A.; Lichiello, P.; Forehand, M.; Mahoney, E.; Snyder, S.; Yarrow, J. A framework for disseminating evidence-based health promotion practices. *Prev. Chronic Dis.* **2012**, *9*, 110081. [CrossRef]
16. Matthews, L.; Kirk, A.; Macmillan, F.; Mutrie, N. Can physical activity interventions for adults with type 2 diabetes be translated into practice settings? A systematic review using the RE-AIM framework. *Transl. Behav. Med.* **2014**, *4*, 60–78. [CrossRef] [PubMed]
17. Estabrooks, P.A.; Glasgow, R.E. Translating effective clinic-based physical activity interventions into practice. *Am. J. Prev. Med.* **2006**, *31*, S45–S56. [CrossRef] [PubMed]
18. Rogers, E.M. *Diffusion of Innovations*, 5th ed.; Free Press: New York, NY, USA, 2003.
19. Healy, G.N.; Goode, A.; Schultz, D.; Lee, D.; Leahy, B.; Dunstan, D.W.; Gilson, N.D.; Eakin, E.G. The BeUpstanding Program: Scaling up the Stand Up Australia workplace intervention for translation into practice. *AIMS Public Health* **2016**, *3*, 341–347. [CrossRef] [PubMed]
20. Kuehl, H.; Mabry, L.; Elliot, D.L.; Kuehl, K.S.; Favorite, K.C. Factors in adoption of a fire department wellness program: Champ-and-chief model. *J. Occup. Environ. Med.* **2013**, *55*, 424–429. [CrossRef] [PubMed]
21. Olson, R.; Elliot, D.; Hess, J.; Thompson, S.; Luther, K.; Wipfli, B.; Wright, R.; Buckmaster, A.M. The COMmunity of Practice And Safety Support (COMPASS) Total Worker Health study among home care workers: Study protocol for a randomized controlled trial. *Trials* **2014**, *15*, 411. [CrossRef] [PubMed]
22. Olson, R.; Wright, R.R.; Elliot, D.L.; Hess, J.A.; Thompson, S.; Buckmaster, A.; Luther, K.; Wipfli, B. The COMPASS pilot study: A Total Worker Health intervention for home care workers. *J. Occup. Environ. Med.* **2015**, *57*, 406–416. [CrossRef] [PubMed]
23. Toseland, R.W.; Rossiter, C.M.; Labrecque, M.S. The effectiveness of peer-led and professionally led groups to support family caregivers. *Gerontologist* **1989**, *29*, 465–471. [CrossRef] [PubMed]
24. Delbecq, J.; DeSchryver Mueller, C. The Ignatian Faculty Forum: A transformative faculty formation program. *Connections* **2012**, *12*, 5–9.
25. Elliot, D.L.; Goldberg, L.; Moe, E.L.; DeFrancesco, C.L.; Durham, M.B.; Hix-Small, H. Preventing substance use and disordered eating: Initial outcomes of the ATHENA (Athletes Targeting Healthy Exercise & Nutrition Alternatives) program. *Arch. Pediatr. Adolesc. Med.* **2004**, *158*, 1043–1049.
26. Elliot, D.L.; Goldberg, L.; Kuehl, K.S.; Moe, E.L.; Breger, R.K.R.; Pickering, M.A. The PHLAME (Promoting Healthy Lifestyles: Alternative Models' Effects) firefighter study: Outcomes of two models of behavior change. *J. Occup. Environ. Med.* **2007**, *49*, 204–213. [CrossRef]
27. Goldberg, L.; Elliot, D.L.; Clarke, G.N.; MacKinnon, D.P.; Zoref, L.; Moe, E.; Green, C.; Wolf, S.L. The adolescents training and learning to avoid steroids (ATLAS) prevention program: Background and results of a model intervention. *Arch. Pediatr. Adolesc. Med.* **1996**, *150*, 713–721. [CrossRef] [PubMed]
28. Kuehl, K.S.; Elliot, D.L.; Goldberg, L.; MacKinnon, D.P.; Vila, B.J.; Smith, J.L.; Miocevic, M.; O'Rourke, H.P.; Valente, M.; DeFrancesco, C. The safety and health improvement: Enhancing Law Enforcement Departments Study: Feasibility and findings. *Front. Public Health* **2014**, *2*, 38. [CrossRef] [PubMed]
29. Cadiz, D.; Sawyer, J.E.; Griffith, T.L. Developing and validating field measurement scales for absorptive capacity and experienced community of practice. *Educ. Psychol. Meas.* **2009**, *69*, 1035–1058. [CrossRef]
30. Buxton, O.M.; Quintilliani, L.M.; Yang, M.H.; Ebbeling, C.B.; Stoddard, A.M.; Pereira, L.K.; Sorensen, G. Association of sleep adequacy with more healthful food choices and positive workplace experiences among motor freight workers. *Am. J. Public Health* **2009**, *99*, S636–S643. [CrossRef] [PubMed]

31. Ware, J.E.J.; Kosinkski, M.; Keller, S.D. A 12-item short-form health survey: Construction of the scales and preliminary tests of reliability and validity. *Med. Care* **1996**, *34*, 220–233. [CrossRef] [PubMed]
32. Dugan, A.G.; Punnett, L. Dissemination and implementation research for occupational safety and health. *Occup. Health Sci.* **2017**, *1*, 29–45. [CrossRef] [PubMed]

© 2018 by the authors. Licensee MDPI, Basel, Switzerland. This article is an open access article distributed under the terms and conditions of the Creative Commons Attribution (CC BY) license (http://creativecommons.org/licenses/by/4.0/).

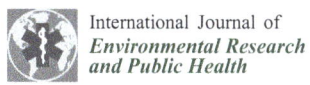

Article

Implementation of the Healthy Workplace Participatory Program in a Retail Setting: A Feasibility Study and Framework for Evaluation

Jaime R. Strickland *[ID], Anna M. Kinghorn, Bradley A. Evanoff and Ann Marie Dale[ID]

Division of General Medical Sciences, Washington University School of Medicine, Saint Louis, MO 63110, USA; akinghorn@wustl.edu (A.M.K.); bevanoff@wustl.edu (B.A.E.); amdale@wustl.edu (A.M.D.)
* Correspondence: jaime.strickland@wustl.edu; Tel.: +1-314-454-7337

Received: 31 December 2018; Accepted: 14 February 2019; Published: 18 February 2019

Abstract: Participatory methods used in Total Worker Health® programs have not been well studied, and little is known about what is needed to successfully implement these programs. We conducted a participatory health promotion program with grocery store workers using the Healthy Workplace Participatory Program (HWPP) from the Center for the Promotion of Health in the New England Workplace. We recruited a design team made up of six line-level workers and a steering committee with management and union representatives; a research team member facilitated the program. Using a formal evaluation framework, we measured program implementation including workplace context, fidelity to HWPP materials, design team and steering committee engagement, program outputs, and perceptions of the program. The HWPP was moderately successful in this setting, but required a substantial amount of worker and facilitator time. Design team members did not have the skills needed to move through the process and the steering committee did not offer adequate support to compensate for the team's shortfall. The evaluation framework provided a simple and practical method for identifying barriers to program delivery. Future studies should address these barriers to delivery and explore translation of this program to other settings.

Keywords: Total Worker Health; participatory methods; program implementation; organizational readiness; process evaluation; logic model

---

1. Introduction

More than one-third of current U.S. workers suffer from at least one chronic disease, including heart disease, cancer, diabetes, stroke, and musculoskeletal disorders [1,2]. Working adults with chronic disease are more likely to have a reduced working capacity and greater difficulty staying at work than their healthy peers [3,4]. These chronic health conditions have an enormous impact in the lives of workers, but they also place a burden on their employers [3,5]. Healthy behaviors can reduce the effects of chronic conditions for better work (fewer missed days, increased productivity) and health (less musculoskeletal pain, improved mental health) outcomes [5–10].

The workplace is an ideal place for supporting healthy behaviors, since workers spend a large portion of their day in the work environment and coworkers and supervisors can provide substantial support. Traditionally, worksite health promotion programs have been separate from other occupational health and safety efforts, and usually target only the individual, ignoring work organization and work environment factors that affect worker behavior. The National Institute for Occupational Safety and Health (NIOSH's) Total Worker Health® (TWH) approach highlights the need for "policies, programs, and practices that integrate protection from work-related safety and health hazards with promotion of injury and illness prevention efforts to advance worker well-being" [11]. The TWH approach recognizes that work is a social determinant of health, and that workplace factors such as work hours, relationships with coworkers and supervisors, and access to health and wellness programs have important effects on worker health and well-being. Further, TWH principles recognize the Hierarchy of Controls framework to illustrate that system-level interventions are more effective than individual-level interventions [12].

Regardless of the level of intervention, the most effective interventions are those that take into consideration the unique characteristics and perspectives of the end users [13,14]. Participatory methods such as Participatory Action Research and Participatory Ergonomics promote the inclusion of end users in the intervention development process [14–20]. These end users may be line-level workers who directly benefit from the intervention, managers or others who implement and monitor interventions, or others who are impacted by the interventions in some way. Including these users in the process allows their perspectives to be considered in identifying both workplace health hazards and possible barriers to adopting or participating in the planned interventions. Participatory methods are increasingly being used in Total Worker Health research and practice [14,17,21–28]. The most thoroughly studied participatory program in the TWH literature to date is the Healthy Workplace Participatory Program (HWPP) developed by the Center for the Promotion of Health in the New England Workplace (CPH-NEW). The HWPP is a worker-management participatory program designed to develop solutions for workplace problems that involve front-line workers. The freely available online program includes step-by-step guidance for assembling the participants, identifying problems, and developing and implementing solutions. The developers note the importance of organizational readiness and leadership support, and have recently developed a checklist to measure organizational readiness as well as a Process Evaluation Rating Sheet (PERS) and Management Dashboard [18,29]. This promising and relatively new program has been used in various work settings including corrections facilities, real estate, non-profit healthcare and social assistance agencies, and state government executive offices [28,30]. Publications to date provide little practical advice for implementing the HWPP program (e.g., characteristics most important for success, total time commitment, expectations of the design team, facilitator role). Further, the TWH literature as a whole discusses the utility of participatory approaches, but offers little guidance on how to comprehensively evaluate both implementation and efficacy of these programs while simultaneously considering the contexts in which they are delivered [12,13,31,32].

We sought to evaluate the feasibility of conducting a participatory health promotion program in a retail grocery store setting. We partnered with a regional grocery store chain who expressed interest in supporting their workers' health. Using the HWPP as a facilitation guide, we formed a team of grocery store workers and evaluated their ability to create meaningful and relevant workplace health activities that promote and support healthy behaviors in their workforce. The purpose of this paper is twofold: (1) to inform others considering a participatory intervention by describing the implementation of this HWPP program, and (2) to describe a framework for evaluating complex TWH interventions, such as the HWPP.

2. Materials and Methods

2.1. Overview and Employer Context

This study was an extension of a partnership with a labor union and several regional grocery store chains who had participated in a preliminary study examining workplace factors related to health behaviors and obesity [33,34]. Upon completion of that study, we approached our partners about piloting the HWPP in one store. We explained that the goal of the program was to develop and implement health and wellness initiatives to promote health in the workplace setting and support workers' efforts to make positive health changes; one of the grocers agreed to participate.

The study period was from September 2014 to June 2016, during which time we piloted the HWPP program, collected process measures, and collected baseline and follow-up worker assessments by surveys and focus groups. The Institutional Review Board at Washington University approved all research activities and all participants provided informed consent.

2.2. Program Description

2.2.1. HWPP Model and IDEAS Tool

The HWPP model includes a design team made up of front-line workers and a steering committee comprised of multiple management levels [35]. These two teams work together, with the help of a program facilitator, to create health and wellness activities for their workplace. The model uses the Intervention Design and Analysis Scorecard (IDEAS Tool) which includes seven steps: (1) identify problems and contributing factors, (2) develop intervention objectives and activities, (3) set selection criteria, (4) apply selection criteria, (5A) rate intervention activities, (5B) select intervention activities, (6) plan and implement intervention activities, and 7) monitor and evaluate intervention activities [21,36]. With the guidance of the facilitator, the design team works through these steps using worksheets to create intervention options (Steps 1–5A) to present to the steering committee (Step 5B); both teams work together to implement and monitor the intervention activities (Steps 6–7).

2.2.2. Planning & Roles

At study initiation, the research team met with the grocer's management to describe the study and outline the project's goal: To trial a participatory process as a method to generate ideas that promote worker health. They outlined the rationale for participatory programs and discussed the expectations and roles of both the employer (i.e., grocer) and research team. The grocer was willing to trial the program in one store and agreed to: (1) help form a representative steering committee and design team; (2) assist with scheduling design team meetings and allowing design team members to meet during work hours, provided they clock out for meetings; (3) provide a meeting space; and (4) provide access to store workers for data collection. It was expected that the research team would assume responsibility and costs for program facilitation and data collection. The research team also made the decision to pay design team members for their time to attend meetings since they were not able to meet on paid work time; they were paid $25 per meeting.

A research team member with experience in workplace interventions and group facilitation served as the facilitator; two additional research team members assisted in program development and attended meetings to collect process measures. The facilitator's role was to guide the Design Team through the IDEAS Tool by teaching them the process, planning and running team meetings, and acting as a liaison between the Design Team & Steering Committee. Along with the research team, the facilitator created an agenda and timeline based on the IDEAS Tool and activities from the HWPP toolkit [36]. The initial program plan consisted of seven, one-hour meetings over the course of nine weeks, with two optional meetings scheduled if needed to complete steps 1–5A of the IDEAS Tool. Considering that the program was initiated within the context of a time-limited research study, the facilitator's goal was to complete one or two cycles of the IDEAS Tool with the Design Team and identify a leader from among the group who could assume the facilitator role and thus ensure program sustainability beyond the study period. Additionally, the HWPP model suggests that employers collect baseline data on the workforce characteristics and health status, and environment or work processes that would aid the design team to creating meaningful interventions [35]. The research team took responsibility for collecting this data; we conducted worker surveys (n = 120) and focus groups (n = 19) to gather information about current health status, behaviors, and health beliefs of store workers, as well as information about existing workplace supports for health [37–44]. The Design Team's main role was to complete the IDEAS Tool worksheets, creating intervention options relevant to their work environment to present to the Steering Committee for consideration. After Steering Committee approval, the Design Team was to work together with the Steering Committee to finalize and implement intervention activities. While the majority of the program was designed to take place during team meetings, design team members were expected to complete 'homework' tasks between meetings in order to increase productivity during meeting time; these homework tasks were to take approximately 30–60 min to complete each week.

2.2.3. Experience Map

The research team used experience mapping as way to present the baseline data to the design team in a simple and meaningful way. To complement the survey and focus group data already collected, design team members were asked to complete a store mapping activity in which they drew their store layout and mapped their routes throughout the workday, noting their perceptions of the positive, neutral, and negative impacts on their health. The totality of the formative research was synthesized by the research team and used to create an experience map (Figure 1) that was presented to the design team to use throughout the program [45].

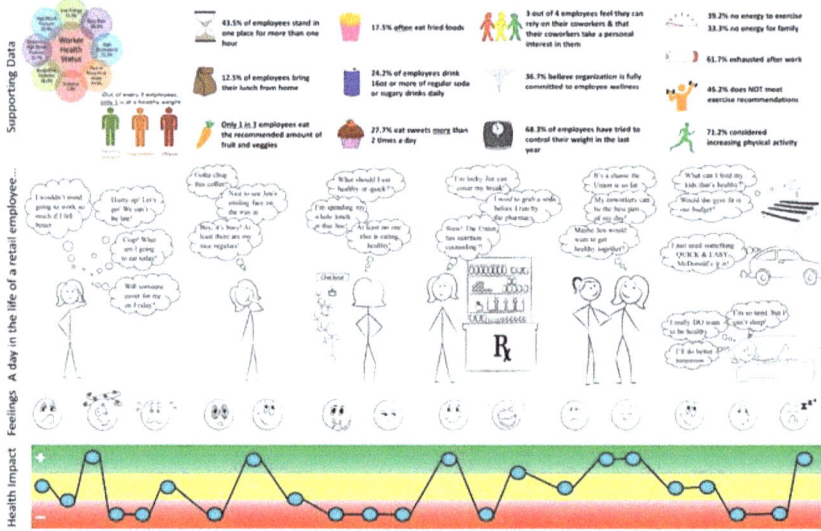

Figure 1. Experience Map.

The experience map's central focus was a persona describing "a day in the life of a grocery store employee." This story included both work and non-work time to highlight the importance of examining both workplace and personal factors to understand health behaviors and outcomes. Also included in the map was quantitative data from the surveys as supporting evidence for the persona, including disease and symptom rates (e.g., obesity, diabetes, back pain), information about current health behaviors (e.g., diet and exercise), and perceptions of workplace influences on health and organizational commitment to employee health. We used a variety of graphics and images to convey ideas and emotions that are not easily expressed in words and numbers. This enabled the research team to present complex information back to the design team in simple graphic format which they could easily digest and utilize to efficiently identify health priorities and goals, workplace barriers to health, and opportunities for intervention.

2.2.4. Design Team and Steering Committee Recruitment

Store workers volunteered for the design team at the time they completed their baseline survey. Because the program is largely driven by the design team, it was essential that we included workers who were interested in the topic and therefore more likely to remain engaged throughout the process. We used the selection criteria outlined in the HWPP Toolkit as a guide for identifying and selecting six to eight workers with the help of store management [46]. The HWPP suggested that team members should (1) represent all line-level jobs and task environments, (2) represent the demographics of line-level workers, (3) be committed to health and safety and/or improving the workplace, (4) be willing to work together, (5) be open to learning new skills, (6) be able to function as an opinion leader, and (7) be able to meet on a regular basis (missing no more than two meetings). The HWPP also provided guidance on selection of the Steering Committee indicating that they should (1) occupy different levels and roles within the organization, (2) be knowledgeable, or interested, in the area of health promotion/protection, (3) have authority to authorize programs and funding as needed, (4) represent and have the respect of a large number of the workforce, (5) be able to coordinate activities of the Healthy Workplace Project with standing committees. When we formed the steering committee [47], we sought approval and participation from the two larger union locals because eligible, unionized workers received health benefits through their union; a representative from these locals agreed to participate. The steering committee also included the storefront supervisor (as a proxy for the store manager), a representative from corporate labor relations, and a representative from corporate human resources. We did not include representatives from the other unions due to the small number of workers they represented.

2.3. Process Evaluation

2.3.1. Logic Model

We created a logic model to guide our evaluation of the HWPP implementation process (Figure 2). We adapted this model from our previously published work in participatory ergonomics [48,49] and incorporated elements that are common in program evaluation [50–52].

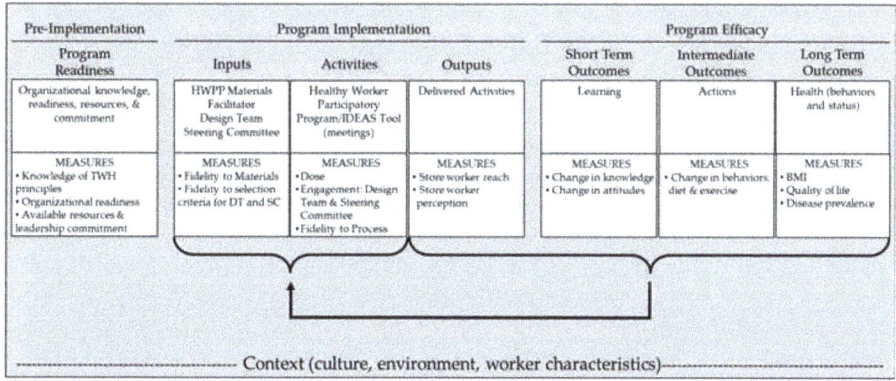

Figure 2. Logic model for evaluating the Healthy Workplace Participatory Program (HWPP).

The logic model begins at the left with "Pre-Implementation" elements (i.e., organizational knowledge, readiness, dedicated resources, and leadership commitment) in order to assess the preparedness of the workplace to initiate a TWH program. This allows the researcher to provide the necessary training and education on TWH before the program begins, creating the foundation for program implementation. The next section shows elements related to the program implementation process, including the inputs (i.e., the resources put into the project), activities (i.e., what the program entails), and outputs (i.e., what was accomplished). The right side of the model shows efficacy measures including the short-term, intermediate, and long-term outcomes the program is indented to produce. All elements are imbedded within the organizational context, which may directly or indirectly influence program or intervention success. Although the model may coincide with time, it is not intended to be a linear evaluation, but rather a continuous, iterative process. As indicated by the brackets, the evaluation of outputs and outcomes will be fed back to inform inputs and activities. This circular process allows periodic evaluation and adjustment of the program as necessary. The evaluation in this paper focuses specifically on the implementation process within the context of a unionized grocery store setting. Due to time and resource limitations, we did not measure pre-implementation elements or program efficacy.

2.3.2. Data Collection

To measure program implementation, the research team collected both qualitative and quantitative data using multiple tools. For each design team meeting, the research team completed field logs and debriefing notes to measure dose (frequency and duration of meetings) and fidelity to the HWPP materials and IDEAS Tool, and rated four dimensions of team member engagement (offered new ideas during meetings, actively participated in meeting, completed homework, and discussed projects with co-workers) on a 3-point scale (0 = no; 0.5 = somewhat; 1 = yes). The design team also rated their own participation and completed meeting reflections [53]. After the completion of the program, the design team members completed semi-structured interviews and a short survey to record final perceptions of both the program and the team's ability to move forward with implementing solutions without the support of the research team. All store workers were surveyed about their awareness and utilization of the implemented activities three months after they were implemented. The survey asked what changes related to health and wellness they had noticed in their store over the study period, and if they had participated in any of the health activities. We asked if any of the activities "helped them improve (their) eating/and or exercise habits," what limitations prevented them from participating in the health activities listed, and if the activities were relevant to their life. We also conducted semi-structured interviews with five store workers to further gauge their perceptions of the activities implemented in their workplace.

2.3.3. Data Analysis

We used SPSS v. 23 (IBM, Armonk, NY, USA) to run descriptive statistics for baseline demographics and with store worker follow up surveys for program reach metrics (i.e., awareness and use of activities). We rated all process components according to the measures described in our logic model. A process measure of design team participation was the average rating of each team member's engagement scores across meetings. Qualitative data was not systematically coded, but each qualitative item was reviewed with consensus by the research team to summarize each process measure. Qualitative data was also used to provide descriptive information to support the quantitative results.

3. Results

3.1. Model Context

The participating grocery store chain offered a large, busy store that was located in a demographically diverse neighborhood. This store was chosen because of the diverse employee and customer demographics, as well as the store manager, who was enthusiastic about the program. After the initiation of the program, this store manager was transferred to another store; the replacement manager was not as invested in the study. During the project planning phase, store management agreed to adjust work schedules of design team members so they would be scheduled to work on meeting days, and could attend meetings immediately before or after their scheduled shift; this did not always happen over the course of the program. Store management provided a space for the design team to meet on site, although it was not always private due to limited space options in the store.

The selected store employed approximately 159 workers, roughly 40% of whom were full-time employees. We obtained baseline surveys from 120 workers (75% response rate); their demographics are presented in Table 1. The majority of the workforce was unionized and represented by one of five different unions/locals within the store.

Table 1. Demographics of the Baseline Survey Respondents.

	Mean (SD)
Age	42 (15.1)
BMI	28.21 (6.3)

	%
Body Mass Index (BMI) Category	
Underweight	1
Normal weight	37.3
Overweight	28.4
Obese	33.3
Gender	
Female	52.4
Race	
African American	37.5
Caucasian	53.8
Other	8.6
Hispanic/Latino	3
Marital Status	
Married	28.6
Member of unmarried couple	14.3
Never married	41.9
Widowed	4.8
Divorced/separated	10.5
1 or more children live in household	40.4
Highest level of education	
Less than high school	1.9
High school graduate or General Education Diploma	35.6
Postsecondary Education	62.5
Health Behaviors	
Often bring lunch from home	12.5
Eat the recommend amount of fruits	34.2
Eat the recommend amount of vegetables	38.7
Often eat fried foods	17.5
Drink 16oz or more of regular soda or sugary drinks daily	24.2
Eats sweets more than 2 times a day	27.7
Does not meet exercise recommendations	45.2
Considered increasing physical activity	71.2
Health Climate	
Believe organization is fully committed to employee wellness	36.7
Tried to control their weight in the last year	68.3
Stand in place for more than one hour	43.5
No energy to exercise	39.2
No energy for family	33.3
Exhausted after work	61.7

3.2. Model Inputs

We used all of the IDEAS Tool worksheets, but simplified some of the language to make them more understandable to the design team members. The design team reported that although they understood the program materials when the facilitator guided the process, the worksheets were not intuitive to complete on their own. Thus, the facilitator was a critical part of the team's success in completing the steps of the IDEAS Tool. The facilitator devoted considerable time over the course of the program to prep, plan, and facilitate team meetings. The majority of the facilitator's time was spent between meetings, combing through the design team's materials to condense and simplify the information to help move the team through the program (Table 2). The criteria for recruitment for the design team and steering committee were met. However, store management was not able to consistently schedule team members to work on the day of the meeting as planned so not all team members were able to attend the weekly meetings. Seven workers were initially recruited, but one was unable to regularly attend the meetings. The final design team consisted of six workers with racial and gender diversity. The team was representative of the line-level workers in terms of age, seniority, union membership, and self-reported weight. We recruited a volunteer from six of the store's largest departments. The six departments with design team volunteers represented 52% of the store's workforce.

Table 2. Participatory Health Program Process Evaluation.

Process Measures & Indicators	Results
Inputs	
Fidelity to HWPP materials	
Used IDEAS Tool materials/worksheets as planned	Yes—minor language modifications
Design team members understood the materials/program process	Yes—design team members reported that materials were easy to understand, but didn't always know the best way to move forward through program materials
Facilitator	
Knowledgeable about the HWPP & IDEAS Tool	Yes—thorough review of facilitator guide prior to program initiation
Knowledgeable about the workplace	Partial—external researcher with previous experience in this store
Time expenditure met expectations (~20 h)	No—greater than anticipated (57 h over 10 weeks)
Design Team	
Recruited 6–8 design team members	Yes—6 design team members
Met recruitment criteria	Yes—met all criteria
Design team members scheduled to work on meeting days	No—all design team members scheduled to work on only 2 of 9 meeting days
Steering Committee	
Steering committee represented various levels of authority	Partial—corporate, store supervisor, unions; store manager not involved
Activities	
Fidelity to the IDEAS Tool	
Design team completed IDEAS Steps 1–5A	Yes—completed Steps 1–5A; also partially completed Step 6
Steering committee completed IDEAS Steps 5B–6	Partiall—completed Step 5B; partially completed Step 6
Dose	
Number/duration/frequency of design team meetings	16 meetings; 50–60 min each; met weekly for 10 weeks, then as needed
Number/duration/frequency of steering committee meetings	2 meetings; 60–90 min each; 7 months between meetings
Engagement	
Design team meeting attendance	All present at six of 16 scheduled meetings; one member absent at seven meetings; two or more members absent at three meetings
Steering committee meeting attendance	All present at 1 of 2 scheduled meetings; 2 members present at second meeting
Design team engagement (Facilitator mean rating for each design team members across all meetings; Scale: 0 = No, 0.5 = some/somewhat, 1 = Yes)	Offered new ideas during meetings = 0.86
	Actively participated in meeting = 0.88
	Completed homework = 0.50
	Discussed projects with co-workers = 0.81
	Design team required significant facilitation to further develop and implement activities; facilitator took on a lot of activity development responsibility; team members reported they were not motivated to take initiative, however they often made a point to attend team meetings even when not scheduled to work (15 out of 20 instances)

Table 2. Cont.

Process Measures & Indicators	Results
Design team perception of the process	Team members reported feeling positively impacted by the program and thought the program was innovative and important, but they did not know how to implement activities without help.
Design team perception of support	The team did not feel they received logistical support from store management to implement solutions and response time was slow. They also felt that the steering committee did not follow through on promises and took too long to respond to the team.
Steering committee perception of program	1 of 6 steering committee members continued with the program until completion; one member was vocal about not believing in the program/process.
Activities generated	The design team generated 3 objectives with 15 distinct activities; the steering committee approved 7 activities
Outputs	
Store Worker Reach	
Activities implemented	5 activities were implemented
Awareness of implemented solutions	Surveys: 99 of 105 workers noticed at least one activity implemented by the design team. Awareness varied by activities; Results shown in Table 3.
Utilization of implemented activities	Surveys: Participation in the activities was higher among workers who used the break room, where most of the activities were implemented and communicated to the workforce. Results shown in Table 3.
Store Workers' Perception of Program	Surveys: 39 of 105 workers reported the activities helped them improve their eating and/or exercise habits
	Worker interviews ($n = 5$): 4/5 thought the activities were good for store workers in general, but changes in their own health behaviors were made for other reasons, not due to program

Note: HWPP: Healthy Workplace Participatory Program, IDEAS: Intervention Design and Analysis Scorecard.

3.3. Model Activities

Fidelity to the IDEAS process was met and Steps 1–6 were completed by the design team or steering committee (Table 2). Step 7 (evaluation) was not completed by the design team or steering committee, as formative and follow-up survey data collection was completed by the research team. Design team members were highly engaged during the meetings and attendance was consistent; no design team member missed more than two meetings and they often attended meetings on their days off work. While the level of participation during meetings varied by person, all team members contributed to the discussion and offered new ideas. The members of the design team were not consistent with completing assigned 'homework' tasks outside of meetings, but they did report talking to each other about the program between meetings. Scheduling conflicts and other priorities prevented greater time for discussion and completion of homework activities.

Overall, design team members had positive perceptions of the program. They reported that the program met their expectations and positively influenced their health (i.e., drinking more water, purchasing healthier food options). Five of the six team members felt that the participatory process created opportunities for more open dialogue with management, although they did not feel confident that management would follow-through on implementing proposed activities. In addition, a few design team members were frustrated with being scheduled to work at the time of the team meetings, however they were able to work with their immediate supervisor to attend. Early in the process (Step 1), the design team participated in two rounds of brainstorming which generated a total of 65 ideas grouped into four themes (diet, physical activity, stress, and health awareness). The team referred to these ideas and themes in Step 2 to identify their goal ("Reduce Stress at Work"), develop three objectives ("Improve Diet at Work," "Improve Store Communication," and "Increase Health Awareness"), and create 15 specific activities related to the three objectives. The design team rated these activities during Steps 3 and 4 with the understanding that they would have to "sell" the ideas to management. The team presented their top rated ideas to the steering committee. The steering committee took approximately 7 months to respond to the design team's proposal; they approved five activities without edit; approved two activities with small changes based on current store logistics; requested more information on four activities; and did not approve four activities (Table 3).

Table 3. Proposed activities and implementation outcomes.

Objectives and Activities	Steering Committee Response to Proposal	Implemented (Yes/No)—Responsible Party	Store Workers Noticed ($n = 105$)	Store Workers Used ($n = 105$)
Improve Store Communication				
Utilize email to communicate info	Agreed	No—store mgmt.	-	-
Use TV in break room for announcements	Agreed with modifications	No—store mgmt.	-	-
Develop better process for tracking and ordering supplies (identified as a stressor)	Not approved (said it was not relevant to the project)	N/A	-	-
Improve Diet at Work				
Get a bigger refrigerator for break room	Agreed	Yes—store mgmt.	78%	43%
Healthier options near checkout	Agreed	Yes (partial)—store mgmt.	30%	16%
Bottled water in break room	Agreed	Yes—design team	81%	47%
"Healthy choices" section	Wanted more details	No—design team	-	-
Include healthy options in $5 meals	Wanted more details	No—steering committee	-	-
Offer healthier premade meals and offer discount	Not approved (not profitable)	N/A	-	-
Add nutrition info and healthy recipes to recipe kiosks	Not approved (kiosks no longer used)	N/A	-	-
Reward workers for eating healthy	Wanted more details	No—design team	-	-
Increase Health Awareness				
Walking challenge with incentives	Agreed	Yes (Completed one 12-week challenge)—design team	50%	13%
Health focused newsletter	Agreed	Yes (2 delivered during study period)—design team	45%	25%
Gym/Exercise class discounts	Need details from unions	No—steering committee	-	-
Add more health topics to the "Meet the Expert" class schedule & increase the number of classes	Not approved (no longer offer classes)	N/A	-	-

3.4. Model Outputs

Of the seven activities that were agreed upon by the steering committee, five were implemented by the design team by the end of the study period; two were not completed because they needed other resources to implement (i.e., waiting on information technology department to complete tasks). Surveys at follow up from 105 store workers (67% response rate) showed the activities noticed most often by workers were ones that were implemented in the breakroom: the new employee refrigerator and discounted bottles of water. Activities that were delivered in other areas of the store were implemented intermittently, and not noticed by many workers. Only six workers said they did not notice any of the implemented program activities. Similarly, utilization of the activities was higher for those implemented in the breakroom and for the activities that did not require much extra effort by the workers. During store worker interviews, workers either were excited about the new health activities and wanted to see more implemented or they had not heard of them. Those that had not heard of the activities indicated that direct communication from store management about new health opportunities may be more useful than printed materials placed throughout the store. Only one of the five workers reported health behavior changes based on an implemented program activity; other workers said that they appreciated the effort, but that none of the implemented activities impacted their personal behaviors.

4. Discussion

Implementation of the HWPP was moderately successful in the grocery store setting as demonstrated by good fidelity to program materials, design team engagement in the IDEAS process, and the number of and uptake of program activities in a relatively short time period. This success can be attributed mostly to the design team's interest in the program and the extra time spent by the facilitator to move the team along; leadership support, including lack of active participation by the store management, was the main barrier to further success. The logic model provided an effective and simple framework for evaluating program implementation and allowed us to better understand the workplace factors necessary for success, as well as challenges or barriers that might be overcome with program modifications or additional resources. The HWPP offers multiple tools that can be used in conjunction with this model including the organizational readiness checklist to evaluate Pre-Implementation and the Management Dashboard and PERS tools to evaluate the Inputs, Activities, and Outputs under Program Implementation.

The program inputs (i.e., HWPP program, design team, steering committee, and facilitator) provided a good structure for the program. The HWPP materials were extremely helpful for the facilitator, although the language was somewhat confusing to the design team. High fidelity to the recruitment criteria led to high engagement and enthusiasm of design team members. The design team's interest in health and improving their store was vital to their success. The design team members had strong and consistent attendance and participation during meetings, yet seemed to lack the skills needed to progress through all steps of the program. They proceeded well with the initial steps to assess the workplace, identify problems, and come up with solutions, but struggled with the subsequent steps required to create a realistic plan to present to the steering committee. It is likely the design team members had not previously had the need nor opportunity to use these skills in their jobs. Employees may develop these skills through their jobs or by participating in employee-management teams for other business reasons. However, teams consisting of employees without these skills may be unable to effectively design and implement workplace changes without additional external support or training [18,19,54,55].

As a result, the team required substantial assistance from the facilitator to organize information and develop plans to complete each step of the process. The time demands on the facilitator far exceeded our expectations. It is possible that the steering committee or store management could have assisted the design team with some steps. We were careful to include various levels of leadership (including union representation) on the steering committee; however, there was a discrepancy between the stated support (i.e., help with scheduling design team members and help rolling out solutions) and the actual support received (i.e., design team members often not scheduled to work on meeting days and steering committee took little responsibility for implementing activities). Earlier and more frequent involvement from the steering committee in the design team meetings may have mitigated the need for substantial facilitator resources.

The main program activity, the IDEAS Tool, was delivered as intended. With support from the facilitator, the design team was able to meet, agree on a goal, and develop specific activities for each objective to propose to the steering committee (Steps 1–5A). The team's inability to meet outside of scheduled meetings and the steering committee's prolonged delay in responding to the design team's proposal left no time in the study period to complete IDEAS Step 7 (i.e., Evaluation), or initiate another cycle of the IDEAS process. Without this entire action-feedback cycle, the potential for organizational learning was decreased. This long delay also affected morale and enthusiasm, which resulted in two members leaving the design team. Additionally, the design team's meeting location may have been a problem for some team members. The onsite meeting space was not private; store managers and other employees frequently passed through the meeting space, causing the design team to feel uncomfortable sharing information. Despite these challenges, the program produced worthwhile outputs, demonstrating program success and a positive design team-steering committee collaboration. Overall, the design team had a positive impression of the process noting an increased comradery with team members and healthier behaviors as a result of the intervention. Some team members reported a sense of self-efficacy for continuing the program, while others did not think they could continue without the research team there to facilitate and hold management accountable. Further, data from surveys and interviews showed that store workers were aware of and utilized the workplace activities developed by the design team, indicating relevance to the target audience. Feedback about the methods used for communicating the activities was helpful in explaining possible reasons for non-awareness.

We encountered several challenges during the program that are best described and understood in the pre-implementation and context elements of the logic model. Most importantly, this pilot project grew out of an existing collaboration with a union and three regional grocers. During the planning phases, because only one grocer volunteered to participate and then offered only one store as the test site, we did not have the opportunity to assess organizational readiness at the corporate or the store levels, nor were we able to choose a site that demonstrated readiness to change. While the initial store manager was enthusiastic, he was transferred to another store early in the study and the manager who replaced him was not as invested. The new store manager's lack of interest in the program filtered down to the design team who felt that their efforts were not appreciated. Over time, the design team's level of enthusiasm and engagement in the process decreased. Many previous studies have shown that lack of organizational readiness and leadership support are critical factors to program success [18,19,28,55–57]. The HWPP program materials describe the importance of organizational readiness but do not provide guidance on how to prevent or remediate diminishing leadership support during the course of implementing the program. In our study, we found that the steering committee and store management were less supportive of interventions that focused on addressing workplace problems (e.g., supply order process and communication) and had fewer concerns about those that focused on changing individual behaviors (e.g., walking program). It is possible that the steering committee did not fully understand the purpose of the program and therefore were less willing to support the design team's ideas. Assessing organizational and leadership knowledge of the Total Worker Health approach may be an important part of determining program readiness and the need for education or training before and during program implementation.

We also faced obstacles related to the labor-management structure and agreements and differences between the different unions. The design team was challenged to find activities that applied to employees from the various unions, since the health benefits varied between different unions. This made it difficult for the design team to promote or build upon existing health resources. Due to labor contracts, design team members were not allowed to meet on paid work time. The research team addressed this by paying team members for their time to attend meetings; we do not know if the team's attendance and engagement would have been different had they been allowed to meet on paid work time. Scheduling design team members to work on meeting days also proved to be difficult, which meant that design team members were asked to come in on their days off. These payment and scheduling challenges made some design team members question management's support and willingness to follow through on proposed activities. The issue of paid time to participate on a design team is a problem when trying to implement a participatory program in hourly-paid workers. Management support should include compensating design team members for their time, and ensuring protected time for team members to develop their ideas.

Research has demonstrated a clear link between worker health and productivity, and investing in employee health has become a popular strategy for improving business outcomes [19,55,56,58]; however, many organizations struggle with supporting worker health initiatives when they compete with business objectives [59]. The design team members in this project recognized the need to fit their ideas into the broader business purpose and were thoughtful in creating activities that capitalized on existing resources or that could be marketed to retail customers in addition to store workers (e.g., premade healthy meals, healthy items near the checkout). While some activities were initially supported by the steering committee, they were not maintained over time because other initiatives, such as holiday product placement, took priority. Additionally, management put little effort into making the existing healthy options for customers more accessible to employees, suggesting that business needs were more important than worker health. This issue of competing interests between business and health is an important contextual factor to consider in interpreting the outcomes of TWH interventions and programs. Other contextual factors that we encountered in this study included seasonality of the work, skill level of employees, rotating employee schedules, and need to put customers first. All of these factors likely influenced the result of the participatory process used in this study, and may impact health and safety initiatives in the retail industry.

Our research study had several limitations. As described, workers were not able to attend meetings during work time and therefore were paid by the research team to attend. The collection of data for the process evaluation may have had an impact on the program's delivery. It is not known if the successful delivery of the program in one store will be generalizable to other retail locations, with different workers, management, facilities, and culture. In addition, we have limited data on whether the observed program implementation had an effect on the health behaviors of workers.

There were also several strengths to the study, including our relationship with the store that allowed us access to employees and support for the research, in addition to the facilitator's strong rapport with the design team. The detailed process measures allowed us to evaluate the fidelity of the program implementation and note which components were problematic and should be improved in future trials. The HWPP materials provided a useful structure and guide to make decisions throughout the process.

Participatory methods like those used in the HWPP may be useful in developing TWH interventions that address a variety of work factors that affect worker health. Our recommendations for those who may choose to use this program are: (1) Assess organizational knowledge, readiness, resources, and commitment; build in time prior to implementation to educate leadership and ensure that they understand the program goals, processes, and expectations; (2) Include and budget for a knowledgeable facilitator who has good communication, planning, and organizational skills; (3) Choose team members who are enthusiastic and have good communication, planning, and organizational skills (or ensure that the steering committee can assist); (4) Schedule in-person meeting time to complete the activities for each step (rather than assume the team will complete things outside of meetings); (5) Customize the worksheets for the audience and add materials as necessary to aid the team through the process; (6) Involve the steering committee early in the process and ask them at the onset of the program to play an active role in planning and implementing solutions; and (7) Build in time and resources for periodic evaluation and modifications that may result from the evaluation.

5. Conclusions

Participatory programs such as the HWPP show promise as a methodology for creating effective Total Worker Health interventions. This approach is useful for developing activities that can be used by workers and are relevant to their health. This is particularly important for workers in lower paying jobs or in jobs that have complex or chaotic work environments which present other challenges for good health behaviors. The detailed evaluation showed that substantial resources are needed to deliver the program and that enthusiastic, consistent, and active support from management is a critical determinant of success. The broader workplace context may also present challenges which should not be minimized or ignored. Future research studies should explore creative approaches for addressing organizational/contextual challenges that arise during participatory programs and should examine the efficacy of participatory programs. The logic model in this paper offers a framework for evaluating both implementation and efficacy, while considering the unique organizational contexts in which the intervention occurs.

Author Contributions: Conceptualization, J.R.S., B.A.E. and A.M.D.; Data curation, J.R.S. and A.M.K.; Formal analysis, J.R.S., A.M.K. and A.M.D.; Funding acquisition, A.M.D.; Investigation, J.R.S., A.M.K. and A.M.D.; Methodology, J.R.S., B.A.E. and A.M.D.; Project administration, J.R.S.; Resources, J.R.S. and A.M.K.; Supervision, A.M.D.; Visualization, J.R.S. and A.M.D.; Writing—Original Draft, J.R.S. and A.M.K.; Writing—Review & Editing, B.A.E. and A.M.D.

Funding: This research was funded by Healthier Workforce Center of the Midwest, grant number CDC/NIOSH U19OH008868 and the Washington University Center for Diabetes Translation Research (WU-CDTR), grant number NIH/NIDDK P30DK09295.

Acknowledgments: We wish to thank our union and grocery store research partners, the design team members, and the steering committee for their support and effort during the program. We would also like to thank Jessica Schenk for all of her work on the project.

Conflicts of Interest: The authors declare no conflict of interest. The funders had no role in the design of the study, in the collection, analyses, or interpretation of data, in the writing of the manuscript, or in the decision to publish the results.

References

1. Dale, A.M.; Enke, C.; Buckner-Petty, S.; Hipp, J.A.; Marx, C.; Strickland, J.; Evanoff, B. Availability and Use of Workplace Supports for Health Promotion Among Employees of Small and Large Businesses. *Am. J. Health Promot.* **2018**, *33*, 30–38. [CrossRef] [PubMed]
2. Lerner, D.; Allaire, S.H.; Reisine, S.T. Work disability resulting from chronic health conditions. *J. Occup. Environ. Med.* **2005**, *47*, 253–264. [CrossRef] [PubMed]
3. Meraya, A.M.; Sambamoorthi, U. Chronic Condition Combinations and Productivity Loss Among Employed Nonelderly Adults (18 to 64 Years). *J. Occup. Environ. Med.* **2016**, *58*, 974–978. [CrossRef] [PubMed]
4. Vuong, T.D.; Wei, F.; Beverly, C.J. Absenteeism due to Functional Limitations Caused by Seven Common Chronic Diseases in US Workers. *J. Occup. Environ. Med.* **2015**, *57*, 779–784. [CrossRef] [PubMed]
5. Asay, G.R.B.; Roy, K.; Lang, J.E.; Payne, R.L.; Howard, D.H. Absenteeism and Employer Costs Associated With Chronic Diseases and Health Risk Factors in the US Workforce. *Prev. Chronic Dis.* **2016**, *13*, E141. [CrossRef]
6. National Center for Chronic Disease Prevention and Health Promotion. Using the Workplace to Improve the Nation's Health: At a Glance 2016. Available online: https://www.cdc.gov/chronicdisease/resources/publications/aag/workplace-health.htm (accessed on 21 December 2018).
7. Froehlich-Grobe, K.; Jones, D.; Businelle, M.S.; Kendzor, D.E.; Balasubramanian, B.A. Impact of disability and chronic conditions on health. *Disabil. Health J.* **2016**, *9*, 600–608. [CrossRef]
8. Schopp, L.H.; Bike, D.H.; Clark, M.J.; Minor, M.A. Act Healthy: Promoting health behaviors and self-efficacy in the workplace. *Health Educ. Res.* **2015**, *30*, 542–553. [CrossRef] [PubMed]
9. Loeppke, R.; Taitel, M.; Haufle, V.; Parry, T.; Kessler, R.C.; Jinnett, K. Health and productivity as a business strategy: A multiemployer study. *J. Occup. Environ. Med.* **2009**, *51*, 411–428. [CrossRef] [PubMed]
10. Bauer, U.E.; Briss, P.A.; Goodman, R.A.; Bowman, B.A. Prevention of chronic disease in the 21st century: Elimination of the leading preventable causes of premature death and disability in the USA. *Lancet* **2014**, *384*, 45–52. [CrossRef]
11. National Institute for Occupational Safety and Health. What is Total Worker Health? Available online: https://www.cdc.gov/niosh/twh/default.html (accessed on 19 December 2018).
12. Tamers, S.L.; Chosewood, L.C.; Childress, A.; Hudson, H.; Nigam, J.; Chang, C.-C. Total Worker Health® 2014–2018: The Novel Approach to Worker Safety, Health, and Well-Being Evolves. *Int. J. Environ. Res. Public Health* **2019**, *16*, 321. [CrossRef] [PubMed]
13. Feltner, C.; Peterson, K.; Palmieri Weber, R.; Cluff, L.; Coker-Schwimmer, E.; Viswanathan, M.; Lohr, K.N. The Effectiveness of Total Worker Health Interventions: A Systematic Review for a National Institutes of Health Pathways to Prevention Workshop. *Ann. Intern. Med.* **2016**, *165*, 262–269. [CrossRef] [PubMed]
14. Henning, R.; Warren, N.; Roberston, M.; Faghri, P.; Cherniack, M.; CPH-NEW Research Team. Workplace Health Protection and Promotion through Participatory Ergonomics: An Integrated Approach. *Public Health Rep.* **2009**, *124*, 26–35. [CrossRef] [PubMed]

15. Van Eerd, D.; Cole, D.; Irvin, E.; Mahood, Q.; Keown, K.; Theberge, N.; Village, J.; St Vincent, M.; Cullen, K. Process and implementation of participatory ergonomic interventions: A systematic review. *Ergonomics* **2010**, *53*, 1153–1166. [CrossRef] [PubMed]
16. Hignett, S.; Wilson, J.R.; Morris, W. Finding ergonomic solutions: Participatory approaches. *Occup. Med. Oxf.* **2005**, *55*, 200–207. [CrossRef] [PubMed]
17. Faridi, Z.; Grunbaum, J.; Gray, B.; Franks, A.; Simoes, E. Community-based Participatory Research: Necessary Next Steps. *Prev. Chronic Dis.* **2007**, *4*, A70. [PubMed]
18. Dugan, A.G.; Farr, D.A.; Namazi, S.; Henning, R.A.; Wallace, K.N.; El Ghaziri, M.; Punnett, L.; Dussetschleger, J.L.; Cherniack, M.G. Process evaluation of two participatory approaches: Implementing total worker health(R) interventions in a correctional workforce. *Am. J. Ind. Med.* **2016**, *59*, 897–918. [CrossRef] [PubMed]
19. Cherniack, M.; Dussetschleger, J.; Dugan, A.; Farr, D.; Namazi, S.; El Ghaziri, M.; Henning, R. Participatory action research in corrections: The HITEC 2 program. *Appl. Ergon.* **2016**, *53*, 169–180. [CrossRef] [PubMed]
20. Evanoff, B.A.; Bohr, P.C.; Wolf, L.D. Effects of a participatory ergonomics team among hospital orderlies. *Am. J. Ind. Med.* **1999**, *35*, 358–365. [CrossRef]
21. Robertson, M.; Henning, R.; Warren, N.; Nobrega, S.; Dove-Steinkamp, M.; Tibirica, L.; Bizarro, A.; CPH-NEW Research Team. The Intervention Design and Analysis Scorecard: A planning tool for participatory design of integrated health and safety interventions in the workplace. *J. Occup. Environ. Med.* **2013**, *55*, S86–S88. [CrossRef] [PubMed]
22. Sorensen, G.; Stoddard, A.; Ockene, J.K.; Hunt, M.K.; Youngstrom, R. Worker participation in an integrated health promotion health protection program: Results from the WellWorks project. *Health Educ. Q.* **1996**, *23*, 191–203. [CrossRef]
23. Baker, E.A.; Israel, B.A.; Schurman, S.J. A participatory approach to worksite health promotion. *J. Ambul. Care Manag.* **1994**, *17*, 68–81. [CrossRef]
24. Wallerstein, N.; Duran, B. Community-based participatory research contributions to intervention research: The intersection of science and practice to improve health equity. *Am. J. Public Health* **2010**, *100*, S40–S46. [CrossRef] [PubMed]
25. Punnett, L.; Cherniack, M.; Henning, R.; Morse, T.; Faghri, P.; CPH-NEW Research Team. A conceptual framework for integrating workplace health promotion and occupational ergonomics programs. *Public Health Rep.* **2009**, *124*, 16–25. [CrossRef] [PubMed]
26. Kazutaka, K. Roles of Participatory Action-oriented Programs in Promoting Safety and Health at Work. *Saf. Health Work* **2012**, *3*, 155–165. [CrossRef] [PubMed]
27. Nobrega, S.; Champagne, N.; Abreu, M.; Goldstein-Gelb, M.; Montano, M.; Lopez, I.; Arevalo, J.; Bruce, S.; Punnett, L. Obesity/Overweight and the Role of Working Conditions: A Qualitative, Participatory Investigation. *Health Promot. Pract.* **2016**, *17*, 127–136. [CrossRef] [PubMed]
28. Nobrega, S.; Kernan, L.; Plaku-Alakbarova, B.; Robertson, M.; Warren, N.; Henning, R. Field tests of a participatory ergonomics toolkit for Total Worker Health. *Appl. Ergon.* **2017**, *60*, 366–379. [CrossRef] [PubMed]
29. Center for the Promotion of Health in the New England Workplace. Evaluate your Program. Available online: https://www.uml.edu/Research/CPH-NEW/Healthy-Work-Participatory-Program/Evaluate-Your-Program/default.aspx (accessed on 31 January 2019).
30. Robertson, M.M.; Henning, R.A.; Warren, N.; Nobrega, S.; Dove-Steinkamp, M.; Tibiriçá, L.; Bizarro, A. Participatory design of integrated safety and health interventions in the workplace: A case study using the Intervention Design and Analysis Scorecard (IDEAS) Tool. *Int. J. Hum. Factors Ergon.* **2015**, *3*, 303–326. [CrossRef]
31. Tamers, S.L.; Goetzel, R.; Kelly, K.M.; Luckhaupt, S.; Nigam, J.; Pronk, N.P.; Rohlman, D.S.; Baron, S.; Brosseau, L.M.; Bushnell, T.; et al. Research Methodologies for Total Worker Health(R): Proceedings From a Workshop. *J. Occup. Environ. Med.* **2018**, *60*, 968–978. [CrossRef]
32. Zhang, Y.; Flum, M.; Kotejoshyer, R.; Fleishman, J.; Henning, R.; Punnett, L. Workplace Participatory Occupational Health/Health Promotion Program: Facilitators and Barriers Observed in Three Nursing Homes. *J. Gerontol. Nurs.* **2016**, *42*, 34–42. [CrossRef]

33. Strickland, J.R.; Eyer, A.A.; Purnell, J.Q.; Kinghorn, A.M.; Herrick, C.; Evanoff, B.A. Enhancing Workplace Wellness Efforts to Reduce Obesity: A Qualitative Study of Low-Wage Workers in St Louis, Missouri, 2013–2014. *Prev. Chronic Dis.* **2015**, *12*, E67. [CrossRef]
34. Strickland, J.R.; Pizzorno, G.; Kinghorn, A.M.; Evanoff, B. Worksite Influences on Obesogenic Behaviors in Low-Wage Workers in Saint Louis, Missouri, 2013–2014. *Prev. Chronic Dis.* **2015**, *12*, E66. [CrossRef] [PubMed]
35. Center for the Promotion of Health in the New England Workplace. Intervention Design and Analysis Scorecard (IDEAS): CPH-NEW Intervention Planning Tool and Facilitator's Guide. Available online: http://www.uml.edu/docs/FGuide_Mar3_Website_tcm18-102071.pdf (accessed on 31 January 2019).
36. Center for the Promotion of Health in the New England Workplace. CPH-NEW Healthy Workplace Participatory Program. Available online: http://www.uml.edu/Research/Centers/CPH-NEW/Healthy-Work-Participatory-Program/default.aspx (accessed on 10 October 2016).
37. Kristensen, T.S. Job stress and cardiovascular disease: A theoretic critical review. *J. Occup. Health Psychol.* **1996**, *1*, 246–260. [CrossRef] [PubMed]
38. Gilbody, S.; Richards, D.; Brealey, S.; Hewitt, C. Screening for depression in medical settings with the Patient Health Questionnaire (PHQ): A diagnostic meta-analysis. *J. Gen. Intern. Med.* **2007**, *22*, 1596–1602. [CrossRef] [PubMed]
39. Centers for Disease Control and Prevention. *CDC National Healthy Worksite Program (NHWP) Employee Health Assessment (CAPTURE)*; Centers for Disease Control and Prevention: Atlanta, GA, USA, 2005.
40. Fassi, M.E.; Bocquet, V.; Majery, N.; Lair, M.L.; Couffignal, S.; Mairiaux, P. Work ability assessment in a worker population: Comparison and determinants of Work Ability Index and Work Ability score. *BMC Public Health* **2013**, *13*, 305. [CrossRef] [PubMed]
41. Chau, J.Y.; Van Der Ploeg, H.P.; Dunn, S.; Kurko, J.; Bauman, A.E. Validity of the occupational sitting and physical activity questionnaire. *Med. Sci. Sports Exerc.* **2012**, *44*, 118–125. [CrossRef] [PubMed]
42. Segal-Isaacson, C.; Wylie-Rosett, J.; Gans, K. Validation of a short dietary assessment questionnaire: The Rapid Eating and Activity Assessment for Participants Short Version (REAP-S). *Diabetes Educ.* **2004**, *30*, 774–781. [CrossRef] [PubMed]
43. Ford, E.S.; Giles, W.H.; Dietz, W.H. Prevalence of the Metabolic Syndrome Among US AdultsFindings From the Third National Health and Nutrition Examination Survey. *JAMA* **2002**, *287*, 356–359. [CrossRef] [PubMed]
44. Zweber, Z.M. A Practical Scale for Multi-faceted Organizational Health Climate Assessment. Master's Thesis, University of Conneticut, Storrs, CT, USA, 2012.
45. Strickland, J.; Kinghorn, A.; Evanoff, B.; Dale, A. Experience Mapping to Convey Complex Data and Aid in the Design of Workplace Interventions. In Proceedings of the 12th International Conference on Occupational Stress and Health, Minneapolis, MN, USA, 7–10 June 2017.
46. Center for the Promotion of Health in the New England Workplace. CPH-NEW Healthy Workplace Participatory Program: Select the Design Team. Available online: http://www.uml.edu/Research/Centers/CPH-NEW/Healthy-Work-Participatory-Program/form-design-team/select-team.aspx (accessed on 31 January 2019).
47. Center for the Promotion of Health in the New England Workplace. CPH-NEW Healthy Workplace Participatory Program: Select Steering Committee. Available online: https://www.uml.edu/Research/CPH-NEW/Healthy-Work-Participatory-Program/steering-committee/role.aspx (accessed on 21 December 2018).
48. Jaegers, L.; Dale, A.M.; Weaver, N.; Buchholz, B.; Welch, L.; Evanoff, B. Development of a program logic model and evaluation plan for a participatory ergonomics intervention in construction. *Am. J. Ind. Med.* **2014**, *57*, 351–361. [CrossRef] [PubMed]
49. Dale, A.M.; Jaegers, L.; Welch, L.; Gardner, B.T.; Buchholz, B.; Weaver, N.; Evanoff, B.A. Evaluation of a participatory ergonomics intervention in small commercial construction firms. *Am. J. Ind. Med.* **2016**, *59*, 465–475. [CrossRef] [PubMed]
50. Haines, H.; Wilson, J.R.; Vink, P.; Koningsveld, E. Validating a framework for participatory ergonomics (the PEF). *Ergonomics* **2002**, *45*, 309–327. [CrossRef]

51. Driessen, M.T.; Proper, K.I.; Anema, J.R.; Bongers, P.M.; van der Beek, A.J. Process evaluation of a participatory ergonomics programme to prevent low back pain and neck pain among workers. *Implement. Sci.* **2010**, *5*, 65. [CrossRef] [PubMed]
52. Pehkonen, I.; Takala, E.P.; Ketola, R.; Viikari-Juntura, E.; Leino-Arjas, P.; Hopsu, L.; Virtanen, T.; Haukka, E.; Holtari-Leino, M.; Nykyri, E.; et al. Evaluation of a participatory ergonomic intervention process in kitchen work. *Appl. Ergon.* **2009**, *40*, 115–123. [CrossRef] [PubMed]
53. Pretty, J.; Guijt, I.; Scoones, I.; Thompson, J. *A Trainer's Guide for Participatory Learning and Action*; International Institute for Environment and Development: London, UK, 1995.
54. Gjessing, C.C.; Schoenborn, T.F.; Cohen, A. *Participatory Ergonomic Intervention in Meatpacking Plants*; Department of Health and Human Services, Public Health Service, Centers for Disease Control and Prevention, National Institute for Occupational Safety and Health: Washington, DC, USA, 1994.
55. Burgess-Limerick, R. Participatory ergonomics: Evidence and implementation lessons. *Appl. Ergon.* **2018**, *68*, 289–293. [CrossRef]
56. Dixon, S.M.; Theberge, N. Contextual factors affecting task distribution in two participatory ergonomic interventions: A qualitative study. *Ergonomics* **2011**, *54*, 1005–1016. [CrossRef] [PubMed]
57. Ferraro, L.; Faghri, P.D.; Henning, R.; Cherniack, M.; Center for the Promotion of Health in the New England Workplace Team. Workplace-based participatory approach to weight loss for correctional employees. *J. Occup. Environ. Med.* **2013**, *55*, 147–155. [CrossRef] [PubMed]
58. Parkinson, M.D. Employer Health and Productivity Roadmap strategy. *J. Occup. Environ. Med.* **2013**, *55*, S46–S51. [CrossRef] [PubMed]
59. Goetzel, R.Z.; Ozminkowski, R.J. The Health and Cost Benefits of Work Site Health-Promotion Programs. *Annu. Rev. Public Health* **2008**, *29*, 303–323. [CrossRef]

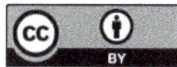

© 2019 by the authors. Licensee MDPI, Basel, Switzerland. This article is an open access article distributed under the terms and conditions of the Creative Commons Attribution (CC BY) license (http://creativecommons.org/licenses/by/4.0/).

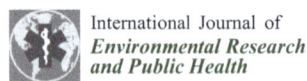

Article

Prospective Evaluation of Fidelity, Impact and Sustainability of Participatory Workplace Health Teams in Skilled Nursing Facilities

Rajashree Kotejoshyer [1,*], Yuan Zhang [1], Marian Flum [1], Jane Fleishman [2] and Laura Punnett [1]

[1] Center for the Promotion of Health in the New England Workplace (CPHNEW), University of Massachusetts Lowell, Lowell, MA 01854, USA; Yuan_Zhang@uml.edu (Y.Z.); Marian_Flum@uml.edu (M.F.); Laura_Punnett@uml.edu (L.P.)
[2] Center for Human Sexuality Studies, Widener University, Chester, PA 19013, USA; janefleishman@gmail.com
* Correspondence: rkotejoshyer@uchc.edu or rajashree_kotejoshyer@student.uml.edu; Tel.: +1-860-679-3857

Received: 5 March 2019; Accepted: 25 April 2019; Published: 27 April 2019

Abstract: Organizational features of work often pose obstacles to workforce health, and a participatory change process may address those obstacles. In this research, an intervention program sought to integrate occupational safety and health (OSH) with health promotion (HP) in three skilled nursing facilities. Three facilities with pre-existing HP programs served as control sites. The intervention was evaluated after 3–4 years through focus groups, interviews, surveys, and researcher observations. We assessed process fidelity in the intervention sites and compared the two groups on the scope of topics covered (integration), program impact, and medium-term sustainability. The intervention met with initial success as workers readily accepted and operationalized the concept of OSH/HP integration in all three intervention facilities. Process fidelity was high at first but diminished over time. At follow-up, team members in two intervention sites reported higher employee engagement and more attention to organizational issues. Two of the three control facilities remained status quo, with little OSH/HP integration. The intervention had limited but positive impact on the work environment and health climate: staff awareness and participation in activities, and organizational factors such as decision-making, respect, communication, and sharing of opinions improved slightly in all intervention sites. Resources available to the teams, management support, and changing corporate priorities affected potential program sustainability.

Keywords: occupational safety and health; workplace health promotion; integration; participatory workplace program; process fidelity; program impact; sustainability

1. Introduction

A number of chronic diseases are known to be associated with psychosocial work stressors, especially low job control, and other organizational factors such as night shift and overtime work [1–5]. It can be argued that because psychosocial job strain is an important predictor of health behaviors, a workplace health promotion (HP) program should seek to improve stressful working conditions in order to support healthy behaviors. Workplace HP programs have traditionally focused instead on trying to modify individual behaviors that increase disease risk. Workplace HP benefits are often unevenly distributed by worker socioeconomic status [6–8]. This may be, at least in part, because low-wage, low-status workers face more conditions at work which are obstacles both to the same health behaviors that are HP targets [8–10] and to HP participation [11].

A newer approach to workplace HP is that of enhancing its effectiveness by combining it with occupational safety and health (OSH) protections. This concept of integrated employee health programs has been put forward by a few researchers [12,13], the World Health Organization [14], and the U.S.

National Institute of Occupational Safety and Health [15]. An integrated strategy has been evaluated empirically by some investigators [16–18] but evidence is still sparse as to its effectiveness [19], in part because implementation approaches differ among investigators and thus are hard to compare [20]. Meanwhile, the norm in most workplaces is still that safety programs and workplace HP programs are managed separately.

Healthcare work is physically and psychologically demanding, exposing workers to many workplace stressors that affect their safety and health and which simultaneously may interfere with effective prevention measures [21–23]. We designed an intervention for the long-term healthcare sector based on a participatory model that engaged employees in examining and improving the physical, organizational, and psychosocial conditions at work that might impact their health and well-being. The program sought to bridge and integrate occupational safety and health with health promotion by identifying higher-level determinants of employee health and safety [24].

We have previously proposed [9,25] that any workplace health program should involve the workers in a decision-making role, both to ensure that obstacles to workers' healthy behaviors are recognized and addressed and to increase workers' decision latitude, a well-known and key health determinant. In a participatory approach, employees are actively engaged in problem identification, program design, implementation and evaluation of the program. The direct involvement of workers in the planning and design of interventions can benefit group and individual self-efficacy, which is consistent with the concept of "sense of coherence" [26], an internal resource for overcoming stress, reducing burnout and other adverse outcomes [27,28]. Participatory ergonomics is one example with demonstrated success as a way to reduce hazardous conditions in the workplace [29,30]. As discussed in depth by Jagosh et al. [31], "partnership synergy" provides a theoretical basis for assessing the links among participatory intervention context, mechanism(s), and outcomes (with elements also commonly utilized in process evaluations).

This article reports our evaluation of process fidelity, extent of OSH/HP integration, health impact, and sustainability of the participatory intervention program. In line with the middle-range "partnership synergy" theory, we have relied on information collected before, during, and after the study to describe the context (institutions and workforce), evidence for posited mechanism of change (e.g., fidelity and amount of intervention), and short- and medium-term outcomes (institutional and individual). The intervention was compared three to four years after initiation in the three participatory intervention program (PIP) sites to three control sites with non-participatory health promotion (NPHP) programs.

2. Materials and Methods

This study, "Promoting Physical and Mental Health of Caregivers through Transdisciplinary Intervention," was carried out through the Center for the Promotion of Health in the New England Workplace (CPH-NEW), a Total Worker Health®Center for Excellence of the National Institute of Occupational Safety and Health. At the time when this study began, "Total Worker Health" was defined by National Institute of Occupational Safety and Health as "a strategy integrating occupational safety and health protection with health promotion to prevent worker injury and illness and to advance worker health and well-being." The study was approved by the University of Massachusetts Lowell Institutional Review Board (protocol # 06-1403).

2.1. Setting and Sample

The project occurred within the context of a multi-year partnership with a large, for-profit long-term care company, which operated over 200 nursing facilities in 12 states within the eastern United States. In 2003–2006, the company had initiated a "safe resident handling" program in all of its skilled nursing facilities. Some sites also had HP activities as of 2006, depending on local initiative; a corporate-sponsored wellness program began in 2011.

Within that context, this project component sought to improve the health and safety of nursing home workers by creating participatory teams of non-supervisory workers to address integrated workplace HP and OSH concerns within their own worksites [32]. The teams were started in three skilled nursing facilities in 2008 with the assistance of university researchers. The participatory program was compared with a corporate-initiated wellness program in three other facilities within the same company and geographical region. None of the six facilities had union representation of their workers. We sought to involve all employees, in various job titles and at different organizational levels. Evaluation of program fidelity, impact, and sustainability was based on data from all employees who answered the surveys. Figure 1 provides an outline of the study process and evaluation activities.

2.2. Intervention Design

Based on the researchers' criteria, the company's regional director for health and safety recommended five skilled nursing facilities that did not yet have active HP programs and whose administrators were expected to be receptive to the participatory intervention process. We selected three of these facilities using a priori criteria to judge which were most organizationally ready for PIP [32]. Another three facilities with pre-existing, corporate-initiated HP programs were recommended by the regional director as control (NPHP) sites on the basis of their current activities and administrator commitment to the program [32].

In the PIP centers, team members were recruited from the entire workforce from volunteers responding to posters and management promotion of the program. Each team started with employees from various departments (clinical, dietary, housekeeping, laundry, maintenance, office/business) who met bi-weekly for one hour with two researchers. Initial team meetings involved identification of key issues in workplace health, psychosocial stress, and work organization.

The intervention began with intensive orientation of the PIP team (2–4 meetings per site over 1–2 months) to worker health and well-being, and Total Worker Health as a comprehensive approach. PIP teams identified issues of importance to members and discussed possible solutions or projects to address these concerns. Team members sought the opinions of their co-workers for program goals and specific activities. PIP team members communicated with individuals at various levels of their facility with updates and available activities (Figure 2).

Initially the researchers facilitated meetings, guided discussions, and assisted in framing presentations to the site administrator regarding a team's proposed project. Active facilitation involved the wellness champion and a research assistant attending all bi-weekly team meetings over 2 to 3 years, followed by monthly team meetings over 1 to 2 years, then quarterly telephone check about the program process with the wellness champion per site. The researchers provided technical assistance on a variety of topics, such as seminars on ergonomics in skilled nursing facilities and a food preferences survey to assist in developing programs for healthier food provision. Meeting minutes and activity logs were maintained by the researchers and utilized for ongoing process evaluation.

The goal was that participatory teams would move over time from co-governance to become independent, with support of the facility wellness champion. Thus, the study plan called for the researchers gradually to reduce our facilitation efforts over time. This was communicated to all participants at the beginning of the project. The phase-out period entailed 1–2 years of quarterly telephone check-ins with the wellness champion.

Pre-intervention (Year 2003-2006)	Baseline (Year 2007-2009)	Study Process	Follow-up (Year 2011-2013)
• Partnership with a long-term care company with prior investment in a safe resident handling program (2003-2006) and health promotion support in some facilities • Researcher site selection process: intervention site criteria = no active HP program, and willingness to support participatory approach; control site = active HP program (2007-2008). Three sites selected in each group.	• Employee focus groups (2007-2008) (6 sites). • Organizational readiness interviews with facility administrators (2008) (6 sites). • Survey of all employees (2008-2009) to assess health and safety, wellness activities, work environment factors, etc. (6 sites) • Survey about current activities by Wellness Champions (six sites). **Three intervention sites only:** Non-supervisory employees from all departments within the skilled nursing facilities were invited to join PIP teams. Ten employees recruited and oriented in each PIP site to serve as members of the "health and wellness" team.	**Three intervention sites only:** • Bi-weekly meetings of the PIP team at each site (3-4 years). • An experienced faculty researcher facilitated the participatory teams at each site, along with 2 trained research assistants. Team members used CPH-NEW worksheets to guide their problem investigations and design of activities and/or facility changes • Meetings usually convened by the facility Wellness Champion • Minutes and other project documentation maintained by the facilitator and research assistant	• Interviews with administrators (6 sites) (2011-2012) • Focus groups with employees not involved in designing wellness activities (6 sites) (2011-2012) • Focus groups with PIP team members (3 sites) (2011-2012) • Follow-up survey of all employees (2012-2013) to assess health and safety, wellness activities, work environment factors, etc. (same questionnaire as at baseline) (6 sites)

Figure 1. Timeline of the participatory intervention process and impact evaluation. HP, health promotion; PIP, participatory intervention program; CPH-NEW, Center for the Promotion of Health in the New England Workplace.

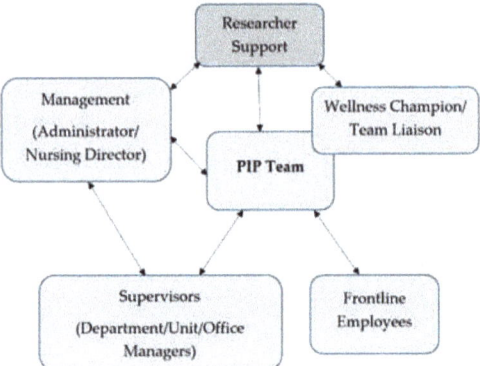

Figure 2. Participatory Intervention Design within Centers.

2.3. Data Collection and Analysis

A mixed-method (convergent parallel strategy) approach utilized qualitative and quantitative data to examine the process and impact of the participatory OSH/HP or NPHP program in each facility. Results from the qualitative and quantitative analyses were triangulated with the researchers' direct experiences and knowledge of the organization to understand the process, impact, and sustainability of the participatory program.

Quantitative data included a brief baseline (pre-intervention) survey of the wellness champions about HP program activities in all six centers. We also conducted employee surveys in the six centers at baseline (2008–2009) and around the fourth year (2012–2013) of the participatory intervention. A self-administered questionnaire collected information on worker chronic disease history, health beliefs and behaviors, and perception of the work environment: physical and psychological job demands, decision latitude, and social support from supervisors and coworkers [8,33,34]. Work environment items included physical exertion, safety climate, psychological demands, decision latitude, and supervisor and coworker support. Psychological demands (two items), decision latitude (two items), physical exertion (five items), and supervisor (two items) and coworker support (two items) were selected from the Job Content Questionnaire (JCQ) [35]. The JCQ subscales have demonstrated good validity and acceptable internal consistency in large study populations from six countries [35]. Safety climate was measured with two items from Griffin and Neal [36] and two items developed by the investigators.

Most analyses compared employees in the pooled intervention (PIP) group to the pooled control (NPHP) group (three centers per group). Baseline ($n = 645$) and post-intervention ($n = 649$) prevalences were compared by cross-tabulation with chi-square statistics and mean values by t-test for independent samples. Cumulative incidence of self-reported chronic diseases was computed from baseline to post-intervention within each group and compared between PIP and NPHP with Fisher exact tests due to small numbers. Within-person changes from baseline to follow-up (limited to workers responding to both surveys) were examined using stratified cross-tabulation and paired sample t-test. All analyses were done with SPSS 22.0 (IBM SPSS, Chicago IL, USA).

Qualitative data included the meeting minutes and activity logs collected throughout the active facilitation period. Follow-up data were collected 3–4 years after the intervention began (2011–2012). Data types included: (1) focus groups with team members; (2) focus groups with other nursing home employees; (3) in-depth interviews with individual team members and wellness champions; (4) in-depth interviews with management (administrators and directors of nursing); and (5) in-depth interviews with supervisors (department heads and unit/office managers) [24].

Other evaluation materials included researchers' field notes on observed indoor spaces (employee lounge, break room, vending machines, and bulletin boards), outdoor spaces (employee picnic areas and gardens), and printed materials (employee newsletters, flyers, and informational literature) devoted to HP, OSH, or related activities or information. Researcher experiences and observations were logged after each field visit and consulted for purposes of this evaluation. Content analysis was performed using NVivo 9.0 software on transcripts from interviews and focus groups. We compared the themes that emerged across and within the six sites, focusing on (1) integration of HP and OSH, (2) comparative effects of the PIP and NPHP programs, and (3) sustainability of PIP as a model.

Metrics for comparison and evaluation included:

- Process: Fidelity, type and number of activities.
- Integration: Extent to which programs and participants understood and adopted the approach of combined attention to HP (weight loss, exercise) and OSH issues (work environment, psychosocial stressors, ergonomics).
- Impact: Evaluated both at the organizational level (characteristics of the work environment and organization); and at the level of individual staff members (program engagement, awareness, opinions, and participation; health outcomes).
- Sustainability: How long the program lasted, indications of future plans or activities.

3. Results

3.1. Baseline Site Comparability

In the six centers, a total of 47 interviews were conducted with management (administrators and directors of nursing), supervisors (department heads and unit/office managers), wellness champions, and individual PIP team members. In addition, qualitative data were obtained from three focus groups of PIP team members, three focus groups of employees engaged in wellness at NPHP sites, and eight focus groups with other employees at the six facilities conducted in 2011 and 2012.

According to the baseline survey of wellness champions, and consistent with the criteria for their selection, the NPHP centers had well-developed programs at that time, whereas the PIP centers had emerging programs, i.e., 1–2 activities loosely organized by staff.

Questionnaires were collected from a total of 645 workers at baseline and 649 workers at follow-up. The PIP and NPHP sites each had more than half of employees in clinical jobs and a predominantly female staff (Table 1). The PIP staff were slightly younger on average. Fewer than 8% in either group indicated fair or poor self-rated health. The average scores were similar for health self-efficacy, prevalence of diabetes and low back problems. Workers in the NPHP centers had slightly higher baseline prevalence of hypertension and elevated cholesterol (Table 1). Decision latitude was higher among PIP staff than NPHP staff at baseline ($p < 0.01$) (Table 2).

Table 1. Baseline characteristics of skilled nursing facility employees (all jobs): 3 participatory intervention program (PIP) and 3 non-participatory health promotion (NPHP) centers.

Baseline Demographics		PIP (n = 360)	NPHP (n = 285)		
Gender	Female	78.3% (282)	85.3% (243)		
	Male	16.9% (61)	11.2% (32)		
Average Age		39.8 ± 12.4	41.8 ± 12.2		
Nursing Aides *		35.8% (124)	54.3% (120)		
Licensed practice nurse/Registered nurses		22.2% (77)	21.3% (47)		
Other jobs (non-clinical)		41.0% (142)	24.4% (54)		
Baseline Health Status		Cumulative incidence (%)	Cumulative incidence (%)	p-value	Difference in rates (NPHP vs. PIP)
Diabetes at baseline		8%	6%	0.77	2%
Hypertension at baseline		18%	20%	0.85	2%
Cholesterol at baseline		13%	25%	0.59	12%

* Jobtitles had missing values of 12.1%.

Table 2. Worker health and working conditions in pre- and post-intervention matched pair surveys: Comparison of PIP and NPHP centers.

Health Status	3 PIP centers (n = 102)		3 NPHP centers (n = 110)		Statistical Significance	
New cases at follow-up:	Cumulative incidence (%)		Cumulative incidence (%)		Difference in rates: NPHP–PIP	p-value [a]
Diabetes	6%		6%		0%	1.00
Hypertension	11%		14%		3%	0.82
High cholesterol	15%		11%		−4%	0.49
Low back problem	8%		8%		0%	1.00
Work Environment	Pre-intervention: mean (SD)	Change in mean value (post-pre)	Pre-intervention: mean (SD)	Change in mean value (post-pre)	Mean group difference, NPHP − PIP, in post-pre change (95% CI) [b]	
Health self-efficacy	26.5	−0.87	26.1	−0.30	0.58 (−0.83–1.99)	
Supervisor support	5.69	−0.07	5.87	−0.35	−0.28 (−0.76–0.20)	
Coworker support	5.88	−0.08	5.99	−0.06	0.02 (−0.34–0.37)	
Safety climate score	2.90	−0.30	2.93	−0.32	−0.03 (−0.16–0.11)	
Decision latitude	5.48 *	−0.22	5.18	0.56	0.77 (0.42–1.13) *	
Psychological demands	5.73	−0.11	5.54	0.00	0.11 (−0.22–0.45)	
Physical exertion	11.21	4.90	11.44	5.69	0.79 (−0.22–1.80)	

[a] from exact test statistic; [b] from t-test of independent samples; * $p < 0.01$.

3.2. Fidelity and Amount of Intervention

The participatory teams were active with the guidance of the researchers. In the intervention sites (I-1, I-2, I-3), the number of regularly attending PIP team members ranged from 4 to 8 of the 10 original members at each site. No NPHP control site (C-1, C-2, C3) had an active team or wellness committee engaging front-line workers.

At the start of this project, not all facilities had a wellness champion appointed. However, by three years after initiation of the program, all six centers had wellness champions, as required under the corporate-sponsored wellness program. Wellness champions were individuals appointed by site administrators to coordinate HP activities in addition to their regular duties. In the PIP centers, these were office staff in ancillary non-supervisory jobs like human resource payroll benefits, medical records manager, and data coordinator. Wellness champions in NPHP centers were all in supervisory positions (assistant admissions director, maintenance manager, and admission director). Interviews and focus groups showed that many staff in the PIP centers knew the identity of their wellness champions. In two of the three NPHP centers, focus group participants were unaware of their wellness champions.

The three PIP teams met every two weeks for one hour. They were planned to involve only non-supervisory personnel, and they began as such. However, at two of the centers, (I-1 and I-3), they were later expanded by managerial decision to include supervisory and administrative employees.

PIP teams were guided to utilize the program planning form and project proposals for approval from center administrators. The use of these forms and proposals became less consistent towards the end of the 5 years as some supervisors and managers became members of these participatory teams.

3.3. Integration of OSH and HP

In each of the PIP centers, the staff members who joined the teams readily voiced acceptance of the integration concept, i.e., that the obstacles to good health resided both in and outside the work environment. Issues related to both OSH and HP were identified in team meetings. These issues largely mirrored the results of the focus groups at the same centers. The discussions within each team, facilitated by the researchers, demonstrated their operational grasp of the connection between work organization, psychosocial stressors, and personal well-being. Many activities that they carried out represented on-going and systemic attempts to address these concerns in the work environment (Table 3). These included improvements in the workplace through mechanisms for enhanced communication, provision or improvement of employee break rooms and relaxation areas, ergonomics training, and provision of healthy food for staff at a reasonable cost.

Table 3. Activities carried out by staff PIP teams (Intervention centers) and wellness champions (Control centers) during the study period, 2008–2012.

Center	Work Organization	Psychosocial Stressors	Musculoskeletal and Ergonomics	Food Environment	Health Improvement
I-1	Communications log	Redesigned employee break room, picnic table	Ergonomics training	Healthy food in vending machine	Yoga, massage
I-2	Employee suggestion box, method to resolve communications problems on units	Picnic tables and lawn furniture	Ergonomics training	Healthy food in vending machine	Nutrition education, walking program
I-3	Staff garden, meetings with certified nursing assistants to discuss health and safety concerns	Staff garden maintenance (for 3 years)	Ergonomics training	Healthy snacks, fruit baskets at each unit, low-cost healthy food options in dining hall	Yoga, weight loss program, nutrition education
C-1	–	–	–	Healthy snacks	–
C-2	–	Softball team	–	Healthy snacks	Annual health fair
C-3	–	–	–	Healthy snacks	–

At intervention center I-3, when the PIP team spearheaded a gardening project, the original motivation was healthy eating. The team members then also used the garden project as a prototype for developing good proposals and presenting them to management for support and funding. Once it began, they discovered that the garden had many other benefits, including team-building, communications, exercise, stress relief, and a potential for fresh produce for residents as well as staff.

In contrast, in the NPHP centers, there were no projects designed to address up-stream work organization, psychosocial stressors, ergonomics, or work environment factors. Activities tended to support individual behavior change, e.g., coping, relaxation, and exercise (such as softball games). Correspondingly, none of the interviewed wellness champions in these centers demonstrated an understanding of how features of the job or workplace might influence health behaviors, or any vision as to what integration of OSH and HP might entail.

3.4. Program Impact

At the organizational level, as discussed above, a markedly larger number of activities was carried out in the PIP centers, compared with the control sites. The PIP teams had a number of positive impacts on their health environment at work. All three, independently, addressed lack of healthy food options as a priority and were able to obtain healthier food choices in vending machines. In one facility, the kitchen agreed to provide soups, salads, and sandwiches at reduced cost to employees. One team initiated the creation of a community garden.

The post-intervention surveys demonstrated slightly more organizational changes in the PIP centers than the NPHP centers (Table 4). These included both better communication and more opportunities to voice opinions and influence decisions. More staff members in the PIP sites (28% versus 16% in NPHP sites) said that they were consulted for program suggestions, and in general they reported slightly more opportunities to participate in decision-making and contribute suggestions. Qualitative data (focus groups and interviews) indicated that staff awareness of and participation in team-sponsored activities were higher in PIP centers. Further, researcher notes confirmed that the participatory teams with non-supervisory staff and administrator involvement generated more wellness activities than supervisor-only teams or those with no administrator involvement.

Table 4. Comparison of post-intervention survey responses between PIP and NPHP centers regarding changes in the work environment since the program began.

Work Environment Changes	3 PIP centers: Prevalence (%) (n = 331)	3 NPHP centers: Prevalence (%) (n = 318)	p-Value [a]
Improved communication between staff and supervisors/management	17% (57)	13% (41)	0.124
Improved communication between co-workers	17% (58)	15% (48)	0.403
More opportunities to participate in decision making	13% (42)	7% (22)	0.014 *
More opportunities to share my opinion (e.g., suggestion box)	13% (43)	9% (28)	0.088
Increased respect	10% (32)	7% (24)	0.336

[a] from chi-square statistic; * $p < 0.05$.

From follow-up survey data, the PIP sites had slightly more employees participating in company exercise (18%) and nutrition programs (25%) than in the NPHP group. There was also notable participation in team-sponsored gardening (9%) and healthy back training (8%), and utilization of outdoor furniture niches set up by the teams for mental relaxation (14%).

At the individual level, there was no within-person difference in self-reported health status (chronic disease diagnosis, musculoskeletal pain, stress levels, etc.) from pre-intervention to post-intervention in either group (Table 2). There were few notable changes in individual health conditions, health self-efficacy, or selected work factors, and all differences were modest. There was a 6% cumulative incidence of self-reported diabetes in both the PIP and NPHP groups. The NPHP group had a slightly higher incidence of new hypertension (14%) compared to the PIP group (11%). In contrast, the PIP group had a higher incidence of elevated cholesterol (15%) than the NPHP group (11%) (Table 2).

Self-efficacy for eating a healthy diet, avoiding fatty foods, and exercise worsened slightly in both groups over time. The NPHP group gained and the PIP group lost self-efficacy for losing weight, compared to their baseline ratings. Neither group had a change in self-efficacy for managing stress, avoiding smoking or alcohol, and there were no statistically significant differences ($p < 0.05$) between groups for any of these metrics (data not shown).

Decision latitude had been slightly higher in the PIP ($p = 0.001$) than the NPHP group at baseline, while it increased slightly in the NPHP group relative to the PIP group (Table 2). In fact, at follow-up decision latitude was (surprisingly) slightly higher in NPHP than in PIP. This was the only statistically significant change over time in group mean ratings of working conditions. Psychological job demands were reported slightly higher in the PIP group than the NPHP group in both surveys. Coworker support was slightly higher in the NPHP group at baseline and remained stable over time. In contrast, supervisor support decreased slightly in both the groups over time but was slightly better in the PIP group than the NPHP group at follow-up. Ratings of physical exertion at work dropped between the time periods in both groups, which might have reflected the impact of the company's safe resident handling program [23,37]. The PIP group improved more and had lower physical exertion than the NPHP post-intervention. Workplace safety climate was similar between the two groups and remained stable over time.

3.5. Sustainability

Sustainability was examined in relation to organizational conditions of leadership, staff participation, resources, and communication.

Leadership was vital for the sustainability of participatory programs. Administrative and supervisor support for wellness towards PIP teams and employees were indicated in many forms within the qualitative data. It included financial support, enabling staff to take time off for meetings and activities, providing meeting space, and verbal encouragement.

Both management and supervisor support were cited in the qualitative data by many employees and managers to be important for program sustainability. The effects of administrator support (and turnover) were mentioned as important in encouraging or discouraging team meetings and activities. Support from management (administrators and nursing directors) and from supervisors (department heads and unit/office managers) were examined separately.

Overall, the NPHP centers demonstrated higher management support than the PIP centers. Administrators in PIP centers discussed HP as part of their everyday work and considered their wellness champions and teams as part of their organizational structure (except in I-2).

Supervisor support was perceived to be higher in two PIP centers, I-1 and I-3, and low at I-2. At the NPHP center C-2, many employees described their supervisors as being supportive to HP by allowing flexibility in their staff schedules and even covering for them while they participated in activities. Other supervisors within this center were described to be supportive by participating in activities themselves and motivating their staff to participate.

PIP teams were able to provide more activities for the staff members with the presence of leadership support. When leadership support was absent, management in these centers talked about being faced with other pressures, needing to make decisions in favor of other more urgent projects and programs.

Management changes in two PIP centers led to combining the existing PIP teams with other, previously inactive committees ("staff appreciation committee" in site I-1, and "fun committee" in I-3). In both cases, the non-supervisory PIP teams were converted to administrator-directed committees with different agendas and priorities.

Staff participation in programs and activities is obviously a key measure of program impact as well as likely sustainability. Perceived lack of staff participation in PIP teams and activities was evaluated from the PIP team member interviews and focus groups.

All PIP team members stated in the focus groups that clinical staff had difficulty in getting time to attend team meetings or activities. Staff participation in team-sponsored activities was poor within center I-2. Researcher experience and logs showed that participation in PIP teams had been quite high at the start of the project, yet involvement of clinical staff diminished due to frustrations with their decision-making process and clinical responsibilities.

Employee participation in all three PIP teams dropped to a low number of non-supervisory clinical staff at the end of year 3 of the intervention. Low participation of clinical staff in activities were attributed to staffing shortages, time constraints, and clinical care responsibilities.

Resources mentioned in the interviews and focus groups included financial support from the corporation, in-house/in-kind personal effort, and outside support. Although wellness was a stated goal for both the PIP and NPHP centers, no funds were allocated in any of the facilities' budgets for employee wellness except in the first year (2008), when the corporation provided $700 per year for each facility. After this line item was dropped, most facilities engaged in regular fund-raising for their programs and many of the key informants expressed frustration at the lack of funds for their programs.

In the PIP centers, several projects and especially the higher cost projects simply could not be implemented without adequate resources. At one PIP site (I-2), much of their past activity had focused on fund-raising, which detracted from effort and time that could otherwise have been spent on health and wellness activities.

Using existing in-house resources was an opportunity for the PIP teams to benefit from the knowledge and skills of individual staff members. At Center I-1, one of the nurses offered yoga classes and another offered massages; at I-3, the dietitian offered many in-house programs and services including a weight loss program, potlucks, and healthy recipes.

Team members in the PIP centers identified researcher involvement and guidance as a key outside resource and a vital link to sustainability of the teams. At center I-2, most members believed that the PIP team would not continue without researcher support. The research team provided material support to all three PIP centers, including ergonomic training sessions to staff members, tools and seedlings for the garden, and an exercise class instructor.

Among NPHP centers, the primary forms of outside support cited were discounts for gym membership, health information, and free health screenings by group health insurance companies. In Center C-2, respondents also cited outside support from community programs along with insurance company services.

Communication was mentioned in the qualitative data as factors that are essential for sustaining a participatory health program.

Communication between the PIP teams or wellness champions with management as well as with the employees was uneven in both the PIP and NPHP centers. Employees in the PIP centers reported having good communication except at the I-2 center, where both the employees and managers expressed lack of communication as one of the largest stressors and most critical barriers to successful program implementation. The administrator at center I-2 concurred about the lack of communication between the PIP team and management. There appeared to be a trend towards better communication in centers where there was focused attention on work organization issues. In centers where closed-door management meetings were opened to staff or where the wellness champion utilized several methods of communication (e.g., memos, flyers, announcements during meetings, etc.), it was viewed as a smaller problem or not a problem at all.

3.6. Differences Among Non-Intervention Centers

Despite the overall group differences, one NPHP center (C-2) exhibited some characteristics and activities similar to the two positive PIP centers from the qualitative data from this center. Even with no official team at this center, the few employees involved in planning the activities had positive management support and were successful in obtaining high staff participation. The administrator, supervisors, and employees appeared to see wellness as a part of their organizational culture. The employee focus group indicated that most of the employees at this center had very few complaints. Most people agreed that good communication existed between management and employees and between the people planning the wellness activities and the rest of the management and staff. While employees at other NPHP facilities appeared uncertain about the idea of integration, the facility manager at C-2 (with previous knowledge about ergonomics and musculoskeletal training) led the safety committee and demonstrated interest in wellness. This manager shared ideas with the researchers about opportunities for integrating OSH and HP within the center.

4. Discussion

This study evaluated a participatory, integrated OSH/HP intervention in three skilled nursing facilities compared to three others with more traditional, non-participatory HP programs. Mixed qualitative and quantitative data collected over a four-year follow-up period demonstrated program feasibility, good process fidelity while the researchers were actively involved, meaningfulness of the integration concept to worker representatives, and moderate program impact on some organizational conditions of work. Sustainability, however, suffered due to lack of resources and inconsistent manager support.

4.1. Process Fidelity

Process fidelity was high initially in all three intervention sites; the program was introduced in a uniform manner by the researchers and proceeded as intended for the first two years or so. Members of the PIP teams were highly motivated and responsive to the organizing principles of worker priority-setting and a combined focus on both work and non-work obstacles to health. The center administrators permitted front-line staff to volunteer for the teams and assisted with the logistics of scheduling meetings, although use of paid work time for meetings was inconsistent. Involvement of non-supervisory clinical employees in the planning of workplace HP projects was high in the PIP centers at the start of the research project, although it diminished subsequently.

4.2. Integration

Compared to the traditional wellness programs in the control sites, the participatory teams in the three PIP centers were far more likely to develop activities with a broad scope, encompassing elements of both OSH and HP. Over time, the teams in the PIP centers addressed work organization, psychosocial stressors, physical ergonomics, in addition to taking an organizational approach to HP goals such as improving the food environment at work. In contrast, the NPHP centers primarily supported individual behavior change, with minimal attention to psychosocial stressors or the work environment. Consistent with our findings, a previous intervention study reported higher blue-collar worker participation with OSH/HP interventions compared to standard HP interventions [16]. In particular, when management's efforts to reduce workplace hazards were apparent, the workers were more likely to participate [16]. In our study, administrative changes and logistical challenges appeared to cause worker participation in the teams to dwindle gradually.

4.3. Impact

The number and variety of workplace HP activities initiated during the study period were higher in the PIP centers than the NPHP centers. Two of the three PIP centers indicated improvement in organizational factors. There were no larger corporate influences that would have produced these positive changes specifically in the three PIP centers, so it seems reasonable to consider them at least partially as outcomes of the integrated participatory program.

There was no evidence of major change in chronic illness incidence or the perception of health status or behaviors following this participatory intervention, but the four-year follow-up period was too short for any such difference to be expected.

The study hypothesis was that the PIP teams would have more impact than the NPHP programs. In a participatory approach, employees are actively engaged in problem identification, decision making, implementation, and evaluation of the program [38]. This approach has been argued to benefit intervention effectiveness because employees are well-qualified to identify opportunities and obstacles present in their work environment [25], and also because participating in intervention design and implementation could reduce perceived lack of decision latitude [9,39]. Intervention study with assembly workers has demonstrated improved health and work performance in the participatory group compared to controls [40]. While there is substantial literature on participatory workplace interventions, the literature is more consistent about short-term and process benefits than longer-term ones. It remains challenging to compile the evidence in such a way as to identify patterns that explain differences in impact.

4.4. Sustainability

Overall leadership support is widely recognized as crucial factors for a sustainable workforce health program of any type [16,32,41] and were so endorsed in the qualitative interviews in our study. Two PIP centers exhibited positive indicators with the participatory approach including essential factors such as support from the center that favored the continuation of meetings and activities.

Unfortunately, the initially high level of administrator supports and staff participation in project planning diminished somewhat over time. One of our goals was to incorporate the teams into other active committees with similar interests, in order to increase their long-term sustainability. In the two centers where this occurred, the teams were absorbed into committees without responsibility for employee health.

Administrator changes also negatively impacted management support, financial resources, and time release for program participation—all identified as important for progress of the participatory program [32]. Challenges to long-term PIP sustainability included communication barriers among employees, especially in different units, shifts, and job groups; excessive reliance on individual program champions at both site and regional levels; inconsistent corporate commitment to employee HP; and lack of a reward system for champions' or administrators' efforts. These mostly pre-dated the participatory teams, although we had sought to screen centers for favorable conditions.

All six centers lacked financial resources to sustain even basic wellness programs, such as paying for instructors in yoga, meditation, or fitness. It did not appear that employee health (other than safe resident handling, which had received a substantial investment) was perceived to generate a high enough return on investment to be sustained in this company.

4.5. Study Strengths and Limitations

A major strength of this study is the detailed information obtained from various data sources and the triangulation of qualitative and quantitative data. Mixed methods research is valuable because it captures the information from various perspectives and can support qualitative and quantitative findings [42]. This process evaluation is rich in detail and provides a comprehensive picture of the program. Further, the long follow-up period permits a reasonable understanding of the dynamics over time.

On the other hand, evaluation of the PIP's impact was limited by the fact that the sites were not selected at random. The three PIP sites were volunteered by their administrators in response to a recruitment effort by the investigators through a key regional staff member. The three NPHP sites were also selected by the same regional representative, in response to the research team's specified criteria, and then approached for management agreement to permit data collection. As a consequence, there were some anticipated baseline differences between the two groups, both in prior HP activity and possibly in administrator interest in and initiative toward workforce well-being. A further issue is that the study results are not expected to be generalizable, except to other nursing homes with similar management interest and willingness. Nevertheless, the results do demonstrate the feasibility of conducting a participatory change process in this sector, despite (in the U.S.A., at least) tight staffing and scheduling, coupled with low union representation to protect job security for those who voice their opinions about root causes of health and safety problems.

In theory, the gold standard for an intervention study is the randomized controlled trial. However, the benefits of randomization in reducing confounding are not realized except with a large sample. In this case, the intervention was carried out at the level of the entire facility (PIP). In practice, it was not logistically or economically feasible for us to enroll a large number of facilities for such an intervention. Even with some alternative designs, such as the stepped-wedge [43], there is still concern about potential confounding and often a randomization element, thus the number of intervention units remains important. One alternative is to compare the treatment groups on baseline characteristics that might influence the outcome, which we have done here. In fact, perceived working conditions were quite similar except for decision latitude; since that decreased later rather than increasing in the PIP group, the change in time was unlikely to be an artifact of a difference at baseline.

The other advantage of a randomized controlled trial is that with double-blinding, the possibility of information bias can be greatly reduced. However, blinding of participants and researchers is also infeasible for organizational-level interventions. In turn, randomization and blinding may have disadvantages for organizational-level interventions, such as limited capacity to assess multi-dimensional interventions or evaluate process, quality, or performance, and incompatibility with community trust, choice, and participation often needed for successful program design and evaluation [44–46].

Another limitation of this study is the difficulty to show the actual impact of the participatory program due to constant changes in the organization. For example, turnover in leadership in the study sites appeared to affect program success with administrator changes in the PIP sites during the study period. Similarly, employee turnover limited our ability to examine within-person changes over time, through reduced statistical power.

Participatory programs can be challenging to implement and evaluate in a research context because key elements cannot be controlled by the investigators; for example, interventions are selected and designed by workers after the program is already underway, and interventions addressing higher-level organizational obstacles may provoke institutional resistance that might not have been visible or even present at the beginning of the project. These issues were known in advance and cannot be prevented even when they are anticipated. It will always be the case that many organizations and workplaces will refuse voluntary worker health improvement efforts, even when resources are offered to facilitate the program. The criteria for selection of participatory intervention sites have been revised on the basis of this experience, in an attempt to better inform decision-makers in advance about the expected process and its potential benefits and costs.

5. Conclusions

The intervention program had some positive impacts on work organization in the intervention centers. The fundamental Total Worker Health concept of integrating OSH and HP was intuitive to many workers; they enthusiastically envisioned and sought to carry out integrated programming, and a number of activities improved the health climate in these workplaces. Active involvement of non-supervisory employees in program design and conduct appeared to benefit the work environment and employee morale and engagement. Actively engaged leadership was no less important: program intensity and success fluctuated noticeably with changes in management. Both managers and employees cited the importance for success of factors such as employee program ownership, empowerment, and skill-building (setting appropriate goals, balancing of costs and benefits when weighing intervention alternatives, etc.).

Unfortunately, our planned reduction in researcher facilitation efforts was followed by an erosion of the previously high level of staff participation in project planning. It was disappointing to observe the decline in company commitment to the participatory employee teams despite their demonstrated feasibility and robust worker engagement, in contrast to the company workplace health promotion program.

Participatory OSH/HP is challenging in the long-term care sector due to highly demanding jobs and tight staffing. Managers and front-line workers have different perceptions of the long-term care environment [21], likely arising naturally from their positions in the occupational hierarchy and their consequent exposures to health and safety hazards. Improved systems of communication between levels and program design are needed that support front-line workers to participate in identifying and resolving problems.

PIP team resources, breadth of worker participation, and management support were important preconditions for potential program sustainability. Future efforts should incorporate more robust organizational structures to enhance these factors for program success. Lessons from this study may guide other long-term care facilities to build a sustainable, integrated, and participatory program.

Author Contributions: Conceptualization, L.P., R.K.; methodology, R.K., L.P., M.F., Y.Z.; formal analysis, R.K., J.F.; investigation, L.P., M.F., R.K., Y.Z., J.F.; writing—original draft preparation, R.K., L.P., Y.Z., M.F.; writing—review and editing, R.K., L.P., Y.Z.; supervision, L.P.; funding acquisition, L.P.

Funding: The Center for the Promotion of Health in the New England Workplace is supported by Grant Number 1 U19 OH008857 from the National Institute for Occupational Safety and Health (CDC). This work is solely the responsibility of the authors and does not necessarily represent the official views of NIOSH.

Acknowledgments: Sandy Sun, project administration; Michelle Holmberg, Lara Blais, Jennifer Russell, and Shpend Qamili, workplace program implementation and facilitation; ProCare research team and numerous students who assisted with survey data collection, and Wing Hung Yuen for manuscript formatting.

Conflicts of Interest: The authors declare no conflict of interest. The funders had no role in the design of the study; in the collection, analyses, or interpretation of data; in the writing of the manuscript, or in the decision to publish the results.

References

1. Sara, J.D.; Prasad, M.; Eleid, M.F.; Zhang, M.; Widmer, R.J.; Lerman, A. Association Between Work-Related Stress and Coronary Heart Disease: A Review of Prospective Studies Through the Job Strain, Effort-Reward Balance, and Organizational Justice Models. *J. Am. Heart Assoc.* **2018**, *7*. [CrossRef]
2. Caruso, C.C. Negative impacts of shiftwork and long work hours. *Rehabil. Nurs.* **2014**, *39*, 16–25. [CrossRef] [PubMed]
3. Chandola, T.; Brunner, E.; Marmot, M. Chronic stress at work and the metabolic syndrome: Prospective study. *BMJ (Clinical research ed.)* **2006**, *332*, 521–525. [CrossRef] [PubMed]
4. Wang, X.S.; Armstrong, M.E.; Cairns, B.J.; Key, T.J.; Travis, R.C. Shift work and chronic disease: The epidemiological evidence. *Occup. Med.* **2011**, *61*, 78–89. [CrossRef] [PubMed]
5. Magnusson Hanson, L.L.; Westerlund, H. Job strain and loss of healthy life years between ages 50 and 75 by sex and occupational position: Analyses of 64 934 individuals from four prospective cohort studies. *Occup. Environ. Med.* **2018**, *75*, 486–493. [CrossRef] [PubMed]
6. Harris, J.R.; Huang, Y.; Hannon, P.A.; Williams, B. Low-socioeconomic status workers: Their health risks and how to reach them. *J. Occup. Environ. Med.* **2011**, *53*, 132–138. [CrossRef] [PubMed]
7. Thompson, S.E.; Smith, B.A.; Bybee, R.F. Factors influencing participation in worksite wellness programs among minority and underserved populations. *Fam. Community Health* **2005**, *28*, 267–273. [CrossRef]
8. Miranda, H.; Gore, R.J.; Boyer, J.; Nobrega, S.; Punnett, L. Health Behaviors and Overweight in Nursing Home Employees: Contribution of Workplace Stressors and Implications for Worksite Health Promotion. *Scientific World J.* **2015**, *2015*, 915359. [CrossRef] [PubMed]
9. Punnett, L.; Cherniack, M.; Henning, R.; Morse, T.; Faghri, P.; Team, C.-N.R. A conceptual framework for integrating workplace health promotion and occupational ergonomics programs. *Public Health Rep.* **2009**, *124* (Suppl. 1), 16–25. [CrossRef]
10. Nobrega, S.; Champagne, N.; Abreu, M.; Goldstein-Gelb, M.; Montano, M.; Lopez, I.; Arevalo, J.; Bruce, S.; Punnett, L. Obesity/Overweight and the Role of Working Conditions: A Qualitative, Participatory Investigation. *Health Promot Pract.* **2016**, *17*, 127–136. [CrossRef]
11. Jorgensen, M.B.; Villadsen, E.; Burr, H.; Punnett, L.; Holtermann, A. Does employee participation in workplace health promotion depend on the working environment? A cross-sectional study of Danish workers. *BMJ Open* **2016**, *6*, e010516. [CrossRef] [PubMed]
12. Baker, E.; Israel, B.A.; Schurman, S. The integrated model: implications for worksite health promotion and occupational health and safety practice. *Health Educ Q.* **1996**, *23*, 175–190. [CrossRef] [PubMed]
13. DeJoy, D.M.; Parker, K.M.; Padilla, H.M.; Wilson, M.G.; Roemer, E.C.; Goetzel, R.Z. Combining environmental and individual weight management interventions in a work setting: Results from the Dow chemical study. *J. Occup. Environ. Med.* **2011**, *53*, 245–252. [CrossRef] [PubMed]
14. World Health Organization. *Healthy Workplaces: A Model for Action: for Employers, Workers, Policymakers and Practitioners*; World Health Organization: Geneva, Switzerland, 2010.
15. Schill, A.L.; Chosewood, L.C. The NIOSH Total Worker Health program: An overview. *J. Occup. Environ. Med.* **2013**, *55*, S8–S11. [CrossRef]
16. Hunt, M.K.; Lederman, R.; Stoddard, A.M.; LaMontagne, A.D.; McLellan, D.; Combe, C.; Barbeau, E.; Sorensen, G. Process evaluation of an integrated health promotion/occupational health model in WellWorks-2. *Health Educ. Behav.* **2005**, *32*, 10–26. [CrossRef] [PubMed]
17. Sorensen, G.; Stoddard, A.; Hunt, M.K.; Hebert, J.R.; Ockene, J.K.; Avrunin, J.S.; Himmelstein, J.; Hammond, S.K. The effects of a health promotion-health protection intervention on behavior change: The WellWorks Study. *Am. J. Public Health* **1998**, *88*, 1685–1690. [CrossRef] [PubMed]
18. Tveito, T.H.; Eriksen, H.R. Integrated health programme: A workplace randomized controlled trial. *J. Adv. Nurs.* **2009**, *65*, 110–119. [CrossRef] [PubMed]

19. Anger, W.K.; Elliot, D.L.; Bodner, T.; Olson, R.; Rohlman, D.S.; Truxillo, D.M.; Kuehl, K.S.; Hammer, L.B.; Montgomery, D. Effectiveness of total worker health interventions. *J. Occup. Health Psychol.* **2015**, *20*, 226–247. [CrossRef]
20. Feltner, C.; Peterson, K.; Palmieri Weber, R.; Cluff, L.; Coker-Schwimmer, E.; Viswanathan, M.; Lohr, K.N. The Effectiveness of Total Worker Health Interventions: A Systematic Review for a National Institutes of Health Pathways to Prevention Workshop. *Ann. Intern. Med.* **2016**, *165*, 262–269. [CrossRef] [PubMed]
21. Zhang, Y.; Flum, M.; Nobrega, S.; Blais, L.; Qamili, S.; Punnett, L. Work organization and health issues in long-term care centers. *J. Gerontol. Nurs.* **2011**, *37*, 32–40. [CrossRef]
22. Kurowski, A.; Gore, R.; Buchholz, B.; Punnett, L. Differences among nursing homes in outcomes of a safe resident handling program. *J. Healthc. Risk Manag.* **2012**, *32*, 35–51. [CrossRef]
23. Kurowski, A.; Buchholz, B.; Punnett, L. A physical workload index to evaluate a safe resident handling program for nursing home personnel. *Hum. Factors* **2014**, *56*, 669–683. [CrossRef] [PubMed]
24. Zhang, Y.; Flum, M.; Kotejoshyer, R.; Fleishman, J.; Henning, R.; Punnett, L. Workplace Participatory Occupational Health/Health Promotion Program: Facilitators and Barriers Observed in Three Nursing Homes. *J. Gerontol. Nurs.* **2016**, *42*, 34–42. [CrossRef]
25. Henning, R.; Warren, N.; Robertson, M.; Faghri, P.; Cherniack, M.; Team, C.-N.R. Workplace health protection and promotion through participatory ergonomics: An integrated approach. *Public Health Rep.* **2009**, *124* (Suppl. 1), 26–35. [CrossRef]
26. Antonovsky, A. *Unraveling the Mystery of Health: How People Manage Stress and Stay Well*; Jossey-Bass: San Francisco, CA, USA, 1987.
27. Bauer, G.; Jenny, G. *Development, Implementation and Dissemination of Occupational Health Management (OHM): Putting Salutogenesis into Practice*; Houdmont, J., McIntyre, S., Eds.; Springer: Dordrecht, The Netherlands, 2007.
28. Kahonen, K.; Naatanen, P.; Tolvanen, A.; Salmela-Aro, K. Development of sense of coherence during two group interventions. *Scand. J. Psychol.* **2012**, *53*, 523–527. [CrossRef] [PubMed]
29. Laing, A.C.; Frazer, M.B.; Cole, D.C.; Kerr, M.S.; Wells, R.P.; Norman, R.W. Study of the effectiveness of a participatory ergonomics intervention in reducing worker pain severity through physical exposure pathways. *Ergonomics* **2005**, *48*, 150–170. [CrossRef] [PubMed]
30. Haro, E.; Kleiner, B.M. Macroergonomics as an organizing process for systems safety. *Appl. Ergon.* **2008**, *39*, 450–458. [CrossRef]
31. Jagosh, J.; Macaulay, A.C.; Pluye, P.; Salsberg, J.; Bush, P.L.; Henderson, J.; Sirett, E.; Wong, G.; Cargo, M.; Herbert, C.P.; et al. Uncovering the benefits of participatory research: Implications of a realist review for health research and practice. *Milbank Q.* **2012**, *90*, 311–346. [CrossRef]
32. Zhang, Y.; Flum, M.; West, C.; Punnett, L. Assessing Organizational Readiness for a Participatory Occupational Health/Health Promotion Intervention in Skilled Nursing Facilities. *Health Promot. Pract.* **2015**, *16*, 724–732. [CrossRef]
33. Zhang, Y.; Punnett, L.; Gore, R. Relationships among employees' working conditions, mental health, and intention to leave in nursing homes. *J. Appl. Gerontol.* **2014**, *33*, 6–23. [CrossRef]
34. Zhang, Y.; Punnett, L.; McEnany, G.P.; Gore, R. Contributing influences of work environment on sleep quantity and quality of nursing assistants in long-term care facilities: a cross-sectional study. *Geriatr. Nurs.* **2016**, *37*, 13–18. [CrossRef] [PubMed]
35. Karasek, R.; Brisson, C.; Kawakami, N.; Houtman, I.; Bongers, P.; Amick, B. The Job Content Questionnaire (JCQ): An instrument for internationally comparative assessments of psychosocial job characteristics. *J. Occup. Health Psychol.* **1998**, *3*, 322–355. [CrossRef]
36. Griffin, M.A.; Neal, A. Perceptions of safety at work: A framework for linking safety climate to safety performance, knowledge, and motivation. *J. Occup. Health Psychol.* **2000**, *5*, 347–358. [CrossRef]
37. Gold, J.E.; Punnett, L.; Gore, R.J. Predictors of low back pain in nursing home workers after implementation of a safe resident handling programme. *Occup. Environ. Med.* **2017**, *74*, 389–395. [CrossRef] [PubMed]
38. Baum, F.; MacDougall, C.; Smith, D. Participatory action research. *J. Epidemiol. Community Health* **2006**, *60*, 854–857. [CrossRef] [PubMed]
39. Punnett, L.; Warren, N.; Henning, R.; Nobrega, S.; Cherniack, M. Participatory ergonomics as a model for integrated programs to prevent chronic disease. *J. Occup. Environ. Med.* **2013**, *55*, S19–S24. [CrossRef]

40. Tsutsumi, A.; Nagami, M.; Yoshikawa, T.; Kogi, K.; Kawakami, N. Participatory intervention for workplace improvements on mental health and job performance among blue-collar workers: A cluster randomized controlled trial. *J. Occup. Environ. Med.* **2009**, *51*, 554–563. [CrossRef]
41. Weiner, B.J.; Lewis, M.A.; Linnan, L.A. Using organization theory to understand the determinants of effective implementation of worksite health promotion programs. *Health Educ. Res.* **2009**, *24*, 292–305. [CrossRef]
42. Curry, L.A.; Krumholz, H.M.; O'Cathain, A.; Plano Clark, V.L.; Cherlin, E.; Bradley, E.H. Mixed methods in biomedical and health services research. *Circ. Cardiovasc. Qual. Outcomes.* **2013**, *6*, 119–123. [CrossRef]
43. Schelvis, R.M.; Oude Hengel, K.M.; Burdorf, A.; Blatter, B.M.; Strijk, J.E.; van der Beek, A.J. Evaluation of occupational health interventions using a randomized controlled trial: Challenges and alternative research designs. *Scand. J. Work Environ. Health* **2015**, *41*, 491–503. [CrossRef] [PubMed]
44. Chaulk, C.P.; Kazandjian, V.A. Moving beyond randomized controlled trials. *Am. J. Public Health.* **2004**, *94*, 1476. [CrossRef] [PubMed]
45. Griffiths, A. Organizational interventions: Facing the limits of the natural science paradigm. *Scand. J. Work Environ. Health.* **1999**, *25*, 589–596. [CrossRef] [PubMed]
46. Simmons, R.K.; Ogilvie, D.; Griffin, S.J.; Sargeant, L.A. Applied public health research—Falling through the cracks? *BMC Public Health* **2009**, *9*, 362. [CrossRef] [PubMed]

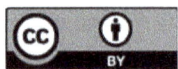

© 2019 by the authors. Licensee MDPI, Basel, Switzerland. This article is an open access article distributed under the terms and conditions of the Creative Commons Attribution (CC BY) license (http://creativecommons.org/licenses/by/4.0/).

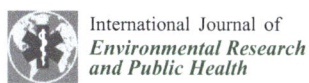

Article

Generalizability of Total Worker Health® Online Training for Young Workers

Ashamsa Aryal [1,*], Megan Parish [2,3] and Diane S. Rohlman [1,2]

1. Department of Occupational and Environmental Health, University of Iowa, Iowa City, IA 52242, USA; diane-rohlman@uiowa.edu
2. Oregon Institute of Occupational Health Sciences, Oregon Health & Science University, Portland, OR 97239, USA; megan.parish@confluencehealth.org
3. Confluence Health, Wenatchee, WA 98801, USA
* Correspondence: ashamsa-aryal@uiowa.edu

Received: 18 January 2019; Accepted: 12 February 2019; Published: 16 February 2019

Abstract: Young workers (under 25-years-old) are at risk of workplace injuries due to inexperience, high-risk health behaviors, and a lack of knowledge about workplace hazards. Training based on Total Worker Health® (TWH) principles can improve their knowledge of and ability to identify hazards associated with work organization and environment. In this study, we assessed changes to knowledge and behavior following an online safety and health training between two groups by collecting information on the demographic characteristics, knowledge, and self-reported behaviors of workplace health and safety at three different points in time. The participants' age ranged from 15 to 24 years. Age adjusted results exhibited a significant increase in knowledge immediately after completing the training, although knowledge decreased in both groups in the follow-up. Amazon Marketplace Mechanical Turk (MTurk) participants demonstrated a greater increase in knowledge, with a significantly higher score compared to the baseline, indicating retention of knowledge three months after completing the training. The majority of participants in both groups reported that they liked the Promoting U through Safety and Health (PUSH) training for improving health and safety and that the training should be provided before starting a job. Participants also said that the training was interactive, informative and humorous. The participants reported that the PUSH training prepared them to identify and control hazards in their workplace and to communicate well with the supervisors and coworkers about their rights. Training programs based on TWH improves the safety, health and well-being of young workers.

Keywords: young workers; training; Total Worker Health®; MTurk; health; safety; likeability; behavior change

1. Introduction

In 2016, there were approximately 19.3 million workers in the United States under the age of 24, representing 13% of the total workforce [1]. For 2016, incidence rates for non-fatal injuries and illnesses were 101.9 per 10,000 Full Time Employment (FTE) compared to 100.4 for all ages [2]. Similarly, in 2014, the rates of work-related injuries treated in emergency departments for workers, aged 15–19 and 20–24 were 2.18 times and 1.76 times greater than the rate for workers 25 years of age and older [3]. According to the Census of Fatal Occupational Injuries, the average rate of fatal injuries among workers less than 18 years was 47 deaths per year from 1994 to 2013 [4]. Inexperience, lack of knowledge about workplace hazards, and a reluctance to speak up have been associated with the increase in injury rates in young workers [5–7]. Young workers do not mention safety as their main priority at work and are often not aware of their legal rights and the tasks prohibited by labor laws [8]. They are eager to please their supervisors and may be reluctant to report injuries leading to underreporting [7,9,10], which might lead to an underestimation of the injury rates.

The Occupational Safety and Health Administration (OSHA) requires training to be a part of every employer's safety and health program to protect workers from injury and illness (OSHA, 2015). Training programs have been found to improve knowledge and awareness of workplace safety [8,11]. However, most young workers report not receiving training on worker safety and health [12]. Those that receive training state that most trainings are brief and inadequate [13] and may not include information addressing both health and safety topics [14].

Recognizing these issues among young workers, the National Institute for Occupational Safety and Health (NIOSH) developed the Youth@Work: Talking Safety classroom-based curriculum to address the needs of young workers [15]. Promoting U through Safety and Health (PUSH), a Total Worker Health® (TWH) training, expands the content of the Youth@Work curriculum to include information addressing health, safety, and communication in an online format. PUSH was developed through the Oregon Healthy Workforce Center, a NIOSH Total Worker Health® Center of Excellence [12,14,16]. Total Worker Health® is a strategy that integrates health promotion with injury prevention by looking at work as a social determinant of health. TWH focuses on job-related factors such as wages, hours of work, workload and stress levels, interactions with coworkers and supervisors, access to paid leave, and health promoting workplaces to have an impact on the wellbeing of workers [17]. Interventions addressing TWH improve workplace health effectively and more rapidly than wellness programs solely focused on health promotion [18–20].

Previously evaluated among parks and recreation workers, PUSH was found to be effective in increasing the safety and health knowledge among young workers [12]. The current study assessed the generalizability of the program among an expanded group of young workers. The main goal of the study was to assess the effectiveness of the PUSH training to increase knowledge about hazard identification, control selection, and communication between two groups of young workers using a pretest-posttest design. A second goal was to assess the likeability of the online training and to examine the impact on behavior to prepare workers to address hazards in the workplace (i.e. preparedness).

2. Materials and Methods

2.1. Participants

The study was conducted in the United States in 2016. Two groups of young workers were recruited for the study: young workers employed at a city park and recreation program (Park and Rec) in the Pacific Northwest and young workers who were members of Amazon Marketplace Mechanical Turk (MTurk) who were located throughout the US. In order to be eligible for the study, the participants in both groups had to be less than 25 years of age and living in the United States. At baseline, 57 Parks and Rec workers agreed to participate after receiving a letter with details on the study during orientation. A second group of young workers were recruited online via Amazon Marketplace Mechanical Turk (MTurk): an open online marketplace for work that requires human intelligence [21]. Around 1000 MTurk workers answered a series of five questions as part of an eligibility screener. One hundred sixty-seven young workers between 18 and 24 years of age who met the eligibility criteria were recruited at baseline.

Park and Rec participants received $25 for completing the initial survey and training, and another $25 for completing the follow-up survey in the form of an Amazon gift card sent via email. MTurk workers received $0.02 to complete the initial screener, $20.00 to complete the training, and $4.00 to complete the follow-up survey through the MTurk platform. MTurk participants were paid less based on the time and difficulty of the task and because of the culture of the platform, where requestors (i.e., researchers) were discouraged from inflating payments to promote responses. The Oregon Health & Science University institutional review board approved the study materials and procedures.

2.2. Survey Instruments

Questionnaires were used to collect information at three time points: immediately prior to completing the training (Baseline), immediately after completing the training (Post-training), and 3-months after the training (Follow-up). Participants completed the questionnaire and the training online after they received a link to the materials either through their email or through the MTurk platform.

At baseline, participants provided demographic information along with information on work history and previous safety trainings. Health and safety knowledge was assessed immediately before and after the training by twenty-one multiple choice questions that were categorized into topics: hazard identification (e.g., "Sarah works at a bakery where her responsibilities are to take orders from customers, make sandwiches, and tidy up. Sometimes the morning rush is so overwhelming that she gets very distracted. What type of hazard is a distraction?"), control selection (e.g., "What is the least effective way of controlling a hazard?"), communication including workers' rights, health behaviors, and safety questions, (e.g., "Regarding workplace violence, it is your responsibility to ... ").

At the three-month follow-up, participants answered survey questionnaires about their current job, whether they liked the training and if they changed their behavior as a result of completing the training. Along with this, participants answered twenty-one knowledge questions and completed items addressing their general health and other health behaviors. Open-ended questions were used to assess the participants' reaction to the training. Likeability and acceptability were assessed using the question "Did you like the PUSH training? Why or Why not?" and the impact of the training on behavior change was assessed through the question "Did you see or experience any behaviors over the last three months that you felt prepared to handle because of the PUSH training program? If so, please explain."

2.3. PUSH Training

The PUSH training is comprised of topics from the NIOSH Youth@Work: Talking Safety curriculum and two evidence-based curricula on health promotion [22,23], with additional topics addressing protection from workplace hazards, promotion of health and well-being, and workplace communication [12,16]. It was delivered through an online training format that had been used to teach skills using behavioral education principles among workers in different industries [14,24–26]. This format has also been effective in disseminating information on occupational health and safety for diverse worker groups [27–29].

Content experts in the field of occupational health and safety, and health promotion developed the original PUSH training. The videos and content used in the training were pilot tested with young workers on the MTurk platform as a part of the development process. Questionnaire items (e.g., demographics, work history, and likeability/acceptability) had been used previously by researchers in other studies with young workers [12,16]. The team used validated measures to assess general health, health behaviors, and job content [12,16].

PUSH is a self-paced online training that uses videos and real-life examples to teach young workers about safety, communication, and health. Participants were directed to a series of content screens with videos by an icon-based navigation system. Multiple choice questions were followed by brief videos that needed to be correctly answered to progress through the training [12]. Additional details in regard to the study are available at a separate study by the same co-author [12].

2.4. Statistical Analysis

Data was analyzed using SAS 9.4 (SAS Institute, Cary, NC, USA). *t*-Tests and chi-square tests were used to examine differences in the demographic characteristics between the two groups at baseline. A mixed linear model with time-group interaction was used to evaluate the change in knowledge score at baseline, post-training and at follow-up. Responses to the twenty-one knowledge questions were marked "correct" and "incorrect", denoted by 1 and 0, respectively, to create a cumulative score used to analyze change in knowledge among the participants. Due to the differences in age of the participants in the two groups, age was adjusted as a covariate in the model. To evaluate likeability and preparedness, responses to the open-ended questions were grouped into positive, neutral and negative categories for each group and were further coded to identify common themes.

3. Results

3.1. Demographics

We started the study with 219 participants who completed the demographic information. There were 118 participants at baseline and post-training and 70 participants at follow-up. Participants in the MTurk group were significantly older ($\bar{X}$ = 22 years, ranging from 19 to 24 years) compared to the participants in the Park and Rec group ($\bar{X}$ = 16 years, ranging from 15 to 19 years). The highest level of education in the MTurk group was a graduate degree and technical school in the Park and Rec group (Table 1). There were a greater number of female participants in the Park and Rec group. The majority of participants were Caucasian. The MTurk group had also been in the workforce longer than the participants in the Park and Rec group (1.9 vs 1.3 years, respectively). Park and Rec workers perceived their health to be better compared to the MTurk participants. The seasonal Park and Rec workers were employed at a single location and participated in regular safety meetings. Whereas, the MTurk workers were employed in a range of workplaces such as retail, food service, construction, health care, public utilities, manufacturing and agriculture with a variety of employers with and without regular safety meetings. Similar to the results in previous studies [5,30], young workers in both groups reported the need for safety training before starting a job: 95% in the MTurk group and 86% in the Park and Rec group.

Table 1. Demographic Data.

	Mturk (N = 39)	Park and Rec (N = 31)
	Mean (SD)	Mean (SD)
Age ***	22.4 (1.4)	16.03 (1.3)
Total years worked ***	1.9 (1.9)	1.3 (0.5)
	n (%)	n (%)
Gender		
Female	17 (43.6)	16 (51.7)
Ethnicity		
White/Caucasian	24 (61.5)	21 (67.6)
Asian/Pacific Islander	11 (28.2)	7 (22.6)
Others	4 (10.2)	3 (9.7)
Education ***		
High School	6 (15.4)	27 (87.1)
Technical school	15 (38.5)	4 (12.9)
College 4 years or more	6 (15.4)	0
College graduate or above	12 (30.8)	0

*** p-Value < 0.0001.

3.2. Knowledge

Participants in the Park and Rec group had higher knowledge scores at baseline than the MTurk participants (Figure 1). The scores significantly increased immediately after the training for both groups (post-training). Compared to post-training, the scores significantly decreased at the 3-month follow-up. However, the scores at follow-up were still higher than the baseline scores for both groups. Even though the Park and Rec group started with higher knowledge scores at baseline, the MTurk group had higher scores post-training and at follow-up. However, the group difference was not significant at baseline and post-training (p-value at follow-up: <0.05). The participants in both groups scored the lowest on the questions addressing hazard identification and control selection at each time point. Cronbach's alpha values measured at each time point for internal consistency of the questionnaires were 0.39, 0.55, 0.56 for baseline, post-training and follow-up, respectively.

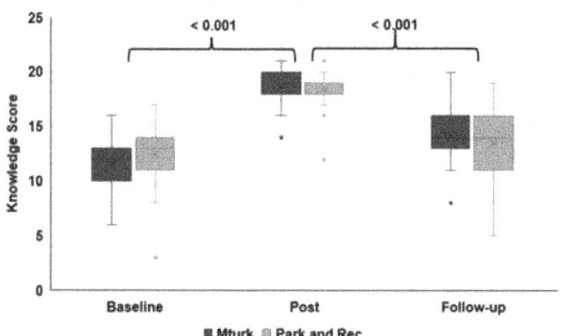

Figure 1. Box and Whisker plot showing change in knowledge score for the groups over time.

3.3. Likeability and Preparedness

Two open-ended questions were used to assess the likeability of the training and whether or not the training led to changes in behavior or responses to situations in the participant's workplace.

3.3.1. Likeability of the Training

All participants completed the open-ended question about whether they liked the training. Most (63%) replied positively, while 15% answered neutral and 22% had a negative response. These responses were coded and grouped into categories that addressed the content of the training, the delivery format, or specific skills that were learned as a result of taking the training.

- Content

Thirteen percent of the MTurk participants and thirteen percent of Park and Rec participants found the content of the training to be informative and stated that it provided useful information. For example, *"I liked the PUSH training because it was very informative in teaching the workers about looking out for those around them and also for their own wellness too."* [MTurk, Restaurant Cashier] and *"Yes because it was informative and useful for future reference."* [Park and Rec].

A few participants (8%) compared PUSH to other safety trainings they had taken in the past. The MTurk participants preferred the PUSH training, *"Yeah, I really liked it. Most job trainings are really boring, but the PUSH training was engaging. I remember enjoying it."* [MTurk, Service manager]; whereas the participants in the Park and Rec group mentioned that they had learned most of the safety information in the PUSH training from their prior onsite training, *"I thought it had good intentions but I learned more about safety procedures from my on-site training at work."* [Park and Rec worker].

- Delivery format

The training is self-paced and divided into topics that include pictures and videos. Several participants (19%) felt the training was interactive and engaging and that they liked the training interface, *"I really enjoyed it. It presented information in an interesting, concise way. The time it took to take really went by quickly because the videos and interaction were so engaging."* [MTurk, Childcare Provider] and *"I liked it because it was very interactive."* [Park and Rec]. Participants' comments identified the engaging/interactive nature (36%), the humor in the training (29%), and reported that it was easy to understand (21%), "*I did. I really enjoyed the way that it was formatted and felt as though it was helpful and funny without being corny or boring.*" [MTurk, Admissions counselor] and "*I enjoy the PUSH program because it's both friendly and easy to understand.*" [MTurk, Office assistant].

- Specific skills

Several of the participants (17%) mentioned that they liked the training because it increased their knowledge and provided specific skills for their job. For example, "*. . . . . I think it was useful, especially the parts about legal rights.*" [Park and Rec].

- Negative and Mixed Findings

In contrast to the MTurk group, some participants in the Park and Rec group felt that the training was repetitive and boring and they had learned this information in previous trainings, "*I didn't like it because it seemed repetitive to the safety training I underwent in order to get my job with PP&R.*" [Park and Rec] and "*It was fine, long but I understand why it was long*" [Park and Rec]. Other participants indicated mixed impressions of the training. They felt that although it was not useful to them, it could be useful to others, "*It was fine. I didn't learn a whole lot, but I can imagine it being useful for others.*" [Park and Rec]

3.3.2. Preparedness

Although the majority of participants did not indicate any change in behavior when asked how they felt prepared to handle real life issues after completing the PUSH training, about 30% did provide an example. These responses were coded into categories that described an increase in awareness of safety and health hazards or identified specific changes in behavior. Most of these responses (67%) came from participants in the MTurk group.

- Increased awareness

Twenty percent of the participants mentioned that the PUSH training increased their awareness of the hazards in their workplace and were able to apply information from the training in certain situations, "*Yes, I am more aware of the dangers that I may face in the working area.*" [MTurk]; "*I experienced/noticed things that had been put in place to help keep us safe.*" [Park and Rec], and "*There were times where I reflected on the push training to help me in certain situations.*" [Park and Rec].

- Behavior changes

Participants in the MTurk group provided more examples of behavior change than participants in the Park and Rec group. Many described a specific change in their behavior as a result of completing the training. For example, thinking about potential hazards prior to starting a task, "*I am able to think through tasks and situations more effectively before starting them. Anticipating potential danger is very important in my workplace.*" [MTurk] and "*I made sure to create a safer workplace for myself. I start by cleaning my work space more often by removing pins and empty plastic bags that may cause me to slip and injury myself.*" [MTurk]. Other participants indicated reporting or "speaking up" about workplace hazards, "*I noticed chemicals were not being stored correctly and I made sure to tell my boss about the issue and correct the problem.*" [MTurk, Customer service representative], "*I thought it was easier to talk to people I manage about safety and how to take care of themselves on the job.*" [MTurk], and "*I have asked for help in a few situations where I thought I may have gotten injured from carrying something I wasn't meant to carry by myself such as large tables.*" [MTurk].

Several described specific instances of where they changed their behavior, "*I was able to handle hostile patients over the phone better to the PUSH training.*" [MTurk], "*There was a fire near our office that forced us to put an evacuation plan into action that was inspired by me after participating in the PUSH program.*" [MTurk, Office assistant], "*I felt I knew how to better assert myself towards healthful choices.*" [MTurk],

"Within the past 3 months, I realized that I was more cautious with my actions especially when I was working with other people." [MTurk], and *"I used all my protective equipment when cleaning up the pool."* [Park and Rec].

4. Discussion

Approaches focusing on education and training have shown improvement in workplace safety [8,11]. As a result of completing the PUSH training, knowledge increased significantly from baseline to post-training for both groups. Although knowledge decreased at follow-up, it still remained elevated compared to baseline. The training was received positively by an overwhelming majority of participants in both groups, with most of the participants reporting the training to be interactive and informative and compared it with other training programs:

"Yes, because it provided me with lots of insightful information that I did not learn on my job. I was able to know how to quickly respond to emergencies on the job after using the training program." [MTurk, Cashier].

Several participants in the Park and Rec group mentioned that the PUSH training was repetitive. This is likely due to the fact that participants in the Park and Rec group receive mandatory safety training before starting their job and have regular safety meetings throughout the season. These meetings address many of the topics presented in the PUSH training and could be the reason for these negative responses. On the other hand, MTurk participants were from diverse workplaces including restaurants and retail stores. Few of these participants reported receiving safety training. The majority of the MTurk participants liked the training and felt the training prepared them for workplace hazards.

The questions evaluating participants' reaction to the training included multiple choice on a Likert scale with items as well as open-ended questions. All the participants entered a response to the question on likeability, and many gave specific reasons why they liked/did not like the training. The majority of participants answered the questions about preparedness and several (21%) provided specific examples. These responses stated that the training prepared them to handle workplace hazards by increasing awareness and led to specific changes in their behavior. One participant in the Park and Rec group indicated, *"I felt empowered to take action in my workplace environment when I saw something that violated my workplace rights or somebody else's."* [Park and Rec]. Raising awareness about working rights and building confidence in young workers to "speak up" about hazards is extremely important in promoting health and safety. It is not uncommon for participants to leave open-ended questions unanswered [31]. However, everyone in the study at follow-up provided their response to the open-ended question on how the PUSH training prepared them for behavior change with majority providing specific examples.

The goal of the current study was to assess the generalizability of the online training among different groups of young workers. The current study included young workers in a range of occupations, including cashiers, accountants, service managers, counselors, and lifeguards. The changes in knowledge in the current study replicated previous findings reported in parks and recreation workers [12]. This study provided additional feedback about the training including a generally positive response about the format of the training and the need for training for young workers. In addition, many participants provided examples in the open-ended questions describing situations where they felt empowered to speak up about safety hazards or specific changes to their behavior they made in their workplace.

One of the study's strengths is that it is the first study to include two groups of young workers that were diverse in terms of their work experience. Young workers hired as summer employees at a city parks and recreation center were recruited along with a diverse group of workers selected via an announcement placed on Amazon Mechanical Turk. However, participants in both groups reported the need for training on health and safety. They liked the training and reported that the PUSH training prepared them to handle health and safety hazards at the workplace. The prospective nature of the study provides information on retention of information among young workers. Although knowledge scores at the three-month follow-up showed a decline from the immediate post-test, the scores were still greater than baseline for both groups with non-seasonal workers getting better scores compared to the seasonal workers. The decline in scores can indicate a need for frequent reminders or trainings on safety and health. Another strength of the PUSH training is the online format and interactive content. Young workers are familiar and comfortable with technology [11], which makes the online format of the training an appropriate dissemination technique for younger adults [16].

Studies have reported the need for training workers on the identification and control of workplace hazards [5,11,30]. A survey of Latino youths under the age of 21 working in construction found that the majority of participants reported that the training they received did not include information on controlling workplace hazards [13]. The results from the current study also emphasize the need to include topics on hazard identification and control selection as part of training for young workers, as evidenced by a higher number of hazard identification and control selection questions missed at each time point by participants in both groups.

One limitation of the study is that several participants were lost to follow up. Only participants who completed all three surveys were included in the analysis. However, the participants who were lost to follow-up had similar knowledge scores compared to the participants in the study at baseline and post-training. Another potential limitation of the study might be its generalizability outside of the US. Hence, there is a need for additional research to identify if the training can be utilized and to understand how young workers outside the US will receive it.

5. Conclusions

PUSH is an online training program utilizing a Total Worker Health® approach to address occupational safety and health for younger workers [12]. These results suggest the usefulness of online-training to improve the safety, health and well-being of young workers, which prepares them to better prevent workplace hazards. Due to its inclusion of comprehensive topics on health and safety and its acceptance by young workers in diverse work environments, the PUSH training could be expanded to young workers in other industries to increase their awareness on workplace rights and responsibility, health communication in order to promote health and safety, and improve well-being.

Author Contributions: Conceptualization, D.S.R. and M.P.; data curation, A.A.; formal analysis, A.A.; funding acquisition, D.S.R.; investigation, D.S.R. and M.P.; methodology, D.S.R. and M.P.; project administration, D.S.R. and M.P.; resources, D.S.R. and M.P.; software, A.A.; supervision, D.S.R. validation, A.A., D.S.R. and M.P.; visualization, A.A.; writing—original draft, A.A.; writing—review & editing, A.A., D.S.R. and M.P.

Funding: The project was funded by the Oregon Healthy Workforce Center: [NIOSH, grant number U19OH010154] and the Healthier Workforce Center of the Midwest [NIOSH, grant number U19OH008868].

Acknowledgments: We thank our colleagues at Portland Park and Recreation center for their strong support. We greatly appreciate the constructive feedbacks and suggestions of our colleagues at the Healthier Workforce Center of the Midwest at the University of Iowa, especially Kevin M. Kelly, Megan R. TePoel.

Conflicts of Interest: Rohlman has a significant financial interest in Northwest Education Training and Assessment, LLC, a company that may have a commercial interest in the results of this research and technology. This potential conflict of interest was reviewed, and a management plan approved by the OHSU and the University of Iowa Conflict of Interest in Research Committees was implemented.

References

1. National Institute of Occupationa Health and Safety (NIOSH). *Analysis of the Current Population Survey*. Morgantown, WV: U.S. Department of Health and Human Services, Centers for Disease Control and Prevention; National Institute for Occupational Safety and Health: Washington, DC, USA, 2017.
2. Bureau of Labor Statistics (BLS). *2016 Survey of Occupational Injuries and Illnesses Charts Package*; BLS: Washington, DC, USA, 2018.
3. National Institute for Occupational Health and Safety (NIOSH). *The Work-Related Injury Statistics Query System (Work-RISQS)*; NIOSH: Washington, DC, USA, 2017.
4. NIOSH. *2017 Young Worker Injury Deaths: A Historical Summary of Surveillance and Investigative Findings*. U.S. Department of Health and Human Services, Centers for Disease Control and Prevention; Perritt, K.R., Hendricks, K.J., Goldcamp, E.M., Morgantown, W.V., Eds.; NIOSH: Washington, DC, USA, 2017.

5. Holizki, T.; McDonald, R.; Foster, V.; Guzmicky, M. Causes of work-related injuries among young workers in British Columbia. *Am. J. Ind. Med.* **2008**, *51*, 357–363. [CrossRef] [PubMed]
6. Mujuru, P.; Mutambudzi, M. Injuries and seasonal risks among young workers in West Virginia—A 10-year retrospective descriptive analysis. *AAOHN J.* **2007**, *55*, 381–387. [CrossRef] [PubMed]
7. Bowling, J.; Runyan, C.; Miara, C.; Davis, L.; Rubenstein, H.; Delp, L.; Arroyo, M.G. Teenage workers' occupational safety: Results of a four school study. In Proceedings of the Fourth World Conference on Injury Prevention and Control, Amsterdam, The Netherlands, 17–20 May 1998.
8. Lavack, A.M.; Magnuson, S.L.; Deshpande, S.; Basil, D.Z.; Basil, M.D.; Mintz, J.J.H. Enhancing occupational health and safety in young workers: The role of social marketing. *Int. J. Nonprofit Volunt. Sector Mark.* **2008**, *13*, 193–204. [CrossRef]
9. Bush, D.; Baker, R. *Young Workers at Risk: Health and Safety Education and the Schools*; Labor Occupational Health Program, University of California: Berkeley, CA, USA, 1994.
10. Castillo, D.N. *Occupational Safety and Health in Young People: Young Workers: Varieties of Experience*; Barling, J., Kelloway, E.K., Eds.; American Psychological Association: Washington, DC, USA, 1999.
11. Loughlin, C.; Barling, J. Young workers' work values, attitudes, and behaviours. *J. Occup. Org. Psychol.* **2001**, *74*, 543–558. [CrossRef]
12. Rohlman, D.S.; Parish, M.; Elliot, D.L.; Hanson, G.; Perrin, N. *Addressing Younger Workers' Needs: The Promoting U through Safety and Health (PUSH) Trial Outcomes. in Healthcare*; Multidisciplinary Digital Publishing Institute: Basel, Switzerland, 2016.
13. O'Connor, T.; Loomis, D.; Runyan, C.; dal Santo, J.A.; Schulman, M. Adequacy of health and safety training among young Latino construction workers. *J. Occup. Environ. Med.* **2005**, *47*, 272–277. [CrossRef] [PubMed]
14. Anger, W.K.; Rohlman, D.S.; Kirkpatrick, J.; Reed, R.R.; Lundeen, C.A.; Eckerman, D.A. cTRAIN: A computer-aided training system developed in SuperCard for teaching skills using behavioral education principles. *Behav. Res. Methods* **2001**, *33*, 277–281. [CrossRef]
15. National Institute for Occupational Health and Safety (NIOSH). *Teaching Young Workers about Job Safety and Health*; NIOSH: Washington, DC, USA, 2017.
16. Rohlman, D.S.; Parish, M.; Elliot, D.L.; Montgomery, D.; Hanson, G. Characterizing the needs of a young working population: making the case for total worker health in an emerging workforce. *J. Occup. Environ. Med.* **2013**, *55*, S69–S72. [CrossRef] [PubMed]
17. National Institute for Occupational Health and Safety (NIOSH). *Fundamentals of Total Worker Health Approaches: Essential Elements for Advancing Worker Safety, Health, and Well-Being. On Behalf of the NIOSH Office for Total Worker Health. Cincinnati, OH: U.S. Department of Health and Human Services, Centers for Disease Control and Prevention*; Lee, M.P., Hudson, H., Richards, R., Chang, C.C., Chosewood, L.C., Schill, A.L., Eds.; National Institute for Occupational Safety and Health DHHS (NIOSH): Washington, DC, USA, 2016.
18. Anger, W.K.; Elliot, D.L.; Bodner, T.; Olson, R.; Rohlman, D.S.; Truxillo, D.M.; Kuehl, K.S.; Hammer, L.B.; Montgomery, D. Effectiveness of Total Worker Health Interventions. *J. Occup. Health Psychol.* **2015**, *20*, 226. [CrossRef] [PubMed]
19. Feltner, C. *Total Worker Health®*; Agency for Healthcare Research and Quality: Rockville, MD, USA, 2016.
20. Carr, L.J.; Leonhard, C.; Tucker, S.; Fethke, N.; Benzo, R.; Gerr, F. Total worker health intervention increases activity of sedentary workers. *Am. J. Prev. Med.* **2016**, *50*, 9–17. [CrossRef] [PubMed]
21. Buhrmester, M.; Kwang, T.; Gosling, S.D. Amazon's mechanical turk: A new source of inexpensive, yet high-quality, data? *Perspect. Psychol. Sci.* **2011**, *6*, 3–5. [CrossRef] [PubMed]
22. Elliot, D.L.; Goldberg, L.; Moe, E.; Defancesco, C.; Durham, M.; Hix-Small, H. Preventing substance use and disordered eating: initial outcomes of the ATHENA (athletes targeting healthy exercise and nutrition alternatives) program. *Arch. Pediatr. Adolesc. Med.* **2004**, *158*, 1043–1049. [CrossRef] [PubMed]
23. Goldberg, L.; MacKinnon, D.P.; Elliot, D.L.; Moe, E.L.; Clarke, G.; Cheong, J. The adolescents training and learning to avoid steroids program: Preventing drug use and promoting health behaviors. *Arch. Pediatr. Adolesc. Med.* **2000**, *154*, 332–338. [CrossRef] [PubMed]
24. Anger, W.K.; Tamulinas, A.; Uribe, A.; Ayala, C. Computer-based training for immigrant Latinos with limited formal education. *Hisp. J. Behav. Sci.* **2004**, *26*, 373–389. [CrossRef]
25. Eckerman, D.A.; Abrahamson, K.; Ammerman, T.; Fercho, H.; Rohlman, D.S.; Anger, W.K. Computer-based training for food services workers at a hospital. *J. Saf. Res.* **2004**, *35*, 317–327. [CrossRef]

26. Eckerman, D.A.; Lundeen, C.A.; Steele, A.; Fercho, H.L.; Ammerman, T.A.; Anger, W.K. Interactive training versus reading to teach respiratory protection. *J. Occup. Health Psychol.* **2002**, *7*, 313. [CrossRef]
27. Anger, W.K.; Patterson, L.; Fuchs, M.; Will, L.L.; Rohlman, D.S. Learning and recall of worker protection standard (WPS) training in vineyard workers. *J. Agromed.* **2009**, *14*, 336–344. [CrossRef] [PubMed]
28. Glass, N.; Bloom, T.; Perrin, N.; Anger, W.K. A computer-based training intervention for work supervisors to respond to intimate partner violence. *Saf. Health Work* **2010**, *1*, 167–174. [CrossRef] [PubMed]
29. Olson, R.; Anger, W.K.; Elliot, D.L.; Wipfli, B.; Gray, M. A new health promotion model for lone workers: Results of the safety & health involvement for truckers (SHIFT) pilot study. *J. Occup. Environ. Med.* **2009**, *51*, 1233–1246. [PubMed]
30. Loughlin, C.; Frone, M.R. *Young Workers' Occupational Safety. The Psychology of Workplace Safety*; American Psychological Association: Washington, DC, USA, 2004.
31. Reja, U.; Manfreda, K.L.; Hlebec, V.; Vehovar, V. Open-ended vs. close-ended questions in web questionnaires. *Dev. Appl. Stat.* **2003**, *19*, 159–177.

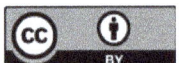

© 2019 by the authors. Licensee MDPI, Basel, Switzerland. This article is an open access article distributed under the terms and conditions of the Creative Commons Attribution (CC BY) license (http://creativecommons.org/licenses/by/4.0/).

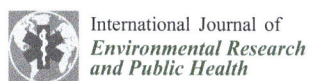

Article

Moral or Dirty Leadership: A Qualitative Study on How Juniors Are Managed in Dutch Consultancies

Onno Bouwmeester [1],[*] and Tessa Elisabeth Kok [2]

[1] School of Business and Economics, Vrije Universiteit Amsterdam, 1081 HV Amsterdam, The Netherlands
[2] PwC Amsterdam, 1066 JR Amsterdam, The Netherlands; tessa.kok@hotmail.com
[*] Correspondence: o.bouwmeester@vu.nl; Tel.: +31-020-598-6079

Received: 4 October 2018; Accepted: 7 November 2018; Published: 9 November 2018

Abstract: Professional service firms in Western Europe have a reputation for putting huge pressures on their junior employees, resulting in very long work hours, and as a consequence health risks. This study explores moral leadership as a possible response to the stigma of such dirty leadership. We conducted semi-structured interviews with 12 consultant managers and with each one of their juniors, and found that managers put several pressures on their juniors; these pressures bring high levels of stress, lowered wellbeing and burnout. Society considers such a pressuring leadership style morally dirty. To counteract the experience of being seen as morally dirty, we found that consultant managers were normalizing such criticisms as commonly assumed in dirty work literature. However, they also employed several moral leadership tactics to counteract the negative consequences criticized in society. However, in addition to the well-known individual-level tactics, consultant managers and their juniors also reported moral leadership support at the organizational level, like institutionalized performance talks after every project, trainings, specific criteria for hiring juniors, and policies to recognize and compliment high performance. Still, we cannot conclude these moral leadership approaches are moral by definition. They can be used in an instrumental way as well, to further push performance.

Keywords: work organization; dirty work; moral leadership; taint normalization; management consulting

1. Introduction

> "Consulting overall is a stressful lifestyle. Travel does suck, and it doesn't get any better. You're at the demand of your manager. . . . at all times, and deadlines are seemingly impossible to meet".
> (www.wallstreetoasis.com, entry 2014)

When Hughes introduced the concept of dirty work, he claimed that "dirty work of some kind is found in all occupations" [1] (p. 319). High-status professions are no exception. For instance, recently, bankers' dirty image has been studied, due to their risky management style, lack of customer care and extreme bonus culture, leading to a financial crisis and public scandals [2,3]. Accountants are in the news as well for big accounting errors and they self-report shame for dirty tasks like providing "ritualized information" and producing "ignored documents", which they consider "dirty work" [4] (p. 235). Popular criticisms also target consultants for their lack of expertise and overly high fees, lack of independence, and a focus on rationalization over human values [5,6]. Mostly consultants' clients are identified as victims of such morally dirty practices [7–9]. Such public criticisms undermine the reputation of consultants and contribute to the occupation's dirty image [10,11]. Despite the profession's high status in general, society disapproves certain dirty aspects of the work, like "laying off" people in client organizations [12] (p. 599).

A different moral problem criticized in society is that managers in professional service industries like banking [13] and law firms [14,15] put quite strong pressures on their employees. The pressures go far beyond standards of social desirability, even to the extent of violating labour laws. The consulting industry, for instance, is known for burnout, mental problems, stress, and disturbed work–life balance due to demanding clients and managers [16–21]. As a consequence, manager criticisms abound in consultant jokes, cartoons and on Internet fora (see for instance managementconsulted.com or www.wallstreetoasis.com). Members and former members of the occupation point at the moral dirtiness of such pressuring leadership, and of the manager job.

The constructs of dirty work and occupational stigma have initially been developed in sociology by Goffman and Hughes. Society stigmatizes in particular low-status occupations like hangman or janitors, similar to groups like drunks or ex-convicts [22,23]. Ashforth et al. [24] have added a social psychological perspective. They have explored how dirty workers and their managers respond to the pressure of feeling stigmatized, and found in their empirical studies that dirty workers respond by normalizing the taint experience in order to protect their self-esteem, and to reduce the stress caused by the feeling of being stigmatized. They also found that managers were helping employees with normalizing the experience of stigma. Luyendijk [25] finds such a phenomenon of creating a "protective bubble" to be quite prominent in the banking industry.

However, whereas insiders are assumed to reduce feelings of stress caused by a critical public opinion [26], outsiders produce such stress for a reason. In case of moral taint, they want to influence the immoral behaviour. Bankers are stigmatized for their extremely high bonuses or irresponsible profit seeking. Moral stigma targets the profession's responsibility and assumes agency. That means a banker can, and should do things differently according to public opinion. Additionally, when greedy bankers start normalizing what they do, public opinion stigmatizes them even more, to make clear their behaviour is still not acceptable. This is illustrated by the Ralph Hamers case in the Netherlands. In March 2018, ING Bank proposed a salary increase of 50% for its CEO, but the bank had to reverse the decision due to public disapproval. Newspapers had headers like: "One million extra? We do not accept." (NRC, 14 March 2018). It was considered very inappropriate behaviour, thus adding to the moral stigma the bank carried already for its role during the financial crisis, and ING Bank lost many clients that month.

Whereas normalization seems helpful when work is dirty due to physical hardship and toxic elements as experienced by miners and firefighters, normalization seems less effective for morally tainted managers due to their assumed agency and responsibility. As a consequence, managers might feel inclined to cope with moral taint differently than only by normalization. While normalization might serve individuals in the short run by reducing their own experience of stress, society could see normalization as a variant of moral disengagement [27], thus adding fuel to the fire, and reinforcing the stigma of morally dirty leadership.

To explore the puzzle around the appropriateness of normalization as response to moral taint, we drew on moral leadership literature, which has studied the dynamics between moral leadership and reputation. Scholars like Rhode [28], Schminke et al. [29] and Zhu et al. [30] have explored how moral leadership can prevent a bad reputation. However, despite the fact that dirty work and moral leadership literature both study responses to moral taint, these responses have not been related (cf. [24,26,28,30]). As the effects of normalization can be counterproductive in situations of tainted leadership, we expected to find moral leadership responses in such cases as alternative response to normalization. However, it assumes that managers have sufficient agency to be able to make a difference in their institutional context, and that they intentionally try to prevent the creation of moral stigma. Following up on these assumptions, we explored how consultant managers cope with the morally dirty aspects of their overly demanding leadership style by studying both their normalization and moral leadership responses. To answer our question, we performed interviews with 12 consultant managers and with each one of their juniors about their common leadership experiences.

The study makes two contributions. First, we found that consultant managers illustrate several moral leadership tactics in their work, in addition to normalization. When talking about the existing social constructions of morally dirty leadership, they stress their moral leadership behaviour. This adds a new coping repertoire to the current dirty work literature (cf. [12,24,26,31–34]). Our research design does not allow conclusions about how effective this new coping repertoire might be in reducing moral stigma, or the stress caused by such stigma. Still, moral leadership is theoretically a more adequate response than normalizing as it does not imply moral disengagement, while normalization often does. As moral taint assumes agency, and responsibility for violating accepted moral standards, moral leadership is the response actually expected by society. When consultant managers meet this expectation better, it could reduce their feelings of stress together with the contempt in society. However, the agency of managers, and even more juniors, is limited, so both do still benefit from self-protection by normalization, and we found such responses as well.

Second, we have identified organization-level support for the moral leadership attempts of consultant managers. Currently, moral leadership literature heavily focuses on what a manager can do as an individual [28,30], but this ignores the limited agency of consultant managers. They need to respond to deadlines, client demands, top management expectations and other institutional constraints. The organization can offer support to counterbalance such constraints. Both junior consultants and their managers mention high-frequency performance reviews to monitor juniors, standard training and coaching sessions for juniors and policies to better select candidates for the job. The latter policies aim at what Ashforth et al. [35] call congruence work. We also found acknowledgement and compensation policies, such as ad-hoc time compensation, increased time off after periods of intense work, and flowers or other reward symbols, to say "thank you" after extraordinary performances. The institutionalized character of these support measures make them quite visible, which responds to the stressful image of consulting work and its pressuring management. The support measures imply visible acknowledgement that the work context challenges consultant leadership more than direct managers can handle on their own with individualized arrangements [18]. A similar multi-level management approach to improving employee wellbeing and to reducing stress has been developed in Australian universities [36].

1.1. Morally Tainted Work

Occupations are regarded as "dirty" in society when they defy accepted societal norms and values and therefore become stigmatized [26] (p. 414). The dirtiness can be physical, leading in extreme cases to disgust and repugnance, but it can also be social and moral [1], leading to a less physical form of social disapproval, but still loss of dignity. The dirtiness becomes more a metaphor then. In that sense, we disapprove the work of morally tainted occupations like used-car salespeople, tabloid reporters, exotic dancers, sex-shop workers or correctional officers (see [24,26,31–34]). It also does not imply everyone avoids these services, as some might even like them. High-status professions can be morally tainted as well: for instance, lawyers [14,15], healthcare professionals doing abortion work [37] and after the 2008 financial crisis, we can add bankers to the list [2,3].

Some scholars argue that moral stigma gives the "dirtiest" taint [31] (p. 100), [33] (p. 32). That is because physically or socially tainted work is usually protected by a necessity shield: garbage needs to be collected although it is dirty [38], we really need AIDS workers even though many could feel uncomfortable in their work context [39], and we also need firefighters although the work is dangerous [33]. In contrast, society sees more evil than necessity in morally dirty work. Morally stigmatized occupations can therefore experience high levels of entitativity, inducing a division of "them" versus "us" [40], (p. 626), which poses a strong "identity threat" [31], (p. 86).

In most dirty work studies, society is assumed to stigmatize a profession as with one voice. However, specific interest groups may be most active in socially constructing a stigma. For instance, these who like to smoke and are still healthy will most likely not actively co-construct the tobacco industry as morally tainted, but the anti-tobacco lobby will certainly do. Next to different interests, time has its effects. For instance, public opinion turns more and more to the acceptance of abortion work in spite of the downsides, thus softening the stigma, whereas the stigma around bankers shows opposite dynamics. While dirtiness of an occupation is reflected in the public eye, we still need to ask who really cares. For instance, the paying client of consultants does not seem to be very concerned about their more dubious virtues, as consultant services continue to be in demand. In contrast, client employees do identify with the popular criticism that consultants lack expertise [5]. Therefore, compared to the Western societies of the fifties and sixties where Hughes [1,23] and Goffman [22] published their seminal work, in our more diverse societies, some more nuance seems required in identifying which groups construct work as dirty and how widespread a stigma becomes.

1.2. Normalizing Morally Tainted Work

Feeling stigmatized usually leads to stress, and thus loss of "coping resources" [41] (p. 572). Hobfoll found that people can respond to such stress by trying "to retain, protect, and build" [42] (p. 516) their coping resources such as a positive sense of themselves, self-esteem, and socioeconomic status. Ashforth et al. [24] have found several tactics that workers and their managers utilize to protect their self-esteem, by normalizing a dirty work experience. They characterize the tactics as occupational ideologies, social buffers, confronting clients or public, and defensive tactics. In later work, Ashforth and Kreiner [31] assume some variation in the applicability of these tactics in relation to physically, socially and morally tainted work. Not all tactics appear equally useful to normalize moral taint.

Occupational ideologies help reframe, recalibrate or refocus the meaning attached to a dirty profession [26]. Reframing heightens the positive side(s) of an occupation. Recalibration revaluates the standards used to assess the "dirtiness" of the work by emphasizing that standards have changed. Refocusing shifts attention from tainted aspects of a profession to non-tainted ones. Occupational ideologies apply very well to moral taint, as Vaast and Levina [3] (p. 84) found in their study on retail bankers, Tyler [34] (p. 1490) identified in her study on sex shop workers and Tracy and Scott [33] (p. 26) revealed in their study on correctional officers.

Social buffers help to gain validation from people who affirm the social worth of the tainted profession. However, for a morally stigmatized group, it might be hard to gain social support from people outside the group; therefore, the tendency will be to turn to in-group members. Ashforth and Kreiner [31] (p. 92) expect this to happen most often in cases of moral taint, but the tactic is not reported in the study by Vaast and Levina [3], maybe due to the high status of bankers. Tyler [34] (p. 1491) does find the tactic in her study on sex shop workers.

Confronting critical clients or the general public occurs when dirty workers actively indicate society's perceptions of the occupation are wrong, by referring to opposite facts. Other methods to mitigate taint include "confrontational humour" and "counter-stereotypical behaviour" [24] (p. 162). However, Ashforth and Kreiner [31] do not mention confrontation tactics as effective in relation to moral taint, and also Vaast and Levina [3] explicitly wrote they do not find them. Thus, confronting outsiders seems less effective for normalizing moral taint, but the reason still remains an open question.

Finally, defence is a normalization tactic that appears very suitable in case of moral taint. Ashforth et al. [24] distinguish seven methods. The first is *avoidance* or the refusal to mention or observe dirty aspects of stigmatized work. The second is *gallows humour*, which is used to relieve the stress caused by the taint itself. The third is *accepting* and involves lowering one's expectations. The fourth is *social comparison* in which the tainted profession is compared to jobs or previous times that are or were even worse. The fifth, *condemning condemners*, is a reversal of the criticism towards those who are judging the dirty workers. The sixth is *blaming and/or distancing from clients*, who are criticized for being the cause of the taint. The last, *distancing from role*, occurs when stigmatized workers separate their personal identity from their work identity. Ashforth and Kreiner [31] (pp. 93–100) suppose that condemning condemners and organization-level defences are most effective in case of moral taint. In contrast, Vaast and Levina [3] (p. 84) find that retail bankers heavily utilize the tactic of social comparison, and they find some new defensive tactics as well: *passing the blame on to other groups* (most often found tactic), *circumstantiating* (there are many reasons that can explain what happened), *diverting conversations*, and *conceding negative changes in the occupation* (thus claiming the essentials remain untainted). The list of tactics suitable for normalizing moral taint might be even longer, as research in this field is still nascent.

It is specific for moral dirtiness that society assumes responsibility and agency for harming accepted values and principles. Moreover, the more agency a worker or manager has, the dirtier moral taint becomes. For instance, Roca [43] (p. 139) argues, "the chief executive officer (CEO) of a tobacco company, who gains riches by endangering others' health, might be perceived even more negatively than a blue-collar worker employed by the same company." This aspect of agency in triggering the construction of moral taint is currently underexplored, as the focus has been more on how those who feel the stigma—the victims—can protect themselves against the stigmatizing outsiders [24]. Additionally, in the case of banking, agency and occupational stigma are clearly linked and the same applies to used-car salespeople consciously concealing flaws of the cars they sell. We expect to find this agency also for over-demanding managers in stressful service industries such as consulting or law firms [13–17,20,44]. When moral taint is socially constructed, it is a response to intentional behaviours: bankers who cause the financial crisis, and continue to demand their bonuses, or managers in law and consultancy firms who earn more money by consciously pressuring their employees beyond their limits. We wonder why literature on dirty work has not explored this agency, and the possibilities suggested by moral leadership theory to do things differently, and maybe even to prevent or moderate the taint.

1.3. Can Moral Leadership Moderate a Dirty Leadership Reputation?

While normalization focuses on how stress due to perceptions of dirty work can be reduced, not much attention has been given to acting on moral stigma as a social construction (cf. [3,24,33,34]). However, in some work, this seems quite well possible, and if it concerns moral taint, it is even demanded by society: the bonus culture in the banking industry is no necessity, and in consulting and law firms, management has sufficient agency to decrease the pressures they impose on their workers. There is not the kind of necessity as with physically tainted jobs like firefighting or cleaning [31]. Further, even in these jobs, we have acted on the dirtiness with technology, which has made several blue-collar jobs less dirty over time. For instance, technological innovations improving protective suits have reduced health risks for firefighters, or for those cleaning up asbestos. As health risks reduce, the reasons for socially constructing dirtiness lose impact as well.

Still, do middle managers also have these possibilities in case of dirty leadership, when performance standards are high, and clients and top management are very demanding? Howard discusses some options, starting from the assumption that leadership is a "process of communication, verbally and non-verbally, which involves coaching, motivating/inspiring, directing/guiding and supporting/counselling others" [45] (p. 385). Following up on similar studies as for instance by Stone et al. who argue that "the most effective leaders pay most attention to employees" [46] (p. 356), moral leadership aims at giving such attention [30].

The first option discussed in moral leadership literature is setting a moral example [29,30,47]. Aronson [48] (p. 245), for instance, argues that if leaders set "moral examples", it fosters high levels of true motivation and morality overall, as employees look for an example they can follow. Applied to a high-performance setting, a lower-level manager could show his employees how to say no to a higher-level manager when managing own work pressures. However, in itself, a pressuring middle manager does not easily qualify for being a moral example. A second option often discussed is giving support, compassion and actively caring about others [29,30,49–51]. Treating employees with dignity and humanity will likely have positive effects on their performance [28]. Especially when management puts high pressures on employees, an open eye for their wellbeing and a supportive attitude might help not to overburden them. A third option of moral leadership is increasing your approachability [29,49]. That is considered to be crucial for establishing an "open environment" [50] (p. 164). When pressures are high, approachability in an open environment invites employees to speak up when they feel they reach their limits. Approachable, forgiving management leads to more employee wellbeing, more trust, and more sharing of interests between managers and their employees [49,52]. Fourth, in an open work environment, employees are more likely to engage in social control [49–52]. This results in more positive relationships among co-workers [29]. Co-workers could then feel more responsible to signal that colleagues get overstretched. Finally, when employees get the responsibility of performing tasks independently, psychological empowerment takes place [28,48]. Employees are being intrinsically stimulated to perform well and feel less commanded [30]. However, this is a risk as well, as you can easily push yourself too far in a high-performance culture, out of commitment. The five approaches are discussed as mutually supportive. For instance, if employees do not feel support from their manager, it is difficult for them to bring up their issues and to take responsibility [28,49].

Moral leadership approaches can potentially help to prevent or moderate a dirty work reputation originating from over demanding management. That is important, as high stress levels over extended periods can lead to emotional instability and decreased wellbeing at work [53] (p. 338). If then management is not approachable and does not foster an open culture, burnout and other stress-related diseases follow more easily, especially in the context of knowledge-intensive industries [54] (p. 166). That moment the dirty work image gets reconfirmed as well, with managers carrying the moral stigma. However, if and how middle managers in a high-performance context can execute moral leadership has not been researched yet. It is an open question if for instance consultant managers have sufficient agency to influence their morally dirty image this way, as they themselves are under high pressures as well. However, if some of these moral leadership approaches would work in their high-performance context, it might offer a more sustainable and more effective solution to the problem of their tainted leadership than only normalizing for themselves a situation society still considers dirty. If the agency of lower-level managers falls short, normalization is still the most likely thing left to do. Therefore, we expect a combination of normalization and moral leadership tactics when middle managers try to cope with the dirtiness of their leadership.

Based on our review of the literature, our main proposition is that the more agency a worker or manager has, the more likely it is that moral leadership tactics will be added to normalization tactics in order to cope with moral taint. Normalization is only a short-term solution for the worker and the morally tainted manager, whereas moral leadership can offer more fundamental answers to the problems that create a morally tainted leadership image.

2. Materials and Methods

2.1. Research Context

We chose management consulting as our research setting because it is well known that consulting managers put a lot of pressure on their employees. Alvesson and Robertson observed, for instance, that consultants frequently work more than 60 h a week [55] (see p. 221). Additionally, Gill found that promotions can only occur through high commitment, so workers constantly feel anxious about their current status and performance [44] (see p. 309). It makes consulting an extremely demanding profession with high levels of stress and burnout [17,20,56]. Society views such high demands and their negative health effects on consultants as "defying morality" [57] (p. 807). In fact, anonymous critiques indicating morally dirty leadership in consulting abound on public Internet forums (see a summary of these critiques in Table 1).

Table 1. Moral taint indications of over-demanding managers on Internet forums.

Critiques on Consulting Forums Found on Different Websites:	Threads/Entries	Period	Illustrative Quotes
Pressure of long working hours http://forum.top-consultant.com/ http://forums.whirlpool.net.au/ http://postgraduateforum.com/ http://www.wallstreetoasis.com/ (last assessed on 22 March 2017)	14/79	2006–2015	Forget work/life balance. Any big 4 [consultancy] you go to, **you'll be overworked**. (User #41779, forum.whirlpool.net.au, entry 2007)
Heavy workload; deadlines http://forum.top-consultant.com/ http://forums.whirlpool.net.au/ (last assessed on 22 March 2017)	12/69	2004–2015	Your start-off salary will be excellent. **For the brain damage resulting over the years there**, they will not compensate. (User, forum.top-consultant.com, entry 2004)
Fear of boss; not supportive http://lynntaylorconsulting.com/ http://managementconsulted.com/ http://socialanxietysupport.com/ (last assessed on 22 March 2017)	11/50	2008–2015	I'm in a bad place at work. It's in a high stakes consultancy firm, and my boss is a la Glen C. in Devil Wears Prada. Anyway, **my fear has just gotten worse**. (User, socialanxietysupport.com, entry 2009)
No empathy; focus on results http://forum.top-consultant.com/ http://lynntaylorconsulting.com/ (last assessed 22 March 2017)	8/24	2007–2013	The most heard story is about the boss who thinks that you can do anything in Excel with just a couple of clicks. **Never understands why everything takes so much time**. Also, never really knows what doing a job entails, and how all that analyst work on is done. (User, forum.top-consultant.com, entry 2007).

Thus, in the public eye, consulting managers are seen as very demanding in several ways. Such socially constructed dirtiness is also visible in the television series House of Lies, loosely based on a novel by Kihn [58], and we see leadership in consulting criticized in autobiographical accounts of ex-consultants as well [59,60]. These worries are confirmed in several academic studies on consultants' work life [16,17,19,21,44,55].

2.2. Research Design and Sample

In order to explore moral taint assigned to consulting managers, we performed 24 semi-structured interviews. The interviews were conducted with 12 consultant managers, sometimes also called senior consultants, and one associated junior consultant each. The dyadic design helped to compare interpretations between juniors and managers on leadership experiences and its dirty nature. More than half of the interviewed consultants work at big international firms, the others at consulting firms mainly working for the Dutch market (small- and medium-sized). Specializations are diverse, as indicated in Table 2.

Table 2. Interviewee characteristics.

Consultant	Gender	Age	Years in Company	Own Hours per Week	Branch of Firm	Size of Firm *
Junior 1	Male	24	1	50–55	Marketing	Small
Manager 1	Male	46	9	45–50	Marketing	Small
Junior 2	Female	25	1.5	45–55	Healthcare	Medium
Manager 2	Male	46	15	45–50	Healthcare	Medium
Junior 3	Male	27	1.5	40–50	IT	Large
Manager 3	Male	42	13	70	IT	Large
Junior 4	Male	27	2.5	50–55	Corporate Finance	Medium
Manager 4	Male	35	11	50	Corporate Finance	Medium
Junior 5	Male	25	1	60	Strategy	Large
Manager 5	Male	30	5	50–70	Strategy	Large
Junior 6	Male	27	1.5	50–60	M&A	Large
Manager 6	Male	34	8	50–80	M&A	Large
Junior 7	Male	26	1.5	45–60	IT	Large
Manager 7	Male	30	6	40–80	IT	Large
Junior 8	Female	25	1.5	40–45	Strategy	Small
Manager 8	Female	28	4	45–60	Strategy	Small

Table 2. *Cont.*

Consultant	Gender	Age	Years in Company	Own Hours per Week	Branch of Firm	Size of Firm *
Junior 9	Female	25	1	45–60	Human Resources	Medium
Manager 9	Female	35	8	40–60	Human Resources	Medium
Junior 10	Female	28	3	40–80	Innovation & Change	Medium
Manager 10	Female	35	6	40–80	Innovation & Change	Medium
Junior 11	Male	27	1	50–70	Strategy & Operations	Large
Manager 11	Male	37	9	50–60	Strategy & Operations	Large
Junior 12	Male	28	1.5	55	Strategy & Operations	Large
Manager 12	Male	48	4	50–60	Strategy & Operations	Large

* Number of employees in consulting departments based on http://www.vault.com/. Last accessed: 18 May 2016). Small: <100 employees; Medium: 100–500 employees; Large: >500 employees.

We selected respondents through "convenience and snowball sampling" [61] (p. 127), with the first few interviewees recommending possible candidates at other firms, mostly starting with the juniors and then connecting to their managers. Juniors and managers with the same number work together.

2.3. Interview Procedure

The interviews lasted an average of 45 min, ranging from 30 to 60 min. We offered anonymity, requested permission to record and started with a short personal introduction of interviewers and interviewees. All interviewees were informed about the study beforehand and gave their informed consent for inclusion before they participated in the study. The study was conducted in accordance with the guidelines of the School of Business and Economics at Vrije Universiteit Amsterdam. We explained to the interviewees that we would talk about tensions in the manager–employee relationship, based on three jokes (two of them were cartoons, and one was a text joke). The aim was to explore how consultant managers and their juniors experience the dirtiness of the management pressures. The three jokes were a starting point for doing very open interviews, in which we discussed each joke (see Table 3) for 5–15 min. The first one resonated most with the experiences of consultants resulting in long conversations, with the last one being the least.

Table 3. Three consultant manager jokes indicating moral taint.

Manager A in his office: What are they complaining about .... The work is challenging, interesting, demanding! *Manager B:* AND we let them do it 80 h per week! Fran (2009) Retrieved from: https://www.cartoonstock.com/, accessed: 23 March 2017
Manager A to Manager B when walking through the office: Naturally our workers look happy. The penalty for not being happy is instant dismissal *Financial Times,* 20 May 2013. Retrieved from: https://www.ft.com/content/41f990f0-b955-11e2-bc57-00144feabdc0#axzz2U2zMvxmp, accessed: 23 March 2017
Please don't tell my mother I'm a consultant. She thinks I play guitar in a strip joint. Consultant Jokes Retrieved from: http://www.weitzenegger.de/en/to/jokes.html, accessed: 23 March 2017.

As jokes do not present the truth literally, it helped us to introduce our topic in a stimulating, but when reflecting on it, not a leading, but rather a very open way [62]. Interviewees were first asked to interpret the jokes (for instance junior 9 said, "cartoon 1 is exaggerated."), then they could explain if or how the jokes related to their work contexts ("this (80 h a week) rarely happens here"), and what further associations they had. Most respondents recognized aspects of the dirty management style illustrated in cartoon 1. Related to cartoon 2, the first response of junior 1 was: "What do they mean by this? That you always need to be happy at work? Or that you should pretend you are happy? With that I agree, as you don't want to show your boss you don't feel happy." Many respondents recognized aspects of cartoon 2 due to their own personality or an "up or out" culture in their consultancy. For the same reasons of personality and company culture, others felt less connection to this cartoon. The third joke was hardly representing how respondents felt about what they have to do, and they did not recognize this dirty image of the job, like manager 2, who said, "I would put banker here instead of consultant." All consultants stated they were proud enough to tell what they do, and did not recognize the suggested shame for being a consultant. However, some did refer to other "sick stereotypes" they encountered, like junior 9 who went on holiday, introduced herself as a consultant, getting the question in return, and said, "where is your lease car and credit card?" The quoted interpretations illustrate that respondents made sense of all three jokes in their own way, by referring to their own experiences.

After this free interpretation, the interviewer facilitated a broad discussion including probing questions concerning over-demanding managers, observed critical evaluations of the behaviour of consultant managers, the experienced effects of their leadership style, and how managers and juniors where coping with the situation of pressuring leadership and its morally tainted nature. None of such coping was suggested in the jokes, with only the pressures and the reputation proposed. Starting a conversation with a respondent by asking for interpreting three jokes is new, but doing open explorative interviews aligns with prior research on dirty work (cf. [3,24,33,34]). It is a good way to explore experiences with work pressures, leadership and dirtiness, and it fits our nascent field of research as outlined by Edmondson and McManus [63] (p. 1170).

2.4. Data Analysis

To analyse the interviews, we worked mostly abductive. We applied elements of a grounded theory approach in our coding [64] but also used existing dirty work and moral leadership tactics to interpret the data. We kept an eye out for any codes that did not fit the existing theoretical labels. To do so, the transcribed interviews were coded with the qualitative data analysis tool Atlas.ti (ATLAS.ti Scientific Software Development GmbH, Berlin, Germany). This resulted in 814 relevant codes with data-driven summarizing labels mostly connected to one quote only, and incidentally to two. Both authors coded iteratively and pointed upon which they disagreed with were discussed and then aligned. An overview of all codes can be found below in Table 4. In the results section we present codes related to dirty leadership pressures and related effects in Table 5, codes related to normalization tactics in Table 6 and codes related to moral leadership tactics in Table 7.

The leadership pressures and their effects on juniors were coded as morally dirty based on two ethical perspectives: deontology (pressures) and consequentialism (effects). Criticized stressors, such as long working hours and high work pressure, were coded as morally dirty from a deontological point of view. For example, demanding more hours than allowed by law does not conform to duty [65]. Codes identifying criticized negative effects, such as burnout, decreased wellbeing, or high turnover rates caused by health problems, were coded as immoral from a consequentialist perspective [66]. Normalization and moral leadership tactics were labelled with existing concepts from the discussed literature, except for the new ones that emerged from the data. Our findings suggest that moral taint experienced by consultant managers is not only mitigated by taint normalization, but also by known and lesser known moral leadership tactics. A process model summarizing the main codes and sub codes (in the boxes) and their relationships (arrows) is presented at the start of the results section (see Figure 1).

Table 4. Parent, child and grandchild codes.

Parent Codes	Child Codes	Grandchild Codes
Morally dirty leadership	Dirty pressures	Long working hours and high workload No support; barriers to request help Focus on results instead of wellbeing
	Dirty effects	Burnout Decreased wellbeing & performance High turnover rate due to pressure
Normalization tactics	Defence	Social comparison Condemning condemners Acceptance Gallows humour
	Confronting	–
	Occupational ideology	Reframing Recalibrating Refocussing
	Social buffers	–
Moral leadership tactics	Individual tactics	Personal support by compassionate managers Open culture for social control Approachability of managers Responsibility given to employees Being a moral example
	Institutionalized tactics	Institutional support through selection of the right candidates, performance reviews & training Compensation time & acknowledgement policies

3. Results

Figure 1 presents a conceptual model representing our coded categories. The model illustrates how pressures due to leadership are experienced as morally dirty by both junior consultants and their managers, and how this experience of moral taint invites on the one hand normalization responses as predicted by dirty work literature, but on the other hand also moral leadership initiatives to prevent or moderate the negative effects of leadership pressures. The reported forms of moral leadership we found require different levels of agency, and are relate to juniors, managing consultants and those who can design institutions at consultancies. We first reported leadership pressures experienced as dirty, second normalization tactics as coping response and third moral leadership practices as an alternative response, as seen from the perspective of managers and junior consultants.

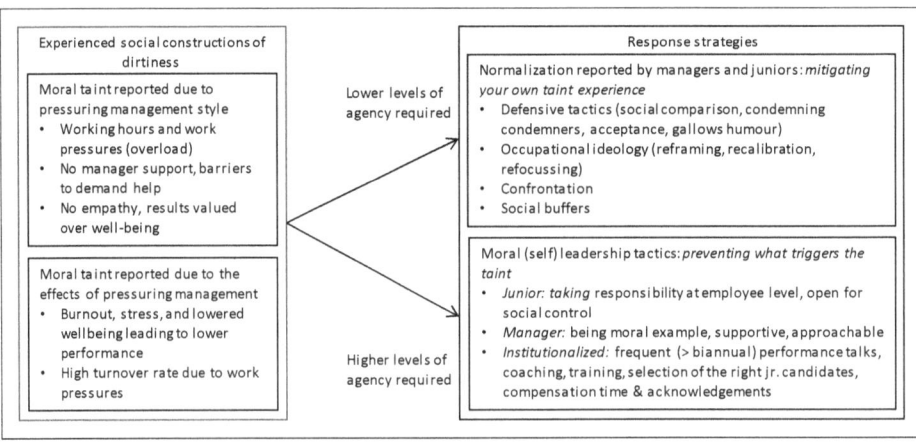

Figure 1. Moral taint constructions linked to management, and response strategies.

3.1. Moral Taint Due to Pressuring Management

The interviews revealed stressors and effects due to pressuring management that interviewees perceived as morally tainted. Respondents expressed their interpretations of moral taint quite explicitly through negative judgments or more implicitly: facts were given and the audience was left to pass judgment. Table 5 summarizes the shared interpretations of managers and junior consultants, and gives for each of the codes their groundedness (how many quotes we could label with the same code) and an illustrative quote of both managers and juniors. It is important to note that the pressuring management style is criticized substantially more often than its negative effects.

Statements from both junior 7 and manager 12 in Table 5 indicate it is quite common in consulting to be asked to work up to 60 h a week and incidentally up to 80 h a week. This is substantially longer than the Dutch maximum of 40 h a week. For a period no longer than 16 weeks, Dutch labour law allows workers to work up till 48 h a week on average [67], but consultants are asked to work much longer. Because of projects with overlapping deadlines, pressuring managers and demanding clients, junior 11 (Table 5) compares his work environment to that of a "pressure cooker", suggesting the pressures are far from comfortable. Of all dirty leadership pressures, required work hours are criticized most by the juniors, and managers admit the pressures are as high as the juniors indicate. It makes the management style morally tainted; for instance, junior 10 said (laughs while looking at cartoon 1), "This is anonymous? Yes, this applies to my manager! This is quite bad indeed. But I need to add some nuance. I recognize this, but it is also something I want to do. I chose to work the 60, 70, 80 h. And I seek challenges, new clients, personal development, etc. This works bi-directional."

While the pressures mentioned above can also be attributed to the work context, and not only to the manager, juniors specifically mention the formal distance they can feel between themselves and their demanding managers. When facing difficulties, juniors can feel "ashamed" for opening up, sensing it is better not to "lose face" by admitting they struggle with the work pressures (see junior 4 in Table 4). Managers recognize the experience of this distance (like manager 3 in Table 4) and admit "you often discover it (overload struggles) later than their direct environment".

Related to this is the focus on results. Consulting firms are organized around meeting productivity and sales targets, causing managers to be primarily concerned with the productivity aspect of their juniors' performances, and the cost of their juniors' wellbeing. As a result, juniors criticize the aspect of being treated as a source of profit. Junior 10 (Table 5) explains it is key that the "client is happy", and feels that it is a "dangerous criterion", as it can push you too far. Managers confirm this, and admit that "consulting is a hard environment" (manager 9), which adds to the list of morally dirty aspects in the leadership style.

Table 5. Management-induced pressures perceived as morally tainted.

Category	Groundedness			Illustrative Quote
	Tot 283	Jr 153	M 130	
Dirty pressures	246			
Long working hours and high workload	111	63	48	"Yes, juniors work long hours. There are projects where they work for longer periods **about 60 h a week**."—Manager 12. "Consulting is working from deadline to deadline. And if a deadline requires a lot, then **working 80 h occurs easily**."—Junior 7. "Working here is working in a **pressure cooker**. It is just hard work. You have deadlines."—Junior 11.
No support; barriers to request help	78	50	28	"**Often juniors are ashamed**, like, I am so young, why does it happen to me? As a manager you often discover it [overload struggles] later than their direct environment, and that it does not go well."—Manager 3. "I know myself. I sure have my issues here. But **I would never go with those to my boss**. . . . opening up could be seen as a loss of face."—Junior 4.
Focus on results instead of wellbeing	57	26	31	"**Consulting is a hard environment**. As a junior you have to satisfy your project managers. Failing to satisfy your manager can only happen 1 or 2 times. Then they look for someone else."—Manager 9 "The key rule is: as long as the client is happy. And that can be a really **dangerous criterion**, in which you can easily go too far."—Junior 10.
Dirty effects	37			
Burnout	18	5	13	"What I do see, is the age at which people come down with long-term illness is rapidly declining. I have an **increasing number of people under 30 coming to me with such symptoms**."—Manager 3. "If you struggle with boundaries, and want to do everything perfectly, working as a consultant is not sustainable. And that's what happened to me. **I made myself sick**."—Junior 10.
Decreased wellbeing & performance	10	4	6	"If you are not handling them [the stressors of consulting] well, you see that in your performance. Then you **don't even like working here, and you couldn't care less about performance**."—Manager 5. "If it is not your own choice to work 80 h a week. It is also not constructive, **for either you or your results**."—Junior 10.
High turnover rate due to pressure	9	5	4	"In the moment you are like 'Okay, we have to get through this'. But you know it's not sustainable. **You can't let juniors work that many hours for several weeks on projects**. You know that they will leave after a year or so. It's not sustainable."—Manager 12. "If people are really unhappy with their projects, they will ask if this is the right job for them, **and then they leave**."—Junior 11

Tot = Total; Jr = Junior consultant; M = Manager.

The juniors and managers not only criticize the moral dirtiness of the cold management style with the focus on results and low tolerance for personal failure. To a lesser extent, they also criticize the immoral effects of such high pressures. Burnout is mentioned most often, and also qualified as the most negative consequence. Manager 3 (Table 5) indicates that increasingly young colleagues suffer from burnout. In addition, junior 10 admitted that she had suffered from a burnout herself. Although we cannot quantify based on our interview data, literature on consultants does indicate a high prevalence of burnout, stress and related psychological problems among consultants, in line with our findings [17,19,20,56].

Some workers, rather than having a burnout, share that they become mentally imbalanced, feel depressed, or have negative emotions. The quote from manager 5 in Table 5 illustrates how stress reduced his performance and work satisfaction. At times that too many stressors escalated "you couldn't care less about performance", a finding also observed by Espeland [68] (see p. 180).

A related effect criticized by our interviewees is the high turnover rate among juniors. It is seen as response to the extreme demands they face. The quotes from manager 12 and junior 11 in Table 5 indicate this, as you "cannot let juniors work that many hours" (manager 12). "They will ask if this is the right job for them, and then they leave." (junior 11). These critiques again indicate dirty leadership, and question the sustainability of the work for juniors.

Juniors and consultant managers are surprisingly aligned in their judgements of when and where their occupation crosses the borders of acceptable work demands. They clearly articulate which leadership pressures and effects are unacceptable against the norms and laws in society. These internalized critical social judgements give stress, as discussed in the dirty work literature, in addition to the work pressures themselves. Therefore, the motivation to normalize an experience of moral taint will be higher, the more conscious you are about the critical public and peer judgements. Both the juniors might normalize (they do not like to be seen as a victim) as well as the pressuring managers (who do not like to be seen as over-demanding).

3.2. Normalizing Morally Tainted Management

If members of an occupation feel aspects of their work are perceived as morally dirty, they are found to engage in normalization to protect their self-image [24,31]. The occurrence of normalization signals foremost a perception of taint. By using normalization tactics, the interviewees tried to mitigate their own experience of being seen as morally tainted, as this causes stress. Our interviewees applied several normalization tactics when discussing their leadership experiences. Table 6 shows that the normalization tactics are well grounded. Remarkably, juniors illustrate normalization more than managers.

Table 6. Taint normalizing tactics that mitigate the experience of moral taint in consulting.

Category	Groundedness			Illustrative Quote
	Tot 171	Jr 101	M 70	
Defence: mainly social comparison, also condemning condemners, etc.	64	40	24	"I think the reputation problem for consultants has become less over the years. **Bankers have a bigger problem.** . . . Lawyers as well, and medical specialists. . . . , why should the latter earn so much?"—Manager 2. "Yes, I don't work from 9 to 5. . . . **These people have a mentality like, whatever.** That does not fit me. So, I don't work from 9 to 5. But I would hate that. . . . Actually, I think that working 9 to 5 is more of a regime than working 80 h."—Junior 10.
Confronting	51	23	28	"I made the calculations myself. Look, I work from 8 A.M. till 7 P.M. That is 55 h. To make it 80 h would mean I could not sleep anymore. **That is not how it works.**"—Manager 5. "I understand that cartoon saying we work 80 h, **but it is exaggerated.** Who is working 80 h . . . ?"—Junior 1
Occupational ideology	46	31	15	"I really like consulting. What I like is to help others and explicate things. **The way I see consulting, is that it helps others.** So no way am I ashamed of that."—Manager 4. "There are people here that can't say no; they can't stop. **But they really like that and do great work because of that.** They are actively seeking such pressure."—Junior 6
Social buffers	10	7	3	"My wife and I, we both work as consultants, so **we understand each other** in terms of work and our careers."—Manager 3. "When I told my uncle that I wanted to become a consultant, he. . . . was very negative. But I think, **among the young professionals, among us, consultancy is being highly appreciated.**"—Junior 8.

Tot = Total; Jr = Junior consultant; M = Manager.

Instances of taint normalization illustrated in the interviews were most often defensive, with social comparison applied the most. Other forms of defence included condemning condemners, acceptance, and a few instances of gallows humour. Manager 2 in Table 6 demonstrated the use of social comparison by relating the moral reputation of consultant managers to, in his eyes, the worse reputation of some other professions: "Bankers have a bigger problem. . . . Lawyers as well." Condemning condemners was used to normalize consultants' long working hours. Compared to her own schedule junior 10 considered working from 9 to 5 "more of a regime". This defensive normalization intends to mitigate the feeling of moral stigma due to leadership pressures put on you: with long working hours, you can still feel better off than the 9-to-5 employee.

Confronting public opinion was a second normalization tactic repeatedly used by juniors and managers. With this tactic, someone proactively confronts the public's perception of occupational taint, intending to change the view. Junior 1 and manager 5 in Table 6 tried this by correcting the stereotypical belief that consultants always work 80 h a week, as suggested in one of the cartoons. Junior 1 argued this is exaggerated and manager 5 stated that it is impossible: "Look, I work from 8 a.m. till 7 p.m. That is 55 h. To make it 80 h would mean I could not sleep anymore." We thus find opposite opinions: many consultants complain about workweeks up till 80 h, as illustrated in Table 4, while manager 5 denies it even as a possibility. Still, he does admit a 55-h average workweek (not counting the weekend)! Another theme for confronting public opinion is the lack of humanity in consultant leadership due to the results-oriented work culture (see Table 5). Consultants are confronting the universality of this tainted aspect of their work suggested in the second cartoon, but less so than the 80-h figure from the first cartoon.

Third, occupational ideology tactics were practiced. Consultants transformed negative opinions about their profession into more positive ones, by reframing, recalibrating and refocusing. Junior 6 recalibrated long working hours and high workload when he stated people "do great work because of that"; this recalibrated the extra effort as simply needed to reach the intended effects. Furthermore, manager 4 reframed the harsh conditions juniors face by emphasizing that they are "helping others", thus presenting the efforts of juniors in a different light. Examples of refocusing included shifting attention to aspects of the work that made consultants proud or happy, like their impact, their pay or their status.

Although creating social buffers supports in-group protection, we found it rarely used to normalize the high-pressure work context. Manager 3 and junior 8 made a distinction between "us" versus "them" as outsiders: "us, young professionals, we appreciate it", or "my wife and I, both consultants, we understand" (see Table 6).

While we interviewed an equal number of managers and junior consultants, the juniors illustrate normalization tactics more. As juniors could be seen as victims with a low degree of agency, normalizing can help. They need to give their best efforts in order to survive. Still, they have a responsibility for their own health, actually more so than their managers. They also have the agency to choose for the job, and they can quit. Managers have more influence: although they have to play their part in the up or out performance system, they are also the ones pressuring their juniors. Managers can make a difference, but their agency to prevent an output oriented and pressuring form of leadership has limits as well, which makes normalization still a convenient way out.

3.3. Moral Leadership to Prevent Moral Taint

Whereas normalization mitigates the experience of stress caused by the feeling that you have a dirty job, interviewees also tried to prevent a morally dirty image by influencing the effects of high work pressures and the extreme focus on results. We have coded many of these prevention tactics as moral leadership because they exactly match the tactics mentioned in this literature. However, institutionalized forms of support for juniors, like frequent performance talks, acknowledgement policies and tailored selection procedures (italicized in Table 7), were new to moral leadership literature. Still, they fit the same rationale of preventing the criticized consequences like burnout or emotional imbalance, and of counteracting the impression of immoral values in the leadership style like the strong output orientation and lack of humanity. Additionally, they help managers to execute traditional moral leadership tactics by organizing how and when they give attention to juniors.

Table 7. Moral leadership tactics used to prevent moral taint.

Category	Groundedness			Illustrative Quote
	Tot 350	Jr 181	M 168	
Personal support by compassionate managers	96	30	66	"I always **ask them a lot of questions**, like 'What does your day look like? What are your responsibilities? What costs too much energy?'. With that, you intend to start something, and make the junior rethink himself."—Manager 8. "I work around 60 h now.... They monitor that you do not work too much. ... You have conversations like 'you leave the project too late every time'. **That is your manager who talks to you individually**."—Junior 8.
Open culture for social control	61	34	27	"It is very important to ensure that your employees dare to speak up, to create an environment in which people **feel safe**."—Manager 10. "There are people that I see three times a week, who could assess my feelings better (than my manager). So I think it is the role of everyone: **social control**."—Junior 9.
Approachability of managers	59	40	19	"I surely am **approachable**. And I am definitely open to those conversations (about stressors)."—Manager 10. "There is no barrier to approach my manager. If there were something bothering me, I could tell him. I also know other stories .... **Here the doors are always open**."—Junior 4
Responsibility given to employees	58	42	16	"Everybody has their own responsibilities. Of course, I will have the final responsibility, but I don't manage their daily activities .... **We give them free reign**."—Manager 4. "In the beginning you get a lot of guidance.... Now, after 1.5 years, I am much more pro-active. I say I want to do this or that. **I organize and plan myself**."—Junior 6
Institutional support through selection of the right candidates, performance reviews & training	48	25	22	"The other day, I conducted some job interviews, in which I explicitly asked: "What do you think of working over night?".... **So I test them**, to see if they need structure or not."—Manager 9. "We have an **HR (Human Resource) cycle**, in which we have a talk about performance, a talk on development and several training courses."—Junior 2. "We recently got a case about work-life balance.... Here we got taught **how to say 'no'** to managers."—Junior 9.
Compensation time & acknowledgement policies	22	9	13	"'If we require our employees to work on the weekends, we **compensate** for that. We send a gift coupon to the family, especially if it happens more often, or we send flowers. And if we require our employees to work hard for an extended period, we send them on a weekend trip with their family."—Manager 3. "We often hear '**thanks for your help, you did really well**' .... After every project we go out for dinner .... Sometimes there also is an event and you get some award for your contribution (he shows an award), awards like that."—Junior 6
Being a moral example	6	1	5	"People try to guard their image. But people should let that guard go. Saying 'Okay, this is who I am; I am putting it on the table'. And then it's easier for people to open up also. So, **if you open up, they open up**."—Manager 11.

Tot = Total; Jr = Junior consultant; M = Manager.

3.3.1. Traditional Moral Leadership Approaches

Managers most often mention the importance of compassion and support for their juniors, which aligns with moral leadership theory [29,30,49–51]. It implies managers not only try to be actively aware of the stressors they put on juniors, but also make them discussable. In our interviews, managers emphasized the importance of actively approaching juniors, especially those who seem stressed. Manager 8 claimed she "always asks them a lot of questions". Her junior (junior 8 in Table 7) confirmed this.

A second aspect, also mentioned in moral leadership literature, is an 'open culture for social control', as it creates positive social effects [29] (p. 139). This is relevant, as consultants mostly work together in project teams [69] (p. 559). Our interviewees illustrated how managers help to establish an open culture, in which peers are encouraged to express their feelings to each other. Manager 10 (Table 7) stated how important it is to create an environment in which everybody can 'speak up'. Her junior (10) confirmed the open culture and the social control: "I experience the social control. It means there is sufficient attention for the persons themselves, and how they really feel, instead of only a result focus, this extreme focus." Junior 9 (see Table 7) has a similar experience of social control, and mentions that colleagues take care of each other.

Third, managers try to be approachable and to react with understanding and forgiveness if juniors approach them. Manager 10 stated that if a junior dared to approach her, she would definitely listen and then try to manage the problem. Manager 4 illustrated a similar attitude: "You try to find out what is the matter, and then seek for a solution together. That cartoon suggesting to dismiss them immediately is not our approach, and I would not support it." His junior confirmed the approachable "the doors are always open" and the forgiving approach of his manager (junior 4, Table 7), but he knows other stories as well, where you "first need to book your appointment".

The impact of acting as a moral example is sufficiently discussed in the literature, as documented in our theory section. However, the tactic was hardly mentioned by our interviewees, indicating it is a difficult one in the context of consulting. Manager 11 (Table 7, bottom row) acknowledged that juniors find it difficult to open up about stressors, and yet he expressed that if he became open about himself, "it is easier for people to open up also". Only one junior (junior 9) referred to exemplary behaviour of one manager who did not respond to an email she had sent on a Sunday. That manager explained later that the weekend should be weekend. However, this does not seem to be standard practice in this occupation.

3.3.2. Juniors' Role in Making Moral Leadership Work

The fourth moral leadership tactic we found (based on groundedness) was giving responsibility to the employee, a practice most often expressed by juniors. By making the juniors more responsible for how they perform their tasks, their feelings of helplessness and lack of control can decrease [30]. Manager 4 (Table 7) stated that he tries to foster autonomy of juniors by not getting involved in their daily tasks. Giving autonomy to plan his or her own schedule and projects reduces the negative impact of workload and deadline stress. Juniors are supported to develop this autonomy, as mentioned by junior 6, and such autonomy is indeed expected. Manager 6 explains: "If they have a problem, they should call me. Sometimes at the end of a call, they just thank me for the talk. It can help to better make sense of a difficult situation. But they have to approach me, as we discussed before. And that does not always happen."

3.3.3. Institutional Approaches to Moral Leadership

Respondents also referred to institutionalized practices, such as the monitoring of juniors through monthly or quarterly performance reviews next to the annual talk. Junior 2 mentions that her consultancy organizes different types of formal evaluations every year (see Table 7), and elsewhere in the interview she refers to evaluations "after every project". It gives juniors a platform to speak up, and this way it is institutionalized that they receive sufficient attention from their managers. Trainings are institutionalized as well, as illustrated in the quotes from juniors 2 and 9 in Table 7. Examples are work–life balance workshops and personal development courses that better prepare juniors to handle the work stress.

Additionally, consultancies make use of an extensive selection process, aimed at hiring these juniors who are sturdy enough to handle the stress of being a consultant, as explained by manager 9 in Table 7. Some people like a challenging work environment and are able to handle the lack of structure for many years. However, the work is too demanding for many others, so consultancies are aware of the importance to pick the right people, in order to protect their reputation as an employer and to manage the consequences of the severe work pressures up front.

A second group of institutionalized practices to counter the moral taint of pressuring management includes compensation and acknowledgment. Overwork or high pressure is not compensated by additional pay, because it is seen as part of the job. However, managers often give juniors visible recognition after a stressful period. For instance, juniors are given dinners, social events, flowers, a couple of days off and even vacations. The quote from manager 3 (Table 7) illustrated this practice. The manager acknowledges the stress, and marks it as out-of-the-ordinary. In addition to acknowledging the stress, he compensates his juniors with time to recover, ultimately also hoping to prevent severe consequences. His junior confirmed his work is quite intense now, heading towards the end of several projects, "but you also know you can slow down after the deadlines. That is quite accepted" (junior 3). Junior 6 illustrated another practice explained by manager 3: "we often hear: 'thanks for your help, you did really well'."

The combination of traditional, more personal, and consultancy-specific institutionalized practices to support juniors demonstrates that the direct managers are not the only ones who take responsibility for supporting juniors. The organization as a whole has taken action to prevent escalation of stress. These institutionalized practices aim at making the consequences of the stressors less severe and the management more humane, at the same time reducing perceptions of moral taint in the eyes of the juniors and their managers. Such multi-level moral leadership is potentially a more effective approach to coping with perceptions of morally tainted leadership than taint normalization. Normalization only targets at the stress due to perceptions of taint, which is symptom management. Moral leadership targets the specific causes behind these perceptions. Additionally, given the fact that the pressuring leadership style is far more criticized than its effects (see Table 5), the multi-level approach seems promising.

4. Discussion

In summary, we found that moral leadership approaches were discussed quite a lot when compared to normalization responses. Twice as many quotes (350 vs. 171) illustrated moral leadership tactics in response to the dirty leadership images. When reflecting on moral leadership approaches, juniors and managers emphasized different options. Managers mentioned their active compassion and support of juniors twice as often as juniors, whereas juniors mentioned the approachability of their managers more often as important to them. Still, juniors and managers referred to the same kind of tactics. This, together with the ample groundedness of the codes, indicates good saturation.

Table 5 shows that the leadership style of managers is more often constructed as dirty (246 quotes) than the resulting effects (37 quotes). However, the number of quotes is not very conclusive regarding this dirtiness as something "essential". The mentioned effects like burnout are really problematic and not mentioning it might even be an avoidance or denial strategy. Still, there is a lot of talk about the dirtiness of the leadership style and this is a big issue in the construction of consultants' dirty leadership.

Moral leadership aims at neutralizing such dirtiness. For instance, the impressions of an output-oriented and pressuring leadership style resulting in long working hours and high workloads is countered by traditional moral leadership tactics. They counter the stigma that managers do not provide support and have no empathy, as these traditional tactics are targeting exactly these aspects of dirtiness in the leadership style. Institutionalized moral leadership tactics, like regular performance talks, training, selective hiring and various compensation tactics, are also discussed a lot, which indicates their social visibility, with the construction of a better leadership impression. These institutionalized approaches seem specific for our high-performance setting, and might be relevant to other high-pressure contexts as well, such as investment banks or law firms. The applicability of the individual moral leadership tactics must be much wider, as these tactics have been found in many other work contexts already [29,30,49,50].

The findings of our study contribute to the literature on moral taint and moral leadership. First, we found that moral problems that cause a dirty leadership image can be targeted with moral leadership approaches [29,30,49]. Consulting managers engage in many forms of moral leadership to counterbalance what juniors and managers socially construct as a dirty leadership style. Especially the pressuring leadership style, like focusing on output only and lack of personal attention, is experienced as dirty in the image of consultant management. Traditional moral leadership tactics target such dirty aspects in the leadership style directly. Thus, they socially construct alternative and more ambiguous leadership image: pressuring yes, but also committed. As deeds can speak louder than words, this approach seems quite relevant for influencing a dirty leadership image. Except for confronting public opinion, normalizing mainly has a focus on individual stress reduction due to a dirty image. Our findings add a new repertoire of tactics to the literature on moral taint (cf. [3,24,26,35]). As a consequence, normalization tactics are just one way to respond to the experience of moral taint.

On a more critical note, we found that some of the propositions in Ashforth and Kreiner [31] did not hold very well in the context of consulting. For instance, proposition 4 that morally tainted professions are assumed to mostly engage in group-level defensive tactics, and proposition 10 that such professions create social buffers to normalize taint were not very prominent in our context. We found, similar to findings by Vaast and Levina [3], that the tactic of social buffering is not utilized much, whereas defensive tactics are most frequently applied. Considering defensive tactics Ashforth and Kreiner [31] assume in their proposition 11 that condemning condemners is the most common one to normalize moral taint, however, in our study, social comparison is the most reported normalizing tactic, a result that aligns by and large with the findings of Vaast and Levina [3] situated in the banking industry. Unlike the propositions in Ashforth and Kreiner [31], we found many instances of confronting public opinions about the dirtiness of consultant leadership. Probably, effectively normalizing moral taint largely depends on context, as both banking and consulting belong to the professional service sector. As professional service industries are a growing field of employment in today's societies, future research should address these high-performance sectors more specifically when studying morally tainted leadership and the potentially tainted health consequences for employees, like burnout. It is important to study such consequences, and possible gender, role or seniority differences based on a quantitative research design, to better tease out to what extent normalization attempts cover up such consequences.

Second, we contribute to moral leadership literature by finding that consultant managers not only apply traditional moral leadership approaches like being approachable, compassionate supportive and encouraging. Consultancies also support managers with institutionalized measures that aim at moral leadership, and that are new in this literature (cf. [29,30,49,50]). As the agency of managers is constrained by institutional pressures, we see that the organization also creates counter pressures with several specific HR practices. As these HR practices are quite visible, they help to clean up the dirty leadership image, again with deeds more than words. Therefore, we invite moral leadership literature to better include the organizational and institutional levels in its theorizing. By having frequent performance reviews planned, trainings available, and several non-monetary compensation policies in place, consultant managers mentioned how they are supported in taking responsibility for the wellbeing of juniors. These institutionalized measures might be specific to high-performance occupations with demanding top management, clients and projects, where it is very tempting to satisfy client needs first and think about your juniors second [11]. Therefore, similar institutional support might be relevant to other high-pressure professional service contexts, such as investment banking, law firms and marketing agencies, or even at the more competitive top universities.

Our research has also some practical implications beyond the fields of moral leadership theory and dirty work literature. We consider it a promising and innovative combination to facilitate moral leadership of middle managers with supportive HR practices. Such tailored institutions might help protecting employee health and reduce psychosocial risks at work, especially in settings of knowledge-intensive work. These are high-performance work contexts where employees are often ambitious and willing to give their best, but where burnout risks lure around the corner, especially when employees do not feel they are seen and cared for, or rewarded for taking initiative and for acting responsible towards their organization, often at the cost of their own mental resources. Our research shows that HR institutions can be further developed to support middle management in taking care of their employees, inspired by moral leadership ideas. If organizations create such institutions to give attention, to show compassion and to take responsibility for workers that give their best, it could help to move away from the more bureaucratic, rule-based and one-size-fits-all HR institutions we are so familiar with today.

5. Conclusions

The identified moral leadership approaches on both the levels of individual manager and the organization add to our understanding of how organizations can influence their image of moral dirtiness associated with pressuring, output-oriented management. Similar multi-level approaches to support employees have been identified in Australian universities [36], and they seem promising in empowering middle management to become moral leaders. However, based on our research findings, we cannot answer yet to what extent individual and organizational moral leadership approaches in consulting make life of juniors really better (see [16,17,19,44]). It is possible that they are merely used instrumentally, to push performance of juniors just a little bit further, without irreversible consequences for leadership reputation and employee health and wellbeing. What we can conclude is that the morally dirty reputation of consultancies is not only articulated regarding the consultant–client relationships [7–10]. Moral leadership issues between consultants and their managers are also publicly addressed, and more prominently indeed than their moral leadership approaches.

Author Contributions: Conceptualization, O.B. and T.E.K.; analysis, O.B. and T.E.K.; investigation, T.E.K.; methodology, O.B.; writing of the original draft, O.B. and T.E.K.; writing of review and editing, O.B.

Funding: This research received no external funding.

Conflicts of Interest: The authors declare no conflict of interest.

References

1. Hughes, E.C. Work and the self. In *Social Psychology at the Crossroads*; Rohrer, J.H., Sherif, M., Eds.; Harper and Bros: New York, NY, USA, 1951; pp. 313–323.
2. Stanley, L.; MacKenzie Davey, K.; Symon, G. Exploring media construction of investment banking as dirty work. *Qual. Res. Organ. Manag. Int. J.* **2014**, *9*, 270–287. [CrossRef]
3. Vaast, E.; Levina, N. Speaking as one, but not speaking up: Dealing with new moral taint in an occupational online community. *Inf. Organ.* **2015**, *25*, 73–98. [CrossRef]
4. Morales, J.; Lambert, C. Dirty work and the construction of identity. An ethnographic study of management accounting practices. *Account. Organ. Soc.* **2013**, *38*, 228–244. [CrossRef]
5. Bouwmeester, O.; Stiekema, J. The paradoxical image of consultant expertise: A rhetorical deconstruction. *Manag. Decis.* **2015**, *53*, 2433–2456. [CrossRef]
6. Sturdy, A. Popular critiques of consultancy and a politics of management learning? *Manag. Learn.* **2009**, *40*, 457–463. [CrossRef]
7. Allen, J.; Davis, D. Assessing some determinant effects of ethical consulting behavior: The case of personal and professional values. *J. Bus. Ethics* **1993**, *12*, 449–458. [CrossRef]
8. Poulfelt, F. Ethics for management consultants. *Bus. Ethics Eur. Rev.* **1997**, *6*, 65–70. [CrossRef]
9. Redekop, B.W.; Heath, B.L. A brief examination of the nature, contexts, and causes of unethical consultant behaviors. *J. Pract. Consult.* **2007**, *1*, 40–50.
10. Krehmeyer, D.; Freeman, R.E. Consulting and ethics. In *The Oxford Handbook of Management Consulting*; Clark, T., Kipping, M., Eds.; Oxford University Press: Oxford, UK, 2012; pp. 487–498.
11. O'Mahoney, J. Advisory anxieties: Ethical individualisation in the UK consulting industry. *J. Bus. Ethics* **2011**, *104*, 101–113. [CrossRef]
12. Baran, B.E.; Rogelberg, S.; Carello Lopina, E.; Allen, J.A.; Spitzmüller, C.; Bergman, M. Shouldering a silent burden: The toll of dirty tasks. *Hum. Relat.* **2012**, *65*, 597–626. [CrossRef]

13. Michel, A. Transcending socialization: A nine-year ethnography of the body's role in organizational control and knowledge workers' transformation. *Admin. Sci. Q.* **2011**, *56*, 325–368. [CrossRef]
14. Fortney, S.S. I don't have time to be ethical: Addressing the effects of billable hour pressure. *Idaho Law Rev.* **2003**, *39*, 305–319.
15. Schiltz, P.J. On being a happy, healthy, and ethical member of an unhappy, unhealthy, and unethical profession. *Vanderbilt Law Rev.* **1999**, *52*, 871–951.
16. Meriläinen, S.; Tienari, J.; Thomas, R.; Davies, A. Management consultant talk: A cross-cultural comparison of normalizing discourse and resistance. *Organization* **2004**, *11*, 539–564. [CrossRef]
17. Mühlhaus, J.; Bouwmeester, O. The paradoxical effect of self-categorization on work stress in a high-status occupation: Insights from management consulting. *Hum. Relat.* **2016**, *69*, 1823–1852. [CrossRef]
18. Noury, L.; Gand, S.; Sardas, J.-C. Tackling the work-life balance challenge in professional service firms: The impact of projects, organizing, and service characteristics. *J. Prof. Organ.* **2017**, *4*, 149–178. [CrossRef]
19. O'Mahoney, J. Disrupting identity: Trust and angst in management consulting. In *Searching for the h in Human Resource Management: Theory, Practice and Workplace Contexts*; Bolton, S.C., Houlihan, M., Eds.; Palgrave Macmillan: Bastingstoke, UK, 2007; pp. 281–302.
20. Vahl, R. Hard werken en gezond leven. *Gezond Ondernemen* **2013**, *6*, 6–11.
21. Stein, F. *Work, Sleep, Repeat: The Abstract Labour of German Management Consultants*; Bloomsbury Academic: London, UK, 2017.
22. Goffman, E. *Stigma: Notes on the Management of Spoiled Identity*; Penquin: London, UK, 1963.
23. Hughes, E.C. *Men and Their Work*; Free Press: Glencoe, UK, 1958.
24. Ashforth, B.E.; Kreiner, G.E.; Clark, M.A.; Fugate, M. Normalizing dirty work: Managerial tactics for countering occupational taint. *Acad. Manag. J.* **2007**, *50*, 149–174. [CrossRef]
25. Luyendijk, J. *Swimming with Sharks: My Journey into the World of the Bankers*; Guardian Faber Publishing: London, UK, 2015.
26. Ashforth, B.E.; Kreiner, G.E. "How can you do it?": Dirty work and the challenge of constructing a positive identity. *Acad. Manag. Rev.* **1999**, *24*, 413–434.
27. Bandura, A.; Barbaranelli, C.; Caprara, G.V.; Pastorelli, C. Mechanisms of moral disengagement in the exercise of moral agency. *J. Personal. Soc. Psychol.* **1996**, *71*, 364–374. [CrossRef]
28. Rhode, D. Where is the leadership in moral leadership? In *Moral Leadership: The Theory and Practice of Power, Judgment and Policy*; John Wiley & Sons: San Fransisco, CA, USA, 2006; pp. 1–53.
29. Schminke, M.; Ambrose, M.L.; Neubaum, D.O. The effect of leader moral development on ethical climate and employee attitudes. *Organ. Behav. Hum. Decis. Process.* **2005**, *97*, 135–151. [CrossRef]
30. Zhu, W.; May, D.R.; Avolio, B.J. The impact of ethical leadership behavior on employee outcomes: The roles of psychological empowerment and authenticity. *J. Leadersh. Organ. Stud.* **2004**, *11*, 16–26.
31. Ashforth, B.E.; Kreiner, G.E. Dirty work and dirtier work: Differences in countering physical, social, and moral stigma. *Manag. Organ. Rev.* **2014**, *10*, 81–108. [CrossRef]
32. Bergman, M.E.; Chalkley, K.M. "Ex" marks a spot: The stickiness of dirty work and other removed stigmas. *J. Occup. Health Psychol.* **2007**, *12*, 251–265. [CrossRef] [PubMed]
33. Tracy, S.J.; Scott, C. Sexuality, masculinity, and taint management among firefighters and correctional officers getting down and dirty with "America's heroes" and the "scum of law enforcement". *Manag. Commun. Q.* **2006**, *20*, 6–38. [CrossRef]
34. Tyler, M. Tainted love: From dirty work to abject labour in Soho's sex shops. *Hum. Relat.* **2011**, *64*, 1477–1500. [CrossRef]
35. Ashforth, B.E.; Kreiner, G.E.; Clark, M.A.; Fugate, M. Congruence work in stigmatized occupations: A managerial lens on employee fit with dirty work. *J. Organ. Behav.* **2017**, *38*, 1260–1279. [CrossRef]
36. Pignata, S.; Winefield, A.H.; Boyd, C.M.; Provis, C. A qualitative study of hr/ohs stress interventions in Australian universities. *Int. J. Environ. Res. Public Health* **2018**, *15*, 103. [CrossRef] [PubMed]
37. O'Donnell, J.; Weitz, T.A.; Freedman, L.R. Resistance and vulnerability to stigmatization in abortion work. *Soc. Sci. Med.* **2011**, *73*, 1357–1364. [CrossRef] [PubMed]
38. Hamilton, P.; Redman, T.; McMurray, R. 'Lower than a snake's belly': Discursive constructions of dignity and heroism in low-status garbage work. *J. Bus. Ethics* **2017**, 1–13. [CrossRef]
39. Grandy, G.; Mavin, S. Sinners and Saints: Morally Stigmatized Work. In *Stigmas, Work and Organizations*; Thomson, S.B., Grandy, G., Eds.; Palgrave MacMillan: New York, NY, USA, 2018; pp. 101–121.

40. Kreiner, G.E.; Ashforth, B.E.; Sluss, D.M. Identity dynamics in occupational dirty work: Integrating social identity and system justification perspectives. *Organ. Sci.* **2006**, *17*, 619–636. [CrossRef]
41. Folkman, S.; Lazarus, R.S.; Dunkel-Schetter, C.; DeLongis, A.; Gruen, R.J. Dynamics of a stressful encounter: Cognitive appraisal, coping, and encounter outcomes. *J. Personal. Soc. Psychol.* **1986**, *50*, 992–1003. [CrossRef]
42. Hobfoll, S.E. Conservation of resources: A new attempt at conceptualizing stress. *Am. Psychol.* **1989**, *44*, 513–524. [CrossRef] [PubMed]
43. Roca, E. The exercise of moral imagination in stigmatized work groups. *J. Bus. Ethics* **2010**, *96*, 135–147. [CrossRef]
44. Gill, M.J. Elite identity and status anxiety: An interpretative phenomenological analysis of management consultants. *Organization* **2013**, *22*, 306–325. [CrossRef]
45. Howard, W.C. Leadership: Four styles. *Education* **2005**, *126*, 384–391.
46. Stone, A.G.; Russell, R.F.; Patterson, K. Transformational versus servant leadership: A difference in leader focus. *Leadersh. Organ. Dev. J.* **2004**, *25*, 349–361. [CrossRef]
47. Mendonca, M. Preparing for ethical leadership in organizations. *Can. J. Admin. Sci./Revue Canadienne des Sciences de l'Administration* **2001**, *18*, 266–276. [CrossRef]
48. Aronson, E. Integrating leadership styles and ethical perspectives. *Can. J. Admin. Sci./Revue Canadienne des Sciences de l'Administration* **2001**, *18*, 244–256. [CrossRef]
49. Gini, A. Moral leadership and business ethics. In *Ethics, the Heart of Leadership*; Ciulla, J.B., Ed.; Praeger Publishers: London, UK, 2004; pp. 25–81.
50. Rushton, C.H. Defining and addressing moral distress: Tools for critical care nursing leaders. *AACN Adv. Crit. Care* **2006**, *17*, 161–168. [CrossRef] [PubMed]
51. Brown, M.E.; Treviño, L.K.; Harrison, D.A. Ethical leadership: A social learning perspective for construct development and testing. *Organ. Behav. Hum. Decis. Process.* **2005**, *97*, 117–134. [CrossRef]
52. Covey, S.R. *The 8th Habit: From Effectiveness to Greatness*; Free Press: New York, NY, USA, 2004.
53. Kazi, A.; Haslam, C. Stress management standards: A warning indicator for employee health. *Occup. Med.* **2013**, *63*, 335–340. [CrossRef] [PubMed]
54. Kärreman, D.; Alvesson, M. Cages in tandem: Management control, social identity, and identification in a knowledge-intensive firm. *Organization* **2004**, *11*, 149–175. [CrossRef]
55. Alvesson, M.; Robertson, M. The best and the brightest: The construction, significance and effects of elite identities in consulting firms. *Organization* **2006**, *13*, 195–224. [CrossRef]
56. Morrell, K.; Simonetto, M. Managing retention at deloitte consulting. *Consult. Manag.* **1999**, *10*, 55.
57. Skagert, K.; Dellve, L.; Eklöf, M.; Pousette, A.; Ahlborg, G. Leaders' strategies for dealing with own and their subordinates' stress in public human service organisations. *Appl. Ergon.* **2008**, *39*, 803–811. [CrossRef] [PubMed]
58. Kihn, M. *House of Lies: How Management Consultants Steel Your Watch and Then Tell You the Time*; Business Plus: New York, NY, USA, 2012.
59. Ashford, M. *Con Tricks: The Shadowy World of Management Consultancy and How to Make It Work for You*; Simon & Schuster: London, UK, 1998.
60. Pinault, L. *Consulting Demons: Inside the Unscrupulous World of Global Corporate Consulting*; Wiley: Chichester, UK, 2000.
61. Creswell, J.W. *Qualitative Inquiry & Research Design*; Sage: Thousands Oaks, CA, USA, 2007.
62. Alvesson, M. Beyond neopositivists, romantics, and localists: A reflexive approach to interviews in organizational research. *Acad. Manag. Rev.* **2003**, *28*, 13–33. [CrossRef]
63. Edmondson, A.C.; McManus, S.E. Methodological fit in management field research. *Acad. Manag. Rev.* **2007**, *32*, 1246–1264. [CrossRef]
64. Gioia, D.A.; Corley, K.G.; Hamilton, A.L. Seeking qualitative rigor in inductive research notes on the Gioia methodology. *Organ. Res. Methods* **2013**, *16*, 15–31. [CrossRef]
65. Larry, A.; Moore, M. Deontological ethics. In *The Stanford Encyclopedia of Philosophy*; Zalta, E.N., Ed.; Metaphysics Research Lab, Stanford University: Stanford, CA, USA, 2016.
66. Sinnott-Armstrong, W. Consequentialism. In *The Stanford Encyclopedia of Philosophy*; Zalta, E.N., Ed.; Metaphysics Research Lab, Stanford University: Stanford, CA, USA, 2015.
67. Rijksoverheid. Werktijden. Available online: https://www.rijksoverheid.nl/onderwerpen/werktijden/vraag-en-antwoord/wat-is-er-wettelijk-geregeld-voor-mijn-werktijden (accessed on 13 June 2017).

68. Espeland, K.E. Overcoming burnout: How to revitalize your career. *J. Contin. Educ. Nurs.* **2006**, *37*, 178–184. [CrossRef] [PubMed]
69. Robertson, M.; Swan, J. Modes of organizing in an expert consultancy: A case study of knowledge, power and egos. *Organization* **1998**, *5*, 543–564. [CrossRef]

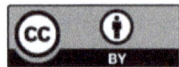

© 2018 by the authors. Licensee MDPI, Basel, Switzerland. This article is an open access article distributed under the terms and conditions of the Creative Commons Attribution (CC BY) license (http://creativecommons.org/licenses/by/4.0/).

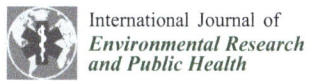

Article

Four Wellbeing Patterns and their Antecedents in Millennials at Work

Tariku Ayana Abdi [1], José M. Peiró [2], Yarid Ayala [3,*] and Salvatore Zappalà [4,5]

1. Department of Psychology, University of Campania, 8100 Caserta, Italy; tarikuayana.abdi@unicampania.it
2. IVIE & IDOCAL, University of Valencia, 46010 Valencia, Spain; jose.m.peiro@uv.es
3. Department of Economics and Management, Pontificia Universidad Javeriana, 110111 Bogotá, Colombia
4. Department of Psychology, University of Bologna, 40126 Bologna, Italy; salvatore.zappala@unibo.it
5. Department of Human Resource Management and Psychology, Financial University under the Government of the Russian Federation, 125993 Moscow, Russia
* Correspondence: ayala.christianyarid@javeriana.edu.co; Tel.: +57-350-347-9920

Received: 15 November 2018; Accepted: 18 December 2018; Published: 22 December 2018

Abstract: Literature suggests that job satisfaction and health are related to each other in a synergic way. However, this might not always be the case, and they may present misaligned relationships. Considering job satisfaction and mental health as indicators of wellbeing at work, we aim to identify four patterns (i.e., satisfied-healthy, unsatisfied-unhealthy, satisfied-unhealthy, and unsatisfied-healthy) and some of their antecedents. In a sample of 783 young Spanish employees, a two-step cluster analysis procedure showed that the unsatisfied-unhealthy pattern was the most frequent (33%), followed by unsatisfied-healthy (26.6%), satisfied-unhealthy (24.8%) and, finally, the satisfied-healthy pattern (14.3%). Moreover, as hypothesized, discriminant analysis suggests that higher levels of job importance and lower levels of role ambiguity mainly differentiate the satisfied-healthy pattern, whereas overqualification and role overload differentiate, respectively, the unsatisfied-healthy and satisfied-unhealthy patterns. Contrary to our expectations, role conflict also characterizes the satisfied-unhealthy pattern. We discuss the practical and theoretical implications of these findings.

Keywords: health; job satisfaction; wellbeing; wellbeing misalignment; Millennials

1. Introduction

Employee wellbeing is a multidimensional construct covering various facets and experiences, and it has no single definition [1–3]. However, probably the most influential narrative on wellbeing and health in the workplace is the seminal review by Danna and Griffin [4]. After a thorough synthesis of the literature, these authors propose a theoretical framework to organize and direct future theory, research, and practice focused on wellbeing and health in the workplace. In their model, wellbeing is proposed as the broader, encompassing construct that includes two main elements of the organizational research arena. First, the model suggests including both generalized job-related experiences (e.g., job satisfaction) and more facet-specific dimensions (satisfaction with co-workers). Second, the model also suggests including general health as a sub-component of wellbeing, including mental (e.g., anxiety) or physical indicators (e.g., blood pressure). Based on this model, we study wellbeing at work by focusing on job satisfaction and mental health as main indicators of employees' wellbeing.

Ceteris paribus, researchers often assume that job satisfaction and mental health are associated with each other in a harmonious way, and this assumption is solidly based on previous meta-analytical evidence. For instance, a meta-analysis of 22 studies of over 4000 workers in Hong Kong [5] and another meta-analysis of 485 studies of over 250,000 individuals [6] show that employees with high job satisfaction also show high levels of mental health. Thus, there is strong evidence that these two indicators of wellbeing may have a harmonious association in which high job satisfaction is correlated with high mental health [5,6], and the opposite may be true, that is, low job satisfaction would be associated with low mental health [6]. However, in this study we consider cases where job satisfaction and mental health are associated in misaligned ways; i.e., high job satisfaction could be associated with low mental health, and vice-versa. We first provide some examples of previous research describing these paradoxical patterns, and then we propose and clarify the aim of this study.

The first misaligned wellbeing pattern is characterized by high levels of job satisfaction and low mental health. For instance, an employee may be satisfied with his/her contribution to a new program launch and, at the same time, stressed because the program unfolds more slowly than expected [7]. Another example of this type of misalignment is an employee who occupies a high-level job position who, although enjoying greater job satisfaction, might also experience low mental health in the form of high levels of job-related anxiety [8]. This type of wellbeing misalignment may also be present when high performing employees with higher-than-average salaries have high job satisfaction but also higher levels of job-demands, leading to emotional exhaustion and low mental health [2].

The second misaligned wellbeing pattern is characterized by low levels of job satisfaction and high mental health. A situation illustrating this second scenario might be the case of overqualification. Researchers have shown that overqualified employees, although reporting low levels of job satisfaction in terms of payment, growth, and promotion opportunities or incentives, also report high levels of life satisfaction, which is an indicator of mental health [9–11]. As such, this is a counterintuitive situation and contrasts with the concept of wellbeing spillover, which suggests that the work-domain and family-domain have similar effects on each other [12], and that low levels of job satisfaction should be related to low levels of life satisfaction or mental health.

Together, these two misaligned wellbeing patterns challenge the concept of wellbeing spillover. At the same time, they also challenge the idea that wellbeing at work should be more responsive to conditions and activities in the work-domain, and that context-free wellbeing should be more responsive to health or family-domains [13]. Paradoxically, what these misaligned wellbeing patterns suggest is that specific conditions, activities, or situations at work may simultaneously and independently impact several work-domain (e.g., job satisfaction) or context-free (e.g., mental health) aspects of wellbeing.

Therefore, the main aim of this study is to make a theoretical contribution to the understanding of misaligned wellbeing patterns. To accomplish this research aim, we propose two specific research objectives. The first objective involves the empirical identification of four wellbeing patterns. We argue that we can identify the four just mentioned wellbeing patterns by combining job satisfaction and mental health; they are: the satisfied-healthy pattern (both job satisfaction and mental health are optimized); the unsatisfied-unhealthy pattern (neither job satisfaction nor mental health are optimized); the satisfied-unhealthy pattern (job satisfaction is optimized, but not mental health); and the unsatisfied-healthy pattern (job satisfaction is not optimized, but mental health is). The second specific research objective involves identifying organizational and personal antecedents that characterize and differentiate each of the four patterns. Based on the model of health and wellbeing in the workplace, proposed by Danna and Griffin [4], we consider organizational stress (in terms of role stress and overqualification) and personal factors (in terms of job importance) as possible antecedents of the four wellbeing patterns. In Table A1, we list the constructs definitions and their relationship with employees' wellbeing. In the following, we argue on the role they may have on the mis/aligned wellbeing patterns.

1.1. Role Stress

Job-related role stress has been a topic of concern across multiple disciplines [14]. Role stress can involve role conflict, role ambiguity, and role overload. Here, we briefly introduce how these components are related to job satisfaction and mental health at work.

Role conflict occurs when an employee receives contradictory or incompatible requests from different parties, or when an employee needs to produce results in different contradictory aspects. Role ambiguity occurs when employees may not have clear information about tasks required by their roles, which makes them feel uncertain about what actions to take. In today's workplace context, role conflict and role ambiguity are salient characteristics in organizational settings. For instance, in complex organizational environments (e.g., digitalization, job redesign, multicultural works), employees are constantly required to fulfill multiple expectations and organizational roles that are ambiguous and/or contradict each other [15–17]. Meta-analytic evidence shows that conflicting and ambiguous roles correlate with low job satisfaction and low health [18], corroborating the role theory, which states that role conflict and role ambiguity will lead to job dissatisfaction and anxiety [19]. However, the strength of the effects of role ambiguity and role conflict on job satisfaction and mental health, although significant, may not be same. Miles [20] indicated that role ambiguity has stronger effects than role conflict on job satisfaction and mental health. Consistent with this finding, we argue that the stronger effect of role ambiguity, compared to role conflict, on the unsatisfied-unhealthy pattern is still pending confirmation. However, we do know that both role ambiguity and role conflict are significantly and negatively related to job satisfaction and mental health.

Role overload occurs when employees have too much work to do within a limited time or with limited resources, which increases the demands they must deal with. Role expansion theory states that multiple roles are beneficial for the individual because the positive effects of strong engagement in both paid work and family life outweigh the possible stressful effects on wellbeing [21]. Thus, engaging in various roles (role overload), although depleting mental health, might have positive outcomes for employee job satisfaction in terms of earning extra income, privilege, and status security [21,22], which would be related to the satisfied-unhealthy wellbeing pattern. However, further research is needed to empirically confirm whether role overload is positively related to job satisfaction, but negatively related to mental health wellbeing.

1.1.1. Job Importance

Some scholars have shown that job importance, as an antecedent of employee wellbeing patterns, is associated with high job satisfaction and life satisfaction [23]. Being satisfied with life may also be related to positive mental health [10], which may predict the satisfied-healthy wellbeing pattern. More specifically, studies have shown that jobs that provide employees with job facets that are important to them can enhance their job satisfaction and decrease stress [24]. Therefore, we argue that jobs that provide employees with intrinsic, extrinsic, and social job importance facets enhance job satisfaction and mental health. Accordingly, based on role theory and empirical evidence on job importance, we hypothesize that:

H1: *Role conflict, role ambiguity, and job importance will mainly differentiate between the unsatisfied-unhealthy and the satisfied-healthy patterns.*

H2: *High role overload will characterize employees with the satisfied-unhealthy wellbeing pattern.*

1.1.2. Overqualification

Nowadays, overqualification is ubiquitous across European job markets, especially in Italy and Spain, and even more so among younger employees [25–27]. Beyond its ubiquity, overqualification raises concerns due to its negative effects on job satisfaction. For instance, studies conducted on young Spanish and Italian employees show that overqualified employees have lower job satisfaction [9,26,28].

Some scholars explain the negative effect of overqualification on job satisfaction based on equity theory. According to equity theory, employees compare the resources they put into work (such as level of education, skills, knowledge, experience) to what they receive in return (e.g., payment, recognition, or responsibility), in order to determine their sense of fairness [9]. When they perceive that their input is greater than what they receive, they develop a sense of unfairness, and as a result, they experience dissatisfaction with their job. However, some studies have shown that, although overqualification has a negative relationship with job satisfaction, at the same time, it has a null or positive indirect relationship with mental health [10,26]. Therefore, we argue that overqualification might negatively affect employees' job satisfaction, but not necessarily their mental health. Furthermore, a study in German firms on the effects of overeducation on productivity, comparing employees working in jobs with similar levels of requirements, observed that overqualified employees are found to be healthier and strongly work- and career-minded [29]. Therefore, we also hypothesize that:

H3: *Overqualification will mainly discriminate employees with the unsatisfied-healthy pattern from the rest of the patterns.*

We test our hypotheses in a sample composed of young employees born between 1980 and 2000, typically called Millennials [30]. Knowledge about individual key outcomes such as wellbeing and health in young employees is still limited and deserves the attention of researchers and practitioners [31]. At the same time, there are approximately 1.8 billion millennials around the world. In 2018, they represent nearly 50% of the global workforce [32]. Therefore, improving outcomes for youth is fundamental to building more inclusive and sustainable societies [33], and one way to this is by promoting full and productive employment and decent work for all [...] including young people [...], which is part of the global agenda of the Sustainable Development Goals [34]. Figure 1 summarizes the four wellbeing patterns resulting from job satisfaction and mental health and the five antecedents we are considering.

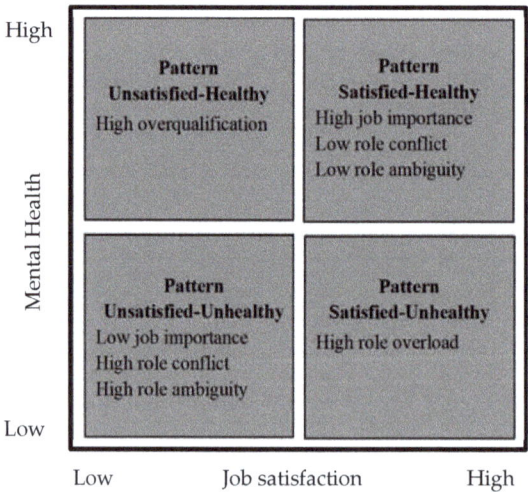

Figure 1. Research Model.

2. Materials and Methods

2.1. Study Design and Procedure

Data were collected from a survey on the transition of young employees to the labor market, which is part of the Valencian Institute of Economic Research (IVIE in Spanish). The survey was designed to facilitate the socioeconomic and psychosocial analysis of young employees' transition to the labor market. Participants between 16 and 30 years old who had been looking for or had found a job in the past 5 years were randomly selected for this study and then contacted by telephone. After two attempted contacts, the researchers replaced non-respondents with a randomly chosen substitute of the same age and gender. Considering the aims of this study, we focused only on respondents who were currently employed. Employees contacted by telephone were always informed of the purpose of the study and assured of the confidentiality of the data. Those who gave their consent to take part in the research were interviewed in their homes using a structured face-to-face procedure.

2.2. Participants

In all, 783 young Spanish respondents were selected for this study. This sample is representative of all the regions in Spain. As mentioned above, the ages of the participants ranged from 16 to 30 years old (M_{age} = 25.21, SD = 3.40), with slightly more females (52%). Most of the participants worked in the private sector (82%), and most of them had a temporary contract (58%).

2.3. Variables/Instruments

Job satisfaction was assessed as the composite of extrinsic, intrinsic, and social job satisfaction [35]. This measure can be applied to a wide range of jobs. Extrinsic job satisfaction was measured with seven items. A sample item is: "Indicate your level of satisfaction with your schedule". Intrinsic job satisfaction was measured with seven items. A sample item is: "Indicate your level of satisfaction with the variety of tasks to perform". Finally, social job satisfaction was measured with five items. A sample item is: "Indicate your level of satisfaction with your coworkers". All items were scored on a 5-point Likert scale (from 1 = *not at all* to 5 = *very much*). The three subscales had good reliability, α = 0.86 (extrinsic job satisfaction), α = 0.91 (intrinsic job satisfaction), α = 0.80 (social job satisfaction), and α = 0.94 (for the composite of the three subscales).

Items measuring health belong to the scale of the General Health Questionnaire, developed by Banks [36] in young community sample. The reliability of the 12 items reported by Banks [36] was α = 0.76. In the current study, we applied four items with higher factor loadings to measure employees' health. A sample item is: "In the last few weeks I have noticed being constantly overwhelmed and under stress". The respondents answered on a 5-point Likert scale (from 1 = *strongly disagree* to 5 = *strongly agree*). The scale showed good reliability (α = 0.76).

Job importance was assessed as the composite of extrinsic, intrinsic, and social job importance [37]. We chose 19 items to measure job importance provided by England and Harpaz [37]. Items were preceded by the phrase "Please, indicate the importance that each of the following aspects of the work has for you"; sample items for each facet are: "Security at work"; "Useful work for society"; "Meaningful work that makes sense to do." The respondents answered on a 5-point Likert scale (from 1 = *nothing* to 5 = *a lot*). The scale showed good reliability (α = 0.89).

Role ambiguity was measured with the scale provided by Rizzo et al. [19]. The original reliabilities, reported by Rizzo and colleagues in two different samples were good (α = 0.82). In the current study, we selected three items with higher factor loadings to measure role ambiguity. A sample item is: "I know how and what my responsibilities and competencies are at work". The respondents answered on a 5-point Likert scale (from 1 = *strongly disagree* to 5 = *strongly agree*). We performed reverse-scoring of the three items. This scale showed good reliability (α = 0.80).

Role conflict was measured with the scale provided by Rizzo et al. [19]. The original reliabilities in two different samples were α = 0.82. In this study, we selected three items with higher factor loadings to measure role conflict. A sample item is: "I receive incompatible requests from two or more people". The respondents answered on a 5-point Likert scale (from 1 = *strongly disagree*, to 5 = *strongly agree*). This scale also showed a good reliability (α = 0.75).

Role overload was measured with the scale of perceived work overload, proposed by Cooke and Rousseau [38]. In the current study, we selected three items with higher factor loadings. A sample item is: "I have too much work to do everything well". The respondents answered on a 5-point Likert scale (from 1 = *strongly disagree* to 5 = *strongly agree*). This scale showed a good reliability score in this study (α = 0.82).

Overqualification was measured with the item: "If an individual had to perform your job, what level of education would you recommend him or her to have?" Participants responded on a 12-point scale of the International Standard Classification of Education—ISCED ((from 1 = no studies (ISCED level 1) to Doctorate (ISCED level 12)). We also considered the individual level of education and transformed both the recommended level of education and the individual level of education into years of education. To determine whether an employee was overqualified, the recommended level of education was subtracted from the level of education achieved. Negative and zero scores were considered indicators of education under-qualification and match, respectively, and positive scores were considered indicators of overqualification [25]. In our study, 21.7% of the participants were overqualified, which is similar to the rate (21.5%) of overqualification across Europe [25].

To eliminate some alternative explanations, we considered some variables that could affect our outcome variables and therefore we controlled for gender (0 = male, 1 = female), type of sector (0 = private, 1 = public), type of employment/contract (0 = temporal, 1 = permanent), and age (in years). We describe in detail the choices and procedures related to the control variables in order to ensure transparency and facilitate the reproducibility of the results [39].

In terms of gender, previous studies show that relatively to men, women tend to report higher levels of depression, but that the positive relationship between the efforts to fulfill work role demands (which interfere with employee's ability to fulfill family demands) and depression is stronger among men [40]. In terms of type of sector and age, previous studies also show that public organizations are good in fulfilling their promises to young employees i.e., their psychological contract, and that this is translated into improved job satisfaction [41]. Considering the type of contract, previous studies also suggest that permanents as compared with temporaries engage more in relational psychological contracting, therefore, when this is violated (e.g., by producing job insecurity), this compromises more the job satisfaction for permanents than for temporaries [42]. Finally, previous research [43] also shows that temporary employees report higher wellbeing (e.g., mental health).

2.4. Data Analysis

To identify the four wellbeing patterns, we performed cluster analyses. One of the advantages of using cluster analysis is that unlike other methods that emphasize the relationship among variables, clustering involves sorting cases or variables according to their similarity in one or more dimensions and producing groups that maximize within-group similarity and minimize between-group similarity [44]. Therefore, to identify the four groups of wellbeing patterns, the 783 employees were clustered based on their individual levels of job satisfaction and mental health, applying a two-step cluster analysis procedure. Loglikelihood measured the distance between job satisfaction and mental health. The clustering criterion was Schwarz's Bayesian Criterion (BIC). Finally, to balance the distribution of responses on the job satisfaction and mental health variables, we standardized these two variables to Z-scores ($M = 0$, $SD = 1$) before performing the cluster analyses.

To test our hypotheses, we employed discriminant analysis to test the unique differentiating role of stress (role ambiguity, role conflict, and role overload), job importance, and overqualification across the four patterns. We conducted a stepwise solution to remove variables that did not make a unique contribution to the predictive and discriminatory function at a probability of 0.05 or less. The stepwise criterion was minimization of Wilks' lambda. Similar studies analyzing wellbeing profiles [45] applied discriminant analysis considering Wilks' lambda stepwise minimization criteria, as we did in the current study. Discriminant analysis is a method used in a multi-group setting to find out if a set of independent variables (nominal and/or continuous) are related to group membership and how they are combined to better understand group differences [46]. In fact, various authors suggest the use of cluster analysis in combination with discriminant analysis for further validation of clusters [47].

3. Results

3.1. Descriptive and Preliminary Analyses

We present the summary of descriptive statistics and bivariate correlations for all the variables included in this research in Table 1. Considering preliminary analyses, missing data, which can occur due to nonresponse to some questions, are a common problem in organizational research [48]. Fichman and Cummings [48] argue that improper treatment of missing data (e.g., listwise deletion, mean imputation) could lead to biased statistical inference using complete case analysis statistical techniques. However, given that we have a reasonably large sample size ($n = 783$), and considering that the percentage of missing data was rather small (less than 1%), we concluded that the missing data had no effect on the results of our study [46].

3.2. Cluster Analysis

With five cases identified as outliers and six cases registered as missing from the system, the two-step cluster analysis efficiently and automatically formed four clusters. Following the recommendations of Aguinis, Gottfredson, and Joo [49] about the best practices for defining, identifying, and handling outliers, we defined them as cluster analysis outliers. We handled them by performing the rest of the analyses (e.g., discriminant) with and without them. We found that they were non-influential outliers because they did not significantly change the rest of our results. Figure 2 depicts the centroids (means) of each cluster, expressed in standardized scores of job satisfaction and mental health measures. The silhouette coefficient (which was approximately 0.5) suggested that a four-cluster solution had fair levels of cohesion and separation. We named the four clusters, considering the centroids of job satisfaction and mental health. Cluster 1 was called unsatisfied-unhealthy and comprised 33% of the sample (258 employees), showing the lowest means on job satisfaction (−0.62) and mental health (−0.97). Cluster 2 was called unsatisfied-healthy and comprised 26.6% of the sample (208 employees), showing low levels of job satisfaction standardized means (−0.56), but high levels of mental health (0.76). Cluster 3 was called satisfied-unhealthy and comprised 24.8% of the sample (194 employees), in this case showing high levels of job satisfaction (0.83), but low levels of mental health (−0.15). Finally, Cluster 4 was called satisfied-healthy and comprised only 14.3% of the sample (112 employees), showing the highest levels of both job satisfaction (1.11) and mental health (1.24). To test whether the clusters were significantly different from one another, we conducted an analysis of variance (ANOVA). The results suggested that there were significant differences in job satisfaction ($F_{(4, 772)} = 276.41$, $p < 0.01$) and health ($F_{(4, 772)} = 477.93$, $p < 0.01$) among the four patterns. Tukey post-hoc analyses also suggested that all the clusters were significantly different from each other. Together, these results reflect different patterns of the relations between job satisfaction and mental health.

3.3. Discriminant Analysis

We present the summary of the results of the discriminant analysis in Table 2. The results show that employees with the unsatisfied–unhealthy pattern (Cluster 1) have systematically higher means on role ambiguity and lower means on job importance, compared to employees with the satisfied-healthy wellbeing pattern (Cluster 4) and the rest of the patterns. Therefore, we partially confirmed hypothesis 1. Thus, role ambiguity and job importance strongly differentiated between the unsatisfied-unhealthy and satisfied-healthy patterns, but we failed to confirm role conflict. Contrary to our expectations, role conflict mainly characterized satisfied-unhealthy employees. Discriminant results also show that employees with the satisfied-unhealthy pattern (Cluster 3), systematically had significantly higher means on role overload (and role conflict), compared to employees with the satisfied-healthy pattern (Cluster 4). Therefore, we confirmed hypothesis 2, which stated that role overload characterized employees with the satisfied-unhealthy pattern. Finally, employees with the unsatisfied-healthy pattern (Cluster 2) have significantly higher means on overqualification (in comparison with the rest of the patterns) and lower means on role conflict, compared to the satisfied-unhealthy pattern (Cluster 3). Therefore, we also confirmed our hypothesis 3; thus, employees with the unsatisfied-healthy pattern perceived themselves as more overqualified for the job/position compared to their satisfied-unhealthy counterparts and the rest of the patterns.

Table 1. Bivariate correlations and descriptive statistics of the job satisfaction-mental health pattern predictors.

Variables	M	SD	1	2	3	4	5	6	7	8	9	10	11
1. Age	25.21	3.40	-	-0.02	0.21 **	-0.00	0.02	0.09 *	0.08 *	0.02	0.07	0.12 **	-0.03
2. Gender	0.48	0.50		-	0.11 **	0.06	-0.09 *	0.04	0.08 *	0.07 *	-0.08 *	0.02	0.00
3. Type of contract	0.58	0.50			-	-0.01	-0.05	0.02	0.01	-0.09 *	0.05	0.14 **	0.05
4. Type of sector	0.18	0.38				-	-0.13 **	0.03	0.01	-0.00	0.07 *	0.09 *	-0.04
5. Overqualification	0.22	0.41					-	-0.02	0.09 *	0.04	-0.03	-0.20 **	-0.04
6. Role overload	2.91	0.97						(0.82)	0.37 **	0.07	0.06	0.05	-0.15 **
7. Role conflict	2.78	0.99							(0.75)	0.25 **	-0.06	-0.12 **	-0.29 **
8. Role ambiguity	2.05	0.80								(0.80)	-0.28 **	-0.46 **	-0.25 **
9. Job importance	4.14	0.51									(0.89)	0.50 **	0.16 **
10. Job satisfaction	3.68	0.73										(0.94)	0.26 **
11. Mental health	3.67	0.83											(0.76)

Internal alpha estimates are in parenthesis * $p = 0.05$; ** $p < 0.01$. (two-tailed).

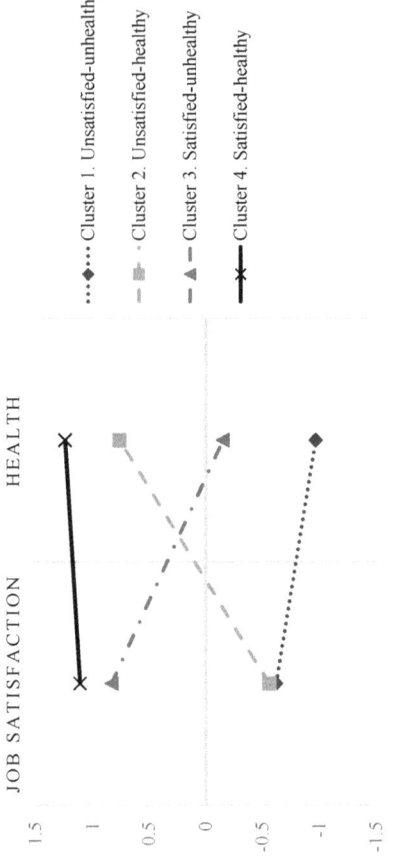

Figure 2. Four-cluster solution: standardized cluster means.

Table 2. Discriminant analysis of the four patterns of relations between job satisfaction and mental health with job importance, role ambiguity, role conflict, role overload, and overqualification as discriminant variables.

Variables/Discriminant Function Statistics	Means (Standard Deviations) of Wellbeing Patterns				Standardized Discriminant Function Coefficients [a]		
	Cluster 1 Unsatisfied-Unhealthy (n = 258)	Cluster 2 Unsatisfied-Healthy (n = 208)	Cluster 3 Satisfied-Unhealthy (n = 194)	Cluster 4 Satisfied-Healthy (n = 112)	Function 1	Function 2	Function 3
Covariates							
Gender [b,c]	0.48 (0.50)	0.44 (0.50)	0.52 (0.50)	0.45 (0.50)	0.10	0.07	−0.03
Sector [c,d]	0.21 (0.41)	0.13 (0.33)	0.17 (0.38)	0.22 (0.42)	−0.07	0.06	−0.04
Type of contract [c,e]	0.54 (0.50)	0.58 (0.50)	0.61 (0.49)	0.64 (0.48)	−0.06	0.08	0.15
Age	24.96 (3.43)	24.99 (3.33)	25.85 (3.31)	24.81 (3.56)	−0.07 (−0.09)	0.21 (0.12)	0.77 (**0.77**)
Discriminant variables							
Job importance	3.96 (0.48)	3.97 (0.50)	4.29 (0.44)	4.52 (0.33)	−0.79 (**−0.73**)	0.25 (0.24)	−0.07 (−0.17)
Role ambiguity	2.33 (0.77)	2.12 (0.78)	1.86 (0.66)	1.51 (0.64)	0.65 (**0.50**)	0.17 (0.03)	−0.12 (−0.13)
Role conflict	3.09 (0.88)	2.53 (0.97)	2.82 (0.93)	2.39 (1.12)	0.29 (0.13)	0.84 (**0.78**)	−0.16 (−**0.43**)
Role overload	3.03 (0.88)	2.77 (0.97)	3.03 (0.93)	2.59 (1.07)	0.14 (0.14)	0.54 (0.23)	0.48 (**0.59**)
Overqualification	0.23 (0.42)	0.30 (0.46)	0.17 (0.38)	0.13 (0.34)	0.19 (0.22)	−0.32 (−**0.41**)	0.15 (0.18)
Significance of function					0.01	0.01	0.05
Canonical correlation					0.50	0.26	0.13
Eigenvalue					0.32	0.07	0.02
Explained variance					79.1%	17.1%	3.9%
Centroid of:							
Cluster 1					0.52	0.20	−0.09
Cluster 2					0.27	−0.39	0.06
Cluster 3					−0.42	−0.22	0.16
Cluster 4					−1.15	−0.13	−0.20

Note: n = 772 after listwise deletion of cases with missing data. [a] In parentheses are the coefficients of a stepwise solution that included only variables entered at the 0.05 significance level (coefficients higher than 0.30 are in boldface). The stepwise criterion was minimization of the overall Wilks' lambda. [b] Gender: Coded 0 = male, 1 = female. [c] The group mean of the dichotomous/dummy variables indicates the proportion of the higher coded category. [d] Sector: Coded 0 = private, 1 = public. [e] Type of Contract: Coded 0 = temporary, 1 = permanent.

Together, the results of the discriminant analyses suggest that job importance, role ambiguity, role conflict, role overload, and overqualification help to differentiate among the four patterns of relations between job satisfaction and mental health. When comparing these variables, job importance and role ambiguity were better at differentiating employees with the unsatisfied-unhealthy pattern from those with the satisfied-healthy pattern. Overqualification and role conflict were better at differentiating between employees with the unsatisfied-healthy and satisfied-unhealthy patterns.

4. Discussion

The main aim of this study was to contribute to the theoretical understanding of misaligned wellbeing patterns by considering the profiles emerging from the combination of different levels of job satisfaction and mental health. To accomplish this aim, we pursued two research objectives. The first was to identify four patterns of employee wellbeing based on a configurational variable that combines job satisfaction and mental health. Second, we examined some antecedents that can discriminate each of the four patterns. The antecedents we considered were role stress (role ambiguity, role conflict, and role overload), job importance, and overqualification.

Results showed that hypothesis 1 was partially confirmed. We confirmed that role ambiguity and job importance strongly differentiate between the unsatisfied-unhealthy and satisfied-healthy patterns and the rest of the patterns. On the one hand, our findings are aligned with previous studies on role ambiguity showing that the strength of relationships between role ambiguity, and job dissatisfaction and tension/anxiety are generally stronger than those for role conflict [20], whereas other studies have also shown that role ambiguity has adverse effects on employee job satisfaction and mental health [18,19,50]. On the other hand, with this hypothesis, we also confirmed that employees who perceive various facets of job importance, such as intrinsic (e.g., learning opportunity), extrinsic (e.g., job security), and social (e.g., societal contribution) facets, have optimal job satisfaction and mental health, compared to employees who have high role ambiguity. This result is consistent with previous studies [24].

Contrary to our expectation that role conflict would differentiate employees with the unsatisfied-unhealthy pattern from those with the satisfied-healthy pattern, our results instead showed that role conflict, along with role overload, characterized employees with the satisfied-unhealthy pattern. This result partly supports our hypothesis 2, confirming that role overload characterizes the satisfied-unhealthy pattern. Thus, role conflict and role overload had negative consequences on mental health, but less on job satisfaction. These results corroborate role expansion theory, which asserts that employees who engage in multiple roles at the same time receive incentives, status security, and position increments, which in turn have a positive effect on job satisfaction [21,22]. Furthermore, this study also confirms that focusing only on negative consequences of role stress is just one side of the issue, as asserted by McGowan et al. [50]. As the Job-Demand Control model indicates, highly demanding jobs can provide high decision latitude, control, and autonomy for employees, which, in turn, may decrease the negative effects of job demands on job satisfaction, although they can still produce negative effects on health [50].

Finally, we confirmed our hypothesis 3. Our argument was that overqualification would characterize employees with the unsatisfied-healthy wellbeing pattern. Results show that employees with higher levels of overqualification were characterized by job dissatisfaction and, at the same time, showed optimal levels of mental health. They may perceive that the salary, incentives, and other resources they receive from their work are not fair, given their qualifications. This argument substantiates equity theory. According to equity theory, employees compare the resources they put into the work (such as level of education, skills, knowledge, experience, etc.) to what they receive in return (such as payment, recognition, responsibility, etc.) in order to determine their sense of fairness [9]. If they perceive unfairness in what they receive, they may be dissatisfied with their job. Previous studies also have shown that overqualified employees have low job satisfaction [9,26] but higher satisfaction with their life and better mental health [6,10].

We also accomplished our first specific research objective, which was to identify these four wellbeing patterns involving job satisfaction and mental health. Surprisingly, the most populated cluster was the unsatisfied-unhealthy pattern, and more than half of our sample had a misaligned pattern i.e., either satisfied-unhealthy or unsatisfied-healthy. Traditionally, job satisfaction and mental health are believed to be harmoniously and positively correlated, with high (or low) job satisfaction positively correlated with high (or low) mental health. However, this might not always be the case. In this research, we focused on a new research paradigm by studying the combinations of different levels of job satisfaction and mental health. By combining different levels of job satisfaction and health, we identified four important wellbeing patterns and their antecedents. We especially focused on the anomalous or misaligned wellbeing patterns (satisfied-unhealthy or unsatisfied-healthy) as new typologies. Therefore, we believe that our research findings may motivate scholars to investigate the wellbeing patterns by using the current model as a framework. Furthermore, future studies could also combine the effects of role ambiguity, role conflict, role overload, job importance, and overqualification to move towards more generalizable empirical findings and theory development.

The results that job satisfaction and mental health together form four wellbeing patterns, indicate the need for theoretical precision; it is in fact important to integrate this complexity into the harmonious relationship between job satisfaction and mental health in order to study a broader taxonomy of relations and the conditions in which these patterns are elicited. For instance, our study questions the model of health and wellbeing in the workplace by Danna and Griffin [4], suggesting that it should be integrated with the four patterns of wellbeing and mental health described here. At the same time, our study questions whether wellbeing spillover always happens. Wellbeing spillover proposes that work and family domains of wellbeing have similar effects on one another [12]; therefore, we would expect low levels of job satisfaction to be related to low levels of mental health. Although our study suggests that this may be the case for the satisfied-healthy and unsatisfied-unhealthy patterns, and their antecedents in terms of role ambiguity and role importance, our results also suggest that this spillover may not always take place because spillover may not be present in the misaligned patterns. The results on their antecedents also suggest that work-related conditions and activities may affect work-domain (e.g., job satisfaction) and context-free (mental health) wellbeing at the same time, which challenges the idea that context-free wellbeing should be more responsive to health or family-domains [13]. We have already described why role conflict, role overload, and overqualification are separately related to the misaligned patterns, but we identified an alternative interaction explanation. For instance, in the introduction of this paper we argued that young employees who are overqualified may not have worse mental health because they may have jobs that do not stress them and that are viewed as stepping-stones to help them achieve higher goals (such as finishing college), all of which lead to the unsatisfied-healthy pattern. Aligned with this idea is that these employees also showed lower levels of job importance, thus confirming previous studies that showed that overqualified employees are more cynical about the meaningfulness of their job [51] and such reduce task importance, or significance, depends on how many other overqualified peers work in the same context [52]. We believe that low levels of importance to one's job may be, for young overqualified employees, a way to reduce the cognitive dissonance between their qualification and skill's usage and this may help in maintaining higher level of mental health. Therefore, future research should study the boundary conditions of the relationship between the antecedents here described (role conflict, role overload, and overqualification) and the misaligned wellbeing patterns.

Future studies might also investigate other potentially relevant antecedents, or moderators, of the mis/alignment between job satisfaction and mental health. In particular, following Danna and Griffin [4] and Nielsen et al. [53], it might be interesting to examine the sector of employment, in particular if it involves hazardous and stressful work settings (requiring for instance, night shifts or traveling), job resources as job autonomy, and also HR practices and social support. Literature has in fact showed that such factors may increase or decrease job satisfaction and wellbeing [4,53], but it should be examined if they differentially affect job satisfaction and mental health, also in relation to the family status of the employees (single, married, with children) and family history of mental health.

Finally, another major point concerns the sample being studied. The sample is composed of so-called millennials, thus, a very specific subgroup. These employees might differ in their general health (both mental and physical), wellbeing, satisfaction, etc., from other employees. As a group, millennials are in between twenties and late thirties, thus they do have a better physical health than older generations. Nevertheless, their lower tolerance to frustrations and their need to deal and face the economic crisis (initiated on 2008), which results in fewer career opportunities, may have as an effect a poorer level of mental health, especially in minor symptoms such as anxiety, life dissatisfaction, etc. Another specific situation of the millennials is that they face the transition from school to work in a situation that is in many cases not favorable. The support from their families, the resignation to have precarious/flexible jobs, to get incomes for subsistence or searching for jobs abroad, are some of the different ways of coping with the complex and difficult situation that millennials are facing during the actual economic crisis period.

5. Limitations and Practical Implications

One of the potential limitations of the current study is related to the sample, which is limited to young Spanish employees. To make better generalizations about the four wellbeing patterns, it is necessary to document their occurrence in other contexts. However, the sample was representative of all the regions of Spain, and the independent variables (role stress, job importance, and overqualification) that we tested in this research might be applicable to millennials in other contexts, which could make the generalization of these research findings more robust. Therefore, this limitation may be at least partially neutralized because the procedures and variables we used are applicable to millennials in other contexts. In addition, to test the external validity of the study, it would be useful to replicate it with millennials in other countries.

Another limitation is related to the measurement of job satisfaction and mental health. In job satisfaction measurement, cognitive/subjective biases may affect employees' evaluations of their satisfaction. Similarly, we assessed mental health by using the General Health Questionnaires (GHQ) in terms of a specific time period: *'during the past few weeks ... '*. However, events occurring "weeks ago" may be poorly recalled, and, therefore, induce some possible inaccuracy in mental processing [3]. However, the measurements of both job satisfaction and mental health are based on well validated and accepted instruments, and so we expect cognitive/personal biases and inaccuracy in mental processing to have little or no impact on the validity of the current research findings.

One of the main aims of organizational psychology is to improve employees' wellbeing. In this regard, our taxonomical approach provides relevant empirical evidence, facilitating the achievement of this endeavor. First, by combining job satisfaction and mental health, this study maps synergistic but also misaligned wellbeing patterns. Second, our study also provides valuable information of some personal and organizational variables related to them. In this way, our study informs organizational psychologists of when they may be improving at the same time job satisfaction and mental health, but also when this might not happen, creating misaligned wellbeing patterns instead. Thus, an important implication of our study is the provision of a useful wellbeing-pattern taxonomy from where to study and improve employees' wellbeing.

We also identify implications for other stakeholders. For instance, our results show that it would be worthwhile for organizations to find mechanisms to track and ensure the fulfillment of their commitments to millennials. Our results show, in fact, that only a small portion of employees are in the optimal job satisfaction and mental health category, whereas larger portions are in the unsatisfied-unhealthy and misaligned patterns. At the same time, organizations should carefully consider HR policies, such as staffing, to establish mechanisms to avoid phenomena such as role ambiguity, role conflict, role overload, and overqualification. These organizational and personal phenomena have been shown to have toxic effects on both job satisfaction and mental health.

Third, the results show that job importance is an important mechanism for a sustainable young workforce. In our study, young employees who reported having high job importance were characterized by being satisfied and healthy. Therefore, we argue that managers and employers should increase job importance by providing incentives related to job satisfaction and mental health. Often the jobs available for youngsters are "poor" overqualified and in some cases precarious. Thus, it is important that the companies enhance the meaning of work for youngsters offering jobs that are valuable and meaningful. This is the type of "incentives" that may make work more meaningful for youth and less toxic, dissatisfying and unhealthy.

6. Conclusions

At the beginning of this paper, we noted that the relationship between job satisfaction and mental health is mainly considered harmonious, and that there is scarce research about the anomalous/misaligned patterns between these two variables. The main aim of this study was to extend the relationship between job satisfaction and mental health by identifying four patterns: satisfied-healthy, satisfied-unhealthy, unsatisfied-healthy, and unsatisfied-unhealthy. This taxonomy seems to provide a valid, interesting, and useful way to study employees' wellbeing by considering their job satisfaction and mental health. It is our hope that addressing this more extended pattern of relationships between the two variables will lead to a possible resolution of the satisfied-healthy conundrum. Thus, the unsatisfied-healthy or satisfied-unhealthy profiles should be the targets of future research. Moreover, this research has contributed to identifying some organizational and personal antecedents that influence and differentiate the four patterns. Future research will need to study how stable or dynamic these patterns are over time, and what their consequences are in the long run. This knowledge will help us to create more effective interventions so that organizations can assist millennials in moving toward a more positive and optimal job satisfaction level and assess its contribution to health and vice-versa.

Author Contributions: T.A.A. performed formal analyses, visualization, and writing–original draft; Y.A. was responsible for the study conception, design, data curation, and writing–review & editing; J.M.P and S.Z. contributed to the conceptualization, project administration, supervision, and writing–review & editing.

Funding: The present study has been prepared with the support of the project PSI2015-64862-R (MINECO/FEDER). It was also supported by the PROGRAM PROMETEO/2016/138 of the GV. The third author has received a pre-doctoral scholarship, CVU 326153, from the National Council on Science and Technology of Mexico (CONACYT).

Acknowledgments: The authors also thank the IVIE for the authorization to use the database from the Spanish Observatory of Youth Labor Market Entry and Employment.

Conflicts of Interest: The authors declare no conflicts of interest.

Appendix A

Table A1. Constructs Definitions and their relationship with employees' wellbeing.

Constructs	Definitions	Relationships with Employees' Wellbeing
Job satisfaction	Job satisfaction is an individual's attitude toward the job, that is, an overall evaluative judgment about one's job that is caused by affective experiences on the job and (cognitive) beliefs about the job [54].	A recent review of quantitative studies show that job satisfaction is the most common conceptualization of employee wellbeing [55]
Mental health	We operationalize the definition of the health sub-dimension of wellbeing proposed by Danna and Griffin [4] in terms of general positive mental health self-reported by employees [36].	Danna and Griffin [4] consider mental health to be a sub-component of wellbeing at work
Role conflict	We define role conflict as parties' contradictory expectations about aspects of a single role or between different roles [15,56].	Studies indicate that when employees are exposed to conflicting and ambiguous roles, they experience job dissatisfaction and low mental health [18,19].
Role ambiguity	We define *role ambiguity* as lack of sufficient information or uncertainty about expectations and actions to fulfill a role/job [15,56]	
Role overload	We define *role overload* as lack of the personal resources that an individual needs to fulfill multiple roles, commitments, obligations, or requirements demanded by the work [15]	Research findings on the impact of role overload on employee job satisfaction and mental health are inconsistent. Some scholars, for instance, show that role overload correlates with low job satisfaction [57] and low mental health (such as experiencing fatigue and tension) [38]. However, in other research, Cooke and Rousseau [38] indicate that role overload does not affect the job satisfaction of employees engaged in multiple roles.
Job importance	Job importance refers to the level of personal significance and value an employee associates with various facets of the job (extrinsic, intrinsic and social) [23,58].	We argue that jobs that provide employees with intrinsic, extrinsic, and social job importance facets enhance job satisfaction and mental health.
Overqualification	We define overqualification as employees' perceptions of having excess education, knowledge, abilities, and skills, compared to the requirements of the job [59]	Scholars indicate that overqualified employees enjoy greater satisfaction with life [28], which correlates with better mental health [10].

References

1. Grant, A.M.; Christianson, M.K.; Price, R.H. Happiness, health, or relationships? managerial practices and employee well-being tradeoffs. *Acad. Manag. Perspect.* **2007**, *21*, 51–63. [CrossRef]
2. Van De Voorde, K.; Boxall, P. Individual well-being and performance at work in the wider context of strategic HRM. In *Well-Being and Performance at Work: The Role of Context*, 95–111; Psychology Press: New York, NY, USA, 2014.
3. Sinclair, R.R.; Wang, M.; Tetrick, L.E. *Research Methods in Occupational Health Psychology: Measurement, Design, and Data Analysis*; Routledge: Abington Thames, UK, 2012.
4. Danna, K.; Griffin, R.W. Health and well-being in the workplace: A review and synthesis of the literature. *J. Manag.* **1999**, *25*, 357–384. [CrossRef]
5. Cass, M.H.; Siu, O.L.; Faragher, E.B.; Cooper, C.L. A meta-analysis of the relationship between job satisfaction and employee health in Hong Kong. *Stress Health* **2003**, *19*, 79–95. [CrossRef]
6. Faragher, E.B.; Cass, M.; Cooper, C.L. The relationship between job satisfaction and health: A meta-analysis. *Occup. Environ. Med.* **2005**, *62*, 105–112. [CrossRef] [PubMed]
7. Fong, C.T. The effects of emotional ambivalence on creativity. *Acad. Manag. J.* **2006**, *49*, 1016–1030. [CrossRef]
8. Warr, P. *Work, Happiness, and Unhappiness*; Psychology Press: New York, NY, USA, 2011.
9. Erdogan, B.; Bauer, T.N.; Peiró, J.; Truxillo, D.M. Overqualified employees: Making the best of a potentially bad situation for individuals and organizations. *Ind. Organ. Psychol.* **2011**, *4*, 215–232. [CrossRef]

10. Headey, B.; Kelley, J.; Wearing, A. Dimensions of mental health: Life satisfaction, positive affect, anxiety and depression. *Soc. Indic. Res.* **1993**, *29*, 63–82. [CrossRef]
11. Johnson, G.J.; Johnson, W.R. Perceived overqualification and dimensions of job satisfaction: A longitudinal analysis. *J. Psychol.* **2000**, *134*, 537–555. [CrossRef]
12. Ilies, R.; Schwind, K.M.; Heller, D. Employee well-being: A multilevel model linking work and nonwork domains. *Eur. J. Work. Organ. Psychol.* **2007**, *16*, 326–341. [CrossRef]
13. Warr, P. How to think about and measure psychological well-being. In *Research Methods in Occupational Health Psychology*; Wang, M., Sinclair, R.R., Tetrick, L.E., Eds.; Psychology Press/Routledge: New York, NY, USA, 2013; Volume 1, pp. 76–91.
14. Babin, B.J.; Boles, J.S. The effects of perceived co-worker involvement and supervisor support on service provider role stress, performance and job satisfaction. *J. Retail.* **1996**, *72*, 57–75. [CrossRef]
15. Peterson, M.F.; Smith, P.B.; Akande, A.; Ayestaran, S.; Bochner, S.; Callan, V.; Francois, P. Role conflict, ambiguity, and overload: A 21-nation study. *Acad. Manag. J.* **1995**, *38*, 429–452.
16. Ashforth, B.E.; Rogers, K.M.; Pratt, M.G.; Pradies, C. Ambivalence in organizations: A multilevel approach. *Organ. Sci.* **2014**, *25*, 1453–1478. [CrossRef]
17. Keller, R.T. Role conflict and ambiguity: Correlates with job satisfaction and values. *Pers. Psychol.* **1975**, *28*, 57–64. [CrossRef]
18. Jackson, S.E.; Schuler, R.S. A meta-analysis and conceptual critique of research on role ambiguity and role conflict in work settings. *Organ. Behav. Hum. Decis. Process.* **1985**, *36*, 16–78. [CrossRef]
19. Rizzo, J.R.; House, R.J.; Lirtzman, S.I. Role conflict and ambiguity in complex organizations. *Adm. Sci. Q.* **1970**, *15*, 150–163. [CrossRef]
20. Miles, R.H. A comparison of the relative impacts of role perceptions of ambiguity and conflict by role. *Acad. Manag. J.* **1976**, *19*, 25–35.
21. Nordenmark, M. Multiple social roles and well-being: A longitudinal test of the role stress theory and the role expansion theory. *Acta Sociol.* **2004**, *47*, 115–126. [CrossRef]
22. Sieber, S.D. Toward a theory of role accumulation. *Am. Sociol. Rev.* **1974**, *39*, 567–578. [CrossRef]
23. Iris, B.; Barrett, G.V. Some relations between job and life satisfaction and job importance. *J. Appl. Psychol.* **1972**, *56*, 301–304. [CrossRef]
24. Thompson, C.A.; Prottas, D.J. Relationships among organizational family support, job autonomy, perceived control, and employee well-being. *J. Occup. Health Psychol.* **2006**, *11*, 100–118. [CrossRef]
25. Agut, S.; Peiró, J.M.; Grau, R. The effect of overeducation on job content innovation and career-enhancing strategies among young Spanish employees. *J. Career Dev.* **2009**, *36*, 159–182. [CrossRef]
26. Di Pietro, G.; Urwin, P. Education and skills mismatch in the Italian graduate labour market. *Appl. Econ.* **2006**, *38*, 79–93. [CrossRef]
27. Pouliakas, K. *Safeguarding Education Investments: Mitigating Overqualification in the EU*; Cedefop: Thessaloniki, Greece, 2015.
28. Peiró, J.M.; Agut, S.; Grau, R. The relationship between overeducation and job satisfaction among young Spanish workers: The role of salary, contract of employment, and work experience. *J. Appl. Soc. Psychol.* **2010**, *40*, 666–689. [CrossRef]
29. Büchel, F. The effects of overeducation on productivity in Germany—The firms' viewpoint. *Econ. Educ. Rev.* **2002**, *21*, 263–275. [CrossRef]
30. De Hauw, S.; De Vos, A. Millennials' career perspective and psychological contract expectations: Does the recession lead to lowered expectations? *J. Bus. Psychol.* **2010**, *2*, 293–302. [CrossRef]
31. Akkermans, J.; Brenninkmeijer, V.; Blonk, R.W.B.; Koppes, L.L.J. Fresh and healthy? Well-being, health and performance of young employees with intermediate education. *Career Dev. Int.* **2009**, *14*, 671–699. [CrossRef]
32. International Labour Organization. *Global Employment Trends for Youth 2013: A Generation at Risk*; International Labour Organization: Geneva, Switzerland, 2013.
33. International Labour Organization (ILO). *World Employment and Social Outlook: Trends 2015*; International Labour Office: Geneva, Switzerland, 2015.
34. Transforming Our World: The 2030 Agenda for Sustainable Development. A/RES/70/1, 70Cong. 2015. Available online: http://research.un.org/en/docs/ga/quick/regular/70 (accessed on 24 October 2018).
35. Warr, P.; Cook, J.; Wall, T. Scales for the measurement of some work attitudes and aspects of psychological well-being. *J. Occup. Organ. Psychol.* **1979**, *52*, 129–148. [CrossRef]

36. Banks, M.H. Validation of the general health questionnaire in a young community sample. *Psychol. Med.* **1983**, *13*, 349–353. [CrossRef]
37. England, G.W.; Harpaz, I. Some methodological and analytic considerations in cross-national comparative research. *J. Int. Bus. Stud.* **1983**, *14*, 49–59. [CrossRef]
38. Cooke, R.A.; Rousseau, D.M. Stress and strain from family roles and work-role expectations. *J. Appl. Psychol.* **1984**, *69*, 252–260. [CrossRef]
39. Bernerth, J.B.; Aguinis, H. A critical review and best-practice recommendations for control variable usage. *Pers. Psychol.* **2016**, *69*, 229–283. [CrossRef]
40. Frone, M.R.; Russell, M.; Barnes, G.M. Work–family conflict, gender, and health-related outcomes: A study of employed parents in two community samples. *J. Occup. Health Psychol.* **1996**, *1*, 57–69. [CrossRef] [PubMed]
41. Ayala, Y.; Silla, J.M.P.; Tordera, N.; Lorente, L.; Yeves, J. Job Satisfaction and Innovative Performance in Young Spanish Employees: Testing New Patterns in the Happy-Productive Worker Thesis—A Discriminant Study. *J. Happiness Stud.* **2017**, *18*, 1377–1401. [CrossRef]
42. Cuyper, N.; Witte, H. The impact of job insecurity and contract type on attitudes, well-being and behavioural reports: A psychological contract perspective. *J. Occup. Organ. Psychol.* **2006**, *79*, 395–409. [CrossRef]
43. Dawson, C.; Veliziotis, M.; Hopkins, B. Temporary employment, job satisfaction and subjective well-being. *Econ. Ind. Democr.* **2017**, *38*, 69–98. [CrossRef]
44. Henry, D.B.; Tolan, P.H.; Gorman-Smith, D. Cluster analysis in family psychology research. *J. Fam. Psychol.* **2005**, *19*, 121–132. [CrossRef] [PubMed]
45. Keyes, C.L.; Shmotkin, D.; Ryff, C.D. Optimizing well-being: The empirical encounter of two traditions. *J. Pers. Soc. Psychol.* **2002**, *82*, 1007–1022. [CrossRef] [PubMed]
46. Raykov, T.; Marcoulides, G.A. *An Introduction to Applied Multivariate Analysis*; Routledge: Abington Thames, UK, 2012.
47. McIntyre, R.M.; Blashfield, R.K. A nearest-centroid technique for evaluating the minimum-variance clustering procedure. *Multivar. Behav. Res.* **1980**, *15*, 225–238. [CrossRef]
48. Fichman, M.; Cummings, J.N. Multiple imputation for missing data: Making the most of what you know. *Organ. Res. Methods* **2003**, *6*, 282–308. [CrossRef]
49. Aguinis, H.; Gottfredson, R.K.; Joo, H. Best-Practice Recommendations for Defining, Identifying, and Handling Outliers. *Organ. Res. Methods* **2013**, *16*, 270–301. [CrossRef]
50. McGowan, J.; Gardner, D.; Fletcher, R. Positive and negative affective outcomes of occupational stress. *N. Z. J. Psychol.* **2006**, *35*, 92–98.
51. Luksyte, A.; Spitzmueller, C.; Maynard, D.C. Why do overqualified incumbents deviate? Examining multiple mediators. *J. Occup. Health Psychol.* **2011**, *16*, 279–296. [CrossRef] [PubMed]
52. Hu, J.; Erdogan, B.; Bauer, T.N.; Jiang, K.; Liu, S.; Li, Y. There are lots of big fish in this pond: The role of peer overqualification on task significance, perceived fit, and performance for overqualified employees. *J. Appl. Psychol.* **2015**, *100*, 1228–1238. [CrossRef] [PubMed]
53. Nielsen, K.; Nielsen, M.B.; Ogbonnaya, C.; Känsälä, M.; Saari, E.; Isaksson, K. Workplace resources to improve both employee well-being and performance: A systematic review and meta-analysis. *Work. Stress* **2017**, *31*, 101–120. [CrossRef]
54. Ziegler, R.; Hagen, B.; Diehl, M. Relationship between job satisfaction and job performance: Job ambivalence as a moderator. *J. Appl. Soc. Psychol.* **2012**, *42*, 2019–2040. [CrossRef]
55. Peiró, J.M. Employees' hedonic and eudemonic well-being and their performance. Do results matter for professional practice? In Proceedings of the 29th International Conference of Applied Psychology (ICAP), Montreal, Canada, 26–30 June 2018.
56. Behrman, D.N.; Perreault, W.D., Jr. A role stress model of the performance and satisfaction of industrial salespersons. *J. Mark.* **1984**, *48*, 9–21. [CrossRef]
57. Beehr, T.A.; Walsh, J.T.; Taber, T.D. Relationships of stress to individually and organizationally valued states: Higher order needs as a moderator. *J. Appl. Psychol.* **1976**, *61*, 41–47. [CrossRef]

58. McFarlin, D.B.; Rice, R.W. The role of facet importance as a moderator in job satisfaction processes. *J. Organ. Behav.* **1992**, *13*, 41–54. [CrossRef]
59. Maynard, D.C.; Joseph, T.A.; Maynard, A.M. Underemployment, job attitudes, and turnover intentions. *J. Organ. Behav.* **2006**, *27*, 509–536. [CrossRef]

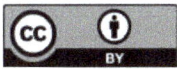

© 2018 by the authors. Licensee MDPI, Basel, Switzerland. This article is an open access article distributed under the terms and conditions of the Creative Commons Attribution (CC BY) license (http://creativecommons.org/licenses/by/4.0/).

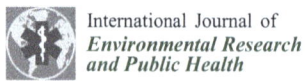

Article

Influence of Work on Elevated Blood Pressure in Hispanic Adolescents in South Texas

Eva M. Shipp [1,2,*], Sharon P. Cooper [3], Luohua Jiang [4], Amber B. Trueblood [1] and Jennifer Ross [5]

1. Texas A&M Transportation Institute, Center for Transportation Safety, 2929 Research Parkway, College Station, TX 77843, USA; a-trueblood@tti.tamu.edu
2. Texas A&M University School of Public Health, Department of Epidemiology & Biostatistics MS 1266, College Station, TX 77843, USA
3. The University of Texas Health Science Center at Houston–San Antonio Regional Campus; sbpcooper@yahoo.com
4. Department of Epidemiology, University of California, Irvine, CA 92697, USA; lhjiang@uci.edu
5. University of Oklahoma, College of Arts & Sciences, 633 Elm Avenue, Norman, OK 73019, USA; jenross@ou.edu
* Correspondence: e-shipp@tti.tamu.edu; Tel.: +1-(979)-458-4398

Received: 5 March 2019; Accepted: 22 March 2019; Published: 27 March 2019

Abstract: Literature supports an association between work and cardiovascular disease in adults. The objective of this study was to examine the relationship between current work status and elevated blood pressure in Hispanic adolescents. Participants were students in Hidalgo County, located along the Texas-Mexico border. Participants enrolled in the cohort study in ninth grade with assessments completed once a year for up to three years. Participants completed a self-report survey, while staff measured height, weight, waist circumference, blood pressure, and were screened for acanthosis nigricans. A generalized linear regression model with a logit link function was constructed to assess current work status and elevated blood pressure. Of the 508 participants, 29% had elevated blood pressure, which was associated with being male and other chronic disease indicators (e.g., acanthosis nigricans, overweight/obesity). The mean probability for elevated blood pressure was higher among currently working adolescents compared to those who were not. Findings were statistically significant ($p < 0.05$) at baseline. The findings illustrate that a large proportion of adolescents along the Texas-Mexico border may have elevated blood pressure and that working may be associated with it. Subsequent research is needed to confirm these findings, as well as to identify the mechanism for how work may increase hypertension in adolescents.

Keywords: adolescent; hypertension; blood pressure; Hispanic; work; farmworker; occupational health

1. Introduction

High blood pressure is among the most important risk factors for cardiovascular disease (CVD), the leading cause of death in adults, and the fifth leading cause of death among those aged 15–24 years in the United States [1–3]. Based on cross-sectional data from the National Health and Nutrition Examination (NHANES) in 2013–2014, an estimated 31.6% of adults aged 18 years and older were hypertensive, which amounted to approximately 75.1 million adults. Only about half of these adults (53.9%) had their blood pressure under control [4], leaving them especially vulnerable to CVD and related health problems.

Hypertension is a critical public health issue that may originate to some extent in childhood or adolescence [1,5–8]. As an example, high blood pressure during adolescence is associated with persistent cardiovascular alterations that can continue into adulthood [1,7,8]. In addition, national survey data illustrate that approximately one in ten adolescents screen positive for elevated blood pressure across the United States. Based on NHANES data from 2011–2012, elevated blood pressure, defined as high or borderline, was reported for 11% of those aged 8–17 years [9]. The prevalence was higher among males (15.4%) versus females (6.8%), Hispanics (11.5%) and non-Hispanic blacks (15.3%) versus non-Hispanic whites (9.4%), and those 13 to 17 years of age (15.0%) versus those 8–12 years of age (6.5%) [9]. In 2017, the American Academy of Pediatrics put forth revised clinical practice guidelines as an update to the 2004 "Fourth Report on the Diagnosis, Evaluation, and Treatment of High Blood Pressure in Children and Adolescent" [10]. Although the new guidelines are not a substantial departure from the prior report, applying the criteria to NHANES and other data suggests that more children would be classified as having elevated blood pressure and that shorter children aged 13 years and younger, and children over 13 years of age of any height may have a greater likelihood of being diagnosed as hypertensive [11,12]. Sharma and colleagues analyzed NHANES data from 1999–2014 and found that the prevalence of elevated blood pressure among children aged 5–18 years was 11.8% under the previous guidelines versus 14.2% under the revised guidelines [12].

Along with age, race and ethnicity, it is well known that socioeconomic status, lifestyle factors, nutrition, exercise, and body composition (e.g., excess body fat) play important roles in the occurrence and prevention of hypertension in adults [13–15]. A growing number of studies provide evidence that adolescents with elevated blood pressure also may be more likely to consume higher levels of sodium, lower levels of potassium, and more dietary fat; be less physically active; have poorer sleep quality; and be from lower socioeconomic levels [9,16–23]. However, the relationships between potential risk factors and the magnitude of their association with elevated blood pressure have not been established conclusively in younger populations.

Work-related factors are also consistently associated with hypertension in adults. Specific issues associated with increased blood pressure include job insecurity, long work hours, low wages, and jobs with poor work organization, as defined by jobs with high demands with low control or jobs that require considerable effort with low reward [24–28]. The exact mechanisms governing how these issues increase blood pressure is not entirely known. In adult workers, work stress may result in repeated activation of the autonomic nervous system, which can contribute to high blood pressure and heart disease based on studies with adult workers [29]. In addition, the time spent working may simply decrease the amount of time available for physical activity or other healthy behaviors (e.g., healthy diet). This may be especially true for adolescents who already contend with notable time demands, including attending school, participating in after school activities including team sports with considerable practice requirements, and helping with family chores and other obligations. Finally, work stress also may increase unhealthy coping behaviors such as excessive food consumption, consuming foods higher in sugar and saturated fat, or consuming alcohol. For example, a study found that fast food restaurant use among adolescents was associated with student employment, television usage, perceived barriers to healthy eating, and availability of unhealthy foods [30]. In addition, studies on working adolescents illustrate that long work hours contribute to the early onset of alcohol use [31–34].

The National Institute for Occupational Safety and Health (NIOSH) has recognized for over a decade that a variety of work-related exposures and issues influence overall health and well-being. From this perspective, whether and how work-related factors including stress, workload, and work hours influence health conditions (such as chronic disease) is as important as ensuring a safe workplace in a more traditional sense (e.g., minimizing physical hazards to address acute injuries). In 2011, NIOSH put forth the Total Worker Health Program to continue elevating this issue, spur further research, and promote workplace wellness programs [35]. In line with this holistic approach to worker health, the objective of the present study was to begin examining the relationship between current work status and elevated blood pressure in adolescents.

2. Materials and Methods

2.1. Study Design

Data for the present study, a secondary analysis, were collected during a prospective cohort study that was designed to estimate the occurrence of chronic disease indicators among students enrolled in a Migrant Education Program (MEP) and a comparison group of non-MEP students [36]. Students qualified for MEP if he or she migrated or had at least one parent who migrated within the prior three years to work in agriculture or fishing as a principal means of employment. "Migrated" was defined as moving temporarily to a different school district or administrative area within the United States [36]. All students enrolled in ninth grade and in MEP in two public high schools in Hidalgo County, Texas (located along the Texas-Mexico border) were recruited to participate and an equal number of students in the ninth grade who were not enrolled in MEP were randomly sampled as a comparison group. Enrollment occurred in 2007 and 2008 with participants followed for up to an additional three years (2008–2010). At the baseline and follow-up assessments, participants completed a survey on demographics, health behaviors, and work characteristics. A minimum clinical examination was also completed, which included measured height, weight, and waist circumference, a noninvasive visual screening for acanthosis nigricans (AN) on the neck, and blood pressure. Prior to partaking in the study, both parental and participant written consent was obtained. Data collection took place each year from January to March to accommodate the migration schedule of MEP students. Data collection took place in a private area in each school during approximately one class period. All interviewers were bilingual, certified in ethical standards for research with human subjects, and retrained in study methods each year to promote adherence to data collection protocols throughout the duration of the study. Additional methodological details are provided by Cooper and colleagues (2016) [36].

This study was approved by the Institutional Review Boards at The University of Texas Health Science Center at Houston (HSC-SPH-07-0284) and Texas A&M University (2010–0878). Written informed consent from parents and written child assent was obtained prior to any data collection.

2.2. Sample

A total of 628 students (n = 297 MEP; n = 331 non-MEP) were asked to complete a baseline assessment during the first and second year of recruitment. Of those, 508 enrolled (257 MEP and 251 non-MEP) and participated in the baseline assessment for a response proportion of 80.9%. For the follow-up assessments, participants with a baseline assessment who were still enrolled in school were eligible to participate. Of those, greater than 90% participated in the follow-up assessments each year. The available sample size for each study year were as follows: baseline (n = 257 MEP, n = 251 non-MEP), follow-up year 1 (n = 209 MEP, n = 220 non-MEP), follow-up year 2 (n = 165 MEP, n = 181 non-MEP), and follow-up year 3, which only included participants who enrolled during the first recruitment year (n = 65 MEP, n = 65 non-MEP). This study focused on the baseline and follow-up years 1 and 2 only.

2.3. Variable Definitions

Variable definitions and data collection protocols included the following. Staff measured blood pressure using an automated device, the Omron HEM-907XL (Omron Healthcare, Lake Forest, IL, USA). This ensured measurement consistency across participants and across survey years. Staff applied the cuff to students' right arm with measurements taken on a single occasion. After five minutes of quiet rest, the automated device took three successive measurements, while the participant sat in a chair with back support, feet flat on the floor, and arm supported with the antecubital fossa at heart level [36]. Staff recorded the first measurement, but it was not included in analysis, since these measurements can be falsely elevated [36]. Consequently, all analyses included only the average of the second and third measurements [36]. The definition of elevated blood pressure was at or above the 90th percentile for age, height, and sex or $\geq 120/80$ mm Hg [36]. Staff recorded height to the nearest 0.1 cm using a Shorr Board stadiometer (Shorr Productions, Olney, MD). Staff measured weight using a portable Tanita BWB-800S digital scale that was certified to be accurate to 400 pounds each year by a professional scale service and maintenance company (Tanita Corporation, Arlington, IL, USA). Overweight or obese categories were based on a body mass index (BMI) at or above the 85th percentile for age and sex, which follows the BMI-for-age- weight status categories provided by the Centers for Disease Control and Prevention (CDC) [37]. BMI was calculated as weight in kilograms divided by the height in meters squared. Waist circumference was measured to the nearest 0.1 cm using a plastic tape measure that was stretch resistant. A waist circumference at or above the 75th percentile for age, sex, and ethnicity was defined as abdominal obesity [36]. AN is a dark discoloration and/or thickening of the skin the back of the neck that is used as an indicator of high insulin levels or resistance. Staff used a similar approach to assess AN as those implemented in a Texas state-wide school- screening program [36,38,39]. The basis of work status was a self-reported annual work history of job type, dates of employment, and number of hours worked with survey items modelled after prior studies with working youth [40,41]. The recall period began from January 1st of the year prior to data collection with data collection occurring between January through March each year. The definition of current work status was working for pay or not for pay. The current work status definition was a student who reported a having a job during the same week when they participated in the survey. The basis of items pertaining to health behaviors was the Youth Risk Behavior Surveillance System YRBSS [42].

2.4. Data Management and Analysis

Data were managed using a Microsoft SQL relational database (Microsoft, Redmond, WA, USA). All data were double entered into the database to minimize data entry errors, as well as computer edited for out-of-range and contradictory values. SAS 9.4 was used for all data analysis (SAS Institute Inc., Cary, NC, USA). Descriptive statistics included means and proportions at baseline and years of follow-up. Appropriate statistical tests including chi-square tests, t-tests, and Fisher's exact tests were used to compare the distribution of variables across the two schools and by elevated blood pressure status. Generalized linear mixed models with a logit link function and binomial distribution were used to estimate the probability of high or high normal blood pressure at each time period by current work status after adjusting for potential confounders, including age, gender, AN, BMI, number of days physically active in the past 7 days, and school enrolled. Random intercepts at the individual level were also included in these models to account for potential correlation of repeated measures from the same student. Statistical significance was set a priori at a level of alpha <0.05.

3. Results

3.1. Participants

Table 1 presents baseline characteristics of participants stratified by school. Overall at baseline, half of participants were male with a mean age of 15.0 years. The place of birth for the majority of participants was the United States (92%). As previously reported in Cooper et al. (2016), a majority of participants self-identified as Hispanic, Latino, or Mexican-American (97%) and used English to complete the survey (79%) (data not shown) [36]. A larger proportion (62%) were enrolled in School 2 than School 1. At baseline, the distribution of demographic and other variables was similar in Schools 1 and 2 with two exceptions. School 2 had a larger percentage of participants who worked in the previous year compared to School 1, 54% and 67%, respectively ($p = 0.01$). However, the prevalence of being currently employed was not statistically different at baseline. School 2 also had a larger percentage of participants who had elevated blood pressure compared to School 1, 33% and 23%, respectively ($p = 0.01$).

Table 1. Baseline characteristics of participants by school.

Characteristics	Total (N = 508) [a] N (%)	School 1 (N = 190) N (%)	School 2 (N = 318) N (%)	p-Value
Gender				0.36 [b]
Female	254 (50)	90 (47)	164 (52)	
Male	254 (50)	100 (53)	154 (48)	
Country of birth				0.95 [b]
US	461 (92)	175 (92)	286 (92)	
Mexico or other	39 (8)	15 (8)	24 (8)	
Years lived in US				0.19 [b]
<14	55 (11)	25 (13)	30 (9)	
≥14	453 (89)	165 (87)	288 (91)	
Work status in the prior year				0.01 [b]
No work	298 (59)	128 (67)	170 (54)	
Any farm work	136 (27)	41 (22)	95 (30)	
Non-farm work only	72 (14)	21 (11)	51 (16)	
Working at the time of survey				0.15 [b]
No	486 (96)	185 (97)	301 (95)	
Yes	22 (4)	5 (3)	17 (5)	
Television (TV) time on average school day				0.27 [b]
None	87 (17)	28 (15)	59 (19)	
1+ hours	421 (83)	162 (85)	259 (81)	
Blood pressure				0.01 [b]
Normal	360 (71)	147 (77)	213 (67)	
High or high normal	148 (29)	43 (23)	105 (33)	
Acanthosis nigricans				0.83 [b]
No	385 (76)	143 (75)	242 (76)	
Yes	123 (24)	47 (25)	76 (24)	
Overweight or obese				0.07 [b]
No	264 (52)	89 (47)	175 (55)	
Yes	244 (48)	101 (53)	143 (45)	
Waist at or above 75th percentile				0.05 [b]
No	264 (52)	88 (47)	176 (56)	
Yes	240 (48)	100 (53)	140 (44)	
Experienced discrimination based on race or ethnicity				0.08 [b]
Never	330 (65)	132 (70)	198 (62)	
Sometimes/often	177 (35)	57 (30)	120 (38)	
Depressive symptoms				0.97 [b]
No	403 (80)	151 (80)	252 (80)	
Yes	102 (20)	38 (20)	64 (20)	
Number of sports teams in previous year				0.45 [b]
None	250 (49)	97 (51)	153 (48)	
1–2 teams	206 (41)	77 (41)	129 (41)	
3+ teams	51 (10)	15 (8)	36 (11)	
Days being physically active				0.43 [b]
None	70 (14)	32 (17)	38 (14)	
1–2 days	87 (17)	32 (17)	55 (17)	
3–6 days	222 (44)	77 (41)	145 (46)	
7 days	127 (25)	48 (25)	79 (25)	
Continuous Variables	Mean (SD)	Mean (SD)	Mean (SD)	p-Value
Age (years)	15.0 (0.8)	14.9 (0.8)	15.0 (0.8)	0.25 [c]
Body Mass Index (BMI)	25.8 (7.1)	26.5 (7.4)	25.4 (6.8)	0.10 [c]
Average waist circumference (cm)	88.5 (17.4)	90.1 (17.7)	87.5 (17.1)	0.12 [c]
Hours sleeping during weekdays	7.7 (1.3)	7.6 (1.4)	7.7 (1.3)	0.21 [c]
Hours sleeping during weekend	8.9 (2.6)	8.8 (2.7)	9.0 (2.6)	0.50 [c]

[a] Characteristics may not sum to 508 due to missing values; [b] chi-square test; [c] t-test.

3.2. Elevated Blood Pressure

Overall, 29% of the participants had elevated blood pressure. Table 2 presents the distribution of baseline characteristics by school and elevated blood pressure status. For School 1 and School 2, elevated blood pressure was more common among males and those with chronic disease indicators including AN, overweight or obesity, and abdominal obesity. Differences were statically significant ($p < 0.05$). Additional statistically significant ($p < 0.05$) differences for School 1 included increasing days physically active in the past seven days and for School 2, increasing participation in the number of sports team during the past 12 months, participation in work in the previous year as well as current employment status.

Table 2. Baseline characteristics of participants by blood pressure status.

Characteristics	School 1			School 2		
	Normal (N = 147)	High or High Normal (N = 43)		Normal (N = 213)	High or High Normal (N = 105)	
	N (%)	N (%)	p-Value	N (%)	N (%)	p-Value
Gender			0.01 [a]			<0.0001 [a]
Female	77 (52)	13 (30)		138 (65)	26 (25)	
Male	70 (47)	30 (70)		75 (35)	79 (75)	
Country of birth			0.80 [a]			0.62 [a]
US	135 (92)	40 (93)		193 (93)	93 (91)	
Mexico or other	12 (8)	3 (7)		15 (7)	9 (9)	
Years lived in US			0.86 [a]			0.21 [a]
<14	19 (13)	6 (14)		17 (8)	13 (12)	
≥14	128 (87)	37 (86)		196 (92)	92 (88)	
Work status in the previous year			0.44 [a]			0.005 [a]
No work	100 (68)	28 (65)		127 (60)	43 (41)	
Any farm work	33 (22)	8 (19)		53 (25)	42 (40)	
Non-farm work only	14 (10)	7 (16)		31 (15)	20 (19)	
Working at the time of survey			0.08 [b]			0.02 [a]
No	145 (99)	40 (93)		206 (97)	95 (90)	
Yes	2 (1)	3 (7)		7 (3)	10 (10)	
Television (TV) time on average school day			0.87 [a]			0.60 [a]
None	22 (15)	6 (14)		37 (17)	22 (21)	
1+ hours	125 (85)	37 (86)		176 (83)	83 (79)	
Acanthosis Nigricans			0.01 [a]			0.01 [a]
No	117 (80)	26 (60)		171 (80)	71 (66)	
Yes	30 (20)	17 (40)		42 (20)	34 (32)	
Overweight or obese			0.0004 [a]			<0.0001 [a]
No	79 (54)	10 (23)		134 (63)	41 (39)	
Yes	68 (46)	33 (77)		79 (37)	64 (61)	
Waist at or above 75th percentile			0.0007 [a]			0.0005 [a]
No	78 (53)	10 (24)		132 (63)	44 (42)	
Yes	68 (47)	32 (76)		79 (37)	61 (58)	
Experienced discrimination based on race or ethnicity			0.26 [a]			0.93 [a]
Never	99 (68)	33 (77)		133 (62)	65 (62)	
Sometimes/often	47 (32)	10 (23)		80 (38)	40 (38)	
Depressive symptoms			0.31 [a]			0.23 [a]
No	119 (82)	32 (74)		165 (78)	87 (84)	
Yes	27 (18)	11 (26)		47 (22)	17 (16)	

Table 2. Cont.

Characteristics	School 1			School 2		
	Normal (N = 147)	High or High Normal (N = 43)	p-Value	Normal (N = 213)	High or High Normal (N = 105)	p-Value
	N (%)	N (%)		N (%)	N (%)	
Number of sports teams in previous year			0.05 [a]			0.03 [a]
None	82 (56)	15 (35)		105 (49)	48 (46)	
1–2 teams	54 (37)	23 (53)		91 (43)	38 (36)	
3+ teams	10 (7)	5 (12)		17 (8)	19 (18)	
Days being physically active in the past 7 days			0.02 [a]			0.06 [a]
None	27 (18)	5 (12)		27 (13)	11 (10)	
1–2 days	26 (18)	6 (14)		38 (18)	17 (16)	
3–6 days	64 (44)	13 (30)		104 (49)	41 (39)	
7 days	29 (20)	19 (44)		43 (20)	36 (34)	
Continuous Variables	Mean (SD)	Mean (SD)	p-Value	Mean (SD)	Mean (SD)	p-Value
Age (years)	15 (0.8)	14.8 (0.7)	0.34 [c]	14.9 (0.8)	15.2 (0.9)	0.01 [c]
Body Mass Index (BMI)	25.7 (7.3)	28.9 (7.6)	0.01 [c]	24.4 (6.4)	27.5 (7.1)	0.0001 [c]
Average waist (cm)	88.3 (17.6)	96.0 (16.8)	0.01 [c]	85.0 (16.4)	92.7 (17.5)	0.0002 [c]
Hours sleeping during weekdays	7.6 (1.4)	7.3 (1.6)	0.23 [c]	7.8 (1.3)	7.6 (1.3)	0.38 [c]
Hours sleeping during weekend	9.0 (2.5)	8.2 (3.1)	0.08 [c]	9.1 (2.6)	8.6 (2.4)	0.07 [c]

[a] chi-square test; [b] Fisher's exact test; [c] t-test.

3.3. Current Work Status

At each survey period, the prevalence of current work status at baseline and first and second years of follow-up was 4.3%, 7.0%, and 6.9%, respectively. At baseline, 26 jobs were held by 22 participants. Job types included farm work (n = 3), adult or child care (n = 7), restaurant waiter or cashier (n = 4), lawn care (n = 3), construction (n = 2), office work (n = 2), fast food cashier or worker (n = 1), general cashier or sales (n = 1), grocery stocker or cashier (n = 1), skilled labor (n = 1), and other (n = 1). During the first and second years of follow-up, similar jobs were held. The most common jobs accounted for 70% of job types and included fast food cashier or worker restaurant waiter or cashier, general cashier or sales, grocery store stocker or cashier, and yard work. On average at their current job, participants engaging in farm work reported working 6.5 hours per day on work days (range: 2–12) and 5.8 days per week (range: 1–7), while participants engaging in non-farm work reported working 5.3 h per day on work days (range: 1–13) and 3.6 days per week (range: 1–7). Work intensity was similar across all three assessment years.

3.4. Work Status and Elevated Blood Pressure

Table 3 presents the results of the statistical model constructed to estimate the association between work status and elevated blood pressure at baseline and the first and second years of follow-up. Based on variables associated with elevated blood pressure at the bivariate level from Table 2, the following were included in the model as potential confounders: school, gender, age, AN, BMI, and number of days physically active in the past seven days. The adjusted mean probability of having elevated blood pressure at baseline among currently working adolescents was approximately twice the probability observed for adolescents who were not currently working. The difference in adjusted mean probability between the two groups was 27% and statistically significant ($p = 0.01$). Although the differences in the adjusted mean probabilities for follow-up year 1 and follow-up year 2 were higher among adolescents who were currently working, the differences were much smaller (4–9%) and not statistically significant ($p > 0.05$).

Table 3. Adjusted [a] mean probability of high or high normal blood pressure at each time point among students who were not working and who were currently working.

Assessment Year	Not Currently Working Mean (95% CI)	Currently Working Mean (95% CI)	Difference Mean (p-Value)
Baseline	0.24 (0.19, 0.29)	0.51 (0.29, 0.73)	0.27 (0.01)
Follow-up Year 1	0.24 (0.20, 0.29)	0.28 (0.15, 0.47)	0.04 (0.63)
Follow-up Year 2	0.32 (0.25, 0.39)	0.41 (0.23, 0.63)	0.09 (0.35)

[a] Adjusted means from generalized linear mixed models with a logit link function, model covariates include: age, gender, AN, body mass index (BMI), number of days physically active in the past seven days, school participant enrolled, work status, year of survey, and the interaction of work status with year of survey.

4. Discussion

A large proportion (29%) of participants had elevated blood pressure in this study of Hispanic adolescents, which was more common among males and those with chronic disease indicators (AN, overweight or obesity, and abdominal obesity). This is consistent with prior studies characterizing hypertension in children and adolescents [43,44]. A major strength of this study is that it is among the first to examine the potential impact of working on blood pressure in adolescents, specifically Hispanics. Working was a significant predictor of elevated blood pressure after adjusting for potential confounders at baseline. In addition, despite not being statistically significant, the mean probabilities of elevated blood pressure were higher for adolescents who were working. This association is also consistent with studies of adult working populations [24–28]. A detailed comparison with literature focusing on adults is difficult given differences in data collection and study variable definitions. The mechanism of how work exposures influence blood pressure could not be examined in this study. However, some of the participants in the study reported long work hours in addition to other demands related to school and home responsibilities. Insufficient time for engaging in healthy and stress relieving behaviors may be a factor. As an example, increased stress and limited time can negatively impact sleep quality and quantity. A recent systematic review indicated evidence of a link between sleep parameters and obesity, hypertension, and insulin sensitivity, but there were an insufficient number of high-quality studies available for assessing causality [45]. With respect to psychosocial job exposures, a study of Brazilian adolescent workers evaluated a connection between job demands, job control, and social support at work on various health indicators. The researchers found associations between psychological job demands and reduced sleep quantity during the week as well as work injury and body pain [46]. In the present study, self-reported sleep quantity was not associated with elevated blood pressure. The lack of association could be due to under or misreporting of sleep parameters since the data were self-reported. Furthermore, the outcome was elevated blood pressure rather than diagnosed hypertension. In addition, work-related as well as general stress may increase unhealthy coping behaviors in adolescents such as excessive food consumption, consuming foods higher in sugar and saturated fat, or consuming alcohol [30–34]. Many of these unhealthy coping mechanisms are associated with hypertension and coronary heart disease [47,48].

Additional strengths of this study included using an existing migrant education program infrastructure to access a hard-to-reach population [36]. Partnering closely with the school administrators and staff allowed for maintaining contact over time with a young, Hispanic population who are clearly at risk for chronic disease. Additional strengths included response proportions that were over 80% at baseline and during each assessment. Over 90% of eligible participants continued to participate in each follow-up assessment.

The key limitations of this study include a low prevalence of students currently engaged in work. While the use of pre-existing data made it possible to examine an under-researched topic with few resources, the low number of current workers also could have restricted the study's statistical power, while also prohibiting the examination of specific types of work and work-related exposures, both physical and psychosocial. Examples of areas of interest for future studies include increased time demands and long work hours combined with other non-work demands on time, psychosocial job stress, and physical job exposures. Future research is needed that addresses other populations beyond Hispanics and that which is designed and powered specifically to examine specific work exposures within the context of nutritional and other risk factors. Another important limitation is a high rate of attrition due to school drop-out, relocating to another school district, and early graduation. Approximately 25% of those in the baseline assessment were no longer eligible to participant in the second follow-up assessment. A subsequent pilot study examined the impact of this loss to follow-up. Blood pressure levels were higher in those who dropped out; however levels were not significantly different when compared to those who remained in the study [36]. This loss to follow-up may have contributed to only a minimal average difference in elevated blood pressure levels comparing those currently working with those who were not in the follow-up assessments. Beyond the potential impact of loss to follow-up, the reason for the lack of an association across all years is not clear. It also could be that participants learned better skills for coping with stress and time demands as they aged. The variables collected for this study along with the sample size were not sufficient for examining these relationships further. The study design also did not allow diagnosis of high blood pressure in any single year. Guidelines recommend observing elevations in blood pressure on three separate occasions prior to making a diagnosis [10]. Finally, this study did not include an in-depth dietary assessment, which is a limitation given the known associations between diet and elevated blood pressure. This would be of particular concern if the working students ate a poorer diet than non-working students.

5. Conclusions

As CVD remains the leading cause of death in adults and the fifth leading cause of death for those aged 15–24 years old, there is a critical need for additional research and interventions to address CVD risk factors, such as high blood pressure [1–3]. In addition, as literature supports that CVD may originate during childhood or adolescence, it is vital to address these risk factors at this critical period [1,5–8]. In this study, working may have increased the risk of high blood pressure in adolescents, specifically those who are in their early high school years. Future studies based on a larger sample of workers are needed to confirm the present study's findings and estimate the association between specific work-related exposures and elevated blood pressure, while accounting for nutritional and other potential risk factors. Future research could also identify the specific mechanism of how work status may increase hypertension in adolescents. The findings from this study provide a motivation for subsequent research in the areas of working youth and high blood pressure.

Author Contributions: E.M.S. assisted in design of the original study and served as the project manager. She oversaw data collection and data management for the study and assisted in the data analysis and interpretation of findings. She was responsible for overall manuscript development. S.P.C. was the principal investigator for the study. She was responsible for its design and overall conduct. She assisted in the interpretation of study findings and edited the manuscript. L.J. developed the analysis plan and was responsible for executing the data analysis. A.B.T. assisted in the literature review and overall manuscript development. J.R. assisted in the literature review, development of the manuscript, and final manuscript review.

Funding: This paper was supported by CDC/NIOSH under Cooperative Agreement No. U50 OH07541 to the Southwest Center for Agricultural Health, Injury Prevention, and Education at the University of Texas Health Science Center at Tyler. Its contents are solely the responsibility of the authors and do not necessarily represent the official views of CDC/NIOSH.

Acknowledgments: We would like to especially thank Yolanda Morado from Texas A&M AgriLife Extension for supporting this project and her dedication toward improving the health of families along the Texas-Mexico border. We would like to thank the students who participated and the school administrators, teachers and staff who made this study possible, specifically Linda Taormina.

Conflicts of Interest: None of the authors have a financial or non-financial competing interest with respect to the study and information presented in this manuscript.

References

1. Bloetzer, C.; Bovet, P.; Joan-Carles Suris Simeoni, U.; Paradis, G.; Chiolero, A. Screening for cardiovascular disease risk factors beginning in childhood. *Public Health Rev.* **2015**, *36*. [CrossRef]
2. Leading Causes of Death. Available online: https://www.cdc.gov/nchs/fastats/leading-causes-of-death.htm (accessed on 25 March 2019).
3. National Center for Health Statistics. *Health, United States, 2016: With Chartbook on Long-Term Trends in Health*; National Center for Health Statistics: Hyattsville, MD, USA, 2016.
4. Zhang, Y.; Moran, A.E. Trends in the prevalence, awareness, treatment, and control of hypertension among young adults in the United States, 1999 to 2014. *Hypertension* **2017**, *70*, 736–742. [CrossRef]
5. Berenson, G.S.; Srinivasan, S.R.; Bao, W.; Newman, W.P.; Tracy, R.E.; Wattigney, W.A. Association between multiple cardiovascular risk factors and atherosclerosis in children and young adults. *N. Engl. J. Med.* **1998**, *338*, 1650–1656. [CrossRef]
6. Berenson, G.S.; Wattigney, W.A.; Tracy, R.E.; Newman, W.P.; Srinivasan, S.R.; Webber, L.S.; Dalferes, E.R.; Strong, J.P. Atherosclerosis of the aorta and coronary arteries and cardiovascular risk factors in persons aged 6 to 30 years and studied at necropsy (The Bogalusa Heart Study). *Am. J. Cardiol.* **1992**, *70*, 851–858. [CrossRef]
7. Chen, X.; Wang, Y. Tracking of blood pressure from childhood to adulthood: A systematic review and meta-regression analysis. *Circulation* **2008**, *117*, 3171–3180. [CrossRef]
8. Lai, C.C.; Sun, D.; Cen, R.; Wang, J.; Li, S.; Fernandez-Alonso, C.; Chen, W.; Srinivasan, S.R.; Berenson, G.S. Impact of long-term burden of excessive adiposity and elevated blood pressure from childhood on adulthood left ventricular remodeling patterns: The Bogalusa Heart Study. *J. Am. Coll. Cardiol.* **2014**, *64*, 1580–1587. [CrossRef]
9. Kit, B.K.; Kuklina, E.; Carroll, M.D.; Ostchega, Y.; Freedman, D.S.; Ogden, C.L. Prevalence of and trends in dyslipidemia and blood pressure among US children and adolescents, 1999–2012. *JAMA Pediatr.* **2015**, *169*, 272–279. [CrossRef]
10. National High Blood Pressure Education Program Working Group. The fourth report on the diagnosis, evaluation, and treatment of high blood pressure in children and adolescents. *Pediatrics* **2004**, *114*, 555–576. [CrossRef]
11. Bell, C.S.; Samuel, J.P.; Samuels, J.A. Prevalence of hypertension in children: Applying the new American Academy of Pediatrics Clinical Practice Guideline. *Hypertension* **2019**, *73*, 148–152. [CrossRef]
12. Sharma, A.K.; Metzger, D.L.; Rodd, C.J. Prevalence and severity of high blood pressure among children based on the 2017 American Academy of Pediatrics Guidelines. *JAMA Pediatr.* **2018**, *172*, 557–565. [CrossRef]
13. Leng, B.; Jin, Y.; Li, G.; Chen, L.; Jin, N. Socioeconomic status and hypertension: A meta-analysis. *J. Hypertens.* **2015**, *33*, 221–229. [CrossRef]
14. Stringhini, S.; Carmeli, C.; Jokela, M.; Avendaño, M.; McCrory, C.; d'Errico, A.; Bochud, M.; Barros, H.; Costa, G.; Chadeau-Hyam, M.; et al. Socioeconomic status, non-communicable disease risk factors, and walking speed in older adults: Multi-cohort population based study. *BMJ* **2018**, *360*, k1046. [CrossRef]
15. Robles-Romero, J.M.; Fernández-Ozcorta, E.J.; Gavala-González, J.; Romero-Martín, M.; Gómez-Salgado, J.; Ruiz-Frutos, C. Anthropometric measures as predictive indicators of metabolic risk in a population of "Holy week costaleros". *Int. J. Environ. Res. Public Health* **2019**, *16*, 207. [CrossRef]
16. Setayeshgar, S.; Ekwaru, J.P.; Maximova, K.; Majumdar, S.R.; Storey, K.E.; McGavock, J.; Veugelers, P.J. Dietary intake and prospective changes in cardiometabolic risk factors in children and youth. *Appl. Physiol. Nutr. Metab.* **2017**, *42*, 39–45. [CrossRef]
17. Lazarou, C.; Panagiotakos, D.B.; Matalas, A.L. Lifestyle factors are determinants of children's blood pressure levels: The CYKIDS study. *J. Hum. Hypertens.* **2009**, *23*, 456–463. [CrossRef]
18. Simons-Morton, D.G.; Obarzanek, E. Diet and blood pressure in children and adolescents. *Pediatr. Nephrol.* **1997**, *11*, 244–249. [CrossRef]
19. De Moraes, A.C.; Carvalho, H.B.; Siani, A.; Barba, G.; Veidebaum, T.; Tornaritis, M.; Molnar, D.; Ahrens, W.; Wirsik, N.; De Henauw, S.; et al. Incidence of high blood pressure in children—Effects of physical activity and sedentary behaviors: The IDEFICS study: High blood pressure, lifestyle and children. *Int. J. Cardiol.* **2015**, *180*, 165–170. [CrossRef]

20. He, F.J.; MacGregor, G.A. Importance of salt in determining blood pressure in children: Meta-analysis of controlled trials. *Hypertension* **2006**, *48*, 861–869. [CrossRef]
21. McGrath, J.J.; Matthews, K.A.; Brady, S.S. Individual versus neighborhood socioeconomic status and race as predictors of adolescent ambulatory blood pressure and heart rate. *Soc. Sci. Med.* **2006**, *63*, 1442–1453. [CrossRef]
22. Javaheri, S.; Storfer-Isser, A.; Rosen, C.L.; Redline, S. Sleep quality and elevated blood pressure in adolescents. *Circulation* **2008**, *118*, 1034. [CrossRef]
23. Chmielewski, J.; Carmody, J.B. Dietary sodium, dietary potassium, and systolic blood pressure in US adolescents. *J. Clin. Hypertens.* **2017**, *19*, 904–909. [CrossRef]
24. Cuffee, Y.; Ogedegbe, C.; Williams, N.J.; Ogedegbe, G.; Schoenthaler, A. Psychosocial risk factors for hypertension: An update of the literature. *Curr. Hypertens. Rep.* **2014**, *16*, 483. [CrossRef]
25. Guimont, C.; Brisson, C.; Dagenais, G.R.; Milot, A.; Vezina, M.; Masse, B.; Moisan, J.; Laflamme, N.; Blanchette, C. Effects of job strain on blood pressure: A prospective study of male and female white-collar workers. *Am. J. Public Health* **2006**, *96*, 1436–1443. [CrossRef]
26. Trudel, X.; Brisson, C.; Milot, A.; Masse, B.; Vezina, M. Adverse psychosocial work factors, blood pressure and hypertension incidence: Repeated exposure in a 5-year prospective cohort study. *J. Epidemiol. Community Health* **2016**, *70*, 402–408. [CrossRef]
27. Trudel, X.; Brisson, C.; Milot, A.; Masse, B.; Vezina, M. Effort-reward imbalance at work and 5-year changes in blood pressure: The mediating effect of changes in body mass index among 1400 white-collar workers. *Int. Arch. Occup. Environ. Health* **2016**, *89*, 1229–1238. [CrossRef]
28. Mucci, N.; Giorgi, G.; De Pasquale Ceratti, S.; Fiz-Perez, J.; Mucci, F.; Arcangeli, G. Anxiety, Stress-Related Factors, and Blood Pressure in Young Adults. *Front. Psychol.* **2016**, *7*, 1682. [CrossRef]
29. Chandola, T.; Britton, A.; Brunner, E.; Hemingway, H.; Malik, M.; Kumari, M.; Badrick, E.; Kivimaki, M.; Marmot, M. Work stress and coronary heart disease: What are the mechanisms? *Eur. Heart J.* **2008**, *29*, 640–648. [CrossRef]
30. French, S.A.; Story, M.; Neumark-Sztainer, D.; Fulkerson, J.A.; Hannan, P. Fast food restaurant use among adolescents: Associations with nutrient intake, food choices and behavioral and psychosocial variables. *Int. J. Obes.* **2001**, *25*, 1823–1833. [CrossRef]
31. Liu, X.C.; Keyes, K.M.; Li, G. Work stress and alcohol consumption among adolescents: Moderation by family and peer influences. *BMC Public Health* **2014**, *14*, 1303. [CrossRef]
32. Steinberg, L.; Fegley, S.; Dornbusch, S.M. Negative impact of part-time work on adolescent adjustment: Evidence from a longitudinal study. *Dev. Psychol.* **1993**, *29*, 171–180. [CrossRef]
33. Brody, G.H.; Flor, D.L.; Hollett-Wright, N.; McCoy, J.K. Children's development of alcohol use norms: Contributions of parent and sibling norms, children's temperaments, and parent-child discussions. *J. Fam. Psychol.* **1998**, *12*, 209–219. [CrossRef]
34. Safron, D.J.; Schulenberg, J.E.; Bachman, J.G. Part-time work and hurried adolescence: The links among work intensity, social activities, health behaviors, and substance use. *J. Health Soc. Behav.* **2001**, *42*, 425–449. [CrossRef]
35. National Institute for Occupational Safety and Health. *Research Compendium: The NIOSH Total Worker Health®Program Seminal Research Papers*; DHHS (NIOSH) Publication No. 2012-146; NIOSH: Washington, DC, USA, 2012.
36. Cooper, S.P.; Shipp, E.M.; Del Junco, D.J.; Cooper, C.J.; Bautista, L.E.; Levin, J. Cardiovascular Disease Risk Factors in Hispanic Adolescents in South Texas. *South Med. J.* **2016**, *109*, 130–136. [CrossRef] [PubMed]
37. Healthy Weight: About Child & Teen BMI. Available online: https://www.cdc.gov/healthyweight/assessing/bmi/childrens_bmi/about_childrens_bmi.html (accessed on 25 March 2019).
38. King-Tryce, K.; Garza, L.; Ozias, J.M. Acanthosis nigricans and insulin resistance. *Dis. Prev. News* **2002**, *62*, 1–4.
39. Office UoT-PABH. *The Texas Risk Assessment for Type 2 Diabetes in Children Program: A Report to the Governor and 82nd Legislature of the State of Texas*; The University of Texas-Pan American Border Health Office: Edinburg, TX, USA, 2011.
40. Cooper, S.P.; Burau, K.E.; Frankowski, R.; Shipp, E.M.; Del Junco, D.J.; Whitworth, R.E.; Sweeney, A.M.; Macnaughton, N.; Weller, N.F.; Hanis, C.L. A cohort study of injuries in migrant farm worker families in South Texas. *Ann. Epidemiol.* **2006**, *16*, 313–320. [CrossRef] [PubMed]

41. Shipp, E.M.; Cooper, S.P.; del Junco, D.J.; Cooper, C.J.; Whitworth, R.E. Acute occupational injury among adolescent farmworkers from South Texas. *Injury Prev.* **2013**, *19*, 264–270. [CrossRef] [PubMed]
42. Youth Risk Behavior Surveillance System (YRBSS). Available online: https://www.cdc.gov/healthyyouth/data/yrbs/index.htm (accessed on 25 March 2019).
43. Din-Dzietham, R.; Liu, Y.; Bielo, M.V.; Shamsa, F. High blood pressure trends in children and adolescents in national surveys, 1963 to 2002. *Circulation* **2007**, *116*, 1488–1496. [CrossRef]
44. Urrutia-Rojas, X.; Egbuchunam, C.U.; Bae, S.; Menchaca, J.; Bayona, M.; Rivers, P.A.; Singh, K.P. High blood pressure in school children: Prevalence and risk factors. *BMC Pediatr.* **2006**, *6*, 32. [CrossRef]
45. Fobian, A.D.; Elliott, L.; Louie, T. A Systematic Review of Sleep, Hypertension, and Cardiovascular Risk in Children and Adolescents. *Curr. Hypertens. Rep.* **2018**, *20*, 42. [CrossRef]
46. Fischer, F.M.; Oliveira, D.C.; Nagai, R.; Teixeira, L.R.; Lombardi Júnior, M.; Latorre, M.D.; Cooper, S.P. Job control, job demands, social support at work and health among adolescent workers. *Revista de Saúde Pública* **2005**, *39*, 245–253. [CrossRef]
47. DiNicolantonio, J.J.; Lucan, S.C.; O'Keefe, J.H. The Evidence for Saturated Fat and for Sugar Related to Coronary Heart Disease. *Prog. Cardiovasc. Dis.* **2016**, *58*, 464–472. [CrossRef] [PubMed]
48. Know Your Risk Factors for High Blood Pressure. Available online: http://www.heart.org/HEARTORG/Conditions/HighBloodPressure/UnderstandSymptomsRisks/Know-Your-Risk-Factors-for-High-Blood-Pressure_UCM_002052_Article.jsp#.Wk0zvVVKthE (accessed on 25 March 2019).

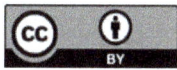

© 2019 by the authors. Licensee MDPI, Basel, Switzerland. This article is an open access article distributed under the terms and conditions of the Creative Commons Attribution (CC BY) license (http://creativecommons.org/licenses/by/4.0/).

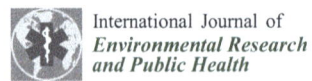

Article

The Happy-Productive Worker Model and Beyond: Patterns of Wellbeing and Performance at Work

José M. Peiró [1,*], Malgorzata W. Kozusznik [2], Isabel Rodríguez-Molina [3] and Núria Tordera [3]

1. IDOCAL (Institut d'Investigació en Psicologia del RRHH, del Desenvolupament Organitzacional i de la Qualitat de Vida Laboral), Universitat de València & IVIE, Avda. Blasco Ibáñez 21, 46010 Valencia, Spain
2. Research Group for Work, Organizational and Personnel Psychology (WOPP), Katholieke Universiteit Leuven, Dekenstraat 2, 3000 Leuven, Belgium; gosia.kozusznik@kuleuven.be
3. IDOCAL (Institut d'Investigació en Psicologia del RRHH, del Desenvolupament Organitzacional i de la Qualitat de Vida Laboral), Universitat de València, Avda. Blasco Ibáñez 21, 46010 Valencia, Spain; isabel.rodriguez@uv.es (I.R.-M.); nuria.tordera@uv.es (N.T.)
* Correspondence: jose.m.peiro@uv.es; Tel.: +34-963-864-689

Received: 27 December 2018; Accepted: 3 February 2019; Published: 6 February 2019

Abstract: According to the happy-productive worker thesis (HPWT), "happy" workers perform better than "less happy" ones. This study aimed to explore the different patterns of relationships between performance and wellbeing, synergistic (i.e., unhappy-unproductive and happy-productive) and antagonistic (i.e., happy-unproductive and unhappy-productive), taking into account different operationalizations of wellbeing (i.e., hedonic vs. eudaimonic) and performance (i.e., self-rated vs. supervisors' ratings). It also explored different demographic variables as antecedents of these patterns. We applied two-step cluster analysis to the data of 1647 employees. The results indicate four different patterns—happy-productive, unhappy-unproductive, happy-unproductive, and unhappy-productive—when performance is self-assessed, and three when it is assessed by supervisors. On average, over half of the respondents are unhappy-productive or happy-unproductive. We used multidimensional logistic regression to explain cluster membership based on demographic covariates. This study addresses the limitations of the HPWT by including both the hedonic and eudaimonic aspects of wellbeing and considering different dimensions and sources of evaluation. The "antagonistic" patterns identify employees with profiles not explicitly considered by the HPWT.

Keywords: occupational wellbeing; performance; happy-productive worker

1. Introduction

Wellbeing at work can be conceptualized from two distinct perspectives based on different philosophical traditions: the hedonic view of pleasure and experience of positive affect [1] and the eudaimonic view of wellbeing as personal growth and a sense of meaning [2]. Therefore, wellbeing can be understood as having both pleasurable (or hedonic) and meaningful (or eudaimonic) components [3–6]. However, the majority of the research has studied wellbeing from the hedonic perspective, conceptualizing wellbeing as judgments and evaluations of satisfaction with some of life's facets (e.g., job satisfaction).

According to the happy-productive worker thesis, "happy" workers should have better performance than "less happy" ones [7,8], and the quality of task performance can be influenced by the coexisting affective states [9]. This thesis has produced a series of studies [10,11] and meta-analytic research, often providing ambiguous and inconclusive results [8,12].

On the one hand, some research shows that wellbeing can predict performance. For example, studies show that when people are more satisfied with their jobs, they show higher performance [13,14].

In addition, higher positive affect has been shown to predict performance quality [15]. Furthermore, when people are more satisfied with their jobs, they show higher productivity [16] over time. People who feel better than usual at work have been found to make more effort on their tasks [17,18] and achieve a higher level of task performance [19]. In this direction, feeling active and enthusiastic in the morning has been shown to increase levels of creativity during the day [20]. Finally, positive affect has been shown to predict performance quality [21]. All these results support the HPWT, which posits that workers with higher levels of wellbeing also tend to show better performance at work, compared to workers with lower levels of wellbeing.

On the other hand, empirical studies and meta-analyses have found the relationships between performance and job satisfaction to be spurious [22] or weak [23]. Some scholars view the connections between happiness and job performance as questionable [7], suggesting an apparently low and non-significant satisfaction–performance relationship [24]. This can be reflected by the fact that most studies that consider job satisfaction and job performance treat them as separate variables that are not directly related to each other [24]. For example, Greenberger, Strasser, Cummings, and Dunham [25] studied the causal relationship between personal control and job satisfaction, and between personal control and job performance, but they did not assume or investigate the relationship between job satisfaction and job performance [24]. There is a need to address this ambiguity in the research, and for this reason we consider it necessary to revisit and expand the happy-productive worker thesis.

Some Limitations of the Happy-Productive Worker Thesis

The ambiguity in the studies on the HPWT can be explained in part by the limitations of these studies [26]. First, they focus on hedonic constructs of wellbeing at the expense of eudaimonic wellbeing. In fact, most of the research has studied wellbeing from the hedonic perspective, understanding it as global evaluations of satisfaction (e.g., job satisfaction). More recently, valuable studies have revisited the thesis of the happy and productive worker, studying the possibility of expanding it conceptually to include affect [7] or alternative relationships between satisfaction and performance [8] by evaluating affective wellbeing, both as a state and a trait [19]. However, this thesis has not been extended to consider key wellbeing constructs, such as its eudaimonic dimension, which involves purpose and personal growth. Wellbeing has also been conceptualized as an eudaimonic experience of meaning at work and purpose in life [27]. This conceptualization of subjective wellbeing can be reflected in the recent progress in its measures [28], which distinguish between activities that people consider 'pleasurable' as opposed to the 'worthwhileness' or meaning at work associated with these activities [2,29,30]. Although few studies have investigated the relationship between eudaimonic wellbeing and performance [31], some research suggests that this relationship exists. For example, Niessen et al. [32] demonstrated that, on days when employees had increased perceived meaning at work, they reported being more focused on tasks and behaving in a more exploratory way, compared to days when they evaluated their work as less meaningful to them.

A second limitation is that, in the study of the relationship between happiness and productivity, little attention is paid to a precise operationalization of productivity, and even its operationalization as job performance is far from systemic and comprehensive in terms of its dimensions or facets (e.g., in-role performance, extra-role performance, creative performance). Job performance can be understood as "a function of a person's behavior and the extent to which that behavior helps an organization to reach its goals" [33] (p. 187). However, there is considerable debate about what work performance is. Koopmans and colleagues [34], in their systematic review, observe that, according to different studies on work performance, it can be conceptualized using the following broad dimensions: task performance, contextual performance, and counter-productive behavior. Task or in-role performance is intrinsically related to the activities included in the job description. Contextual performance refers to behaviors that are not directly related to the activities included in the job description. Organizational citizenship overlaps with the definitions of contextual performance and refers to helping others at work in the social and psychological context, thus promoting task performance [35]. Counterproductive work behaviors include behaviors such as absenteeism, theft, and substance abuse. Furthermore, creativity [36] and innovation [37] have been pointed out as another important aspect of job performance. Several authors suggest conceptualizing job performance using a broader theoretical framework, in order to mitigate error sources and find relationships between performance and job satisfaction [38]. In the present study, we incorporate different aspects of performance (in-role, organizational citizenship, and creative performance) in a global measure. Performance evaluations may come from different sources (e.g., self-assessed, supervisor, peers, customers, etc.). It is necessary to complement the employees' self-rated performance assessment with the supervisors' evaluation of their performance in order to avoid employee leniency or self-deception in self-ratings, which has been shown to be particularly prominent in overall or general performance assessments [39]. By including supervisors' evaluations of their employees' performance levels, we make sure that we are using evaluations that have been shown to have the highest mean reliability, as found in a meta-analysis by Conway and Huffcutt [40]. Therefore, the present study, in addition to employees' self-ratings of their own performance, includes information about their performance from their direct supervisors.

A third limitation lies in the fact that most organizational research has studied "happiness" as an antecedent of "productivity", and only a few studies have looked for the inverse relationship [24,31]. However, there is evidence suggesting that work performance can explain wellbeing indicators. For example, evidence shows that self-rated performance predicts an increase in dedication and a decrease in emotional exhaustion over time [41]. Moreover, performance [42,43] and the experience of making progress toward one's goals at work [44–46] have been shown to predict positive affective states. Additionally, studies have shown that personal initiative is positively related to an increase in work engagement over time [47]. Along the same lines, there is evidence that on days when employees were strongly focused on tasks at work, they also exhibited more vitality and learning than on days when they were weakly focused on their tasks [32].

A fourth limitation is that the studies from both the happy-productive and productive-happy approaches have assumed positive linear relationships, although other patterns of relations may exist, especially those that establish negative relationships between these two variables. These complex and alternative relations between these constructs require taking into consideration different configurations or patterns of these relationships, instead of analyzing them sequentially. In fact, the studies carried out within the happy productive thesis emphasize the results that confirm this thesis. These studies tend to especially explore the synergistic side of the model that produces a win-win situation for employers and employees (happy and productive), while disregarding the antagonistic or win-lose relations (happy and unproductive or unhappy and productive). However, some studies suggest that we should pay more attention to these antagonistic relations, showing, for instance, that difficulty in remembering information and poor task performance can be considered negative consequences of being "happy" at work [48]. Furthermore, other authors provide evidence of the benefits of negative affect on creative performance [49]. Based on this research, Peiró et al. [26] proposed the need to attend to not only the synergetic relations between performance and wellbeing, but also to the antagonistic ones, thus extending the propositions of the HWPW. They proposed the coexistence of four patterns of relationships between performance and wellbeing: "happy-productive", "unhappy-unproductive", "happy-unproductive", and "unhappy-productive". In fact, Ayala et al. [50] found support for these different types of patterns when considering job satisfaction and innovative performance in young employees. Moreover, they found that almost 15% of a sample of Spanish young employees fell in the group of unhappy-productive (about 9%) or the group of happy-unproductive (more than 5%). Acknowledging that the correlations between happiness and productivity are moderated, it is important to focus on the different groups of workers according to their profiles. In order "to learn more about individuals who are outside the hypothesized pattern ... , it is now desirable to investigate additional measures of wellbeing and performance and identify situational and personal features associated with membership in each cluster" [51] (p. 12).

In order to overcome the limitations of the research mentioned above, in the present study, we address them by revisiting the happy-productive worker, incorporating both the hedonic and eudaimonic components of wellbeing and considering different aspects of job performance as well as different evaluation sources. In addition, in this study, we consider wellbeing and performance simultaneously, instead of analyzing the sequence between these two constructs. To this end, we study patterns of wellbeing and performance that serve to integrate these two constructs, taking into account different operationalizations where neither of them is an antecedent of the other, in order to identify different patterns of employees, both synergistic (i.e., happy-productive) and antagonistic (i.e., unhappy-unproductive, happy-unproductive and unhappy-productive). In this way, we aim to further advance our knowledge in the direction pointed out by Warr and Nielsen [51] when they proposed identifying situational and personal features associated with membership in each cluster. More specifically, we formulate the following research questions:

- Research Question 1: Do employees show different patterns of relationships between performance and wellbeing, synergistic (i.e., unhappy-unproductive and happy-productive) and antagonistic (i.e., happy-unproductive and unhappy-productive), taking into account different operationalizations of wellbeing (i.e., hedonic vs. eudaimonic) and performance (i.e., self-rated vs. supervisor ratings)?
- Research Question 2: Will the employees remain in the same profile of wellbeing and performance in their different operationalizations?
- Research Question 3: Are there any demographic variables that may play a role as antecedents of the profiles in the different operationalizations of the "happy-productive" worker?

2. Materials and Methods

2.1. Sample and Procedure

The members of the research team contacted several organizations, inviting them to participate in the project. Convenience sampling was used, focusing mainly on the services and production sector. The first contact was made with the general manager or the director of human resources. In a first meeting, the project, the objectives, the time required, and the procedure were explained to them. Then, if they agreed, all the workers in the organizations were invited to participate by completing the questionnaire voluntarily and confidentially.

The sample was composed of 1647 employees (52% women, 43% men, 5% information not available) from the services (81%) and production/construction (19%) sectors, working in 239 work units in different Spanish companies. With regard to age, 26% percent of participants were under 35 years old, 55% were between 35 and 50, and 16% were over 50 years old. The majority of the sample had a university degree (46%) and high school or professional training (37%). The majority were technicians/administrative workers (46%) and highly qualified professionals (24%). In addition, 62% were permanent workers, and 30% were temporary workers. The majority of the employees had worked for more than 5 years in their current position (53%). Members of the research team informed the participants on the purpose of the study, the guarantee of confidentiality and the willfulness of their participation. Participants expressed their consent to participate. The research protocol was approved by the Ethics Committee of the University of Valencia.

In this study, we used two types of informants to assess employee performance. First, we asked the employees to self-evaluate their performance. These ratings were obtained for all the employees. Second, we asked employees' direct supervisors to rate the performance of their subordinates. In this case, performance evaluated by the direct supervisor was only obtained for 915 employees. Confidentiality of the data was guaranteed.

2.2. Measures

Hedonic wellbeing. Hedonic wellbeing was conceptualized as the employee's job satisfaction, and it was measured by a 10-item reduced version of the Job Satisfaction Scale (IJSS) by Cooper, Rout and Faragher [52], referring to intrinsic job satisfaction and extrinsic job satisfaction, and one additional item measuring general job satisfaction. The score for hedonic wellbeing was the global mean score for the three types of job satisfaction. It includes items such as "Opportunity to use your skills". The items have a seven-point Likert response format, ranging from 1 (quite dissatisfied) to 7 (very satisfied). Cronbach's alpha for the global score of Hedonic Wellbeing was 0.87.

Eudaimonic wellbeing. Eudaimonic wellbeing was conceptualized as a feeling of meaning and purpose at work, and it was measured by an 8-item reduced version of the scale constructed by Ryff [53], with two subscales: purpose at work and personal growth. The score for eudaimonic wellbeing was obtained by computing the global mean score for the two dimensions of the scale. It includes items such as "For me, life has been a continuous process of learning, changing, and growth". The items have a seven-point Likert response format, ranging from 1 (strongly disagree) to 7 (strongly agree). Cronbach's alpha for the global score of eudaimonic wellbeing was 0.72.

Performance—rated by the employee. Employees' self-rated work performance was operationalized as in-role performance (carrying out tasks required by the job), extra-role performance (carrying out tasks that are not required in the job description, e.g., helping others), and creative performance (carrying out tasks that are both creative and useful at work). In-role performance was measured by 3 items from a scale constructed by Williams and Anderson [54], extra-role performance was measured by 3 items from a scale by Mackenzie and colleagues [55], and creative performance was measured by a 3-item method constructed by Oldham and Cummings [36]. The composite score for performance was obtained by calculating the global mean score for the in-role, extra-role, and creative performance scales. It includes items such as: "I adequately complete assigned duties" (in-role performance); "I do not hesitate to challenge the opinions of others who I feel are leading the store/company in the wrong direction" (extra-role performance); and "How original and practical am I in my work?" The items have a seven-point Likert response format, ranging from 1 (strongly disagree) to 7 (strongly agree). Cronbach's alpha for the global work performance score was 0.71.

Performance—rated by the supervisor. Employee work performance evaluated by the supervisor was also operationalized as a general measure of performance quality. We measured these three aspects using three items: "What is his/her performance like?"; "What is the quality of his/her work?"; and "What was his/her level of goal achievement in the past year?" The items have a five-point Likert response format, ranging from 1 (very bad) to 5 (very good). Cronbach's alpha for the global work Performance score was 0.89.

Demographic variables included. Organization's sector: dummy variable (0 service, 1 production/construction). Gender: dummy variable (0 female, 1 male). Age: under 35 years old, between 35 and 50, and over 50 years old. The highest educational level achieved: no education or compulsory education, professional training or high school, advanced university degree. Occupational category: unqualified manual work, technician or administrative work, highly qualified professional, manager. Type of contract: dummy variable (0 = temporary, 1 = permanent). Seniority in the position: dummy variable (0 = less than 5 years, 1 = more than 5 years).

2.3. Statistical Analysis

The sample was divided into clusters using the two–step cluster analysis method developed by Chiu and colleagues [56] in SPSS v.22 (IBM Corp., Armonk, NY, USA). The SPSS two-step cluster method is a scalable cluster analysis algorithm designed to handle large datasets, such as those analyzed in the present study. The algorithm is based on a two–stage approach: in the first stage, it undertakes a similar procedure to the k-means algorithm. In the second step, based on these results, a modified hierarchical agglomerative clustering procedure is carried out that combines the objects sequentially to form homogenous clusters [57].

The two-step clustering algorithm output offers fit information, such as the Bayesian Information Criterion (BIC), as well as information about the importance of each variable for the construction of a specific cluster [57], which is an additional attractive feature of the two-step cluster method in comparison with traditional clustering methods. Empirical results indicate that the two-step clustering method shows a near-perfect ability to detect known subgroups and correctly classify individuals into these subgroups [58]. Based on these analyses, the sample was classified into groups reflecting different configurations of wellbeing and performance dimensions.

After finding cluster solutions for each of the combinations of variables of interest, we applied multidimensional logistic regression to explain cluster membership based on the demographic covariates described. Multinomial logistic regression is a statistical technique that specifies the dependent variable as a categorical variable that can take more than two values (in our case, the number of clusters). In multinomial logistic regression, one of the responses is chosen to serve as reference. Switching the reference group allowed us to compare the effects on all the groups. The independent variables are also categorical, with K categories. They are introduced in the model coded as k-1 binary variables. When the variables have two categories, they have been introduced as a dummy variable with a value of 0 or 1. In this case, the exponential beta coefficient represents the change in the odds of the dependent variable, associated with a one-unit change in the corresponding independent variable. When the variables have more than two categories, the coding system used is deviation coding. In this case, because there is no clear reference category, the reference category is coded as -1. This coding system compares the mean of the dependent variable for a given level to the mean of the dependent variable for the other levels of the variable. The exponential beta coefficient estimates the magnitude at which the probability of the occurrence of the event varies, comparing that category to the average of all the subjects in the study. Because the analysis does not show results for the reference group, we have repeated the analysis using the coding system with a different group as reference. With this system, we can obtain the coefficients for all the categories, which are presented in the results tables.

3. Results

3.1. Descriptive Analysis

The descriptive results are shown in Tables 1 and 2.

Table 1. Descriptive statistics (demographic variables).

Variables	%
Sector	
service	81
production	19
Gender	
female	52
male	43
Age	
<35 years	26
35–50 years	55
>50 years	16
Educational level	
No education or compulsory	14
Professional training or high school	37
University degree	46

Table 1. *Cont.*

Variables	%
Occupational category	
Unqualified manual work	10
Technician or administrative	46
Highly qualified professional	24
Manager	
Type of contract	
temporary	30
permanent	62
Seniority in the position	
<5 years	40
>5 years	53

Table 2. Descriptive statistics.

Feature	Mean	Standard Deviation (SD)
Hedonic wellbeing	5.25	0.91
Eudaimonic wellbeing	5.78	0.76
Performance rated by the employee	5.65	0.69
Performance rated by the supervisor	4.17	0.68

3.2. Cluster Analyses: Different Operationalizations of the Wellbeing-Performance Patterns.

As mentioned above, we used cluster analysis to find different patterns of relationships between performance and wellbeing, taking into account different operationalizations of wellbeing (i.e., hedonic vs. eudaimonic) and performance (i.e., self-rated vs. supervisor ratings). The results are shown below. Models 1 and 2 consider self-rated performance by the employee (hedonic wellbeing in Model 1 and eudaimonic wellbeing in Model 2). Models 3 and 4 consider performance evaluated by the supervisor (hedonic wellbeing in Model 3 and eudaimonic wellbeing in Model 4).

When performance is evaluated by the employee, there are four clusters: (1) employees who are high in both wellbeing and high performance; (2) employees who are medium low in wellbeing and medium high in performance; (3) employees who are medium high in wellbeing and medium low in performance; and (4) employees who are low in both wellbeing and performance.

When performance is evaluated by the supervisor, there are three clusters: (1) employees who are high in both wellbeing and performance; (2) employees who are high in wellbeing and low in performance; and (3) employees who are low both in both wellbeing and performance.

The results show that there are antagonistic patterns of wellbeing and performance (i.e., happy-unproductive, and in some cases, unhappy-productive). In fact, the results indicate that, on average, over 50% of the respondents belong to these clusters.

3.2.1. Model 1: Hedonic Wellbeing vs. Self-Rated Performance (H-PE).

In Model 1, we consider two variables: hedonic wellbeing and self-rated composite performance rated by the employee. The auto-clustering algorithm indicated a four–cluster solution as the best model because it minimized the BIC value (BIC = 1060.892, BIC change from the previous cluster = −228.184). The average silhouette measure of cohesion and separation was 0.5, indicating fair to good cluster quality. The importance of both predictors was 1.00.

Four clusters emerged (see Figure 1): (1) employees high in hedonic wellbeing ($M = 6.17$, SD = 0.35) and high in self-reported performance ($M = 6.29$, SD = 0.36), i.e., "hH-hPE" ($n = 411$; 24,95%); (2) employees medium low in hedonic wellbeing ($M = 4.97$, SD = 0.49) and medium high in self-reported performance ($M = 6.10$, SD = 0.31), i.e., "mlH-mhPE" ($n = 383$; 23,25%); (3) employees medium high in hedonic wellbeing ($M = 5.45$, $SD = 0.46$) and medium low in self-reported performance ($M = 5.26$, $SD = 0.34$), i.e., "mhH-mlPE" ($n = 578$; 35,09%); and (4) employees low in hedonic wellbeing ($M = 3.82$, $SD = 0.71$) and low in self-reported performance ($M = 4.88$, $SD = 0.69$), i.e., "lH-lPE" ($n = 274$; 16,67%).

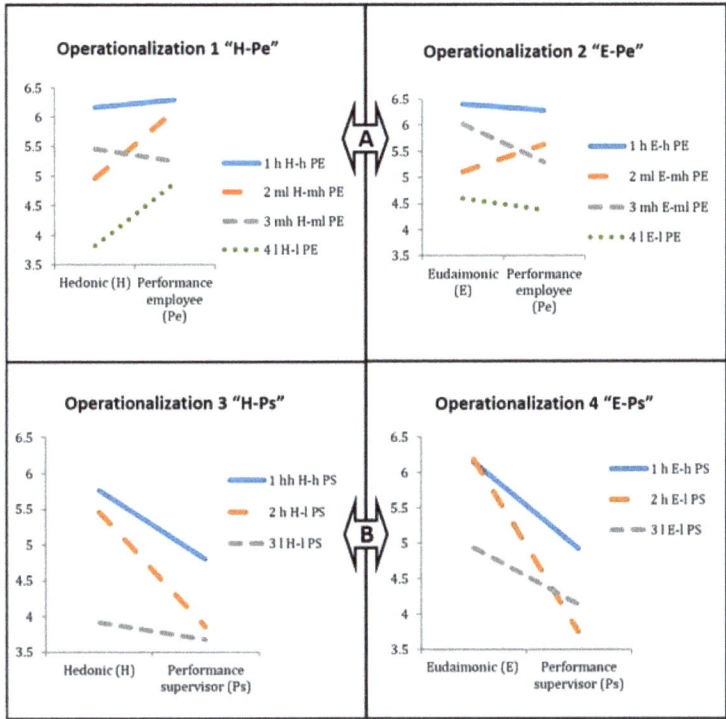

Figure 1. Four cluster analyses of different combinations of well-being dimensions and performance from two sources. h stands for high level; mH stands for medium high level; ml stands for medium low level; l stands for low level. H-Pe stands for Hedonic-Performance (self-rated by the Employee); E-Pe stands for Eudaimonic-Performance (self-rated by the Employee); H-Ps stands for Hedonic-Performance (evaluated by the Supervisor); E-Ps stands for Eudaimonic-Performance (evaluated by the Supervisor); A and B inside the arrows denote different types of comparisons that can be made among the different operationalizations of well-being and performance within the "happy-productive" worker framework.

3.2.2. Model 2: Eudaimonic Wellbeing vs. Self-Rated Performance (E-PE).

In Model 2, we consider the following variables: eudaimonic wellbeing and self-rated performance. Although the auto-clustering algorithm indicated a two-cluster solution as the best model, we decided to opt for a four-cluster solution to maintain a similar cluster structure to Operationalization 1, and because the four-cluster solution also presented fair to good quality (BIC = 1067.114, BIC change from the previous cluster = -197.159, average silhouette measure of cohesion and separation = 0.5). The importance of both predictors was 1.00.

Four clusters emerged (see Figure 1): (1) employees high in eudaimonic wellbeing ($M = 6.39$, $SD = 0.41$) and high in self-reported performance ($M = 6.27$, $SD = 0.34$), i.e., "hE-hPE" ($n = 596$, 36%); (2) employees medium low in eudaimonic wellbeing ($M = 5.10$, $SD = 0.40$) and medium high in self-reported performance ($M = 5.63$, $SD = 0.43$), i.e., "mlE-mhPE" ($n = 425$, 26%); (3) employees medium high in eudaimonic wellbeing ($M = 6.02$, $SD = 0.35$) and medium low in self-reported performance ($M = 5.28$, $SD = 0.36$), i.e., "mhE-mlPE" ($n = 474$, 29%); and (4) employees low in eudaimonic wellbeing

($M = 4.60$, $SD = 0.61$) and low in self-reported performance ($M = 4.38$, $SD = 0.45$), i.e., "lE-lPE" ($n = 152$, 9%).

3.2.3. Model 3: Hedonic Wellbeing vs. Performance Evaluated by the Supervisor (H-PS).

In Model 3, we consider two variables: hedonic wellbeing and performance assessed by the supervisor. The auto-clustering algorithm indicated a three-cluster solution as the best model because it minimized the BIC value (807.301, BIC change from the previous cluster = -172.428). The average silhouette measure of cohesion and separation was 0.5, indicating fair to good cluster quality. The importance of the predictors of hedonic wellbeing and performance evaluated by the supervisor is 1.00 and 0.91, respectively.

Three clusters emerged (see Figure 1): (1) employees high in hedonic wellbeing ($M = 5.76$, $SD = 0.57$) and high performance evaluated by the supervisor ($M = 4.80$, $SD = 0.26$), i.e., "hH-hPS" ($n = 334$, 37%); (2) employees high in hedonic wellbeing ($M = 5.46$, $SD = 0.56$) and low in performance evaluated by the supervisor ($M = 3.86$, $SD = 0.36$), i.e., "hH-lPS" ($n = 402$, 44%); and (3) employees low in hedonic wellbeing ($M = 3.91$, $SD = 0.83$) and low in performance evaluated by the supervisor ($M = 3.67$, $SD = 0.86$), i.e., "lH-lPS" ($n = 179$, 20%).

3.2.4. Model 4: Eudaimonic Wellbeing vs. Performance Evaluated by the Supervisor (E-PS).

In Model 4, we consider two variables: eudaimonic wellbeing and performance evaluated by the supervisor. Although the auto-clustering algorithm indicated a four–cluster solution as the best model, we decided to opt for a three-cluster solution to maintain a similar cluster structure to operationalization 3, and because the three-cluster solution also presented fair to good quality (BIC = 786.235, BIC change from the previous cluster = -242.320, average silhouette measure of cohesion and separation = 0.5). The importance of the predictors of eudaimonic wellbeing and performance evaluated by the supervisor was 1.00 and 0.81, respectively.

The three clusters identified are (see Figure 1): (1) employees high in eudaimonic wellbeing ($M = 6.14$, $SD = 0.52$) and high performance evaluated by the supervisor ($M = 4.92$, $SD = 0.14$), i.e., "hE-hPS" ($n = 240$, 26%); (2) employees high in eudaimonic wellbeing ($M = 6.19$, $SD = 0.45$) and low in performance evaluated by the supervisor ($M = 3.75$, $SD = 0.56$), i.e., "hE-lPS" ($n = 416$, 46%); and (3) employees low in eudaimonic wellbeing ($M = 4.93$, $SD = 0.52$) and low in performance evaluated by the supervisor ($M = 4.14$, $SD = 0.55$), i.e., "lE-lPS" ($n = 259$, 28%).

3.3. Profiles of (un)Happy-(un)Productive Workers in Different Operationalizations of Wellbeing and Performance

In the following section, we try to reveal on whether it is helpful to obtain different profiles of (un)happy–(un)productive workers on the basis of different operationalizations of wellbeing and performance. If the individuals remain in the same or an equivalent category regardless of the variables considered to create the groups, it would be sufficient to consider only one operationalization. In order to analyze this, we compare Models 1 and 2 (both with four clusters) and Models 3 and 4 (both with three clusters). Other comparisons do not make sense because the number of clusters is different. In fact, a different number of clusters depending on the performance measure (self-rated or evaluated by the supervisor) would mean that this operationalization is important.

In order to shed light on this issue, we present the results of the analysis of how many individuals belonging to a specific cluster in one operationalization (e.g., hH-hPE) belong to the same cluster in a different operationalization (e.g., hE-hPE), as well as how many participants belonging to one cluster in one operationalization (e.g., hH-hPS) belong to a different cluster in another operationalization (e.g., hE-lPS). The clusters found with the four types of operationalizations of the variables (dimensions of wellbeing and two sources of information about performance) can be found in the Figure 1. The results show that a large number of employees do not belong to analogous clusters in different operationalizations of wellbeing and performance. This result means that some employees are classified as both unhappy in a hedonic way and, simultaneously, happy in an eudaimonic way (and vice-versa).

3.3.1. Comparison A (Model 1–Model 2): Hedonic–Employee-Rated Performance (H-PE) vs. Eudaimonic–Employee-Rated Performance (E-PE).

If the whole sample is considered, 50.6% of the respondents belong to a homologous cluster in both the H-PE and E-PE models. This means that about half of the employees had comparable wellbeing and performance profiles in both models. They have similar profiles in terms of both kinds of wellbeing. Interestingly, the other half of the employees (49.4%) do not belong to homologous clusters, which means that they belong to a cluster that suggests that they are unhappy in a hedonic way and, simultaneously, to a cluster that suggests that they are happy in an eudaimonic way, or vice versa.

3.3.2. Comparison B (Model 3–Model 4): Hedonic–Supervisor-Rated Performance (H-PS) vs. Eudaimonic–Supervisor-Rated Performance (E-PS)

Almost two thirds of the respondents (63.9%) belong to a homologous cluster in the H-PS and E-PS models, whereas 36.1% of the respondents belong to clusters with different profiles depending of the operationalization of wellbeing. This means that almost a third of the participants could be simultaneously happy in a hedonic way and unhappy in an eudaimonic way, or vice-versa, at a certain level of performance evaluated by the supervisor.

3.4. Demographic Variables as Significant Antecedents of the Wellbeing—Performance Classification.

As indicated previously, we used multidimensional logistic regression to explain cluster membership based on the demographic covariates. The odds ratios for all the models are displayed in Tables 3–6. An odds ratio greater than 1 implies that a person in a given category has greater odds of belonging to a cluster than a person in the reference category (in the case of variables with 2 categories) or than the average of all the subjects in the study (in the case of variables with more than 2 categories). An odds ratio below 1 suggests reduced odds. We identified different demographic predictors when different operationalizations of wellbeing (hedonic-eudaimonic) and performance (self- or supervisor-evaluated) are considered.

Table 3. Multinomial logistic regression analysis of factors associated with the clusters. Model 1: Hedonic (H) Performance employee (PE).

Predictors	(Cluster 1)				(Cluster 2)				(Cluster 3)				(Cluster 4)		
	2 OR (95% CI)	3 OR (95% CI)	4 OR (95% CI)	1 OR (95% CI)	3 OR (95% CI)	4 OR (95% CI)	1 OR (95% CI)	2 OR (95% CI)	4 OR (95% CI)	1 OR (95% CI)	2 OR (95% CI)	3 OR (95% CI)
Sector (0 service / 1 production)		0.55 ** (0.37–0.82)	0.61 * (0.39–0.96)		0.49 *** (0.33–0.73)	0.54 ** (0.34–0.85)	1.8 ** (1.22–2.67)	2.03 *** (1.38–3.01)		1.64 * (1.04–2.58)	1.85 ** (1.17–2.91)	
Gender (0 female / 1 male)			1.61 ** (1.11–2.31)			1.44 * (1.00–2.08)			1.62 ** (1.15–2.28)	0.62 ** (0.43–0.90)	0.69 * (0.48–1.00)	0.62 ** (0.44–0.87)
Seniority (0 <5 years / 1 >5 years)	1.37 * (0.99–1.91)			0.73 * (0.52–1.01)	0.63 ** (0.46–0.85)			1.59 ** (1.17–2.16)	1.4 * (0.99–1.96)			0.72 * (0.51–1.01)
Educational level												
No education or compulsory			1.59 ** (1.13–2.23)		1.36 ** (1.07–1.72)	1.52 * (1.08–2.14)		0.74 ** (0.58–0.94)	1.68 ** (1.22–2.32)			
Professional training or high school												
University degree			0.61 *** (0.46–0.82)			0.54 *** (0.41–0.72)			0.67 ** (0.51–0.87)	1.63 *** (1.23–2.17)	1.83 *** (1.39–2.43)	1.5 ** (1.14–1.95)
Occupational category												
Unqualified manual work												
Technician or administrative	2.04 *** (1.55–2.69)	2.16 *** (1.67–2.80)	2.37 *** (1.69–3.32)	0.49 *** (0.37–0.65)			0.46 *** (0.36–0.60)			0.42 *** (0.30–0.59)		
Highly qualified professional												
Manager	0.53 ** (0.32–0.86)	0.51 ** (0.32–0.81)	0.33 ** (0.16–0.68)	1.89 ** (1.16–3.07)			1.96 ** (1.23–3.13)			3.07 ** (1.48–6.38)		

Reference cluster is in brackets. Cluster 1: h H- h PE; Cluster 2: ml H-mh PE; Cluster 3: mh H-ml PE; Cluster 4: l H-l PE; OR: odds ratio; CI: confidence interval; * $p \leq 0.05$, ** $p \leq 0.01$, *** $p \leq 0.001$.

Table 4. Multinomial logistic regression analysis of factors associated with the clusters. Model 2: Eudaimonic (E) Performance employee (PE).

Predictors	(Cluster 1)			(Cluster 2)			(Cluster 3)			(Cluster 4)		
	2 OR (95% CI)	3 OR (95% CI)	4 OR (95% CI)	1 OR (95% CI)	3 OR (95% CI)	4 OR (95% CI)	1 OR (95% CI)	2 OR (95% CI)	4 OR (95% CI)	1 OR (95% CI)	2 OR (95% CI)	3 OR (95% CI)
Sector (0 service / 1 production)	0.62 ** (0.43–0.90)	0.57 ** (0.40–0.82)	0.29 *** (0.15–0.55)	1.75 ** (1.22–2.50)		0.47 * (0.24–0.90)			0.51 * (0.26–0.99)	3.42 *** (1.81–6.46)	2.14 * (1.11–4.13)	1.96 * (1.01–3.78)
Gender (0 female / 1 male)	1.56 ** (1.16–2.10)		1.69 ** (1.11–2.58)	0.64 ** (0.48–0.86)	0.67 ** (0.49–0.91)			1.49 ** (1.10–2.03)	1.61 * (1.05–2.48)	0.59 ** (0.39–0.90)		0.62 * (0.40–0.95)
Age												
<35 years					1.32 * (1.05–1.68)							
35–50 years						1.37 * (1.02–1.84)		0.75 * (0.60–0.95)			0.73 * (0.54–0.98)	
>50 years	1.4 ** (1.08–1.82)	0.71 ** (0.55–0.92)			0.69 ** (0.43–0.96)	0.64 * (0.43–0.96)	1.44 *** (1.10–1.89)				1.56 * (1.04–2.35)	
Educational level												
No education or compulsory			1.7 ** (1.17–2.46)			1.84 ** (1.25–2.71)			1.82 ** (1.24–2.68)	0.59 ** (0.41–0.85)	0.54 ** (0.37–0.80)	0.55 ** (0.37–0.80)
Professional training or high school												
University degree			0.59 *** (0.43–0.81)			0.60 ** (0.43–0.84)			0.66 ** (0.47–0.92)	1.7 *** (1.23–2.35)	1.66 ** (1.19–2.33)	1.52 ** (1.09–2.12)
Occupational category												
Unqualified manual work	1.85 ** (1.24–2.76)	1.56 * (1.04–2.34)		0.54 ** (0.36–0.80)			0.64 * (0.43–0.96)			0.58 ** (0.39–0.88)		
Technician or administrative	1.3 * (1.01–1.67)	1.31 * (1.02–1.69)	1.71 ** (1.14–2.58)	0.77 * (0.60–0.98)			0.76 ** (0.59–0.98)					
Highly qualified professional	0.47 ** (0.29–0.75)	0.45 ** (0.27–0.74)	0.36 * (0.14–0.91)	2.15 ** (1.33–3.46)			2.22 ** (1.35–3.65)			2.76 * (1.10–6.91)		
Manager												

Reference cluster is in brackets; Cluster 1: h E- h PE; Cluster 2: ml E-mh PE; Cluster 3: mh E-ml PE; Cluster 4: l E-l PE; CI: confidence interval; * $p \leq 0.05$, ** $p \leq 0.01$, *** $p \leq 0.001$.

Table 5. Multinomial logistic regression analysis of factors associated with the clusters. Model 3: Hedonic (H) Performance supervisor (PS).

Predictors	(Cluster 1)		(Cluster 2)		(Cluster 3)	
	2 OR (95% CI)	3 OR (95% CI)	1 OR (95% CI)	3 OR (95% CI)	1 OR (95% CI)	2 OR (95% CI)
Contract (0 temporary / 1 permanent)	1.82 *** (1.26–2.62)		0.55 *** (0.38–0.79)	0.62 * (0.40–0.97)		1.6 * (1.03–2.48)
Occupational category						
Unqualified manual work	1.65 * (1.06–2.57)	2.59 *** (1.55–4.35)	0.61 * (0.39–0.94)		0.39 *** (0.23–0.65)	
Technician or administrative		1.53 * (1.04–2.25)			0.65 * (0.44–0.96)	
Highly qualified professional		0.59 * (0.38–0.93)			1.68 * (1.08–2.63)	
Manager	0.59 * (0.34–1.01)	0.42 * (0.18–0.97)	1.7 * (0.99–2.93)		2.36 * (1.03–5.41)	

Table 6. Multinomial logistic regression analysis of factors associated with the clusters. Model 4: Eudaimonic (E) Performance supervisor (PS).

Predictors	(Cluster 1)		(Cluster 2)		(Cluster 3)	
	2 OR (95% CI)	3 OR (95% CI)	1 OR (95% CI)	3 OR (95% CI)	1 OR (95% CI)	2 OR (95% CI)
Sector (0 service / 1 production)		0.46 ** (0.26–0.81)		0.57 * (0.34–0.94)	2.18 ** (1.23–3.86)	1.76 * (1.07–2.92)
Gender (0 female / 1 male)		1.56 * (1.00–2.44)		1.93 *** (1.30–2.86)	0.64 * (0.41–1.00)	0.52 *** (0.35–0.77)
Contract (0 temporary / 1 permanent)	2.2 *** (1.46–3.31)	2.06 ** (1.29–3.28)	0.45 *** (0.30–0.69)		0.48 ** (0.30–0.77)	
Age						
<35 years						
35–50 years	0.68 ** (0.51–0.91)	0.68 * (0.50–0.93)	1.47 ** (1.10–1.95)	0.72 * (0.54–0.96)	1.46 * (1.07–2.00)	1.39 * (1.04–1.86)
>50 years		1.66 * (1.07–2.58)			0.6 * (0.39–0.94)	
Occupational category						
Unqualified manual work	1.89 * (1.11–3.20)	2.63 *** (1.50–4.63)	0.53 * (0.31–0.90)		0.38 *** (0.22–0.67)	
Technician or administrative						
Highly qualified professional						
Manager	0.55 * (0.30–0.99)	0.44 * (0.22–0.89)	1.83 * (1.01–3.34)		2.28 * (1.13–4.63)	

Reference cluster is in brackets; Cluster 1: h E- h PE; Cluster 2: h E-l PE; Cluster 3: l E-l PE; OR: odds ratio; CI: confidence interval; * $p \leq 0.05$, ** $p \leq 0.01$, *** $p \leq 0.001$.

3.4.1. Multidimensional Logistic Regression: Model 1 (H-PE)

The multinomial logistic regression analyses identified five predictors that explain cluster membership: the organization's sector, gender, seniority in the position, educational level, and occupational category (see Table 3). The results show that the model has a good fit ($-2 \log$ LR = 679.06, X^2 = 129.83, df = 24, $p \leq 0.001$) (with LR being the likelihood ratio). The probability of having high wellbeing and high performance is greater in the production sector and for managers. The probability of having medium low wellbeing and medium high performance is greater in the production sector, for people with more than 5 years of seniority, and for technicians/administrative work. The probability of having medium high wellbeing and medium low performance is greater in the services sector, for people with less than 5 years of seniority, with professional training or high school, and for technicians/administrative workers. Finally, the probability of having low wellbeing and low performance is greater in the services sector, for men, with no education or compulsory education, and for technicians/administrative work.

Comparing Clusters 1 (high levels) and 4 (low levels), the production sector, women, people with a university degree, and managers are more likely to be in Cluster 1, whereas the services sector, men, people with no education or compulsory education, and technicians/administrative workers are more likely to be in Cluster 4.

3.4.2. Multidimensional Logistic Regression: Model 2 (E-PE)

The multinomial logistic regression analyses identified five predictors that explain cluster membership: the organization's sector, gender, age, educational level, and occupational category (see Table 4). The results show that the model has a good fit ($-2 \log$ LR = 777.45, X^2 = 99.68, df = 27, $p \leq 0.001$) The probability of having high wellbeing and high performance is greater in the production sector, women, and managers. The probability of having medium low wellbeing and medium high performance is greater for men, people over 50 years old, and unqualified manual workers or technicians/administrative workers. The probability of having medium high wellbeing and medium low performance is greater for women, and for unqualified manual workers or technicians/administrative workers. Finally, the probability of having low wellbeing and low performance is greater for the services sector, men, people with no education or compulsory education, and technicians/administrative workers.

Comparing Clusters 1 (high levels) and 4 (low levels), results are similar to those in Operationalization 1. The production sector, women, people with university degrees, and managers are more likely to be in Cluster 1, whereas the services sector, men, people with no education or compulsory education, and technicians/administrative workers are more likely to be in Cluster 4.

3.4.3. Multidimensional Logistic Regression: Model 3 (H-PS)

The multinomial logistic regression analyses identified two predictors that explain cluster membership: type of contract and occupational category (see Table 5). The results show that the model has a good fit ($-2 \log$ LR = 68.14, X^2 = 38.70, df = 8, $p \leq 0.001$). The probability of having high wellbeing and high performance is greater for people with a temporary contract and for highly qualified professionals or managers. The probability of having high wellbeing and low performance is greater for people with a permanent contract and people who do unqualified manual work. Finally, the probability of having low wellbeing and low performance is greater for people with a temporary contract and for unqualified manual workers or technicians/administrative workers.

Comparing Clusters 1 (high levels) and 3 (low levels), highly qualified professionals or managers are more likely to be in Cluster 1, whereas unqualified manual workers or technicians/administrative workers are more likely to be in Cluster 3.

3.4.4. Multidimensional Logistic Regression: Model 4 (E-PS)

The multinomial logistic regression analyses identified five predictors that explain cluster membership: the organization's sector, gender, type of contract, age, and occupational category (see Table 6). The results show that the model has a good fit ($-2 \log LR = 358.37$, $X^2 = 60.39$, $df = 16$, $p \leq 0.001$). The probability of having high wellbeing and high performance is greater in the production sector, women, people between 35-50 years old, people with a temporary contract, and managers. The probability of having high wellbeing and low performance is greater in the production sector, women, people under 35 years old, with a permanent contract, and who do unqualified manual work. Finally, the probability of having low wellbeing and low performance is greater for the services sector, men, people over 50 years old, with a permanent contract, and who do unqualified manual work.

Comparing Clusters 1 (high levels) and 3 (low levels), the production sector, women, people with a temporary contract, between 35–50 years old, and managers are more likely to be in Cluster 1, whereas the services sector, men, people with a permanent contract, over 50 years old, and who do unqualified manual work are more likely to be in Cluster 3.

4. Discussion

The aim of the present study was to revisit the happy productive worker model, extending it to consider not just the synergies between happiness and productivity, but also the antagonistic relations between these two constructs. Moreover, we aimed to clarify the implications of different operationalizations of relevant theoretically-based constructs for the model. Finally, we aimed to identify demographic antecedents for each cluster solution. In this way, this work has addressed important limitations of the happy-productive worker model by incorporating both the hedonic and eudaimonic components of wellbeing, considering different aspects of job performance as well as their different sources of evaluation, and focusing not just on the synergies between the two constructs (happiness and productivity), but also on the antagonistic relations, an issue that has hardly been considered in the research based on the model.

The results support a different way to specify and expand the happy-productive worker model. Indeed, by analyzing the relationships between different constructs, we are not taking a positive relationship that leads to being a "happy-productive" or "unhappy-unproductive" worker for granted. The present research has also contemplated a negative relationship between constructs that would appear on a daily basis and that would lead to being "happy-unproductive" or "unhappy-productive" at work. In this study, we provide an affirmative response to Research Question 1, which asks whether "employees show different patterns considering the antagonist relation beyond the traditional synergetic relation between performance and wellbeing (i.e., happy-productive)". In fact, we have found antagonist patterns of wellbeing and performance (i.e., happy-unproductive and, in some cases, unhappy-productive) that are well represented in our sample. We found these alternative patterns by taking into account different operationalizations of wellbeing (i.e., hedonic, eudaimonic) and performance (i.e., self-rated, evaluated by the supervisor). In fact, the results indicate that, on average, over 50% of the respondents belong to the unhappy-productive/happy-unproductive clusters, which suggests that it is important to consider the antagonistic patterns of wellbeing and performance when re-defining the happy-productive worker thesis. Thus, we contribute to filling the gap identified by Warr and Nielsen [51], who pointed out that it is important to learn more about individuals who are outside the happy-productive pattern by considering additional measures of performance and wellbeing.

In fact, Research Question 2 asks whether the same employees belong to the same patterns of wellbeing and performance in their different operationalizations. The results show that a large number of employees do not belong to analogous clusters in different operationalizations of wellbeing and performance, which means that some employees are classified as unhappy in a hedonic way and, simultaneously, happy in an eudaimonic way (and vice-versa). This result draws our attention to the complexity of the phenomenon of wellbeing and the importance of considering both the hedonic and eudaimonic dimensions in studies on wellbeing. It clearly shows that merely considering the hedonic aspect of wellbeing provides only half the picture. We believe future research should more thoroughly investigate the antecedents and outcomes for "hedonically-happy" and "eudaimonically unhappy" employees.

In addition, the results suggest that employees' self-rated performance is often not reflected in their supervisor's evaluation of their performance. This draws our attention to the importance of considering more than one source of evaluation of work performance in order to obtain valid information about the employees' task performance, extra-role performance, and creativity. It is possible that the disparity in the evaluation of the employees' performance level is due to the fact that employees might be more lenient when self-rating their general performance [38]. It is also possible that, when assessing their own performance, employees' responses reflect not only their past behavior, but also their expectations of current and future behavior [58]. We think it would be interesting to investigate more in depth the reasons for the differences between employees' ratings of their own performance and the ratings given by their direct supervisors.

Finally, the results provide an affirmative response to Research Question 3 about whether there are any demographic variables that play a role as antecedents of the clusters in different operationalizations of the "happy-productive" worker. The existence of differences in the demographic variables between clusters provides yet another way to validate the clusters and the different operationalizations of wellbeing and performance. This means that it is reasonable to expand the study of employees and their different outcomes at work to different patterns of wellbeing and performance, and include alternative configurations of "happy-unproductive" and "unhappy-productive" clusters.

Following the recommendations of Warr and Nielsen [51], we identified a number of situational and personal features associated with membership in each profile when additional measures of wellbeing and performance are considered. Our study examines whether personal features, such as gender, age, and educational level, and situational features, such as sector, type of contract, occupational category, and seniority in the position, play a predictor role in the different profiles obtained, based on the operationalizations of wellbeing (hedonic-eudaimonic) and performance (self- or supervisor- evaluated) considered. The exploratory results provide relevant information showing that occupational category is the only variable with a predictor role in the four models studied. Moreover, another situational variable (sector) and a personal variable (gender) significantly predict the profiles in three of the four models studied. Interestingly, the type of contract is a significant antecedent in the two models in which the supervisors' performance assessment is considered, whereas the educational level is a significant antecedent in the two models where self-assessed performance is considered. More specifically, women, workers in the production sector, and management or highly qualified professionals are more likely to be included in the happy-productive profile, whereas men, workers in the services sector, employees with a low education level, and technicians/administrative workers are more likely to be included in the unhappy-unproductive cluster.

We also identified the main features of employees included in the happy-unproductive profiles. These features differ across the four models studied. The "high hedonic/low performance (self-rated)" pattern is populated more by employees from the services sector with professional training and technician-administrative jobs. In the case of the "high eudaimonic/low performance (self-rated)" pattern, it is mostly composed of women and employees in unqualified or technician/administrative jobs. It is interesting to note that, when we look at the two similar profiles generated using supervisor ratings of performance, the employees with a higher probability of belonging to these patterns (both hedonic and eudaimonic) have permanent contracts and are employed in unqualified or manual jobs. Finally, it is interesting to identify the features that more often characterize employees included in the unhappy/productive profiles. The employees included in the "low hedonic/high performance (self-rated)" profile work in the production sector, have seniority (>5 years) and professional education, and work in technician-administrative jobs. The employees included in the "low eudaimonic/high performance (self-rated)" profile are mostly men over 50 years old working in unqualified-manual or technician-administrative jobs. Considering this complex picture of personal and situational characteristics associated with the different profiles obtained with different types of wellbeing and performance, we can conclude that the different models are not redundant, and different types of wellbeing and different sources of performance need to be considered to better understand the happy-productive worker model. Further research is needed to confirm the predictive power of the variables studied and extend the study by including other personal and situational variables, in order to better describe the employees in each profile.

In sum, the present study addresses a number of limitations of the happy productive worker thesis, and it sheds light on a number of issues that may clarify the previous inconsistencies of the model. First, this study included both the hedonic and eudaimonic aspects of wellbeing, coinciding with recent conceptualizations of wellbeing as having both pleasurable and meaningful components [3–5]. The identification of the hedonic "happy-productive" and "unhappy-unproductive" patterns coincides with studies indicating that there is a positive relationship between hedonic wellbeing and performance [13–18]. The identification of the "unhappy-productive" pattern agrees with research that shows a negative relationship between positive affect and the dimensions of performance [48]. Simultaneously, the identification of the eudaimonic "happy-productive" pattern supports research that suggests a synergetic relationship between eudaimonic wellbeing and performance [31]. These patterns support previous research showing that daily increases in perceived meaning at work were related to employees' increased focus on tasks and greater exploratory behavior [31]. Second, this study considers different dimensions and sources of evaluation of employees' performance. On the one hand, we operationalize job performance as consisting of different facets or dimensions (i.e., in-role performance, extra-role performance, creative performance) that can help to capture its manifestations. On the other hand, we consider two sources of information about performance: self-rated performance and performance rated by the direct supervisor. Third, the present research analyzes alternative configurations that have not been considered in the happy-productive worker thesis. It shows the importance of these alternative configurations, reflected by the number of employees who belong to the "happy-unproductive" and "unhappy-productive" clusters (over 50% on average), suggesting that the work reality is built on these antagonistic patterns, as well as on the synergetic ones. Thus, antagonistic patterns should not be neglected in future research. Finally, this study has identified a number of individual and situational features that significantly distinguish the different profiles in each of the operationalizations of the happy-productive worker model.

Limitations

The current paper's findings should be interpreted cautiously in light of several potential limitations. A limitation of the study is that most of the sample belonged to the services sector, although some of the sample is from the production sector, including areas such as construction. This limitation questions the representativeness of the results of underrepresented sectors. Services and production sectors could certainly vary in their different types of procedures and practices, such as performance evaluation or health and wellbeing promotion. The sample is more balanced in terms of gender, age, job category, or type of contract. In any case, this study represents a first approach to understanding the diversity in the patterns of relationships between performance and wellbeing in organizations. A second limitation is the fact that self-rated performance and performance rated by supervisors were not assessed with the same scale, due to the difficulties in obtaining responses from supervisors about all their subordinates (in fact, we had a high reduction in the sample when gathering data). This situation can raise some doubts about the reasons for the differences in performance-wellbeing patterns when each of the measurement methods is used. Thus, these differences could be due to different performance measures rather than to different informants. However, both measures can be considered global performance measures. Self-rated performance is a composite measure that includes the basic components of performance [34]. Performance rated by the supervisor measures global performance considering three global indicators: general performance, quality, and achievement of objectives.

5. Conclusions

This study shows that the relationship between wellbeing and performance is more complex than the HPWT proposes. Different operationalizations of these constructs need to be considered. Moreover, we found that a large percentage of respondents are grouped under the happy-unproductive or the unhappy-productive profiles. The results also indicate that employees can be unhappy in a hedonic way and, simultaneously, happy in an eudaimonic way (and vice versa). Finally, we show that there are several significant antecedents of the patterns, in terms of demographic variables, in different operationalizations of wellbeing and performance.

Future studies on the antecedents and consequences of these patterns of wellbeing and performance can be relevant for organizational practice because they might help to identify a broader scope of employees' profiles regarding their performance and wellbeing and the circumstances in which they experience synergies and antagonisms between these two important constructs.

In conclusion, the results of this study draw our attention to the fact that there can be different typologies of "happy-productive" workers that may take into account both hedonic and eudaimonic dimensions of wellbeing, as well as two different informants about the employees" work performance. As we can see, a large percentage of workers do not pertain to the conventional "happy-productive" or "unhappy-unproductive" patterns, but rather to the antagonistic quadrants of "unhappy but productive" and "happy but unproductive".

Author Contributions: Conceptualization, J.M.P, N.T., I.R.-M. and M.W.K.; data gathering and databases, N.T. and I.R.-M.; methodology, J.M..P, M.W.K. and I.R.-M.; formal analysis, M.W.K. and I.R.-M.; writing—original draft preparation, M.W.K. and I.R.-M.; writing—review and editing, J.M.P. and N.T.; funding acquisition, J.M.P. and N.T.

Funding: The present study was funded by the MINECO/FEDER Research agencies: project PSI2012-36557 funded by DGICYT and the project PSI2015-64862-R (MINECO/FEDER)

Conflicts of Interest: The authors declare no conflicts of interest.

References

1. Diener, E. Subjective well-being. The science of happiness and a proposal for a national index. *Am. Psychol.* **2000**, *55*, 34–43. [CrossRef] [PubMed]
2. Ryff, C.D. Psychological well-being in adult life. *Curr. Dir. Psychol. Sci.* **1995**, *4*, 99–104. [CrossRef]
3. Dolan, P. *Happiness by Design*; Hudson Street Press: New York, NY, USA, 2014.
4. Keyes, C.L.M.; Shmotkin, D.; Ryff, C.D. Optimizing well-being: The empirical encounter of two traditions. *J. Pers. Soc. Psychol.* **2002**, *82*, 1007–1022. [CrossRef] [PubMed]
5. Linley, P.A.; Maltby, J.; Wood, A.M.; Osborne, G.; Hurling, R. Measuring happiness: The higher order factor structure of subjective and psychological well-being measures. *Pers. Individ. Differ.* **2009**, *47*, 878–884. [CrossRef]
6. Ryan, R.M.; Deci, E.L. On happiness and human potentials: A review of research on hedonic and eudaimonic well-being. *Annu. Rev. Psychol.* **2001**, *52*, 141–166. [CrossRef] [PubMed]
7. Cropanzano, R.; Wright, T.A. When a "happy" worker is really a "productive" worker: A review and further refinement of the happy-productive worker thesis. *Consult. Psychol. J. Pract. Res.* **2001**, *53*, 182–199. [CrossRef]
8. Wright, T.A.; Cropanzano, R.; Bonett, D.G. The moderating role of employee positive well being on the relation between job satisfaction and job performance. *J. Occup. Health Psychol.* **2007**, *12*, 93–104. [CrossRef] [PubMed]
9. Beal, D.J.; Weiss, H.M.; Barros, E.; Macdermid, S.M. An Episodic Process Model of Affective Influences on Performance. *J. Appl. Psychol.* **2005**, *90*, 1054–1068. [CrossRef]
10. Baptiste, N.R. Tightening the link between employee wellbeing at work and performance—A new dimension for HRM. *Manag. Decis.* **2008**, *46*, 284–309. [CrossRef]

11. Schulte, P.; Vainio, H.M.D. Well-being at work—Overview and perspective. *Scand. J. Work Environ. Health* **2010**, *36*, 422–429. [CrossRef] [PubMed]
12. Wright, T.; Cropanzano, R. Psychological well-being and job satisfaction as predictors of performance. *J. Occup. Health Psychol.* **2000**, *5*, 84–94. [CrossRef] [PubMed]
13. Mofoluwake, A.; Oluremi, A. Job satisfaction, organizational stress and employee performance: A study of NAPIMS. *IFE Psychol.* **2013**, *21*, 75–82.
14. Fogaça, N.; Junior, F.A.C. Is "Happy Worker" More Productive. *Manag. Stud.* **2016**, *4*, 149–160.
15. Hosie, P.; Willemyns, M.; Sevastos, P. The impact of happiness on managers' contextual and task performance. *Asia Pac. J. Hum. Resour.* **2012**, *50*, 268–287. [CrossRef]
16. Böckerman, P.; Ilmakunnas, P. The job satisfaction-productivity nexus: A study using matched survey and register data. *Ind. Labor Relat. Rev.* **2010**, *65*, 244–262. [CrossRef]
17. Foo, M.-D.; Uy, M.A.; Baron, R.A. How do feelings influence effort? An empirical study of entrepreneurs' affect and venture effort. *J. Appl. Psychol.* **2009**, *94*, 1086–1094. [CrossRef] [PubMed]
18. Seo, M.-G.; Bartunek, J.M.; Feldman Barret, L. Conceptual Model. *J. Organ. Behav.* **2010**, *31*, 951–968. [PubMed]
19. Zelenski, J.M.; Murphy, S.A.; Jenkins, D.A. The happy-productive worker thesis revisited. *J. Happiness Stud.* **2008**, *9*, 521–537. [CrossRef]
20. Binnewies, C.; Wörnlein, S.C. What makes a creative day? A diary study on the interplay between affect, job stressors, and job control. *J. Organ. Behav.* **2011**, *32*, 589–607. [CrossRef]
21. Rothbard, N.P.; Wilk, S.L. Waking up on the right or wrong side of the bed: Start-of-workday mood, work events, employee affect, and performance. *Acad. Manag. J.* **2011**, *54*, 959–980. [CrossRef]
22. Bowling, N.A. Is the job satisfaction-job performance relationship spurious? A meta-analytic examination. *J. Vocat. Behav.* **2007**, *71*, 167–185. [CrossRef]
23. Iaffaldano, M.T.; Muchinsky, P.M. Job satisfaction and job performance: A meta-analysis. *Psychol. Bull.* **1985**, *97*, 251–273. [CrossRef]
24. Judge, T.A.; Thoresen, C.J.; Bono, J.E.; Patton, G.K. The job satisfaction-job performance relationship: A qualitative and quantitative review. *Psychol. Bull.* **2001**, *127*, 376–407. [CrossRef] [PubMed]
25. Greenberger, D.B.; Strasser, S.; Cummings, L.L.; Dunham, R.B. The impact of personal control on performance and satisfaction. *Organ. Behav. Hum. Decis. Process.* **1989**, *43*, 29–51. [CrossRef]
26. Peiró, J.M.; Ayala, Y.; Tordera, N.; Lorente, L.; Rodríguez, I. Sustainable wellbeing at work: A review and reformulation. *Pap. Psicólogo* **2014**, *35*, 7–16.
27. Rosso, B.D.; Dekas, K.H.; Wrzesniewski, A. On the meaning of work: A theoretical integration and review. *Res. Organ. Behav.* **2010**, *30*, 91–127. [CrossRef]
28. OECD. *OECD Guidelines on Measuring Subjective Well-Being*; OECD Publishing: Paris, France, 2013.
29. Dolan, P.; Layard, R.; Metcalfe, R. *Measuring Subjective Wellbeing for Public Policy*; Office for National Statistics: Newport, UK, 2011.
30. White, M.P.; Dolan, P. Accounting for the richness of daily activities. *Psychol. Sci.* **2009**, *20*, 1000–1008. [CrossRef]
31. Sonnentag, S. Dynamics of well-being. *Annu. Rev. Organ. Psychol. Organ. Behav.* **2015**, *2*, 261–293. [CrossRef]
32. Niessen, C.; Sonnentag, S.; Sach, F. Thriving at work—A diary study. *J. Organ. Behav.* **2012**, *33*, 468–487. [CrossRef]
33. Ford, M.T.; Cerasoli, C.P.; Higgins, J.A.; Decesare, A. Relationships between psychological, physical, and behavioural health and work performance: A review and meta-analysis. *Work Stress* **2011**, *25*, 185–204. [CrossRef]
34. Koopmans, L.; Bernaards, C.M.; Hildebrandt, V.H.; Schaufeli, W.B.; de Vet, H.C.W.; van der Beek, A.J. Conceptual frameworks of individual work performance: A systematic review. *J. Occup. Environ. Med.* **2011**, *53*, 856–866. [CrossRef] [PubMed]
35. LePine, J.A.; Erez, A.; Johnson, D.E. The nature and dimensionality of organizational citizenship behavior: A critical review and meta-analysis. *J. Appl. Psychol.* **2002**, *87*, 52–65. [CrossRef] [PubMed]
36. Oldham, G.R.; Cummings, A. Employee creativity: Personal and contextual factors at work. *Acad. Manag. J.* **1996**, *39*, 607–634.
37. Länsisalmi, H.; Kivimäki, M.; Elovainio, M. Is underutilization of knowledge, skills, and abilities a major barrier to innovation? *Psychol. Rep.* **2004**, *94*, 739–750. [CrossRef] [PubMed]

38. Hosie, P.J.; Sevastos, P. Does the "happy-productive worker" thesis apply to managers? *Int. J. Work Health Manag.* **2009**, *2*, 131–160. [CrossRef]
39. Heidemeier, H.; Moser, K. Self-other agreement in job performance ratings: A meta-analytic test of a process model. *J. Appl. Psychol.* **2009**, *94*, 353–370. [CrossRef] [PubMed]
40. Conway, J.M.; Huffcutt, A.I. Psychometric properties of multisource performance ratings: A meta-analysis of subordinate, supervisor, peer, and self-ratings. *Hum. Perform.* **1997**, *10*, 331–360. [CrossRef]
41. Akkermans, J.; Brenninkmeijer, V.; Van den Bossche, S.N.J.; Blonk, R.W.B.; Schaufeli, W.B. Young and going strong? A longitudinal study on occupational health among young employees of difference educational levels. *Career Dev. Int.* **2013**, *18*, 416–435. [CrossRef]
42. Fisher, C.D.; Noble, C.S. A within-person examination of correlates of performance and emotions while working. *Hum. Perform.* **2004**, *17*, 145–168. [CrossRef]
43. Seo, M.; Ilies, R. Organizational Behavior and Human Decision Processes The role of self-efficacy, goal, and affect in dynamic motivational self-regulation. *Organ. Behav. Hum. Decis. Process.* **2009**, *109*, 120–133. [CrossRef]
44. Harris, C.; Daniels, K.; Briner, R.B. A daily diary study of goals and affective well-being at work. *J. Occup. Organ. Psychol.* **2003**, *76*, 401–410. [CrossRef]
45. Hoppmann, C.A.; Klumb, P.L. Daily management of work and family goals in employed parents. *J. Vocat. Behav.* **2012**, *81*, 191–198. [CrossRef]
46. Scott, B.A.; Colquitt, J.A.; Paddock, E.L.; Judge, T.A. A daily investigation of the role of manager empathy on employee well-being. *Organ. Behav. Hum. Decis. Process.* **2010**, *113*, 127–140. [CrossRef]
47. Hakanen, J.J.; Perhoniemi, R.; Toppinen-Tammer, S. Positive gain spirals at work: From job resources to work engagement, personal initiative and work-unit innovativeness. *J. Vocat. Behav.* **2008**, *73*, 78–91. [CrossRef]
48. Baron, R.A.; Hmieleski, K.M.; Henry, R.A. Entrepreneurs' dispositional positive affect: The potential benefits and potential costs of being "up". *J. Bus. Ventur.* **2012**, *27*, 310–324. [CrossRef]
49. Bledow, R.; Rosing, K.; Frese, M. A dynamic perspective on affect and creativity. *Acad. Manag. J.* **2013**, *56*, 432–450. [CrossRef]
50. Ayala, Y.; Peiró, J.M.; Tordera, N.; Lorente, L.; Yeves, J. Job satisfaction and innovative performance in young Spanish employees: Testing new patterns in the Happy-Productive Worker Thesis. A discriminant study. *J. Happiness Stud.* **2017**, *18*, 1377–1401. [CrossRef]
51. Warr, P.; Nielsen, K. Wellbeing and work performance. In *Handbook of Well-Being*; Diener, E., Oishi, S., Tay, L., Eds.; DEF Publishers: Salt Lake City, UT, USA, 2018.
52. Cooper, C.L.; Rout, U.; Faragher, B. Mental health, job satisfaction, and job stress among general practitioners. *Br. Med. J.* **1989**, *298*, 366–370. [CrossRef]
53. Ryff, C.D. Happiness is everything, or is it? explorations on the meaning of psychological well-being. *J. Personal. Soc. Psychol.* **1989**, *57*, 1069–1081. [CrossRef]
54. Williams, L.; Anderson, S. Job Satisfaction and Organizational Commitment as Predictors of organizational citizenship and in-role behaviors. *J. Manag.* **1991**, *17*, 601–617. [CrossRef]
55. Mackenzie, S.B.; Podsakoff, P.M.; Podsakoff, N.P. Challenge oriented organizational citizenship behaviors and organizational effectiveness: Do challenge-oriented behaviors really have an impact on the organization's bottom line. *Pers. Psychol.* **2011**, *64*, 559–592. [CrossRef]
56. Chiu, T.; Fang, D.; Chen, J.; Wang, Y.; Jeris, C. A robust and scalable clustering algorithm for mixed type attributes in large database environment. In Proceedings of the 7th ACM SIGKDD International Conference in Knowledge Discovery and Data Mining, Association for Computing Machinery, San Francisco, CA, USA, 26–29 August 2001; pp. 263–268.
57. Mooi, E.; Sarstedt, M. Cluster analysis. In *A Concise Guide to Market Research*; Mooi, E., Sarstedt, M., Eds.; Springer: Heidelberg, Germany, 2010; pp. 237–284.
58. Kent, P.; Jensen, R.K.; Kongsted, A. A comparison of three clustering methods for finding subgroups in MRI, SMS or clinical data: SPSS TwoStep Cluster analysis, Latent Gold and SNOB. *BMC Med. Res. Methodol.* **2014**, *14*, 113. [CrossRef] [PubMed]

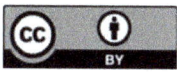

© 2019 by the authors. Licensee MDPI, Basel, Switzerland. This article is an open access article distributed under the terms and conditions of the Creative Commons Attribution (CC BY) license (http://creativecommons.org/licenses/by/4.0/).

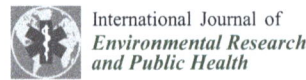

Article

Trust in the Work Environment and Cardiovascular Disease Risk: Findings from the Gallup-Sharecare Well-Being Index

Toni Alterman [1,*], Rebecca Tsai [1], Jun Ju [1] and Kevin M. Kelly [2]

1. Division of Surveillance, Hazard Evaluations and Field Studies, National Institute for Occupational Safety and Health, CDC, (MS-R17), 1090 Tusculum Ave, Cincinnati, OH 45226, USA; vht5@cdc.gov (R.T.); jnj7@cdc.gov (J.J.)
2. UI Healthier Workforce Center, The University of Iowa, UI Research Park, IREH #106, Iowa City, IA 52242, USA; kevin-kelly@uiowa.edu
* Correspondence: talterman@cdc.gov; Tel.: +1-513-841-4210

Received: 30 November 2018; Accepted: 9 January 2019; Published: 15 January 2019

Abstract: This study examined associations between trust, an important aspect of workplace social capital, with seven cardiovascular disease (CVD) risk factors (American Heart Association Life's Simple 7 (LS7)): smoking, obesity, low physical activity, poor diet, diabetes, high cholesterol, and high blood pressure. Data are from the U.S. Gallup-Sharecare Well-Being Index (2010–2012), a nationally representative telephone survey of U.S. workers (n = 412,884). The independent variable was the response to a work environment (WE) question as to whether their supervisor always creates an open and trusting environment. Regression models were adjusted for demographic characteristics with each of the LS7 CVD risk factors as dependent variables. Twenty-one percent of workers reported that their supervisor did not create an open and trusting environment. Trust was associated with increased adjusted odds of having many of the LS7 CVD risk factors. Among those workers whose supervisor created a mistrustful environment, the odds ratios were greatest (>20%) for having four or more of the LS7 CVD risk factors.

Keywords: cardiovascular disease; work environment; social capital; trust; Total Worker Health®; health behaviors; job stress

---

1. Introduction

Cardiovascular disease (CVD) continues to be a costly and significant problem and is the leading cause of death in the United States [1]. Moreover, by 2030, the prevalence of CVD among American adults (20 years of age and older) is expected to increase from 35% to over 40% [2]; direct medical costs of CVD are expected to triple to $818 billion [2,3]. To address these pressing issues, the American Heart Association (AHA) set strategic impact goals to improve cardiovascular health by 20% and achieve a 20% reduction in CVD mortality by 2020 [4–6].

Numerous studies have examined associations between work stress and CVD [7–16]. In addition, many studies have examined associations between work organization and workplace psychosocial factors with CVD and its risk factors [17–24]. However, much of the occupational health literature on CVD has focused on a few select models such as job demand and control [11,19,20]; job demands-resources [25–27]; social support [18]; and effort–reward imbalance [17,23]. In addition, attention has more recently been given to the role of work engagement and cardiovascular reactivity [28] and forms of organizational justice that share some aspects of the effort-reward model [29–33].

Cardiovascular health can be assessed by AHA's My Life Check® Life's Simple 7 (LS7) [4–6]. The AHA defined ideal cardiovascular health by the presence of all four favorable health behaviors (abstinence from smoking within the past year, ideal body mass index (BMI), physically active, and healthy diet) and three favorable health factors (ideal fasting glucose, ideal total cholesterol, and ideal blood pressure). Having ideal levels in all seven components of LS7 can increase life span and reduce healthcare costs [4,5].

Recent literature has focused on the theory of social capital as important in explaining these health behaviors. While there are many definitions of social capital [34–38], this study uses a relational or social cohesion approach suggested by Berkman and Kawachi [39], who define social capital 'as those features of social structures such as levels of interpersonal trust and norms of reciprocity and mutual aid—which act as resources for individuals and facilitate collective actions'. Measures of social capital involve examining elements of a relationship, relational networks, levels of trust, and levels of collaborative activity [40].

In the past, literature on associations between social capital and health focused mainly on community, residential, or geographic areas [36,41–43]. More recently, workplaces have been seen as important social units where social capital may promote well-being and health and as providing a means of understanding relationships in the workplace [44–48]. A number of hypotheses as to how social capital may act on health behaviors have been proposed; these include providing norms and attitudes that influence health behaviors, and psychosocial mechanisms that promote emotional support and enhance self-esteem [39]. For example, Lindström and Giordano [49] suggest that social capital reduces cigarette smoking by (1) deterring socially 'deviant' behavior; (2) increasing dissemination of positive health messages; and (3) providing a buffer against psychosocial stress'.

Some findings of associations between social capital and health behaviors have been mixed [34,50]. A recent systematic review of 14 prospective studies using a variety of definitions of social capital and different contexts found no association among most social capital dimensions and all-cause mortality, CVD, or cancer [34]. However, definitions of social capital varied among the individual studies reviewed, including dimensions of social participation, social network, civic participation, social support, trust, norms of reciprocity, and sense of community [34]. Other empirical research supports associations between social capital and health, including mental health [42,51,52]; diet [53]; alcohol use [54–56]; physical activity [57–59]; hypertension [60]; and smoking [49,61–63]. A recent study by Nieminen et al. [64] found support for an association between social capital and five health behaviors (smoking, alcohol use, physical activity, vegetable consumption, and sleep). Analyses of data from the Finnish Public Sector Study found that low workplace social capital was associated with the co-occurrence of multiple lifestyle risk factors in cross-sectional analyses, but not in longitudinal analyses [65].

The report of the 2017 Total Worker Health® Workshop [66] identified "perceived working conditions and supervisor support," the bases of worker trust, as important worker-level measures for understanding worker health. Trust is acknowledged as a key principle in the supervisor–subordinate relationship, especially as it as it relates to the distribution of rewards, sanctions, and resources [67] including promotions, pay raises, and job security [68]. Moreover, Schill [69] reminds us that "leaders at all levels set the tone (for Total Worker Health) through their shared commitment to safety, health and well-being". There are many definitions of trust, but for the current study, the authors define trust as a multidimensional psychological state that involves cognitive processes as well as affective and motivational components [68]. For trust to develop, there needs to be understanding, fairness, and mutual respect between the supervisor and subordinate.

It is often difficult and expensive to collect data on work environment and workplace psychosocial factors across multiple worksites and regions. In the U.S., a number of ongoing national surveys, such as the Quality of Worklife [70], the Health and Retirement Survey (HRS) [71], and the 2010 [72] and 2015 National Health Interview Survey (NHIS) [73], have included work organization and workplace psychosocial questions. The Gallup-Sharecare Well-Being Index (WBI) [74] collects data from adults

18 years and older living in the United States, including questions on work environment (WE). A number of studies have used the Gallup survey to look at health and well-being [74–78], but few have specifically focused on the work environment questions associated with social capital in relation to health.

The current study examines whether trust, an important aspects of social capital, is associated with the seven CVD risk factors identified in the AHA LS7 screening tool. Increasing social capital may improve health behaviors and outcomes directly, or in conjunction with workplace prevention and intervention programs. Due to the gender differences in the prevalence, progression, and underlying mechanisms in CVD, results are presented separately for women and men [79].

2. Materials and Methods

2.1. Data Source

Data for this study are based on the Gallup-Sharecare Well-Being Index (WBI) survey conducted between 2010 and 2012 in the United States. Every day, the Gallup Organization conducts computer-assisted telephone interviews (in English or Spanish) with 1000 randomly sampled U.S. adults ($\geq$18 years of age) on political, economic, and well-being topics. Random-digit-dial (RDD) to landlines and cell phones was used to reach wireless-only and wireless-mostly households. Although the response rate is low, 9–11%, it is estimated that the Gallup sample covers more than 95% of the U.S. adult population. Gallup weights data daily to account for disproportionate selection in age, sex, geographic region, gender, education level, ethnicity, race, self-reported location, and phone use status [73].

2.2. Study Population

The sample consists of survey participants interviewed between 2010 and 2012 who reported being currently employed by an employer for at least 30 h per week. Only workers who were employed by an employer were selected because this study focuses on supervisor behavior. In addition, full-time workers (i.e., those working 30 or more hours per week) were selected because results from this study would be more relevant to those who spend a greater proportion of their time at work, than those working part time.

2.3. Measures

Life's Simple 7: The WBI included questions that address the seven cardiovascular health components of the LS7, but are not a complete match to the AHA definition. Figure 1 shows how the authors adapted WBI questions to match AHA's LS7 components. For blood pressure, the WBI asks if the respondent had ever been told by a physician or nurse that they had high blood pressure (yes = high blood pressure). The LS7 defines high blood pressure as >120/80 mm Hg. Similarly, the WBI asks if the respondent had ever been told by a physician or nurse that they had high cholesterol, (yes = high cholesterol). The LS7 defines high cholesterol as total cholesterol >200 mg/dL. Diabetes in the WBI is measured by the response to a question about whether the respondent had been told by a physician or nurse that they had diabetes (yes = diabetes). The LS7 defines diabetes as a fasting plasma glucose >100 mg/dL. The study definition for at-risk BMI (based on self-reported height and weight), or obesity, was BMI $\geq$ 30 kg/m^2; the LS7 definition for at-risk BMI is $\geq$25 kg/m^2. For diet, the WBI asks respondents the number of days per week they consumed five or more servings of fruits or vegetables. For this study, a healthy diet was defined as consuming five or more servings of fruits or vegetables seven days per week; adequate consumption on less than seven days was defined as a poor diet. The LS7's dietary assessment requires additional information such as the amount of fish, sodium, whole grains, and sugary beverages consumed daily or weekly. Similarly, for physical activity, the WBI asks about the number of days of exercise for at least 30 min during the past week, but does not ask about the intensity of physical activity. The LS7 definition includes the amount of vigorous and moderate activities per week. In the current study, meeting physical activity guidelines was defined as exercising for at least 30 min five days per week. Performing less than this was defined as insufficient exercise. In the WBI, smoking is defined as a yes response to a question about whether the respondent smokes. In the LS7, smoking is based on whether the person is a current smoker or quit <12 months ago.

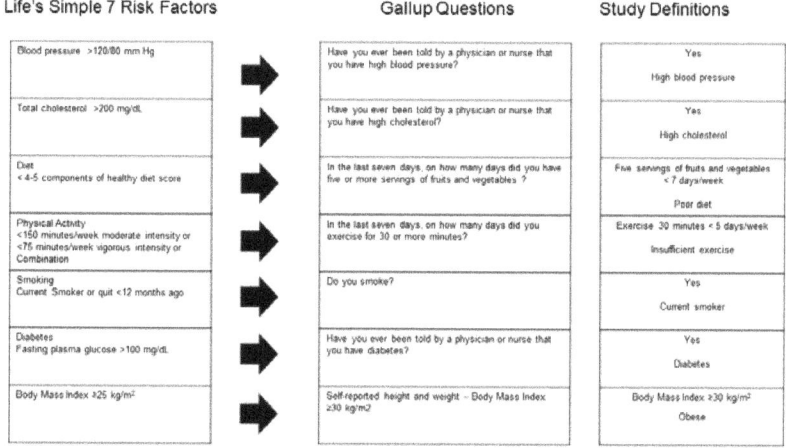

Figure 1. Cross-walk between American Heart Association Life's Simple 7 (LS7) cardiovascular disease (CVD) risk factors and Gallup-Sharecare Well-Being Index.

Work environment: Gallup scientists created a work environment question related to social capital based on their understanding of the literature. Work environment was coded in a negative direction and measured by the question: 'Does your supervisor always create an environment that is trusting and open, or not?' (No = mistrustful environment).

2.4. Data Analysis

All analyses were stratified by gender and calculated using SAS 9.3 (SAS Institute Inc., Cary, NC, USA), using weights provided by Gallup to represent the U.S. population and to account for the complex survey design. Gallup surveyed 1,059,894 individuals between 2010 and 2012, of which 412,884 were full-time employees (working 30 or more hours per week). Responses of 'don't know' or 'refused' were set to missing. Because of a skip pattern, 23,554 (6%) were not asked the open and trusting environment question. Approximately 14% of the sample were missing income data, and 5% or fewer were missing data for the LS7 risk factors. Descriptive statistics were calculated for demographic, LS7, and the trust question. Z-tests for the difference between women and men were calculated. Logistic regression models were run with each of the LS7 CVD risk factors as dependent variables in separate regression models. Odds ratios and 95% confidence intervals were calculated. Confidence intervals excluding 1.0 indicate significance at $p < 0.05$. In addition, a sensitivity analysis was conducted to examine the impact on associations using four or more CVD risk factors as a dependent variable in the regression model. Trust was entered into separate logistic regression models as an independent variable. All models were adjusted for potential confounders including demographic factors: age (years); race/ethnicity (White, Black, Asian, Hispanic, and Other); education (less than high school diploma, high school graduate, technical/some college or associate degree, college degree, and post-graduate degree); marital status (single/never married, married, separated, divorced, widowed, and domestic partner); family income (<$1000/month, $1000–$2999/month, $3000–$4999/month, $5000–$7499/month, and ≥$7500/month) and any health insurance. Due to the large sample size in the current study, we focused on effect sizes (odds ratios) rather than p-values. According to a recent policy statement by the American Statistical Association on *p*-values and statistical significance, any effect, no matter how tiny, can produce a small *p*-value if the sample size is large enough [80].

3. Results

Demographic characteristics: Forty-two percent of the sample were women. Descriptive statistics for workers stratified by gender and trust are presented in Table 1. For both women and men, the largest percent of respondents (72.0% and 72.2%, respectively) were White, Non-Hispanic with a mean age of about 42. More than half of the respondents were married and had either technical training or some college.

Mistrustful environment: Approximately 22% of women and 20.3% of men indicated that their supervisor did not always create an open and trusting environment (Table 1). As shown in Table 1, for both women and men, the highest prevalence of mistrust reported was among workers ages 45–64, (women = 24.4%, men = 23.0%) followed by workers ages 30–44 (women = 22.3%, men = 20.5%). Black women (23.2%), followed by White women (22.4%) had the highest prevalence of reporting that their supervisor does not create an open and trusting environment, compared with women of other races/ethnicities (Asian, Hispanic, Other). White men (21.1%) followed by Black men (20.6%) reported higher prevalence of a mistrustful environment. Prevalence of a mistrustful environment was higher for women with increasing levels of education (highest for those with college or post-graduate education, 25.2%). Men with technical training or some college/associate degree had a slightly higher prevalence (20.9%) of a mistrustful environment. Divorced women (26.8%) and men (24.7%) had the highest prevalence of reporting a mistrustful work environment. Prevalence by income was similar for both women and men, with slightly higher prevalence of a mistrustful environment for those earning $3000–$4999 per month among women (23.0%) and for those earning $5000–$7499 among men (21.7%).

Table 1. Weighted prevalence (%) and standard errors (SE) of open and trusting and open work environment factors by sociodemographic characteristics and gender (Gallup-Sharecare Well-Being Index, 2010–2012).

Characteristics	Total Women	Mistrustful Environment		Total Men	Mistrustful Environment	
	%	%	SE	%	%	SE
Total		22.1	0.1		20.3	0.1
Age						
18–29 *	19.8	17.4	0.3	21.8	15.7	0.2
30–44 *	32.4	22.3	0.2	35.1	20.5	0.2
45–64 *	45.0	24.4	0.2	40.3	23.0	0.2
65+	2.8	17.2	0.5	2.9	15.9	0.5
Race/ethnicity						
White *	72.0	22.4	0.1	72.2	21.1	0.1
Black *	12.9	23.2	0.4	8.8	20.6	0.4
Asian	2.4	17.7	0.8	2.7	17.1	0.6
Hispanic *	9.9	18.7	0.4	12.8	16.3	0.3
Other	2.8	21.9	0.8	3.4	19.5	0.6
Education						
<High school *	4.4	19.3	0.7	7.1	17.3	0.5
High school graduate	21.9	20.0	0.3	26.0	19.8	0.2
Technical/some college or associate degree *	53.5	22.0	0.2	53.4	20.9	0.1
4-year college/post graduate *	20.3	25.2	0.3	16.6	20.4	0.2
Marital status						
Single/ Never married *	22.7	20.8	0.3	23.1	18.0	0.2
Married *	54.2	21.4	0.2	61.8	20.7	0.1
Separated	2.6	23.3	0.8	1.9	21.9	0.9
Divorced	12.1	26.8	0.4	7.0	24.7	0.4
Widowed *	2.9	22.8	0.7	0.8	20.8	1.1
Domestic partner *	5.5	23.2	0.6	5.5	20.1	0.5
Family Income per month						
<$1000 *	3.3	21.0	0.8	2.8	18.6	0.8
$1000–$2999 *	27.0	22.5	0.3	22.9	20.1	0.3
$3000–$4999 *	26.6	23.0	0.3	23.8	21.2	0.2
$5000–$7499 *	21.4	22.5	0.3	21.5	21.7	0.2
≥$7500 *	21.9	21.9	0.3	29.1	19.6	0.2

* Z-test for difference between women and men $p < 0.05$.

Table 2 shows the weighted prevalence of LS7 risk factors by trust. The prevalence of all LS7 risk factors were higher for both women and men who reported working in a mistrustful environment, compared to those whose working environment was not mistrustful.

Table 2. Weighted prevalence (%) and standard errors (SE) for LS7 CVD risk factors by work environment characteristics and gender (Gallup-Sharecare Well-Being Index, 2010–2012).

Mistrustful Environment	High Blood Pressure *				High Cholesterol *				Diabetes				Current Smoker *			
	Women		Men		Women		Men		Women		Men		Women		Men	
	%	SE	%	SE	%	SE	%	SE	%	SE	%	SE	%	SE	%	SE
Yes	21.9	0.3	25.7	0.3	19.7	0.2	24.6	0.2	6.9	0.2	7.0	0.1	18.7	0.3	23.5	0.3
No	18.7	0.1	21.2	0.1	16.6	0.1	20.2	0.1	5.9	0.1	5.8	0.1	17.2	0.1	21.6	0.1

Mistrustful Environment	Poor Diet *				Insufficient Exercise *				BMI $\geq$ 30 *			
	Women		Men		Women		Men		Women		Men	
	%	SE	%	SE	%	SE	%	SE	%	SE	%	SE
Yes	69.3	0.3	76.6	0.2	77.7	0.3	73.2	0.3	26.2	0.3	31.0	0.3
No	67.6	0.2	75.1	0.1	76.1	0.1	71.4	0.1	22.8	0.2	26.9	0.1

* Z-test for difference between women and men significant $p < 0.05$.

Multivariate results for trust with LS7 CVD risk factors, after adjustment for demographic factors and having any health insurance, are shown in Table 3. Confidence intervals excluded 1.0, indicating statistical significance at $p < 0.05$ for each outcome. Trust was associated with the LS7 CVD risk factors in both men and women after adjustment for covariates. Due to the large sample size, we report effect sizes with a focus on those $\geq 10\%$. We found that workers who did not work in an open and trusting environment had greater odds of having high blood pressure (women = 15%, men = 20%), high cholesterol (women = 18%, men = 22%), and diabetes (women = 15%, men = 18%) compared to those who reported having an open and trusting environment with their supervisor. Both women and men workers had greater odds of being a current smoker (both 15%), having a poor diet (women = 10%, men = 11%), and being obese (both women and men = 18%). Women reporting a mistrustful environment also had greater odds of having a low physical activity level (10%). Odds ratios for having four or more LS7 CVD risk factors were elevated for those working in a mistrustful environment (women = 22%, men = 29%).

Table 3. Multivariate associations between LS7 CVD risk factors and open and trusting work environment stratified by gender (Gallup-Sharecare Well-Being Index, 2010–2012) [a].

CVD Risk Factors (Dependent variables)	Models	
	Mistrustful Environment	
	OR (95% CI)	
	Women	Men
High blood pressure	1.15 (1.11, 1.20)	1.20 (1.16, 1.24)
High cholesterol	1.18 (1.13, 1.22)	1.22 (1.18, 1.26)
Diabetes	1.15 (1.09, 1.23)	1.18 (1.12, 1.25)
Current smoker	1.15 (1.10, 1.20)	1.15 (1.11, 1.19)
Poor diet	1.10 (1.07, 1.14)	1.11 (1.07, 1.15)
Insufficient physical activity	1.10 (1.06, 1.14)	1.08 (1.05, 1.11)
Obese	1.18 (1.14, 1.23)	1.18 (1.15, 1.22)
Four or more risk factors	1.22 (1.16, 1.27)	1.29 (1.25, 1.34)

[a] Models are adjusted for age, race/ethnicity, education, marital status, family income, and any health insurance.

4. Discussion

The findings of this study suggest that lower workplace social capital, as measured by the WBI, is associated with higher odds of having one or more of the LS7 CVD risk factors.

Our findings are consistent with others who have found associations between social capital and health [39,46,48,65,81–83]. Previous research reported that working in a negative environment and having low social support could lead to stress and psychosocial distress [84]. Workplace stress can directly increase CVD risk through biological pathways (e.g., inflammation) or CVD risk factors [12,13]. Studies have found that workers experiencing job stress were more likely to have diabetes [85]. Associations between work environment and high blood pressure and high cholesterol are mixed, with some studies reporting results similar to our findings [86,87] and others reporting no association [85].

Furthermore, workplace stress can indirectly affect CVD risk through at-risk health behaviors [85,87]. These behaviors include poor diet, insufficient physical activity [85,86], smoking [85], high alcohol consumption, and lack of sleep [88]. Workers who reported a lack of support from supervisors were more likely to be heavy smokers [89]. In addition, men with low workplace social support were more likely to be obese [90].

Although we adjusted for potential demographic confounders in our models, we examined each of the LS7 CVD risk factors separately. Health behaviors are often interrelated and can affect the presence or absence of other health behaviors. For example, smoking was found to increase caloric intake [91], while a healthy lifestyle (diet and exercise) was negatively associated with smoking [92]. Because of the potential co-occurrence, we conducted sensitivity analyses to see whether the odds ratios increased if we selected having four or more of the LS7 risk factors instead of only one. We used this as the dependent variable in our regression models. Both women (22%) and men (29%) showed an increase in odds for having four or more LS7 risk factors if they indicated that their supervisor did not create an open and trusting environment.

Analyses were presented separately by gender, not only due to the differences in CVD risk between women and men, but also due to the importance of gender in the social capital and managerial psychology literature [93]. Odds ratios were similar for both genders when the LS7 factors were looked at individually, and slightly higher among men when the dependent variable was having four or more LS7 factors.

Improvements to the work environment are needed to reduce CVD risk among workers. Social modification to the work environment, such as adjusting managerial style to create an open and trusting environment, can decrease work stress. Considering managerial trust from a Total Worker Health® framework meets the goals of illness prevention to advance worker well-being. Efforts can also be made to target the health behaviors themselves. There are a range of possible strategies for addressing the LS7 risk factors in the workplace. For example, physical modification to the work environment, such as installing sit/stand desk stations and walking workstations, can reduce sedentary behavior and may increase physical activity. Additionally, increased access to nutritious food in the workplace may improve diet. Supervisors who support workplace wellness may help in reducing CVD risk factor in workers [94].

Strengths and Limitations

This study has several strengths. The WBI is a large, nationally representative survey. Skopec et al. [95] found that the survey provided reasonably similar data when compared to established national surveys, such as the National Health Interview Survey (NHIS) and the Behavioral Risk Factor Surveillance System (BFRSS), on several important health-related measures. However, the Gallup sample was slightly older, had fewer minorities, and a higher educated sample than in other national surveys [95]. Outcomes examined included select health behaviors and health outcomes. Findings in our study are similar to those reported by adults who worked in the past 12 months in the 2010 National Health Interview Survey (NHIS) conducted by the National Center for Health Statistics. Weighted prevalence items were obesity (BMI $\geq$30) (Gallup = 27.7%; NHIS = 28.1%), current smoker (Gallup = 21.9%, NHIS = 19.7%), hypertension (Gallup = 22.3%; NHIS = 19.4%), insufficient exercise (Gallup = 76.3%; NHIS = 88.3%), and diabetes (Gallup = 6.1%; NHIS = 5.8%) [72]. Data on high cholesterol are not available for the 2010 NHIS, but are available for 2015 (Gallup = 21.3%; NHIS = 21.5%) [72].

The work environment question included in this study allows us to examine an important workplace psychosocial factor that is often difficult or expensive to study. It is unclear where the work environment question originated. Documentation provided by Gallup indicated that it was based upon findings from leading scientists in the areas of survey research, behavioral economics, and health. No information on the validity or reliability of the Gallup question is available.

This study also has several limitations. The survey is cross-sectional and therefore no conclusions can be made regarding causality. Data were collected via a telephone survey that has a low response rate, potentially affecting the representativeness of our findings. For each regression model, observations with missing values for included covariates were dropped. All data were self-reported at one point in time and are subject to response biases, such as recall and social desirability. Social desirability bias [96] is the tendency of respondents to present themselves in a socially desirable light, which may deviate from their true behaviors. Social desirability bias has been shown to affect the reporting of health behaviors, including underreporting negative behaviors and over reporting positive ones [97]. However, a recent study by Prather et al. [98] did not find confounding due to social desirability bias. Additionally, although we adjusted for potential confounders in our models, other non-measured confounders may have influenced our results. The WBI survey only touched upon a small number of components of an individual's work environment. Components of social capital and the work environment such as occupation, organizational structure (e.g., work schedule, work arrangements), culture, job autonomy, job resources, job security, work engagement, workplace hostility, additional characteristics of the supervisor, and others are needed for a better-informed study. Findings by Oksanen et al. [45,46] suggest that the effects of low social capital might not be similar in all work units or groups of different socioeconomic structure. However, because social capital and socioeconomic status were measured at the individual level, we are unable to examine the effects of social capital in different work contexts. Additionally, stand-alone, single-item questions may not offer the precision needed to make an accurate assessment of supervisory style, and as Choi et al. [34] suggest, there is a lack of consensus on measurement of social capital. The measure of social capital used in this study deals with leadership trust. Researchers have also included differing measures of social capital that include employee networks and workforce norms [99].

Health behavior questions in the WBI were different from AHA's LS7 definitions, particularly diet that included only one of the five diet variables. The health factor metrics are markedly different in the WBI compared to the AHA's LS7 definitions, noticeably absent are the clinical measurements of blood pressure, blood cholesterol, fasting glucose, and medication used to treat these health factors. Lastly, the study's large sample size increases the probability of finding statistically significant associations; therefore, we focused on effect size rather than p-values. Despite these limitations, results show that more than 20% of workers report that their supervisor does not always create an open and trusting environment. This is associated with a 20% increase in odds for having four or more CVD risk factors, suggesting that this is an important factor when designing interventions to address worker cardiovascular health. Therefore, these results show support for the usefulness of this aspect of social capital to understand the work environment, supervisory behavior, and their association with worker cardiovascular health.

5. Conclusions

This study found that a negative work-environment characteristic representing an aspect of workplace social capital contributed to greater odds of having important CVD risk factors among full-time workers. Results suggest that supervisor behavior can play an important role in improving worker health. Workplace intervention programs for CVD and other chronic health conditions should consider addressing this aspect of workplace social capital, and supervisor competencies and behavior in particular, with proper training as a potential means to improve worker health. Thus, our results reinforce the notion voiced elsewhere [69,100] that supervisor support is essential to a comprehensive approach to worker safety and health; issues of managerial trust are worthy of inclusion in a Total Worker Health® framework.

Author Contributions: T.A. and R.T. contributed equally to the manuscript. T.A., R.T., J.J. and K.M.K. contributed to Writing-Review and Editing.

Funding: This research received no external funding. However, Kelly's effort was supported by Cooperative Agreement No. U19OH008868 from the Centers for Disease Control and Prevention (CDC), National Institute for Occupational Safety and Health (NIOSH) to the Healthier Workforce Center at the University of Iowa.

Acknowledgments: The authors would like to thank Chia-Chia Chang and Casey Chosewood, NIOSH Total Worker Health®, and Melanie Standish of the Gallup organization for their assistance in accessing and understanding the data. We would also like to thank Leslie McDonald and Candice Johnson, Division of Surveillance, Hazard Evaluation and Field Studies, National Institute for Occupational Safety and Health, for their valuable comments regarding the American Heart Association Life's Simple 7. Appreciation is extended to James Grosch, Tara Hartley, Sara Luckhaupt, and Marie Haring Sweeney for their review comments on this manuscript.

Conflicts of Interest: The authors declare that they have no conflict of interest. The findings and conclusions in this report are those of the authors and do not necessarily represent the views of the National Institute for Occupational Safety and Health.

References

1. Centers for Disease Control and Prevention. CDC Heart Disease Facts. 2016. Available online: https://www.cdc.gov/dhdsp/data_statistics/fact_sheets/fs_heart_disease.htm (accessed on 17 April 2018).
2. Heidenreich, P.A.; Trogdon, J.G.; Khavjou, O.A.; Butler, J.; Dracup, K.; Ezekowitz, M.D.; Finkelstein, E.A.; Hong, Y.; Johnston, S.C.; Khera, A.; et al. Forecasting the future of cardiovascular disease in the United States: A policy statement from the American Heart Association. *Circulation* **2011**, *123*, 933–944. [CrossRef] [PubMed]
3. Mozaffarian, D.; Benjamin, E.J.; Go, A.S.; Arnett, D.K.; Blaha, M.J. American Heart Association Statistics, C.; Stroke Statistics, S. 'Heart disease and stroke statistics—2015 update: A report from the American Heart Association. *Circulation* **2015**, *131*, e29–e322. [PubMed]
4. Benjamin, E.J.; Blaha, M.J.; Chiuve, S.E.; Cushman, M.; Das, S.R.; Deo, R.; de Ferranti, S.; Després, J.P.; Fullerton, H.J.; Howard, V.J.; et al. American Heart Association Statistics C, Stroke Statistics S: Heart disease and stroke statistics—2017 update: A reportfFrom the American Heart Association. *Circulation* **2017**, *135*, e146–e603. [CrossRef]
5. Lloyd-Jones, D.M.; Hong, Y.; Labarthe, D.; Mozaffarian, D.; Appel, L.J.; Van Horn, L.; Greenlund, K.; Daniels, S.; Nichol, G.; Tomaselli, G.F.; et al. Defining and setting national goals for cardiovascular health promotion and disease reduction: The American Heart Association's strategic impact goal through 2020 and beyond. *Circulation* **2010**, *121*, 586–613. [CrossRef] [PubMed]
6. Shay, C.M.; Gooding, H.S.; Murillo, R.; Foraker, R. Understanding and Improving Cardiovascular Health: An Update on the American Heart Association's Concept of Cardiovascular Health. *Prog. Cardiovasc. Dis.* **2015**, *58*, 41–49. [CrossRef] [PubMed]
7. Backé, E.M.; Seidler, A.; Latza, U.; Rossnagel, K.; Schumann, B. The role of psychosocial stress at work for the development of cardiovascular diseases: A systematic review. *Intl. Arch. Occup. Environ. Health* **2012**, *85*, 67–79. [CrossRef]
8. Belkic, K.L.; Landsbergis, P.A.; Schnall, P.L.; Baker, D. Is job strain a major source of cardiovascular disease risk? *Scand. J. Work Environ. Health* **2004**, *30*, 85–128. [CrossRef]
9. Choi, B.K.; Schnall, P.; Landsbergis, P.; Dobson, M.; Ko, S.; Gomez-Ortiz, V.; Juárez-Garcia, A.; Baker, D. Recommendations for individual participant data meta-analyses on work stressors and health outcomes: Comments on IPD-Work Consortium papers. *Scand. J. Work Environ. Health* **2015**, *41*, 299–311. [CrossRef]
10. Kasl, S.V. The influence of the work environment on cardiovascular health: A historical, conceptual, and methodological perspective. *J. Occup. Health Psychol.* **1996**, *1*, 42–56. [CrossRef]
11. Kivimäki, M.; Kawachi, I. Work stress as a risk factor for cardiovascular disease. *Curr. Cardiol. Rep.* **2015**, *17*, 630. [CrossRef]
12. Kivimäki, M.; Virtanen, M.; Elovainio, M.; Kouvonen, A.; Vaananen, A.; Vahtera, J. Work stress in the etiology of coronary heart disease—A meta-analysis. *Scand. J. Work Environ. Health* **2006**, *32*, 431–442. [CrossRef] [PubMed]
13. Steptoe, A.; Kivimäki, M. Stress and cardiovascular disease: An update on current knowledge. *Ann. Rev. Public Health* **2013**, *34*, 337–354. [CrossRef]
14. Szerensci, K.; van Amelsvoort, L.; Viechtbauer, W.; Mohren, D.; Prins, M.; Kant, I. The association between study characteristics and outcome in the relation between job stress and cardiovascular disease: A multilevel meta-regression analysis. *Scand. J. Work Environ. Health* **2012**, *38*, 489–502. [CrossRef] [PubMed]
15. Theorell, T. Commentary triggered by the Individual Participant Data Meta-Analysis Consortium study of job strain and myocardial infarction risk. *Scand. J. Work Environ. Health* **2014**, *40*, 89–95. [CrossRef] [PubMed]
16. Toivanen, S. Social determinants of stroke as related to stress at work among working women: A literature review. *Stroke Res. Treat.* **2012**, *2012*, 873678. [CrossRef] [PubMed]
17. Gilbert-Ouimet, M.; Trudel, X.; Brisson, C.; Milot, A.; Vezina, M. Adverse effects of psychosocial work factors on blood pressure: Systematic review of studies on demand-control-support and effort-reward imbalance models. *Scand. J. Work Environ. Health* **2014**, *40*, 109–132. [CrossRef] [PubMed]
18. Johnson, J.V.; Hall, E.M. Job strain, work place social support, and cardiovascular disease: A cross-sectional study of a random sample of the Swedish working population. *Am. J. Public Health* **1988**, *78*, 1336–1342. [CrossRef] [PubMed]

19. Karasek, R. Job demands, job decision latitude, and mental strain: Implications for job redesign. *Adm. Sci. Q.* **1979**, *24*, 285–308. [CrossRef]
20. Karasek, R.; Theorell, T. *Healthy Work: Stress, Productivity, and the Reconstruction of Working Life*; Basic Books: New York, NY, USA, 1990; ISBN 978-0465028979.
21. Nieuwenhuijsen, K.; Bruinvels, D.; Frings-Dresen, M. Psychosocial work environment and stress-related disorders, a systematic review. *Occup. Med.* **2010**, *60*, 277–286. [CrossRef]
22. Schaufeli, W.; Bakker, A.; Salanova, M. The measurement of work engagement with a short questionnaire. A cross-national study. *Educ. Psychol. Meas.* **2006**, *66*, 701–716. [CrossRef]
23. Siegrist, J. Adverse health effects of high-effort/low-reward conditions. *J. Occup. Health Psychol.* **1996**, *1*, 27–41. [CrossRef] [PubMed]
24. Virtanen, M.; Heikkila, K.; Jokela, M.; Ferrie, J.E.; Batty, G.D.; Vahtera, J.; Kivimäki, M. Long working hours and coronary heart disease: A systematic review and meta-analysis. *Am. J. Epidemiol.* **2012**, *176*, 586–596. [CrossRef] [PubMed]
25. Bakker, A.B.; Demerouti, E. The Job Demands-Resources model: State of the art. *J. Manag. Psychol.* **2007**, *22*, 309–328. [CrossRef]
26. Bakker, A.B.; Demerouti, E.; Euwema, M.C. Job resources buffer the impact of job demands on burnout. *J. Occup. Health Psycholol.* **2005**, *10*, 170–180. [CrossRef]
27. Demerouti, E.; Bakker, A.B.; Nachreiner, F.; Schaufeli, W.B. The job demands-resources model of burnout. *J. Appl. Psychol.* **2001**, *86*, 499–512. [CrossRef] [PubMed]
28. Black, J.K.; Belanos, G.M.; Whitikaer, A.C. Resilience, work engagement and stress reactivity in a middle-aged manual worker population. *Int. J. Psychophysiol.* **2017**, *116*, 9–15. [CrossRef]
29. Colquitt, J.A.; Conlon, D.E.; Wesson, M.J.; Porter, C.O.; Ng, K.Y. Justice at the millennium: A meta-analytic review of 25 years of organizational justice research. *J. Appl. Psychol.* **2001**, *86*, 425–445. [CrossRef]
30. De Vogli, R.; Ferrie, J.E.; Chandola, T.; Kivimäki, M.; Marmot, M.G. Unfairness and health: Evidence from the Whitehall II Study. *J. Epidemiol. Community Health* **2007**, *61*, 513–518. [CrossRef]
31. Elovainio, M.; Kivimäki, M.; Vahtera, J. Organizational justice: Evidence of a new psychosocial predictor of health. *Am. J. Public Health* **2002**, *92*, 105–108. [CrossRef]
32. Inoue, A.; Kawakami, N.; Eguchi, H.; Miyaki, K.; Tsutsumi, A. Organizational justice and physiological coronary heart disease risk factors in japanese employees: A cross-sectional study. *Int. J. Behav. Med.* **2015**, *22*, 775–785. [CrossRef]
33. Kivimäki, M.; Ferrie, J.E.; Brunner, E.; Head, J.; Shipley, M.J.; Vahtera, J.; Marmot, M.G. Justice at work and reduced risk of coronary heart disease among employees: The Whitehall II Study. *Arch. Intern. Med.* **2005**, *165*, 2245–2251. [CrossRef] [PubMed]
34. Choi, M.; Mesa-Frias, M.; Nuesch, E.; Hargreaves, J.; Prieto-Merino, D.; Bowling, A.; Smith, G.D.; Ebrahim, S.; Dale, C.E.; Casas, J.P. Social capital, mortality, cardiovascular events and cancer: A systematic review of prospective studies. *Int. J. Epidemiol.* **2014**, *43*, 1895–1920. [CrossRef] [PubMed]
35. Coleman, J. *Foundations of Social Theory*; Harvard University Press: Cambridge, MA, USA, 1990.
36. Hayami, Y. Social capital, human capital and the community mechanism: Toward a conceptual framework for economists. *J. Dev. Stud.* **2009**, *45*, 96–123. [CrossRef]
37. Murayama, H.; Fujiwara, Y.; Kawachi, I. Social capital and health: A review of prospective multilevel studies. *J. Epidemiol.* **2012**, *22*, 179–187. [CrossRef]
38. Putnam, R. *Making Democracy Work: Civic Traditions in Modern Italy*; Princeton University Press: Princeton, NJ, USA, 1993; ISBN 9780691037387.
39. Berkman, L.F.; Kawachi, I. *Social Epidemiology*; Oxford University Press: New York, NY, USA, 2000.
40. Zischka, L. Valuing Social capital by the Resources People Allocate to One Another. *J. Int. Dev.* **2013**, *25*, 609–625. [CrossRef]
41. Giordano, G.N.; Ohlsson, H.; Lindström, M. Social capital and health-purely a question of context? *Health Place* **2011**, *17*, 946–953. [CrossRef]
42. Pattussi, M.P.; Olinto, M.T.; Canuto, R.; da Silva Garcez, A.; Paniz, V.M.; Kawachi, I. Workplace social capital, mental health and health behaviors among Brazilian female workers. *Soc. Psychiatry Psychiat. Epidemiol.* **2016**, *51*, 1321–1330. [CrossRef] [PubMed]
43. Samuel, L.J.; Commodore-Mensah, Y.; Himmelfarb, C.R. Developing behavioral theory with the systematic integration of community social capital concepts. *Health Educ. Behav.* **2014**, *41*, 359–375. [CrossRef] [PubMed]

44. Kawachi, I.; Kennedy, B.P.; Glass, R. Social capital and self-rated health: A contextual analysis. *Am. J. Public Health* **1999**, *89*, 1187–1193. [CrossRef]
45. Oksanen, T.; Kawachi, I.; Kouvonen, A.; Takao, S.; Suzuki, E.; Virtanen, M.; Pentti, J.; Kivimäki, M.; Vahtera, J. Workplace determinants of social capital: Cross-sectional and longitudinal evidence from a Finnish cohort study. *PLoS ONE* **2013**, *8*, e65846. [CrossRef]
46. Oksanen, T.; Kouvonen, A.; Kivimäki, M.; Pentti, J.; Virtanen, M.; Linna, A.; Vahtera, J. Social capital at work as a predictor of employee health: Multilevel evidence from work units in Finland. *Soc. Sci. Med.* **2008**, *66*, 637–649. [CrossRef] [PubMed]
47. Sundquist, J.; Johansson, S.E.; Yang, M.; Sundquist, K. Low linking social capital as a predictor of coronary heart disease in Sweden: A cohort study of 2.8 million people. *Soc. Sci. Med.* **2006**, *62*, 954–963. [CrossRef] [PubMed]
48. Suzuki, E.; Takao, S.; Subramanian, S.V.; Komatsu, H.; Doi, H.; Kawachi, I. Does low workplace social capital have detrimental effect on workers' health? *Soc. Sci. Med.* **2010**, *70*, 1367–1372. [CrossRef]
49. Lindström, M.; Giordano, G.N. Changes in social capital and cigarette smoking behavior over time: A population-based panel study of temporal relationships. *Nicotine Tob. Res.* **2016**, *18*, 2106–2114. [CrossRef] [PubMed]
50. Tsuboya, T.; Tsutsumi, A.; Kawachi, I. Null association between workplace social capital and body mass index. Results from a four-wave panel survey among employees in Japan (J-HOPE study). *Soc. Sci. Med.* **2016**, *150*, 1–7. [CrossRef]
51. Ehsan, A.M.; De Silva, M.J. Social capital and common mental disorder: A systematic review. *J. Epidemiol. Community Health* **2015**, *69*, 1021–1028. [CrossRef]
52. Tsuboya, T.; Tsutsumi, A.; Kawachi, I. Change in psychological distress following change in workplace social capital: Results from the panel surveys of the J-HOPE study. *Occup. Environ. Med.* **2015**, *72*, 188–194. [CrossRef]
53. Johnson, C.M.; Sharkey, J.R.; Dean, W.R. Eating behaviors and social capital are associated with fruit and vegetable intake among rural adults. *J. Hunger. Environ. Nutr.* **2010**, *5*, 302–315. [CrossRef]
54. Lindström, M. Social capital, the miniaturization of community and high alcohol consumption: A population-based study. *Alcohol Alcohol.* **2005**, *40*, 556–562. [CrossRef]
55. Lindström, M. Social capital, political trust and purchase of illegal liquor: A population-based study in southern Sweden. *Health Policy* **2008**, *86*, 266–275. [CrossRef]
56. Weitzman, E.R.; Chen, Y.Y. Risk modifying effect of social capital on measures of heavy alcohol consumption, alcohol abuse, harms, and secondhand effects: National survey findings. *J. Epidemiol. Community Health* **2005**, *59*, 303–309. [CrossRef]
57. Ball, K.; Cleland, V.J.; Timperio, A.F.; Salmon, J.; Giles-Corti, B.; Crawford, D.A. Love thy neighbour? Associations of social capital and crime with physical activity amongst women. *Soc. Sci. Med.* **2010**, *71*, 807–814. [CrossRef] [PubMed]
58. Lindström, M. Social capital, desire to increase physical activity and leisure-time physical activity: A population-based study. *Public Health* **2011**, *125*, 442–447. [CrossRef]
59. Lindström, M.; Moghaddassi, M.; Merlo, J. Social capital and leisure time physical activity: A population based multilevel analysis in Malmo, Sweden. *J. Epidemiol. Community Health* **2003**, *57*, 23–28. [CrossRef] [PubMed]
60. Oksanen, T.; Kivimäki, M.; Kawachi, I.; Subramanian, S.V.; Takao, S.; Suzuki, E.; Kouvonen, A.; Pentti, J.; Salo, P.; Virtanen, M.; et al. Workplace social capital and all-cause mortality: A prospective cohort study of 28,043 public-sector employees in Finland. *Am. J. Public Health* **2011**, *101*, 1742–1748. [CrossRef] [PubMed]
61. Giordano, G.N.; Lindström, M. The impact of social capital on changes in smoking behaviour: A longitudinal cohort study. *Eur. J. Public Health* **2011**, *21*, 347–354. [CrossRef]
62. Kouvonen, A.; Oksanen, T.; Vahtera, J.; Vaananen, A.; De Vogli, R.; Elovainio, M.; Pentti, J.; Leka, S.; Cox, T.; Kivimäki, M. Work-place social capital and smoking cessation: The Finnish Public Sector Study. *Addiction* **2008**, *103*, 1857–1865. [CrossRef] [PubMed]
63. Lindström, M. Social capital, political trust and daily smoking and smoking cessation: A population-based study in southern Sweden. *Public Health* **2009**, *123*, 496–501. [CrossRef]

64. Nieminen, T.; Prattala, R.; Martelin, T.; Harkanen, T.; Hyyppa, M.T.; Alanen, E.; Koskinen, S. Social capital, health behaviours and health: A population-based associational study. *BMC Public Health* **2013**, *13*, 613. [CrossRef]
65. Väänänen, A.; Kouvonen, A.; Kivimäki, M.; Oksanen, T.; Elovainio, M.; Virtanen, M.; Pentti, J.; Vahtera, J. Workplace social capital and co-occurrence of lifestyle risk factors: The Finnish Public Sector Study. *Occup. Environ. Med.* **2009**, *66*, 432–437. [CrossRef]
66. Tamers, S.L.; Goetzel, R.; Kelly, K.M.; Luckhaupt, S.E.; Nigam, J.A.; Pronk, N.P.; Rohlman, D.S.; Baron, S.; Brosseau, L.; Bushnell, P.T.; et al. Research methodologies for Total Worker Health®: Proceedings from a workshop. *J. Occup. Environ. Med.* **2018**, *6*, 968–978. [CrossRef] [PubMed]
67. Werbel, J.; Henriques, P. Different views of trust and relational leadership: Supervisor and subordinate perspectives. *J. Manag. Psychol.* **2009**, *24*, 780–796. [CrossRef]
68. Nienaber, A.; Romeike, P.; Searle, R.; Schewe, G. A qualitative meta-analysis of trust in supervisor-subordinate relationships. *J. Manag. Psychol.* **2015**, *30*, 507–534. [CrossRef]
69. Schill, A.L. Advancing well-being through Total Worker Health®. *Workplace Health Saf.* **2017**, *65*, 158–163. [CrossRef] [PubMed]
70. Centers for Disease Control and Prevention. Quality of Worklife Questionnaire. 2013. Available online: http://www.cdc.gov/niosh/topics/stress/qwlquest.html (accessed on 17 April 2018).
71. University of Michigan. 'Health and Retirement Study'. Available online: http://hrsonline.isr.umich.edu (accessed on 17 April 2018).
72. National Center for Health Statistics. 2010 National Health Interview Survey (NHIS) Public Use Data Release. NHIS Survey Description; 2011. Available online: ftp://ftp.cdc.gov/pub/Health_Statistics/NCHS/Dataset_Documentation/NHIS/2010/srvydesc.pdf (accessed on 13 February 2018).
73. National Center for Health Statistics. National Health Interview Survey (NHIS) Public Use Data Release. NHIS Survey Description; 2015. Available online: ftp://ftp.cdc.gov/pub/Health_Statistics/NCHS/Dataset_Documentation/NHIS/2015/srvydesc.pdf (accessed on 16 April 2018).
74. Gallup. Gallup Daily Methodology 2015. Available online: http://www.gallup.com/poll/195539/gallup-healthways-index-methodology-report-indexes.aspx (accessed on 17 April 2018).
75. Kahneman, D.; Deaton, A. High income improves evaluation of life but not emotional well-being. *Proc. Natl. Acad. Sci. USA* **2010**, *107*, 16489–16493. [CrossRef]
76. Deaton, A.; Stone, A.A. Evaluative and hedonic well-being among those with and without children at home. *Proc. Natl. Acad. Sci. USA* **2014**, *111*, 1328–1333. [CrossRef]
77. Fujishiro, K.; Heaney, C.A. Doing what I do best: The association betweem skill utilization and employee health with healthy behavior as a mediator. *Soc. Sci. Med.* **2017**, *175*, 235–243. [CrossRef]
78. Rentfrow, P.; Mellander, C.; Florida, R. Happy states of America: A state-level analysis of psychological, economic, and social well-being. *J. Pers. Res.* **2009**, *43*, 1073–1082. [CrossRef]
79. Sommers, B.D.; Gunja, M.Z.; Finegold, K.; Musco, T. Changes in self-reported insurance coverage, access to care, and health under the Affordable Care Act. *JAMA* **2015**, *314*, 366–374. [CrossRef]
80. Maric-Bilkan, C.; Arnold, A.P.; Taylor, D.A.; Dwinell, M.; Howlett, S.E.; Wenger, N.; Reckelhoff, J.F.; Sandberg, K.; Churchill, G.; Levin, E.; et al. Report of the National Heart, Lung, and Blood Institute Working Group on Sex Differences Research in Cardiovascular Disease: Scientific Questions and Challenges. *Hypertension* **2016**, *67*, 802–807. [CrossRef]
81. Wasserstein, R.; Lazar, N. The ASA's statement on p-values: Context, process, and purpose. *Am. Stat.* **2016**, *70*, 129–133. [CrossRef]
82. Gilbert, K.L.; Quinn, S.C.; Goodman, R.M.; Butler, J.; Wallace, J. A meta-analysis of social capital and health: A case for needed research. *J. Health Psychol.* **2013**, *18*, 1385–1399. [CrossRef] [PubMed]
83. Giordano, G.N.; Lindström, M. The impact of changes in different aspects of social capital and material conditions on self-rated health over time: A longitudinal cohort study. *Soc. Sci. Med.* **2010**, *70*, 700–710. [CrossRef]
84. Barnay, T. Health, work and working conditions: A review of the European economic literature. *Eur. J. Health Econ.* **2016**, *17*, 693–709. [CrossRef] [PubMed]
85. Nyberg, S.T.; Fransson, E.I.; Heikkila, K.; Alfredsson, L.; Casini, A.; Clays, E.; De Bacquer, D.; Dragano, N.; Erbel, R.; Ferrie, J.E.; et al. Job strain and cardiovascular disease risk factors: Meta-analysis of individual-participant data from 47,000 men and women. *PLoS ONE* **2013**, *8*, e67323. [CrossRef]

86. Chandola, T.; Britton, A.; Brunner, E.; Hemingway, H.; Malik, M.; Kumari, M.; Badrick, E.; Kivimaki, M.; Marmot, M. Work stress and coronary heart disease: What are the mechanisms? *Eur. Heart J.* **2008**, *29*, 640–648. [CrossRef] [PubMed]
87. Janczura, M.; Bochenek, G.; Nowobilski, R.; Dropinski, J.; Kotula-Horowitz, K.; Laskowicz, B.; Stanisz, A.; Lelakowski, J.; Domagala, T. The relationship of metabolic syndrome with stress, coronary heart disease and pulmonary function—An occupational cohort-based study. *PLoS ONE* **2015**, *10*, e0133750. [CrossRef]
88. Hammer, L.B.; Sauter, S. Total worker health and work-life stress. *J. Occup. Environ. Med.* **2013**, *55*, S25–S29. [CrossRef] [PubMed]
89. Väänänen, A.; Kouvonen, A.; Kivimäki, M.; Pentti, J.; Vahtera, J. Social support, network heterogeneity, and smoking behavior in women: The 10-town study. *Am. J. Health Promot.* **2008**, *22*, 246–255. [CrossRef]
90. Jaaskelainen, A.; Kaila-Kangas, L.; Leino-Arjas, P.; Lindbohm, M.L.; Nevanpera, N.; Remes, J.; Järvelin, M.R.; Laitinen, J. Psychosocial factors at work and obesity among young finnish adults: A cohort study. *J. Occup. Environ. Med.* **2015**, *57*, 485–492. [CrossRef]
91. Cundiff, D.K. Diet and tobacco use: Analysis of data from the diabetic control and complications trial, a randomized study. *Medscape J. Gen. Med.* **2002**, *4*, 2.
92. Nomura, K.; Nakao, M.; Tsurugano, S.; Takeuchi, T.; Inoue, M.; Shinozaki, Y.; Yano, E. Job stress and healthy behavior among male Japanese office workers. *Am. J. Ind. Med.* **2010**, *53*, 1128–1134. [CrossRef] [PubMed]
93. Westermann, O.; Ashby, J.; Petty, J. Gender and social capital: The importance of gender differences for the maturity and effectivenss of natural resource management groups. *World Dev.* **2005**, *33*, 1783–1799. [CrossRef]
94. Fonarow, G.C.; Calitz, C.; Arena, R.; Baase, C.; Isaac, F.W.; Lloyd-Jones, D.; Peterson, E.D.; Pronk, N.; Sanchez, E.; Terry, P.E.; et al. Workplace wellness recognition for optimizing workplace health: A presidential advisory from the American Heart Association. *Circulation* **2015**, *131*, e480–e497. [CrossRef] [PubMed]
95. Skopec, L.; Musco, T.; Sommers, B.D. A potential new data source for assessing the impacts of health reform: Evaluating the Gallup-Healthways Well-Being Index. *Healthcare* **2014**, *2*, 113–120. [CrossRef] [PubMed]
96. Crowne, D.P.; Marlowe, D. A new scale of social desirability independent of psychopathology. *J. Consult. Psychol.* **1960**, *24*, 349–354. [CrossRef]
97. Olynk Widmar, N.J.; Byrd, E.S.; Dominick, S.R.; Wolf, C.A.; Acharya, L. Social desirability bias in reporting of holiday season healthfulness. *Prev. Med. Rep.* **2016**, *4*, 270–276. [CrossRef]
98. Prather, A.A.; Gottlieb, L.M.; Giuse, N.B.; Koonce, T.Y.; Kusnoor, S.V.; Stead, W.W.; Adler, N.E. National Academy of Medicine social and behavioral measures: Associations with self-reported health. *Am. J. Prev. Med.* **2017**, *53*, 449–456. [CrossRef]
99. Hauser, C.; Perkmann, U.; Puntscher, S.; Walde, J.; Tappeiner, G. Trust works! Sources and effects of social capital in the workplace. *Soc. Indic. Res.* **2016**, *128*, 589–608. [CrossRef]
100. Hämmig, O. Health and well-being at work: The key role of supervisor support. *SSM Popul. Health* **2017**, *3*, 393–402. [CrossRef]

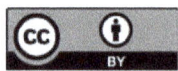

© 2019 by the authors. Licensee MDPI, Basel, Switzerland. This article is an open access article distributed under the terms and conditions of the Creative Commons Attribution (CC BY) license (http://creativecommons.org/licenses/by/4.0/).

MDPI
St. Alban-Anlage 66
4052 Basel
Switzerland
Tel. +41 61 683 77 34
Fax +41 61 302 89 18
www.mdpi.com

International Journal of Environmental Research and Public Health Editorial Office
E-mail: ijerph@mdpi.com
www.mdpi.com/journal/ijerph

www.ingramcontent.com/pod-product-compliance
Lightning Source LLC
LaVergne TN
LVHW071937080526
838202LV00064B/6621